THE CRAFT OF SURGERY

THE CRAFT

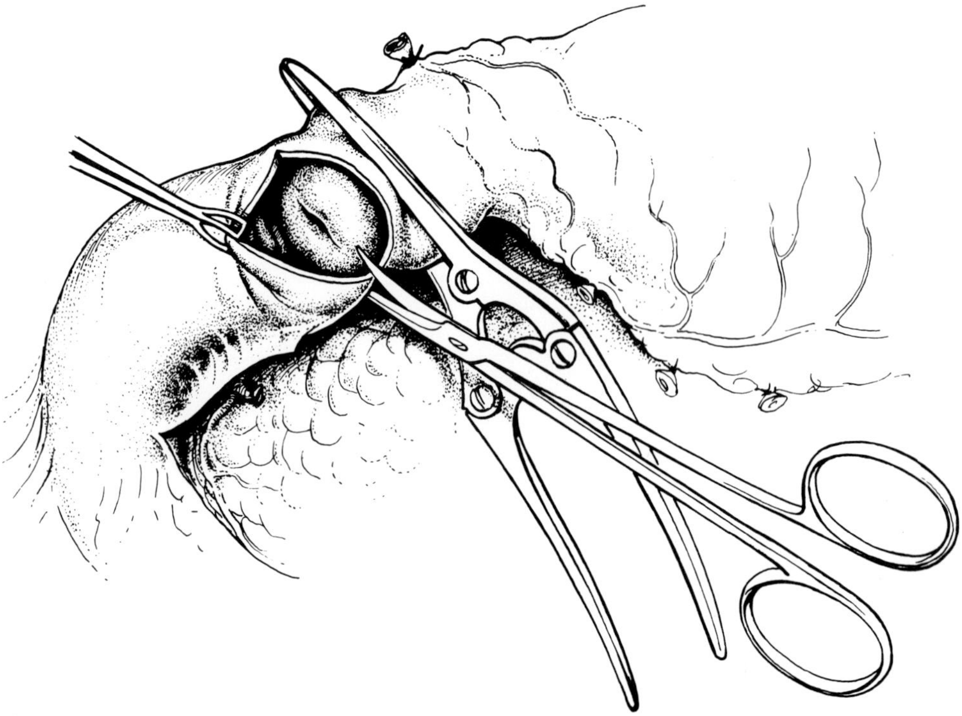

VOLUME II

OF SURGERY

EDITED BY

Philip Cooper, *M.D.*

Professor of Clinical Surgery, Albert Einstein College of Medicine, New York; Chief of Surgical Services, Veterans Administration Hospital, Bronx, New York

FOREWORD BY

LOUIS M. ROUSSELOT, M.D.

97 CONTRIBUTING AUTHORS

1600 ILLUSTRATIONS

LITTLE, BROWN AND COMPANY
BOSTON

LIBRARY OF CONGRESS CATALOG CARD NO. 64-22985

FIRST EDITION

Second Printing

Published in Great Britain by J. & A. Churchill Ltd., London

PRINTED IN THE UNITED STATES OF AMERICA

Contents

VOLUME II

XX. THE EXTREMITIES

XXI. THE KIDNEY, URETER, AND BLADDER

XXII. THE SCROTUM AND PENIS

THE CRAFT OF SURGERY

XI. THE ABDOMEN

68. *Abdominal Incisions and Exploration*

PHILIP COOPER

THE CHOICE of the abdominal incision is influenced by many factors, the most important of which are: (1) the anticipated intraabdominal pathology, (2) the contemplated operative procedure, and (3) the general condition and the habitus or physique of the patient. The incision should allow ready access to and adequate exposure of the operative area. It should be one that can be conveniently extended if necessary, and closed in a satisfactory and secure fashion. It should limit or avoid the sacrifice of nerves supplying the abdominal musculature. It should take into consideration and therefore avoid or incorporate, as indicated, any existing sinuses, fistulas, established colostomies, etc. It should also be placed so that it will not interfere with further stages of planned surgery.

Abdominal incisions may be divided into several basic types: (1) vertical or longitudinal, (2) transverse or oblique, and (3) special, such as the thoraco-abdominal.

Vertical or Longitudinal Incisions

Vertical or longitudinal incisions are good primary incisions and are generally preferred over other basic types by many surgeons. Regardless of any general preference for a specific type of incision, the vertical or longitudinal incision is indicated if the patient is a relatively poor risk or if the operator is uncertain of the intraabdominal pathology or the extent of the final operative procedure. Such incisions are particularly useful for patients with a narrow costal arch. They can be performed rapidly and be readily extended if necessary. However, the pull of the abdominal muscles is predominantly in a lateral direction, due to the oblique muscles (the external and internal oblique and the transversus abdominis), which participate in the formation of the anterior and posterior rectus sheaths. This lateral pull can be readily appreciated if one attempts to close a vertical incision under light anesthesia. In such a situation the closure of the incision may prove difficult.

The midline and paramedian incisions are, in general, preferred to the transrectus, because they preserve the nerve supply to the rectus muscle and produce less bleeding.

Midline Incisions

The midline incision is the simplest abdominal incision. It can be extended upward along the xiphoid, or the xiphoid may be excised. It can also be extended diagonally across the costal border, or extended distally by being curved around the umbilicus and brought back to the midline and then to the pubis. A lateral extension can be made by incising the rectus sheath and retracting or cutting the rectus muscle. Since the blood supply to the linea alba is relatively limited, wound healing may possibly be delayed. It is the impression of some surgeons that postoperative hernia is more common after use of the midline incision than after other vertical incisions.

The midline incision offers adequate exposure to any part of the abdominal cavity. We use it frequently for gastric surgery. It is valuable in the patient with an actively bleeding gastric or duodenal ulcer. It is a good incision for splenectomy. It is a satisfactory approach for biliary or pancreatic surgery. It gives good exposure for pelvic surgery. It is the ideal incision for surgery of the abdominal aorta and its major branches.

Paramedian Incisions

The paramedian incision is probably the most desirable vertical incision, all factors considered. It avoids injury to nerves, limits trauma to the rectus muscle, allows an anatomical and secure closure, and offers good restoration of function. If necessary, it may be extended from the xiphoid to the pubis. When placed on the appropriate side, it can be satisfactorily employed for any intraabdominal surgery. A second paramedian incision placed on the other side of the midline, opposite the original scar, may conceivably cause difficulty in healing due to interference with blood supply from both lateral directions. This precaution is presented for consideration, although on the few occasions when we have disregarded it for specific reasons, no obvious problem arose.

Transrectus Incisions

The transrectus incision must be limited in length; otherwise it results in injury to too many nerves. If the ends of more than two nerves are sacrificed there will be some postoperative relaxation of the abdominal wall. The transrectus incision can be performed more rapidly than the paramedian incision. It gives a more direct lateral exposure than the midline or the paramedian incision since there is less rectus muscle to be retracted laterally. These advantages do not justify its extensive use, because it does result in more tissue injury to both muscle and nerve, and in more bleeding, than the midline or paramedian incision. When a limited incision is adequate, it may prove very satisfactory. An example would be its use in surgery for a perforated duodenal ulcer. It may also be used as a general exploratory incision—about 5 inches in length and centered at the umbilicus. This length is usually enough to allow the insertion of the operator's hand into the abdominal cavity. If a long incision is required to accomplish the indicated surgery, it may be feasible to convert the transrectus to a paramedian incision.

Transverse or Oblique Incisions

Transverse or oblique incisions, in general, follow Langer's skin lines, and therefore give good cosmetic results. Any nerve damage that occurs is usually limited to one or, rarely, two nerves. Since the pull of the abdominal musculature and its aponeurosis is in line with or somewhat parallel to the incision, there is much less tension on the edges of the incision than in a vertical incision. In general, transverse or oblique incisions give only limited exposure if pathology is found both in the upper and the lower abdomen, except possibly in the short person with a wide abdomen and wide costal border. In that type of patient a long transverse incision above the umbilicus gives a satisfactory exposure for most intraabdominal surgery except that for pathology in the region of the pelvis.

Since the extent of exposure with a transverse or oblique incision is restricted, the incision must be appropriately and carefully planned. For example, in exposing the gallbladder through a subcostal incision, the incision is placed at a lower level than usual when the liver edge extends below the costal border. A subcostal incision should never be made too close to the costal border, since, if a hernia develops, enough of the abdominal wall must be available along the upper margin of the wound for satisfactory repair of the hernial defect. The same precautions apply when a transverse incision is made close to the symphysis.

The transverse tendinous inscriptions attach the rectus muscle to the anterior rectus sheath, thereby keeping it from retracting significantly as it is incised. However, tendinous inscriptions are rarely found beyond a certain level below the umbilicus, and there may be some retraction of the incised rectus muscle in that region unless it is sutured to the anterior sheath.

There are many varieties of transverse and oblique incisions, some of which are associated with proper names. These incisions are reviewed in many standard atlases. Transverse incisions may be truly horizontal or may curve to varying degree; similarly, oblique incisions may be straight or curved and vary considerably in angle. The incision may be limited to the oblique muscles or it may involve sectioning of a part or the whole of the entire width of both recti.

Thoracoabdominal Incisions

Thoracoabdominal incisions are usually extensive, and it requires considerable time to open and close them. Sectioning of the costal arch may lead to postoperative discomfort if the arch fails to heal. The patient may also experience pain as a sequel to injury of an intercostal nerve at the time of surgery.

This incision, appropriately placed on the right or left, is indicated for lesions of the lower esophagus and/or cardiac end of the stomach, for resections of the right lobe of the liver, for some portacaval shunts, for large vascular or adherent spleens, and in general, for other large left upper quadrant masses. Certain operations that may be more easily accomplished through thoracoabdominal incisions, for example the repair of diaphragmatic hernia or a total gastrectomy, can usually be adequately handled through an abdominal incision alone.

In making a thoracoabdominal incision, it is not necessary or advisable to resect a rib, because the intercostal approach is satisfactory. Resection of a rib may create a problem, in that the defect resulting from the resection will be difficult to close anteriorly since the costal arch is involved. The abdominal part of the incision may be entirely transverse or oblique, or may be partially oblique and extend vertically down as a midline, a paramedian, or a transrectus incision.

In patients with carcinoma of the stomach, it may be advisable to complete the abdominal part of the incision first to determine resectability before extending the incision over the chest.

Technique

The Incision

The skin incision is usually made by one stroke of the scalpel deep into the subcutaneous tissue. Slight tension on and spreading of the skin by the thumb and index finger of the other hand is helpful. The desired depth of the stroke can usually be determined by the estimated thickness of the subcutaneous tissue and by the response of the tissues as they give way to the scalpel. The amount of pressure on the dorsum of the blade by the index finger and the angle of the scalpel to the skin surface determine the extent and depth of the initial incision. The scalpel edge should be sharp. There may be variation in the quality of the blades delivered to the surgeon. If it appears necessary to apply excessive force to the blade to incise the skin properly, the blade should be discarded.

We do not use the scalpel to make "cross-marks" for orientation during the subsequent skin closure, for they frequently result in persistent fine scars. One can usually approximate the skin properly by observing the usual skin markings and the status of the remaining unapproximated skin edges as the skin is being sutured. If the incision has been curved or angulated, fine silk sutures or "markers" may be inserted at appropriate points superficially in the subcutaneous tissue when the incision is made.

The scalpel is discarded after the initial skin incision, and the wound is draped. The draping can be readily and appropriately done by suturing pads or towels directly to the subcutaneous tissue with interrupted silk sutures. Although the cut silk strands are exposed, they will not be evident or annoying as one proceeds with the surgery. One may dispense with this initial draping if adhesive plastic material has been applied to the skin.

Excessive sponging increases bleeding and traumatizes tissue. Until the wound has been properly draped, a sponge is held in the palm of the hand and applied as needed. The sponge is not wiped or rubbed over the skin. This practice limits contamination of the wound. However, with the new adhesive plastic material this precautionary measure is not necessary.

Next, the index finger and thumb are inserted into the wound, the fingers are spread, and the subcutaneous tissue is further incised down to the aponeurosis. Beveling the scalpel at this time allows one both to incise and to clear fat off the underlying tissue simultaneously. The amount of fat freed by this maneuver should be limited to that required for later approximation of the tissue properly.

Incision of an aponeurosis or sheath is usually done with a scalpel, although a curved Mayo scissors may be used at either end of the wound if it appears more desirable technically. However, with a midline incision, the aponeurosis is opened first in its lowest one-fifth, and a scalpel is used throughout the extent of the incision.

If a muscle, such as the rectus, is incised in the general direction of its fibers, the combination of sharp dissection by scalpel, alternating with blunt dissection using the index finger alone or the index and middle fingers, and the handle of the scalpel, limits the extent of trauma to tissue (Fig. 1A, B). Blunt dissection is used only when the fibers can be readily separated by "gentle persuasion."

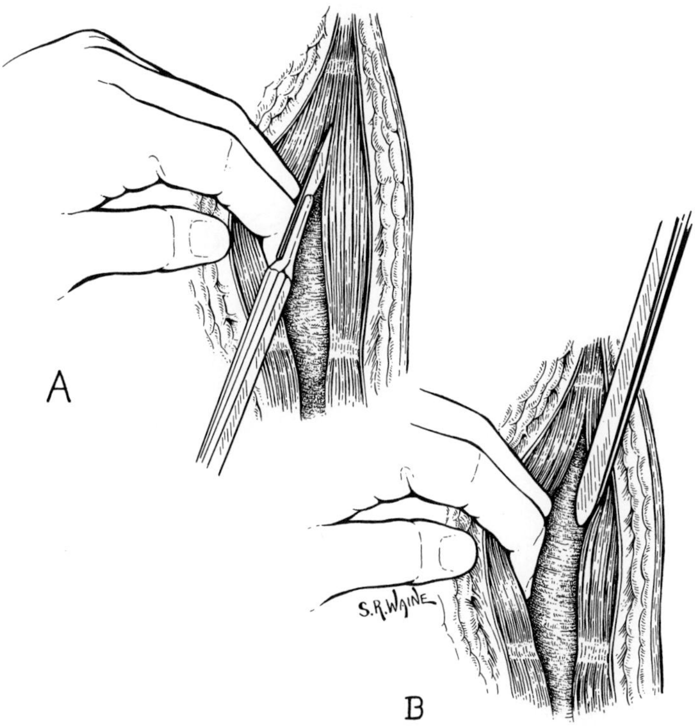

FIGURE 1. Transrectus incision. (A) The muscle is incised by scalpel when gentle blunt dissection fails to separate the fibers. (*B*) The muscle fibers are being separated by blunt dissection, utilizing the fingers of one hand and the handle of a scalpel held in the other hand.

In the paramedian incision, the muscle is freed from the linea alba by small scissor bites, or by short strokes of the scalpel, alternating with blunt dissection (Fig. 2A, B). There will be less shredding of muscle if it is dissected free in a downward direction. Vessels requiring ligation can be dissected, clamped, cut, and ligated without difficulty. They are usually found in the region of the tendinous inscriptions. The rectus muscle is then freed by blunt dissection from the underlying rectus sheath, transversalis fascia and peritoneum. The extent of this dissection should be limited to that required for the opening and the subsequent closure of the peritoneum.

Incision of a muscle obliquely or at right angles to the fibers should usually be done without mobilizing the muscle from underlying tissues. In this way one limits retraction of the cut muscle and reduces the amount of residual "dead space" following wound closure. In incising certain oblique muscles, however, one may

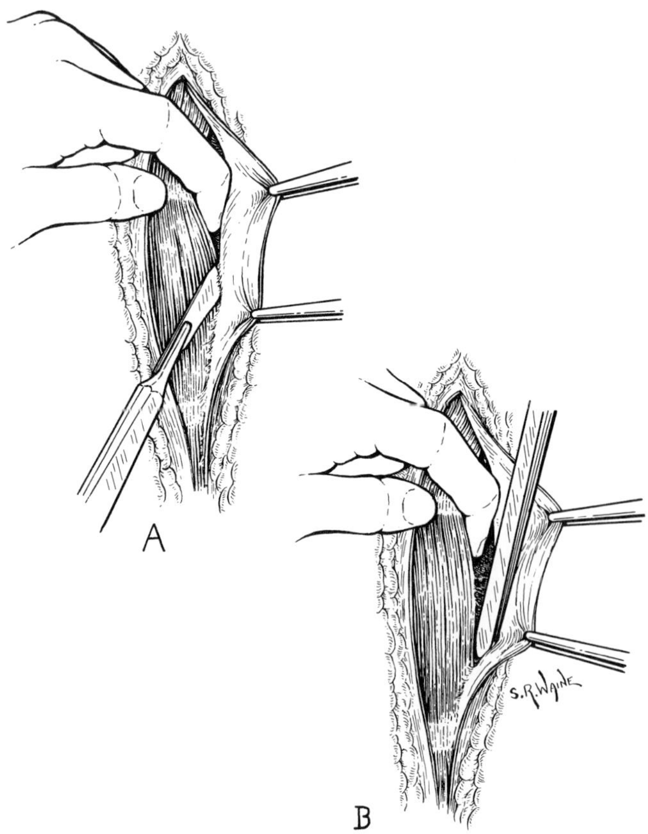

FIGURE 2. (*A*) Paramedian incision. The fibrous tissue bands and areolar tissue which attach the rectus muscle to the anterior sheath are being incised by scalpel. A finger is being used to retract the muscle. (*B*) Blunt dissection further frees the medial border of the rectus muscle. A closed scissors may be substituted for the scalpel handle if a scissors is being used for sharp dissection. Vessels going from the muscle to the rectus sheath or linea alba are not illustrated.

choose to mobilize a narrow border of each cut muscle to allow a better layered closure.

Two Allis clamps, hemostats, or tissue forceps are applied to the peritoneum. The one first applied is then removed and reapplied after slight tension has been placed on the second instrument. This serves as a precaution against the inadvertent incision of an intraperitoneal structure that may have been grasped by the first instrument initially.

In incising the peritoneum, in the midline incision, one should preferably stay to the right or left of the falciform ligament; for if the ligament is opened, extraperitoneal fat in that structure will often obscure the peritoneum. Usually, there is less fat near the umbilicus. In the obese person, therefore, incising the peritoneum first in that area may prove helpful.

If we are concerned about the presence of intraabdominal adhesions in the area of incision, we incise the transversalis fascia as a separate layer over an appropriate distance. We can then better visualize the underlying peritoneum and can determine whether it is adherent to bowel. We always attempt to incise the peritoneum first in an area free of adhesions, particularly if intestine is involved.

The Exploration

The sequence and the extent of abdominal exploration will be determined to some degree by the type and extent of the pathology and the general condition of the patient. The exploration should be as thorough as the circumstances indicate, and should provide assurance that no pathology has been overlooked, as sometimes happens through failure to examine a reasonably accessible organ or region of the abdominal cavity. In general, it is best to complete the exploration before one evaluates the major pathology. The exploration may be restricted by the chosen incision; by finding an acute inflammatory process or an abscess; or by the general condition of the patient, which may demand that the indicated procedure be accomplished as expeditiously as possible.

Before inserting a retractor for exploratory purposes, one should elevate the edge of the wound by hand to see whether the peritoneum is free in that area. A few comments on the respective functions of the operator and the assistant in the use of retractors are pertinent here. Rake retractors (used only in the subcutaneous tissue) may be shifted by the assistant. These are not used widely, because they traumatize tissue and may tear the glove of the operator or an assistant. Other types of small retractors applied *within* the wound may also be shifted by an assistant. In the abdominal cavity, however, *all retractors* are placed by the operator, and should not be shifted or moved by an assistant without instructions or assistance from the operator. The assistant should be aware of the tissues or structure he is retracting. He should be made as comfortable as possible; otherwise the retraction may prove unsatisfactory. Self-retaining retractors usually give good exposure and relieve the assistant of what is often a tiresome effort. However, they cannot be shifted readily by the operator, and are traumatic to the abdominal wall because they maintain continued pressure over a limited area for the duration of a procedure.

Intraabdominal adhesions can be more readily freed if they are placed under tension. This can be achieved by the application of small Ochsner clamps to the peritoneum and transversalis fascia, or to the peritoneum and the posterior rectus sheath; by the use of right-angle retractors; or by the application of a sponge stick or pad. There is usually a relatively avascular zone where adhesions are attached to peritoneum, bowel, or other structures, except where an organ is "fused" or frozen at the site of attachment. When the relatively avascular area is demonstrated, it can usually be dissected and incised without significant bleeding. Adhesions can often be thinned out and lengthened by compressing and spreading them between the index finger and thumb of one hand as sharp dissection is accomplished by a scalpel or scissors held in the other hand.

If one finds a broad attachment of structures to the abdominal wall, one should seek an area of less adhesion, and work around the more involved area. The operator should require the assistant to hold attached clamps on the outside so that the operator can readily disengage them and hasten dissection. The scissors may also be "palmed" when not being used. When adhesions are cut after the application of a clamp, they should be incised slightly beyond the end of the clamp so that there will be no difficulty in applying a secure ligature.

If the serosa of the bowel is torn while one is freeing adhesions, it is best to close the defect with interrupted sutures. If the muscle layer has also given way, the closure should not be delayed, for further traction on the bowel may disrupt the continuity of the mucosa.

There are a few points that may prove helpful in exploring certain organs, structures, or regions in the abdominal cavity.

1. A gallbladder distended with bile may obscure the presence of calculi. In order to rule out their presence more fully, one may *partially* empty the gallbladder (through the cystic duct) by very gentle compression. Then, by tapping the gallbladder on one side and applying the fingers of the other hand on the opposite side, calculi may be felt as they strike the wall of the gallbladder. This maneuver, although unlikely to do so, may conceivably force calculi into the common duct. It is therefore probably preferable to examine a bile-distended gallbladder by partially evacuating its contents by a needle or by a small trocar inserted through the fundus. If the gallbladder is not removed, the opening made by the needle or trocar must be carefully closed by purse-string or Lembert sutures; and a Penrose drain inserted alongside the gallbladder.

The common duct can be palpated by inserting the index finger through the foramen of Winslow while placing the thumb on the anterior surface of the duct. Palpation of the lower part of the duct can often be best performed from the left side of the table.

2. Ulcers on the posterior gastric or duodenal wall may be found only after the gastrocolic omentum has been adequately incised for adequate inspection and palpation. If one is uncertain about the presence of an ulcer, gently rubbing the overlying serosal surface with a dry gauze sponge will usually produce small petechiae when an ulcer is present in that area.

3. The esophageal hiatus should be examined while one is exploring the upper abdomen. The examining finger should not be forced alongside the esophagus,

but should be gently applied to that region. If a hernia is present, it will be readily apparent from the ease with which the finger can be inserted into the hiatus.

4. In general it is safer to limit exploration and palpation of the spleen to its lower and anterior border. This is usually adequate for determination of size and configuration. Ordinarily the spleen is examined through a vertical incision, and visualization of the structure is limited. If extensive palpation is performed, it may result in tearing of the splenic capsule as the result of tension being transmitted through adhesions attached to the splenic capsule. Care must also be taken in placing traction on the stomach or colon, since adhesions to the spleen may be torn and the hemorrhage that follows may make splenectomy necessary.

5. Palpation of the transverse colon and the hepatic and splenic flexures, particularly in the obese patient, is best accomplished by elevating the greater omentum and palpating the bowel from below. The ascending and the descending colon are approached by passing the hand along the parietal peritoneum until the colon is reached. The hand then grasps the bowel and follows it to the splenic flexure and into the pelvis on the left, and to the hepatic flexure and the cecum on the right. The transverse colon, the cecum, and the sigmoid can usually be delivered for more thorough inspection.

6. Careful attention to gross pathology may be very helpful in differentiating an inflammatory from a neoplastic process, and may spare the patient extensive unnecessary surgery. For example, if one has difficulty differentiating diverticulitis from carcinoma of the colon, it is helpful to do a colotomy and inspect the mucosa, since diverticulitis is an intramural or extramural disease, whereas carcinoma is of mucosal origin. This maneuver should rarely be indicated if the patient has had adequate preoperative studies. However, if a colotomy is necessary to evaluate the problem properly, it should be done through essentially normal bowel near the area of involvement. It should not be undertaken if the lesion is causing significant obstruction, unless a resection or a colostomy is to be done.

The Wound Closure

Prior to wound closure there should be a final check of the abdominal cavity for bleeding and for possible retained foreign bodies. A sponge count and instrument count should be made. One should always combine these counts with an adequate survey of the abdomen since it is possible for a nurse to err in reporting a "correct" count.

Closure of the thoracic part of a thoracoabdominal incision will be discussed only briefly. Indicated chest tube or tubes are inserted. The incision in the diaphragm is closed with interrupted 00 silk sutures. To obtain a more secure closure, mattress reinforced with interrupted single stitches should be used. The anterior 1 to 1½ inches of the diaphragm is difficult to close with the chest open. To handle this problem, the final sutures may be inserted through the abdominal side, held toward the abdomen, and drawn up and tied individually from the abdominal side when the chest has been closed. At present we utilize pericostal sutures of doubled No. 1 or 2 chromic catgut for the intercostal incision. Incising the periosteum and freeing it for a short distance from the inferior border of the lower rib allows the pericostal sutures to be inserted without having them encompass the neurovascular structures associated with that rib. The reader is referred to Chapter 20, by Dr. Alley, for other comments on this subject. To close the posterior part of an intercostal incision properly, one has to utilize a segment of the sacrospinalis by suturing it to the adjacent intercostal muscle. The costal arch is usually repaired, after a small wedge has been excised, by suturing with 0 or No. 1 silk.

The abdominal wall should be properly relaxed during wound closure; otherwise sutures may tear through tissue. This is particularly true during the peritoneal closure. Disruption of this closure may be the initiating factor in the subsequent development of a hernia. Also of significance is the fact that the peritoneal cavity is able to tolerate contamination far better than the abdominal wall. Slits or holes around peritoneal sutures permit seepage of contaminated intraabdominal fluid which may be responsible for subsequent deep wound infection.

The use of wire for wound closure will be discussed separately. Cotton, dacron, or other synthetic suture material may be substituted for silk if the surgeon desires.

The peritoneum and transversalis fascia, including the posterior rectus sheath, where present, are closed in one layer with a continuous lockstitch of 0 chromic catgut. The catgut is doubled for the larger incisions. The closure may also be reinforced with interrupted sutures where advisable. If there is inadequate relaxation of the wound because of anesthesia problems, a continuous suture should be avoided and interrupted mattress sutures of 00 silk or 0 catgut employed. Placing four to five mattress sutures, and drawing them taut together, prior to tying, will relieve tension on the individual sutures as they are tied. Since mattress sutures often leave gaps between the individual sutures, interrupted sutures should be inserted at those points.

The oblique muscles are approximated with interrupted 00 chromic catgut or 00 or 000 silk sutures. These may be spaced at intervals of 0.7 to 1 cm. The sutures should be inserted through the overlying aponeurosis, and partially through the thickness of the muscle. The transversely incised rectus muscle is usually not sutured, because suture of the overlying anterior rectus sheath approximates the muscle except when the rectus muscle has been severed well below the umbilicus. If the rectus muscle in that area tends to retract, it can be sutured to the anterior rectus sheath.

The anterior rectus sheath is closed with simple interrupted or figure-of-eight sutures of 0 chromic catgut or 00 silk. These sutures should be placed approximately 0.8 cm. from the fascial edge, and 0.7 cm. apart.

Subcutaneous sutures of catgut or silk add little to the security of a closure but help in obliterating dead space and in achieving a satisfactory cosmetic result.

Tension sutures should in general be limited to patients with nutritional problems or debilitating diseases. They will, however, add security to the closure of wounds in the obese, in patients with respiratory diseases, and in situations in which abdominal distention is likely to persist or develop postoperatively. Tension sutures should preferably be placed through all layers of the abdominal wall approximately 2.5 to 3 cm. from wound edges and 2 cm. apart. They should be carefully approximated but not tied under tension. One should be able to insert a clamp readily under the tied suture. It is best to combine the tension sutures with a layered closure. Tension sutures should be left in at least 12 days. Double 0 or No. 1 silk, No. 26 (0) wire, or dacron or other suitable synthetic suture may be used for this purpose.

Chromic catgut may be used in the contaminated wound, but may not give the security of the nonabsorbable suture, for catgut may be rapidly absorbed, particularly in the presence of wound infection. Silk can be used for wound closure if there is limited contamination. If it is used with significant contamination, one may be faced with a persistent wound infection or with wound sinuses. These may occur years after surgery. If a wound is heavily contaminated, sutures placed through the skin and subcutaneous tissues may be left untied for two to three days.

Wire Closure. The use of buried wire sutures has enjoyed varying popularity over recent years. If properly used, wire gives a secure closure, and there is little likelihood of persistent wound infection or wound dehiscence. Wire may be inserted through all layers, or catgut or silk may be used for the peritoneum, transversalis fascia, and posterior rectus sheath.

In vertical incisions, the wire, usually stainless steel No. 30 (000), may be carried through the anterior rectus sheath alone, or through the sheath and muscle, or through sheath, muscle, and peritoneum. It may also be used in all transverse and oblique incisions. Since it adds little additional security to the closure of small incisions such as the McBurney, it should not be used for them.

When wire is used in the anterior rectus sheath alone, it should be placed as a figure-of-eight suture, similar to that employed with catgut or silk. When the wire is inserted through additional layers it should be placed 1 to 1.5 cm. from the cut edge of the rectus sheath or aponeurosis and continued as a "far-near" stitch with the near part of the stitch inserted 0.3 to 0.4 cm. from the edge (Fig. 3). The sutures are placed 1 to 1.3 cm. apart. In the midline incision one may insert both loops through the various layers of the abdominal wall by placing a so-called "far-near, near-far" stitch (Fig. 4).

It is essential to avoid tying wire sutures too tight, as it may result in shearing of the tissue. Each suture should be tied directly after being inserted. Three knots are used. It is important to keep the wire from kinking. The knots must be tied flat. As they are being tied, the strand should be held longitudinally along the tips of the finger. If it is placed transversely, it may cut through the glove and possibly the finger. Each suture is kept long for retraction purposes until the next suture has been inserted and tied. A clamp is then placed directly beyond the tie, the wire is cut beyond the clamp, and the end of the wire is turned down against the sheath or the aponeurosis. When the wires include the peritoneum the final two sutures are placed in the middle of the wound, or at least away from the ends of the wound. They are inserted as follows. (1) With the "far-near" suture the first loop

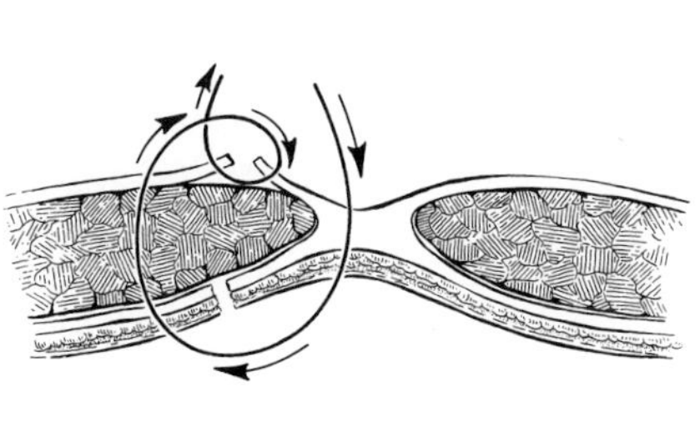

FIGURE 3. "Far-near" buried wire suture encompassing the anterior rectus sheath and the peritoneum, in a paramedian incision.

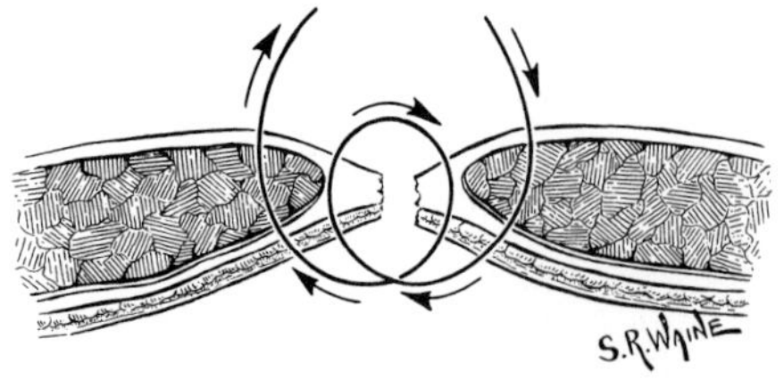

FIGURE 4. "Far-near, near-far" buried wire suture. This is recommended for use only with the midline incision.

of both sutures is inserted; then, with the tied sutures above and below held elevated, the near part of the two final sutures is inserted and they are tied as tension is applied to the other sutures. (2) For the "far-near, near-far" suture the same technique is used except that both loops are inserted at once.

It often proves unnecessary to apply clamps to the peritoneum when it is included in a wire closure. It may be grasped and exposed by mouse-tooth forceps. A finger inserted below the peritoneum as the sutures are being inserted should protect the underlying intestine. A sponge stick is also helpful for exposure purposes as the sutures are being placed. It is of interest that after the "far-near" sutures are placed and tied one can identify very little of the wire on the peritoneal surface.

Other suture materials, both absorbable and nonabsorbable, are easier to use and can be most efficient; and if the basic principles of surgical technique are followed, usually they prove as satisfactory as wire. The newer synthetic materials, such as dacron, Teflon-impregnated dacron, and others, have a low coefficient of friction and, if used, should be tied with at least four throws, all squared.

Drainage with Wire Closure. Although intraabdominal drains are usually brought through stab wounds, when the wound is closed with wire, the drain may be brought directly through the wound. The use of an incisional drain does not appear to increase the incidence of wound infections. It is desirable, nevertheless, to use one or two catgut sutures near the drain, since wire may possibly cut the drain, or may act as a foreign body when close to the drainage tract. Incisional drains frequently allow the drainage to be established more directly over the pathology. Double Penrose drains are used. They should be sutured to the skin and transfixed with a safety pin. Penrose drains made of nonreactive plastics should prove less irritating to tissues than the latex material now being used.

69. *Repair of Inguinal, Femoral, and Incisional Hernia*

JOHN L. MADDEN

Indirect Inguinal Hernia

In the repair of an indirect inguinal hernia, the closure of the V-shaped defect in the transversalis fascia (Fig. 1A) is considered a most important part of the operation. Its omission is believed to be the major factor in the postoperative "recurrences" about the internal ring.

In Figure 1A the origin of the external spermatic (cremaster) and pubic vessels from the deep epigastric vessels is clearly depicted. Following high ligation and excision of the hernial sac the characteristic defect commonly found in the transversalis fascia is closed with interrupted sutures of 3–0 silk, a snug closure being obtained about the internal ring. The ligated neck of the hernial sac in relation to the closure about the internal ring is indicated in dotted outline in Figure 1B.

After suture of the cut margins of the cremaster muscle, the medial leaflet of the aponeurosis of the external oblique muscle is enfolded on itself with interrupted sutures of 3–0 silk and united, "white fascia to white fascia," with the shelving edge of the inguinal ligament (Fig. 1C). More recently, closure of the cremaster muscle over rather than under the cord as depicted is preferred. This change precludes the imbrication of the overlying aponeurosis of the external oblique muscle (Fig. 1D, E) because of the excess tension on the suture line. Accordingly, simple approximation of the cut margins of the aponeurosis is done. This technique is called the anatomical method of repair because it restores the normal anatomical relations of the musculofascial structures in the inguinal canal. We believe that the classic Bassini type of repair is deficient both anatomically and mechanically, and we neither practice nor recommend it.

Direct Inguinal Hernia

In a direct inguinal hernia the protrusion is through a "weakness" in the posterior wall (transversalis fascia) medial to the deep epigastric vessels (Fig. 2A). In

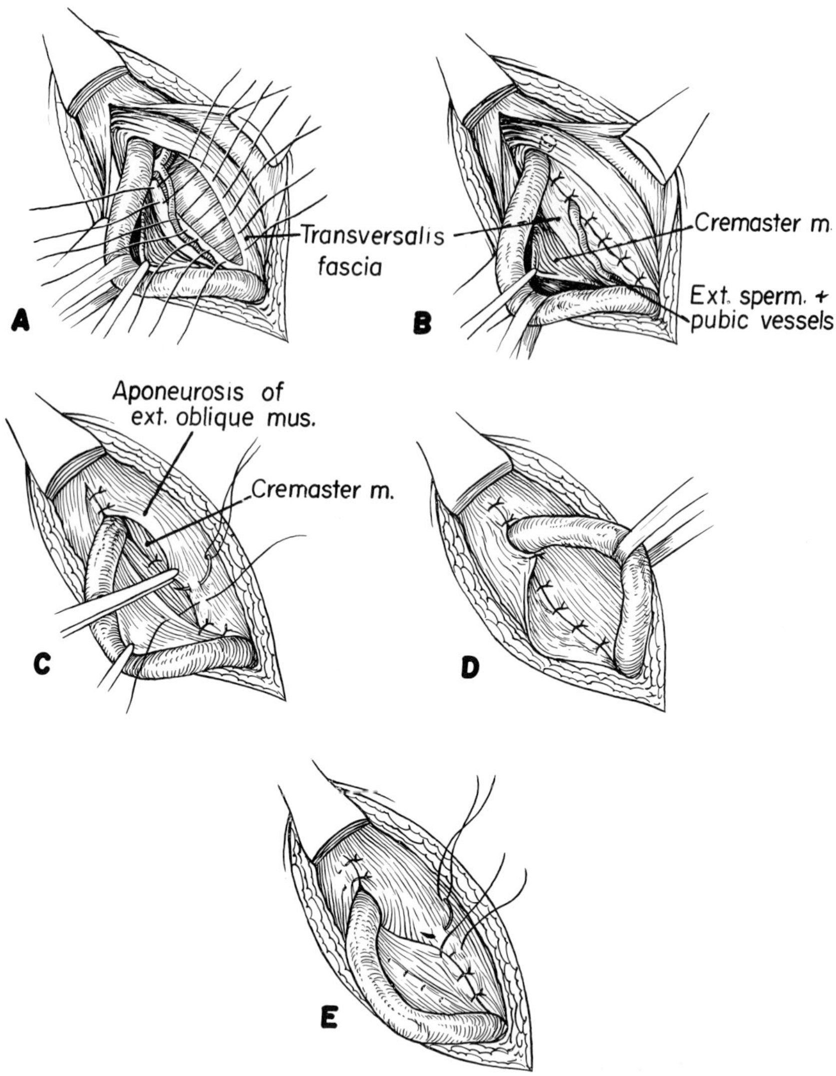

FIGURE 1. Indirect inguinal hernia.

general, the majority of surgeons prefer simple inversion of the hernia and closure of the overlying transversalis fascia. It is argued that a direct hernia is an eventration of the anterior abdominal wall and accordingly there is no formation of a true sac. Admittedly this may be true in small hernial protrusions, but in the large hernias all the morphological characteristics of a sac are present. It has been observed repeatedly that when the sac is exposed, it is always much larger than anticipated. Also, not infrequently, pseudo sliding components of adherent bowel and omentum need to be freed and reposited in the peritoneal cavity. This, in

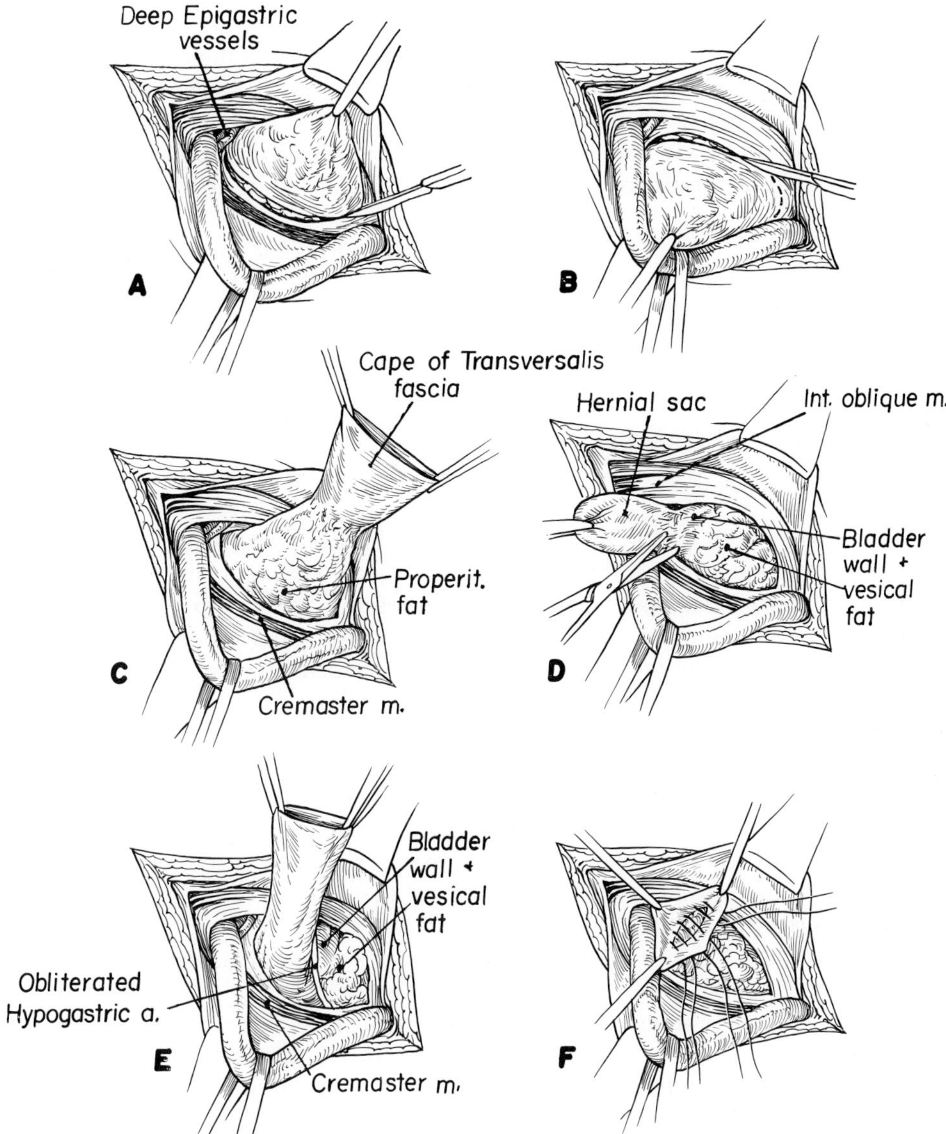

FIGURE 2. Direct inguinal hernia.

conjunction with the excision of the protruded peritoneum (sac), eliminates the perpetual "battering ram" effect of the inverted contents on the line of closure of the transversalis fascia.

In the mobilization of the sac of a direct hernia, a circumferential incision is made at its base, through the transversalis fascia (Fig. 2A, B) and the attenuated cape of transversalis fascia is removed (Fig. 2C). This permits herniation of the properitoneal fat, in which dissection is continued to expose the sac of the direct hernia. The fundus of the sac is grasped in a clamp for traction, and by scissor dissection it is separated from its attachment medially to the wall of the bladder (Fig. 2D). The mobilized sac is opened (Fig. 2E) and any adherent contents are freed and replaced into the peritoneal cavity. A direct hernia is classified as medial or lateral depending upon its relation to the obliterated hypogastric artery (Fig. 2E). The redundant sac tissue is excised and the opening in the peritoneum, because of its size, is closed routinely with interrupted everting mattress sutures of 00 silk (Fig. 2F).

The closure of the defect in the transversalis fascia and the subsequent steps in the reconstruction of the inguinal canal are the same as for the repair of an indirect inguinal hernia.

Sliding Inguinal Hernia

By definition, a true sliding hernia is an irreducible hernia in which a portion of the wall of the sac is formed by the protruding viscus. In the inguinoscrotal region the sliding component may be sigmoid colon, cecum, or bladder. The lack of a thorough understanding of the mechanism of formation and the anatomical basis of repair is believed the main factor for the high incidence (18 to 20 per cent) of postoperative recurrence.

In the smaller type of sliding hernia a modification of the Bevan type of repair is suitable. However, in the large hernia the repair on the La Roque principle as suggested by Carrington Williams is preferred and is the technique illustrated here.

The hernial sac is opened and the sigmoid colon which forms its posterior wall is seen. The medial aponeurotic leaflet of the external oblique muscle is retracted cephalad to expose a broad surface of the internal oblique muscle, which is incised as indicated in Figure 3A. The incision is deepened through the underlying layers (Fig. 3B) and the peritoneal cavity is entered (Fig. 3C). The sigmoid colon is withdrawn through the separate incision (Fig. 3C), and as traction is maintained the whole of the sliding component of the sigmoid colon is reduced (Fig. 3D). It may now be seen that the opening first made in the anterior wall of the sac is essentially an opening in the peritoneal covering of the mesosigmoid (Fig. 3D), which has been separated from the mesosigmoid in the process of formation of the sliding hernia. This opening is closed with a continuous suture of 3–0 silk (Fig. 3E). The separate incision into the peritoneal cavity is closed as depicted (Fig. 3F) and the defect in the transversalis fascia (Fig. 3F) is closed about the external spermatic and pubic vessels (Fig. 3G). A snug fit is obtained about the internal ring, and the remainder of the repair is the same as for an indirect inguinal hernia.

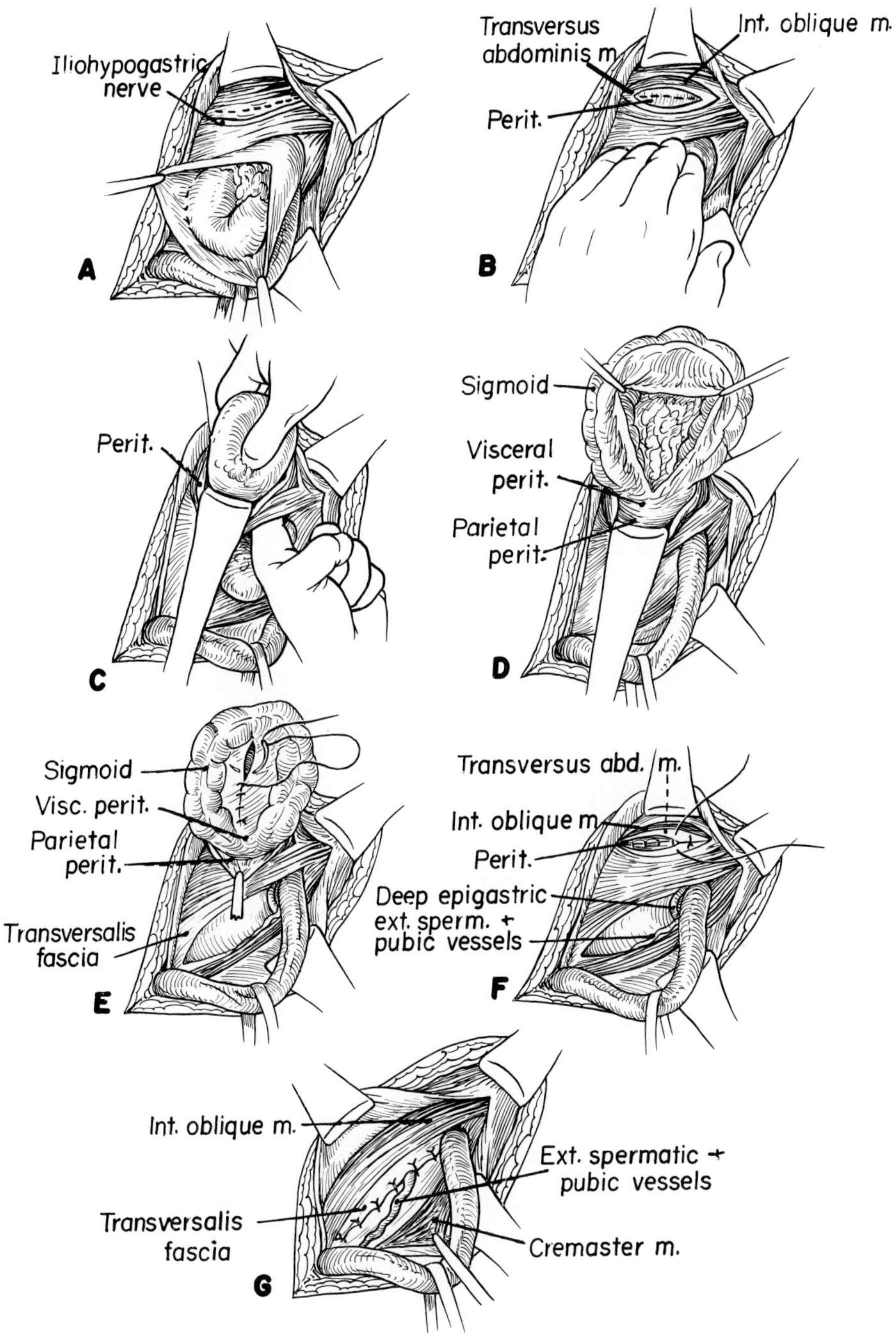

FIGURE 3. Sliding inguinal hernia.

Femoral Hernia

Femoral Approach

In the elective surgical correction of a femoral hernia, either the inguinal (Fig. 4A, a) or the femoral (Fig. 4A, b) approach may be employed. However, when-

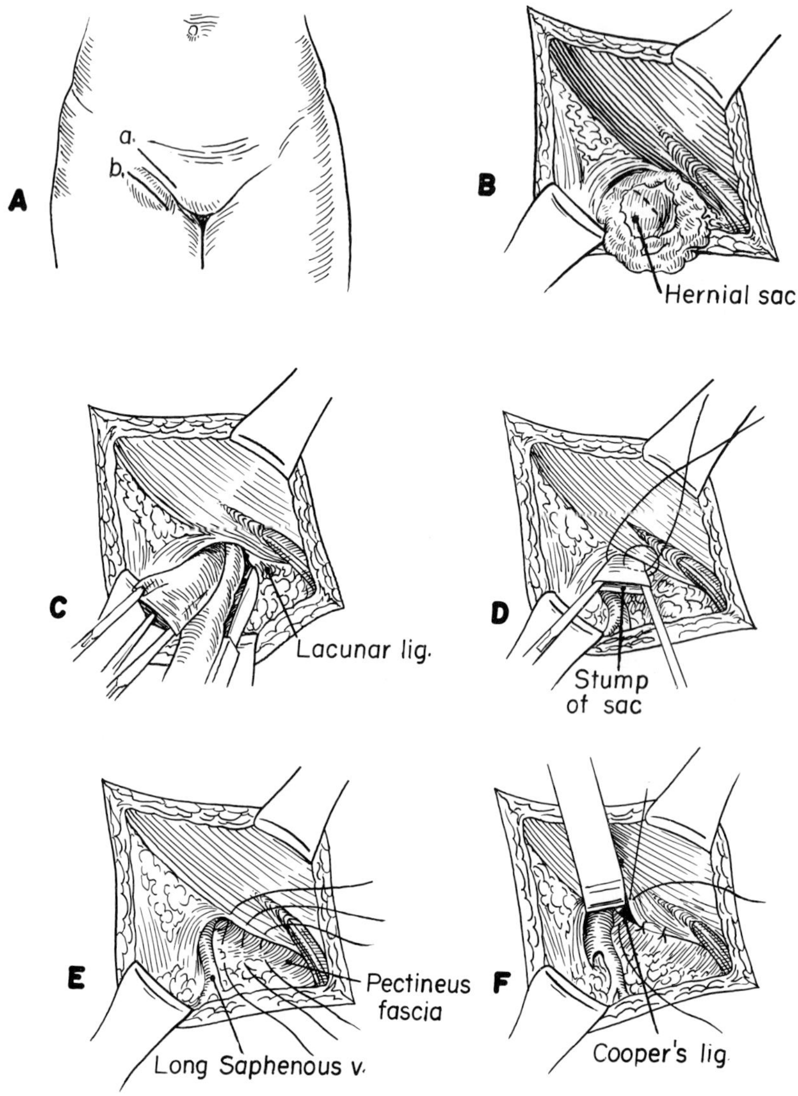

FIGURE 4. Femoral hernia–femoral approach.

ever strangulation is present or suspected, the inguinal approach is used routinely because of the possible necessity of performing a bowel resection.

Following the skin incision, the hernial protrusion within the surrounding fatty areolar tissue is exposed and an incision made in the sac (Fig. 4B). If there is difficulty in reducing the contents of the sac, constriction of its neck may be released by severance of the lacunar (Gimbernat's) ligament (Fig. 4C), which is practically always preferred to transection of the inguinal ligament. In the performance of this part of the operation one must always be cognizant of the possible presence of an anomalous obturator artery, injury to which should be judiciously avoided. After excision of the redundant sac tissue, the neck of the sac is occluded with a transfixion suture of 00 silk (Fig. 4D). In the fascial closure of the femoral canal the inguinal ligament may be sutured (3–0 silk) to either the pectineus fascia (Bassini technique) as in Figure 4E or to Cooper's ligament as in Figure 4F.

Inguinal Approach

The inguinal incision is deepened through the underlying subcutaneous fat and fascia to expose the related structures (Fig. 5A). An opening in the aponeurosis of the external oblique muscle is extended by scissor dissection through the external ring, as shown in Figure 5A. Next the cremaster muscle layer is severed and the mobilized round ligament is retracted laterally to show the incision in the transversalis fascia (Fig. 5B). The properitoneal fat is dissected to expose the peritoneum and the relation of the hernial protrusion to the surrounding structures (Fig. 5C). The peritoneum is incised as indicated in Figure 5C and the peritoneal cavity is entered (Fig. 5D). The afferent and efferent limbs of the incarcerated loop of small intestine are now seen. As in the femoral approach, constriction of the neck of the sac may be released by severance of the lacunar (Gimbernat's) ligament (Fig. 5E), caution being taken to avoid injury to an anomalous obturator artery, which when present should be visible from this approach.

In the event of frank necrosis of the incarcerated hernial contents, the release of the constriction of the neck of the sac should be deferred. The viable afferent and efferent limbs of the gangrenous loop are doubly clamped and transected, and intestinal continuity is restored by proximal end-to-end anastomosis. The remaining attachment of the peritoneum to the sac is severed and the peritoneal cavity closed. The incarcerated gangrenous contents within the isolated hernial sac may then be removed as a unit from below after first transecting the lacunar ligament. This technique, recommended by Varco and Dennis, avoids the potential contamination of either the peritoneal cavity or the wound.

When resection of the bowel is not required, the released loop of intestine is first withdrawn into the wound (Fig. 5F) and reposited into the peritoneal cavity (Fig. 5G). The empty hernial sac is then inverted through the femoral canal (Fig. 5G, H) and the remaining peritoneal attachment of the sac is transected as indicated in Figure 5G. The femoral canal is closed by suturing Cooper's ligament to the inguinal ligament (Fig. 5I). The opening in the transversalis fascia is closed

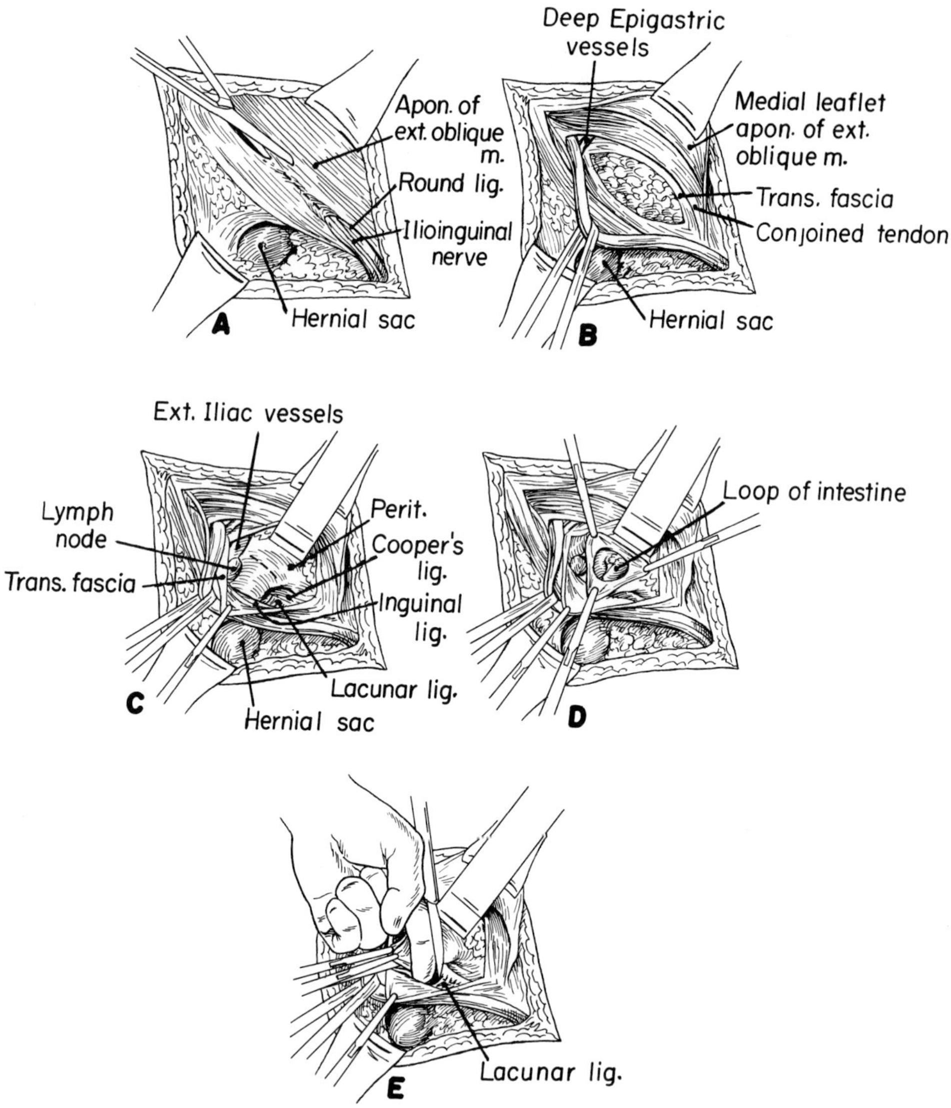

FIGURE 5. Femoral hernia–inguinal approach.

with interrupted sutures of 00 silk (Fig. 5J) and the remainder of the repair is the same as for an indirect inguinal hernia.

Postoperative Incisional Hernia

In the surgical repair of a postoperative incisional hernia an extensive undermining on either side of the hernia in the plane between the subcutaneous fatty tissue layer

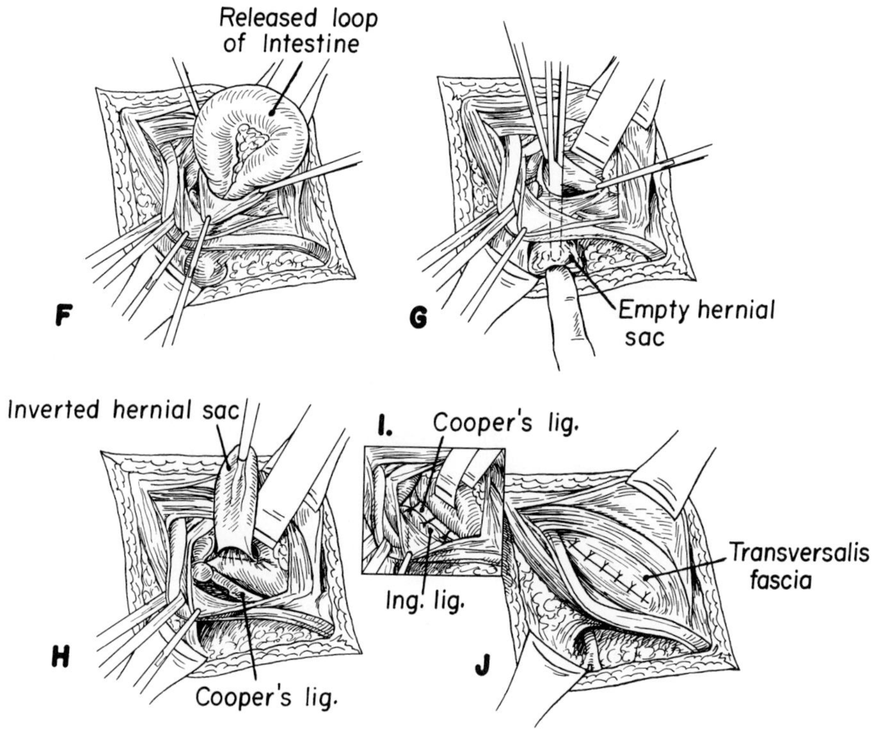

FIGURE 5 (*continued*)

and the musculofascial layer of the anterolateral abdominal wall is required. It is surprising how frequently an adequate repair of a large hernia may be obtained when one is primarily interested in using the patient's tissue in preference to the more expedient artificial devices such as tantalum and stainless steel mesh.

An elliptical incision is made about the previous operative scar (Fig. 6A), which is excised. Toweling is applied to the incised skin margins, and with clamp traction maintained upward the wound margins are widely undermined by scalpel dissection (Fig. 6B) to expose a broad expanse of the surrounding anterolateral abdominal wall (Fig. 6C). An incision is next made at the line of junction of the true and false fascia to expose the free margin of the underlying rectus muscle (Fig. 6D). The rectus muscle on either side is retracted and the line of union of the false sac and peritoneum is defined (Fig. 6E). The false sac is opened, a technique greatly to be preferred to inversion, because frequently a multiplicity of intestinal loops are adherent to the walls of the hernial sac. After reduction of its contents, the sac is excised and the cut margins of the peritoneum are approximated with interrupted sutures of 00 silk (Fig. 6F). The mobilized muscle and fascial layers are similarly approximated with interrupted sutures of 00 silk (Fig. 6G, H). When required—and they often are—lateral relaxing incisions are made in the fascia to relieve tension on the suture line at the site of fascial repair. Penrose drains are inserted beneath the mobilized flaps of the anterolateral abdominal wall and have their exits through separate stab wound drainage incisions lateral to

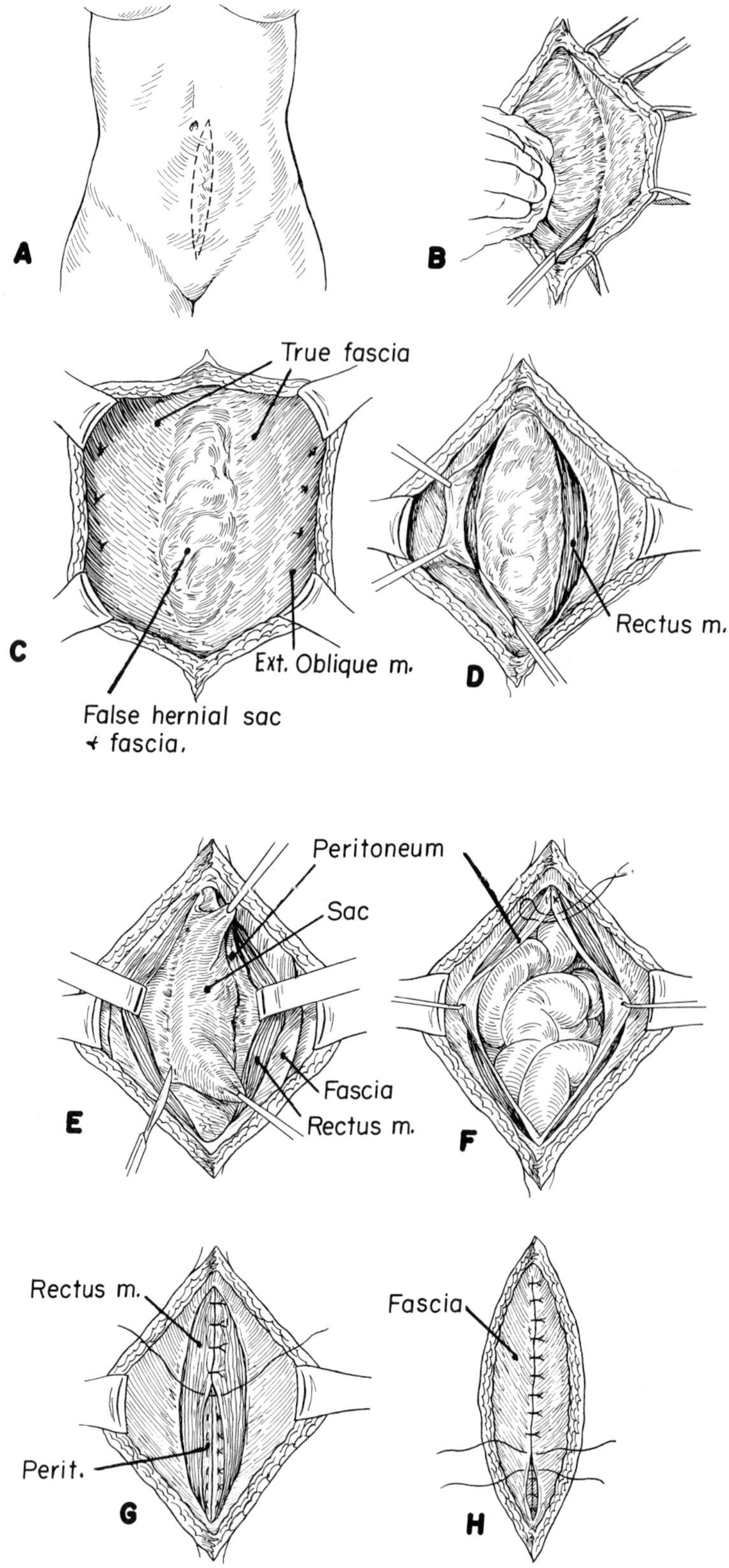

FIGURE 6. Incisional hernia.

the line of skin closure. The drains permit the ready escape of serosanguineous accumulations and are believed to lessen thereby the incidence of wound infection.

References

Bevan, A. D. Sliding hernias of the ascending colon and cecum, the descending colon and sigmoid, and the bladder. *Ann. Surg.* 92:754, October 1930.

Cattell, R. B. Repair of incisional hernia. *S. Clin. North America* 29:787, June 1949.

Lam, C. R., Szilagyi, D. E., and Puppendahl, M. Tantalum gauze in the repair of large postoperative ventral hernias. *Arch. Surg.* 57:234, August 1948.

McVay, C. B., and Anson, B. J. A fundamental error in current methods of inguinal herniorrhaphy. *Surg., Gynec. and Obst.* 74:746, March 1942.

Williams, C. Repair of sliding inguinal hernia through the abdominal (La Roque) approach. *Ann. Surg.* 126:612, October 1947.

Zimmerman, L. M. Inguinal hernia; surgical treatment of direct inguinal hernia. *Surg., Gynec. and Obst.* 66:193, February 1938.

70. *Use of Drains in the Peritoneal Cavity and Abdominal Wall*

NORMAN C. TANNER

BROADLY SPEAKING, drainage may be used either as a main method of treatment or as a preventive of complications. It may be therapeutic or prophylactic.

Therapeutic Drainage

Under this heading comes the drainage of intraabdominal collections of pus; for example, pelvic, subphrenic, and appendix abscesses. Therapeutic drainage may also be required in the treatment of extravasations of bile or pancreatic juice in the peritoneal cavity. In the past it was common to employ stab suprapubic drainage, or even multiple drainage of the peritoneal cavity, for all forms of diffuse peritonitis. This practice has been largely discontinued, because much of the exudate is protective. Mopping out or aspiration of the secretion is usually employed at the time of operation, particularly if a viscus has perforated. Drainage in diffuse peritonitis is placed only to an area where abscess formation has become established, or to an area of active disease from which a flow of purulent or irritant fluid may come. Organ drainage, e.g. gastrostomy, cholecystostomy, will not be considered here.

Prophylactic Drainage

This is required whenever physiological fluid is expected to collect, or when the anastomosis or closure of a viscus could possibly leak. For example, bile may escape after operations on the bile ducts or liver, or pancreatic juice after operations on the pancreas, or urine after operation on or injuries to the kidney. It may be wise to resort to drainage if it is feared that intestinal secretions may escape following intestinal strangulations or injuries, or operations on the bowel; for example, colectomy in obese, infected, or frail patients, particularly if the colon is diverticulous. Drainage of the neighborhood of the closed duodenal stump is advisable if the closure is unsatisfactory. Any surgeon who has a 2 per cent or greater incidence of duodenal stump leakage would be well advised to drain every stump he closes.

After evacuation of certain cysts, it may be advisable to drain in order to prevent re-formation of the cyst. A good example is the pancreatic pseudocyst, when marsupialization is used until the cyst walls have approximated to obliterate the cavity. Drainage was formerly employed almost routinely, too, with hydatid cysts of the liver once the daughter cysts and endocysts had been dealt with. Nowadays it is more customary to fill the cyst with saline and then to close the liver. The cyst walls will approximate slowly as the saline is absorbed.

Drainage may be required if collections of blood are expected to develop; for example, after splenectomy or after hepatic lobectomy or pelvic exenteration. Here a second object is sometimes in mind, diagnosis. One may leave a tube down to an area where it is feared that secondary or reactionary hemorrhage may occur, in order to discover the hemorrhage as soon as possible. This is not an entirely reliable method, for the tube may become occluded by clot and the blood may then escape into the general peritoneal cavity.

Drainage may be established in areas of bacterial or other soiling with the object of insuring that if an abscess develops, the pus will escape via the tube rather than collect and necessitate a further operation for its evacuation or, worse still, produce a generalized peritonitis.

Wound Drainage

Drainage of the deep layers of an abdominal wound rather than the peritoneal cavity may be prudent on occasion. One such occasion is the occurrence of contamination of a wound before closure; for example, in opening an abdominal abscess or through encountering stitch abscesses when reopening an old incision.

A wound in which good hemostasis has not been secured may be drained to prevent hematoma formation, with its risk of disruption of the wound. Perfect hemostasis may be difficult to attain when an old incision is reopened or an incision is made through chronically inflamed parietes, for the vessels in the chronically inflamed or fibrous wound are more difficult to grasp, and multiple small points of bleeding are found rather than the few normal discrete bleeding points.

Most intraperitoneal abscesses *tend* to point toward a previous abdominal incision; hence some surgeons, in dealing with cases in which it is feared that an abdominal abscess may arise, put a drain down to, but not through, the closed peritoneum. This directs and facilitates the passage of pus through the more superficial layers of the wound.

Principles in Peritoneal Drainage

In therapeutic drainage, the pus should be drained by the shortest practical route from the abscess to the skin surface, whenever possible avoiding opening the general peritoneal cavity.

In prophylactic drainage, the drain should be carefully placed down to the site where the fluid is expected to collect; for example, after cholecystectomy the drain should come from Morison's pouch.

Good positioning of a drain is important. On several occasions after cholecystectomy, I have observed that when a drain was placed through a small stab wound lateral to the cholecystectomy incision, a subsequent collection of fluid found its way to and through the upper part of the paramedian scar, rather than through the stab drain.

It is well to consider where intraperitoneal collections escape when they find a way out of the general peritoneal cavity. Such collections have a strong tendency to find their way toward recent operation incisions, or even to old scars or sites of previous peritoneal drainage. If no such scar is present, they find their way to the umbilical cicatrix or, rarely, through weak areas of the abdomen, e.g. the triangle of Petit. Pelvic abscesses tend to point and burst through the rectum or posterior vault of the vagina or into the bladder before they point on the abdominal wall. Abscesses around the gallbladder tend to burst into neighboring viscera, colon or duodenum, before the pus approaches the skin, unless there is a nearby recent incision or scar.

Drainage Materials

The main object of drainage is to establish a track along which secretions from the peritoneum can escape to the exterior. There is a wide range of drainage materials from which to choose. They have three characteristics in common: (1) they are fairly soft and malleable, in order to avoid pressure on important blood vessels or other structures; (2) they are nonirritant to tissues; and (3) they are stable in composition, not decomposing when subjected to prolonged heat and moisture.

Rubber fulfills most of these criteria; also latex and certain plastic materials, e.g. Teflon. Some surgeons prefer a simple soft tube, such as Paul's tubing; others prefer a corrugated material which can be cut to any size. Corrugated latex is probably the most commonly employed drainage material in the British Isles. If stiffer rubber tubing is used, it is possible for bowel or omentum to be sucked into its end, causing difficulties in removal. Such tubes should have a slit 2 cm. or more in length along one or both sides of the peritoneal end of the tube. Somewhat stiffer tubes must be used if suction drainage is to be employed.

A Foley catheter may be used as a drainage tube, though it is of more value as an enterostomy tube. Better suction from the wound, by capillary attraction, is believed by some surgeons to occur if a soft tube is lightly filled with a wick or plug of gauze, as in the Penrose drain. This is not used much in England, although popular in the United States.

Other materials have been used; for example, stainless steel or even glass in particular circumstances.

When a cavity in the abdomen, e.g. a marsupialized pancreatic cyst, is packed with gauze, it is only necessary to withdraw the end of the gauze through the wound to establish a drain. Simple gauze drains are not much employed, however, because of the difficulty and discomfort of extraction.

Risks of Drainage

The presence of a foreign body passing from the exterior to the peritoneal cavity is an obvious situation which could allow the entry of organisms from the exterior toward the peritoneum. The rapid formation of granulation tissue along and around the track usually prevents this. Nevertheless, it is important to maintain scrupulous technique when dealing with the wound and the drain.

Secondary infection is particularly likely to occur if a tuberculous abdominal abscess is drained.

In the days when the Talma-Morison operation was used in the treatment of ascites, it was customary to place a glass drain into the pelvis for a few days to prevent ascitic fluid from accumulating in the upper abdomen. Peritonitis, often fatal, was not uncommon, and originated in the drainage site. The constant flow of ascitic fluid tended to prevent the local concentration of protective fibrinous exudate and impeded the development of adhesions.

I have mentioned the danger of bowel entering the end of a firm rubber tube, and the risks attendant on tubes pressing on blood vessels; for example, the pelvic drain brought out through an iliac fossa incision may press on one of the iliac veins or arteries. If drainage is made through a long laparotomy wound, there is a risk that fluid from the peritoneal cavity, often irritant or infective, may enter the wound and delay healing, or produce a wound abscess, sinus, disruption or, later, a hernia.

Any wound drain may lead to a hernia, particularly if placed in an area where the abdominal wall is fibrous or weak. Drainage made through the linea alba or the linea semilunaris is an example. The insertion of a drainage tube leads to the development of an encircling track of granulations, replaced later by fibrous tissue which may diminish or almost disappear with time. However, this fibrous tissue may kink the bowel, leading to obstruction, or cause a band to form. The tube track, whenever possible, should have omentum wrapped around it. The tubes should not press firmly on bowel, for obstruction has been known to result from such pressure. I have seen obstruction of the ascending colon result from pressure of a cholecystectomy drain from Morison's pouch which was led to a point far out on the flank.

Technique of Drainage

The previous notes will guide the operator in the general principles underlying the technique of abdominal drainage.

Theoretically the drainage should be at a place on the parietes where an abscess would naturally tend to burst, though this is not always the ideal or the most practical site; otherwise we might drain infected gallbladders through the umbilicus!

If an abscess or irritant fluid collection is already present, drainage should be established at a point on the parietes close to the abscess cavity, and where bowel is least likely to be present. It is also desirable, when possible, to avoid opening the general peritoneal cavity.

If the incision is in such a position that gravity helps the drainage, the abscess cavity will tend to remain empty, and as a consequence its walls will come together with more rapid healing.

Nevertheless, an abscess *will* drain against gravity, a common example being the draining of a pelvic abscess through a suprapubic incision. In such cases, the fibrous contraction of the walls of the abscess, together with the intraabdominal pressure, keeps the secretions flowing out and eventually leads to obliteration of the cavity and track.

Peritoneal Abscess

In draining an appendix abscess the incision should be over the tender or indurated area, preferably well over to the right side, away from the small bowel. It is in some cases possible to dissect laterally and extraperitoneally, and to open the abscess without opening the peritoneal cavity. On the rare occasion when a retroperitoneal abscess points over the triangle of Petit, direct drainage through that area is indicated.

If the peritoneal cavity is to be opened in exploring for an abscess, the bowel should first be carefully packed away with moistened gauze packing. The abscess region is tentatively explored with a finger, a good "sucker" being held nearby. The moment pus is seen it is aspirated with the sucker until the cavity is as empty and as dry as possible. An antibiotic may be introduced into the cavity. A wide rubber drain or two drains of the corrugated latex or Penrose type are then introduced. These drains need not be brought out through the wound, but through the nearest parietes, making a separate incision if need be. Then the pack can be removed. Drainage is employed also in closing the wound, a soft fine rubber tube being placed down to the closed peritoneum. Postoperatively, sealing off of the abscess region will be encouraged by nasogastric suction, intravenous feeding, and antibiotics.

Drainage Through the Laparotomy Wound

This is at times desirable, particularly if the wound is in the natural route for drainage, or is nearest to the area to be drained, or is already infected.

If a paramedian wound, perhaps for cholecystectomy, is used, it is wise to bring the drain, usually a strip of corrugated rubber with or without a tube drain from the common duct, through the uppermost part of the incision, just under the liver, so that when the drains are removed the liver tends to descend slightly and protect this area. In such cases it is advisable to place a catgut stitch above and another below the drain, taking all layers of both sides of the incision, excluding the skin. The object is to prevent secretions which escape alongside the tube from entering between the layers of the wound.

Stab Drainage

Stab drains are placed usually in the suprapubic region or flanks, when there is established local infection or when there is soiling which it is impossible to remove adequately; for example, rupture of a stercoral or malignant ulcer of the rectum. It may also be required at points of potential danger, such as an inadequately closed duodenal stump, or colonic anastomosis. In such a case the wound edge is retracted until the peritoneal surface of the intended stab incision is seen, which should be a place free of large arteries. The edge of the peritoneum is grasped by two Kocher forceps to steady it; otherwise the skin and peritoneal incisions may not be in the same line (Fig. 1). An incision is made through the parietes until the

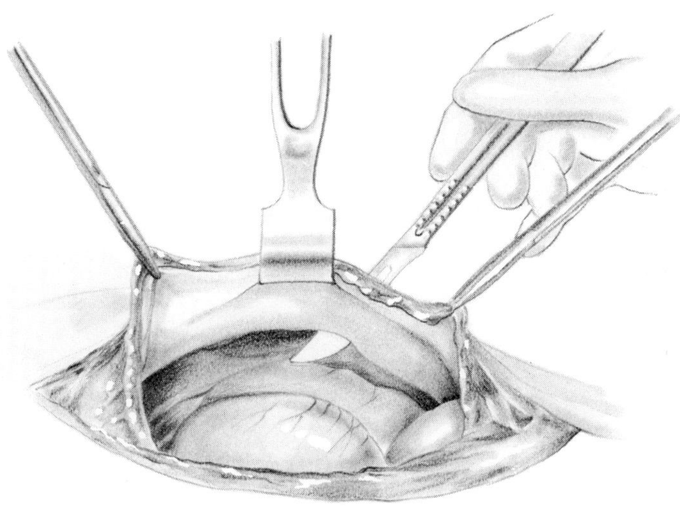

FIGURE 1. The edge of the peritoneum is grasped with two Kocher forceps to steady it, and a retractor is used to obtain a view of the peritoneal surface. An incision is made through all layers of the abdominal wall until the peritoneum is reached.

scalpel is seen to enter the peritoneum, and then a straight or curved forceps, e.g. a long artery or a Moynihan cholecystectomy forceps, is passed through the skin into the peritoneal cavity and made to project through the main abdominal incision. A drainage tube is grasped in the forceps and drawn through the stab incision and fixed at its optimum position (Fig. 2).

At times it is not possible to view the peritoneal surface of the stab incision, in which case the surgeon can make the incision onto a finger guarded with a thimble.

When a stab incision is completed it is important to make sure that no major vessel has been injured. Temporary brisk bleeding is common, but persistent bleeding must be arrested. If hemostasis is not secured, it is possible for bleeding to persist afterward, either to the exterior or into the peritoneal cavity.

Fixation of the Drain

When the drain is properly positioned, it should be fixed to one edge of the skin incision with a nonabsorbable suture. A safety pin is also inserted as an extra safeguard.

If there is a reason to avoid transfixing a drainage tube, the stitch I call the "Anglo-Saxon stocking" can be used. A nonabsorbable, rough (e.g. linen) stitch

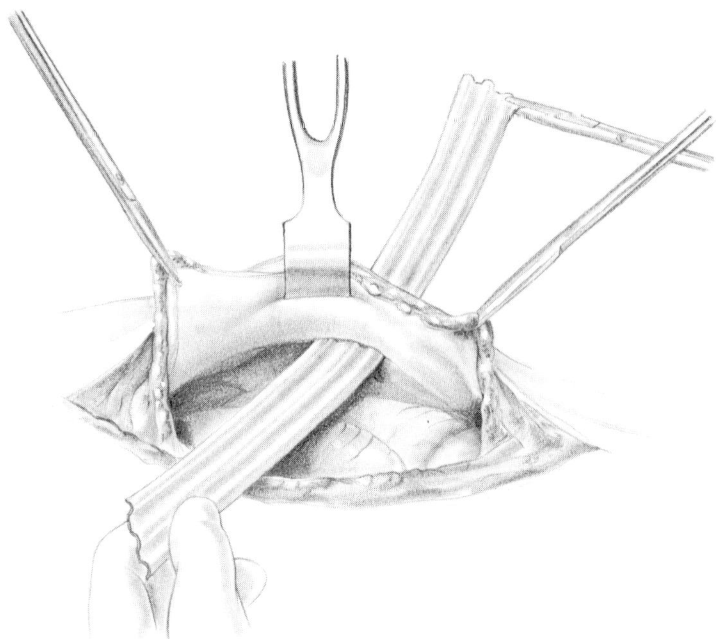

FIGURE 2. A forceps is introduced through the stab wound into the peritoneal cavity and out of the incision. It is made to grasp a tube or a corrugated drain. The drain is drawn into the peritoneal cavity, leaving a part out of the stab wound.

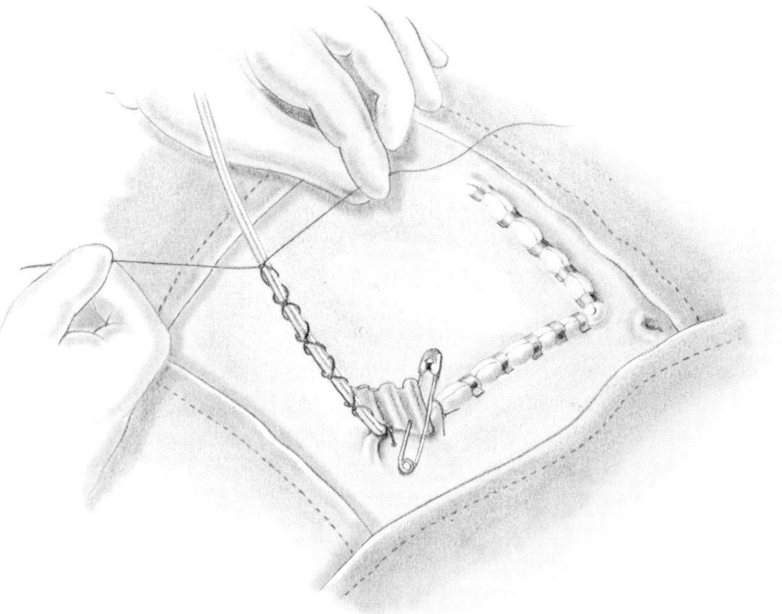

FIGURE 3. Fixation of two drains through one end of an L-shaped (Kehr) incision, following an operation for repair of a divided common bile duct. The corrugated drain leading from Morison's right kidney pouch is fixed to one edge of the wound with a stitch. The tube leading from the common duct is fixed by an "Anglo-Saxon stocking" stitch, and is being finally tied.

transfixes the wound edge and the strands are tied around the tube. The tying continues obliquely around and up the tube, with a half-tie at each crossing. After half a dozen such turns and a final reef knot tie, even a slippery tube will be secure (Fig. 3).

If a drainage tube is rather long or to be attached to a suction bottle on the side of the bed, the occasional or constant drag of the tube on the small area of skin to which it is stitched causes a good deal of discomfort. This can be readily prevented as follows. A suitable length of adhesive is attached to the skin for a third of its length; then it is looped up to surround and fix the drainage tube, leaving a good deal of slack drain between the drain site and the adhesive. The adhesive is in its middle third stuck to itself, and in the final third is applied to the skin again. It will be seen that any drag on the tube cannot be transmitted to the sensitive place where the tube is stitched to the skin.

Postoperative Management of the Drain

A careful aseptic technique is advisable in dealing with the drain, particularly when the drainage is excessive.

Prophylactic drains can usually be extracted after two to four days if there is no notable discharge. By this time a potential track to the exterior exists and any subsequent fluid collection will usually find its way into the track.

Therapeutic drains are shortened and then removed when the drainage diminishes.

Persistence of Discharge

Persistence of discharge may be due to inadequate drainage of an infected and perhaps loculated cavity which is constantly full of fluid. Sometimes it is due to a deep connection with the duct of a secretory organ; for example, the pancreatic duct or an accessory bile duct. No matter which is the cause, some help in diagnosis and management may be obtained, after drainage has persisted for a fortnight or so, by radiography, after the instillation of a radiopaque watery solution into the track (oily solutions are not advised). If radiography discloses that a large persisting abscess cavity is present, then more accurate positioning of the end of the tube in the cavity and low pressure suction may help. If this fails, one must consider the possibility of persisting abdominal disease or the presence of a foreign body, such as a fecolith, an unabsorbed suture, or even a swab.

If a fistula persists because there is a communication with the duct of an abdominal gland, the best hope of closure is slow fibrous contraction of the fistula along its *whole* length, until the secretions can pass more readily into the intestine by their normal route than through the narrowed fistula. Premature tube removal will lead to pooling in the region of the damaged duct. It is better in such cases to insert a slightly loose-fitting tube and apply suction to the depth. In this way the secretions are kept from pooling in the track, the granulation lining of which can contract until it is firm round the tube. A narrower tube is then put in, and this process repeated until even a small tube can hardly be inserted. Then the whole narrowed track usually closes. If it fails to do so, one must suspect obstruction in the duct. For example, a fistula connected with the common bile duct may persist if there is a neoplasm or stone near the lower end of the duct, or a pancreatic duct fistula will persist if a carcinoma or stone blocks the duct of Wirsung.

71. *Intraabdominal Abscesses*

PHILIP COOPER

THE DEVELOPMENT of an intraabdominal abscess postoperatively may to some extent be avoided by a proper peritoneal toilet at the time of surgery. This includes additional draping when a viscus is open, the cleansing of soiled viscera, and the aspiration of bloody fluid and contaminated or infected material from the peritoneal cavity prior to closure of the wound. Instruments used near or on open viscera should be kept within the dirty field—that is, the contaminated area which includes the operative site—and a towel spread over the lower extremities of the patient. To impress the staff with the need to separate the dirty from the clean field, it may be helpful to use a towel of a specified color for the dirty field. The nurse should not handle contaminated instruments with the gloved hands, but should pass them to the operator by grasping them with forceps. Further to reduce contamination, she should place each needle with the suture material into the needle holder held by the operator. The needles should not be returned to the nurse, but should be retained in a basin within the dirty field.

When the operator returns to a clean dissection, the contaminated instruments are removed, or are temporarily covered if a dirty field is to be re-established for later surgery involving an open viscus. Contaminated towels or pads used as drapes are removed before a change of gloves, and clean towels or pads are applied after gloves have been changed by those who worked in the dirty field. All dirty instruments should be removed from the operating table prior to closure of the abdominal incision.

Although it would be preferable to have a tray with unused instruments available for wound closure, this is impractical in many operating rooms, since it may result in an excessive prolongation of operating time because of the shortage and frequent change of trained personnel.

There is evidence that some abscesses in certain areas of the abdominal cavity may respond to antibiotic therapy alone. These include some appendiceal, probably some subphrenic, and possibly some pericolic abscesses. However, it is doubtful whether a well-established collection of purulent material can often be cured without spontaneous or surgical drainage; the contents may become sterile under antibiotic therapy, but the abscess cavity will usually remain.

The hazards of a nonoperative approach must be kept in mind, for an undrained abscess may erode into a blood vessel and cause serious bleeding or generalized dissemination of the infection; or the abscess may rupture into the general peritoneal cavity. Patients on this form of therapy should be closely observed and evaluated frequently. Rarely is indefinite postponement attainable.

Technique of Drainage

General Principles

The technical approach to drainage of an intraabdominal abscess is influenced by the anatomy of the region and by the type and extent of the abscess. Drainage should be established in as dependent an area as possible so that the abscess can readily drain, collapse, and heal. One should avoid, if at all feasible, traversing uninvolved peritoneal cavity to reach the abscess, and should establish drainage through a tract that will remain patent long enough for the abscess to respond fully to treatment. In addition, all pockets of an abscess cavity should be explored digitally or with an instrument, care being taken not to disrupt its outer protective wall.

If drainage necessitates an approach through uninfected peritoneal cavity, the viscera should be well packed off beforehand, and suction should be available for use as soon as the abscess cavity is entered. It is advisable to have two suction tips and two suctions ready in case one unit fails to function properly. After the abscess has been entered and aspirated, definitive drainage should be established by the safest and shortest route through both the peritoneal cavity and the abdominal wall, consideration also being given to the principle of dependent drainage.

When multiple intraabdominal abscesses are present, occasionally more than one may be handled through a major incision. Frequently, however, separate incisions are required to drain multiple abscesses in accordance with the basic principles of drainage here delineated.

Periappendiceal and Pericolic Abscesses

Abscesses that follow appendicitis, or diverticulitis or other inflammatory lesions of the colon, can in most cases be drained "extraperitoneally," that is, without entering uninvolved peritoneal cavity—by making an incision over the mass, often over the most prominent and tender area. This area may be abnormally warm and show some redness, particularly if the abscess is juxtaposed to or involves the overlying abdominal wall. The peritoneum is usually thickened, edematous, and adherent to the adjacent abscess wall. Even if it appears clean, and moves freely over underlying structures, the wise course may be to open the peritoneum to determine if another incision is indicated, and where it should be made. Some surgeons drain the abscess through the initial incision, rather than make a second incision, for they feel that antibiotics will adequately handle limited peritoneal contamination. My recommendation is to avoid such contamination of the general peritoneal cavity if this is at all possible and reasonable.

Abscesses following appendicitis may form in a number of sites, depending on the location of the appendix. Occasionally a mass formed by adhesion of edematous and inflamed omentum to the appendix or/and neighboring structures may give one the impression of an abscess on abdominal examination. However, the diagnosis of abscess can usually be made from the clinical findings. The abscess may be in the iliac fossa, adjacent to the colon, in the pelvis, anterior or posterior to the ileum, in the retroperitoneal space, or in other locations. It may be difficult to drain a periappendiceal abscess located within the vicinity of the ileum without traversing uninvolved peritoneal cavity. Frequently the remnants of the appendix can be removed when the abscess is drained.

One must consider the possibility of a malignant tumor when an abscess occurs in relation to the colon, particularly when the infection does not respond in the usual manner after drainage. Indications for colostomy as part of the treatment of pericolic abscesses secondary to primary colonic disease are discussed in other chapters.

Subphrenic Abscesses

In recent years the increased number and the extent of intraabdominal operations performed on the gastrointestinal tract and on other structures have probably placed surgery in a somewhat defensive position with respect to subphrenic abscesses, in that the number following surgery surpasses the number associated with nonoperative clinical conditions.

It has been shown that the ligaments attaching the liver to the diaphragm are essentially posterior structures, and from an anatomical standpoint, therefore, there are only two superior spaces, the right and the left. The space posterior to the right triangular ligament, the right posterior space, is essentially infrahepatic. Anteroposterior and lateral x-ray films should always be taken preoperatively to assist in localizing abscesses in these regions.

Right superior space abscesses can usually be approached through a right anterior subcostal incision. Some, in a posterolateral position, can often be more readily approached through a low lateral thoracic incision, with the removal of a short segment of one or two ribs. This approach may be used as an extension of an operation when the anterior subcostal approach has been attempted and found to be unsuitable, or as an initial approach when it appears indicated. The right posterior approach is used to drain those abscesses which develop in the right posterior space. It is now rarely used to drain right superior space abscesses.

Left superior space and other left subphrenic abscesses are usually best approached through a left anterior subcostal incision. However, the lateral approach may occasionally prove more direct. The left posterior approach is rarely indicated, and may be hazardous if the spleen is still present.

The surgeon must recognize the possibility that an undrained subphrenic abscess may spread through the diaphragm and produce an empyema, a bronchopleural fistula, or a necrotizing bronchopneumonia. The treatment of these complications is not covered in this chapter.

Anterior Subcostal Approach. If a diagnosis of subphrenic abscess is made by clinical and/or x-ray findings, and if the anterior subcostal approach is indicated and used, the location of the point of maximum tenderness and the results of the x-ray studies should influence and determine the exact site of the skin incision. It is usually made approximately 1 to 1½ inches below and parallel to the costal border, and should be about 4 to 5 inches in length to assure adequate exposure (Fig. 1). All layers of the abdominal wall, including the posterior rectus sheath and the transversalis fascia, should be incised, except the peritoneum, which preferably should be left intact. If it is inadvertently opened, it should be sutured and a pack placed over the repair as the procedure is continued. If the proper plane of dissection is followed, the dissection can be readily continued with the index finger or with a small gauge roll on a clamp ("peanut" or "dissector"), freeing the peritoneum from the diaphragm.

When the abscess wall is reached and the finger or the dissector does not readily penetrate it, it is wise to withdraw the finger or the dissector and cautiously insert a needle through the thickened wall to see if pus can be extracted. If purulent material is found, a small hemostat is carefully inserted alongside the needle, followed by a larger clamp, and finally the surgeon's finger. As the cavity is explored, the opening in the abscess wall is extended, usually by blunt dissection, to allow adequate drainage. During this dissection care is taken to avoid injury to the liver on the right, and to the stomach, spleen, and other structures on the left side of the abdomen. Drainage should be generous and is established by large cigarette or Penrose drains, which usually prove satisfactory. They are brought directly through the wound. Rubber or plastic tubes should be avoided; if used,

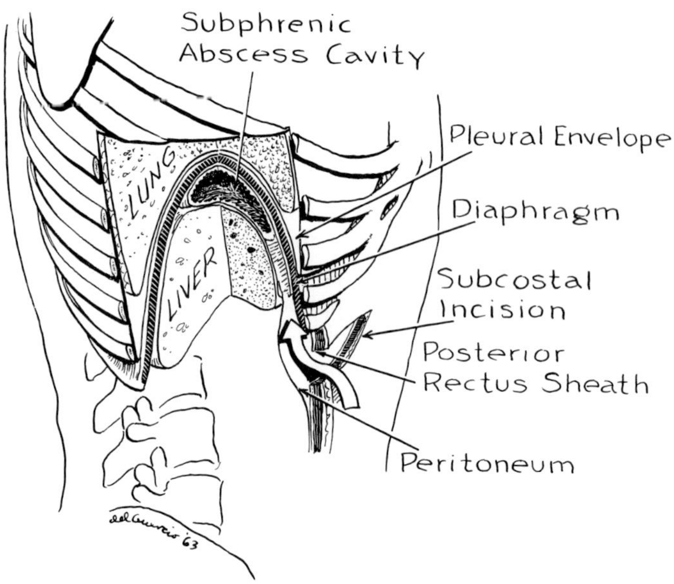

FIGURE 1. Subphrenic abscess: anterior subcostal approach. A diagonal incision is made parallel to and 1½ inches below the costal border. The various layers of the abdominal wall are incised in line with the skin incision, to the peritoneum, which is left intact. The peritoneum is bluntly freed from the diaphragm by finger dissection.

they should be soft but not fragile. A hard tube is contraindicated since it may erode into a viscus. Postoperatively the drains should not be disturbed for about two weeks except to free them from the edges of the abdominal wound, and to advance them for a short distance when indicated to maintain drainage. The drains are then gradually shortened. Drainage is continued until the cavity has filled in properly.

Lateral Thoracic Approach. When the low lateral thoracic approach is used the location of the abscess is determined as carefully as possible by anteroposterior, lateral and other x-ray films of the chest. This is supplemented by needle exploration, percutaneously or/and through the bed of an excised rib. Should the initial needle exploration fail to reveal purulent material, it is reasonable to insert the needle percutaneously at other appropriate levels. The skin incision is made over the appropriate area, and a rib segment is excised subperiosteally (Fig. 2). If the surgeon is convinced that the approach is indicated, in spite of negative needle exploration, or if pus is extracted by needle, the next step after the removal of the segment of rib is to suture the pleura to the diaphragm with a row of interrupted mattress sutures of swaged-on catgut placed in an oval fashion near the periphery of the wound. A second row of sutures is placed beyond the first row to provide a circumscribed area as large as possible for further surgery. The pleura and diaphragm are then incised transversely through the area protected by the surrounding sutures. If an abscess is found, it is opened and explored as described in the preceding section, Anterior Subcostal Approach. If the segment of pleural cavity traversed has been properly sequestrated by the sutures, there is essentially

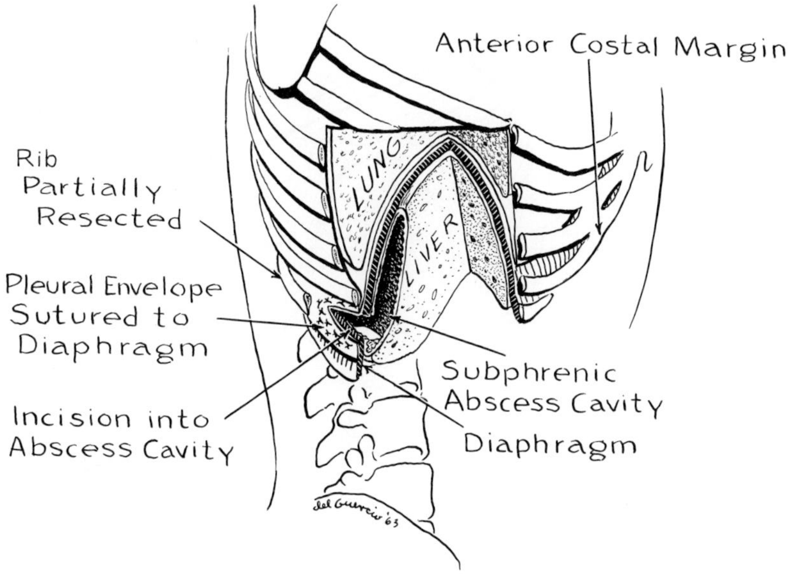

FIGURE 2. Subphrenic abscess: low lateral thoracic approach. The skin incision is made over the rib which is to be excised. A 2½- to 3-inch segment of rib is removed subperiosteally. Two layers of mattress sutures are placed circumferentially and the pleura and diaphragm are incised within the area enclosed by the sutures.

no danger of infecting the general pleural cavity. Further exploration by needle may be advisable after the diaphragm has been opened, and before liver tissue is incised, if the abscess proves to be within rather than on the liver. Penrose drains or soft rubber tubes are used, and brought through the wound.

Posterior Approach. In the posterior approach, a skin incision is made over the twelfth rib on the involved side (Fig. 3). A segment of the rib is excised subperiosteally, and a transverse incision is made through the bed of the rib at the level of the spinous process of the first lumbar vertebra. As one proceeds with the dissection, one should make a determined effort to remain out of the pleural cavity. If this appears improbable, the pleural space in the area of incision should be sequestrated from the general pleural cavity by multiple mattress sutures of swaged-on catgut. Fibers of the diaphragmatic insertion are cut and the retroperitoneal space is entered. If an abscess is present, the fatty tissue over the abscess will probably be found to be edematous and indurated. The abscess cavity is found and entered by finger dissection. Drainage by Penrose drains is established as described with the other approaches.

Anterior Infrahepatic Abscesses

An anterior infrahepatic abscess is drained through an abdominal approach. An anterior subcostal incision is usually made—again the tissue adjacent to the abscess, in this case peritoneum, will often be thickened and edematous—and the abscess is entered by blunt dissection. If the free peritoneal cavity must be traversed, the

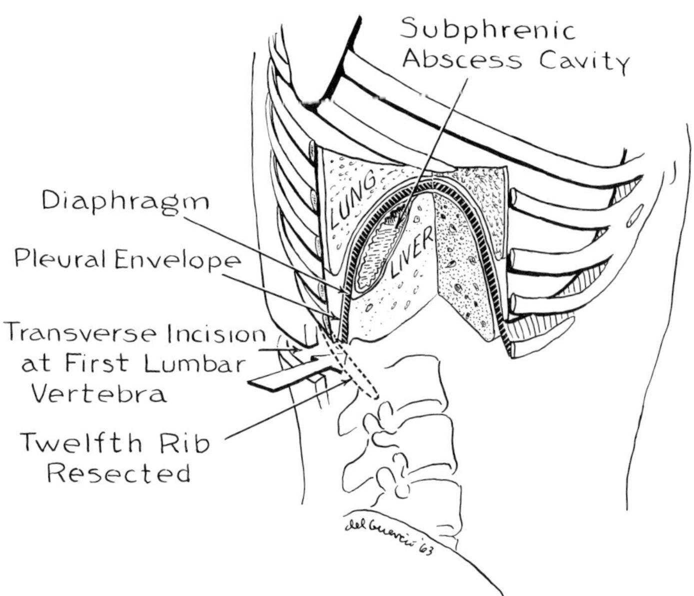

FIGURE 3. Subphrenic abscess: posterior approach. A transverse incision is made over the twelfth rib on the appropriate side. The rib is removed subperiosteally. A transverse incision is made at the level of the spinous process of the first lumbar vertebra, and the retroperitoneal area is exposed.

viscera are packed off thoroughly before the abscess is opened. Drainage is best established through a stab wound. Other surgery for associated pathology in the biliary tract or in other structures should be accomplished as indicated.

Pelvic Abscesses

Pelvic abscesses can be drained from above, through an incision in the abdominal wall, approaching the abscess either extraperitoneally or directly through the peritoneal cavity; or through the rectum or vagina. The abdominal approach employs the principles already outlined for drainage of abscesses in other locations. The rectal approach is of considerable value and is used frequently (Fig. 4). For this type of drainage, spinal anesthesia is preferable because it readily produces good relaxation of the anal sphincter. When the abscess is clinically ready for

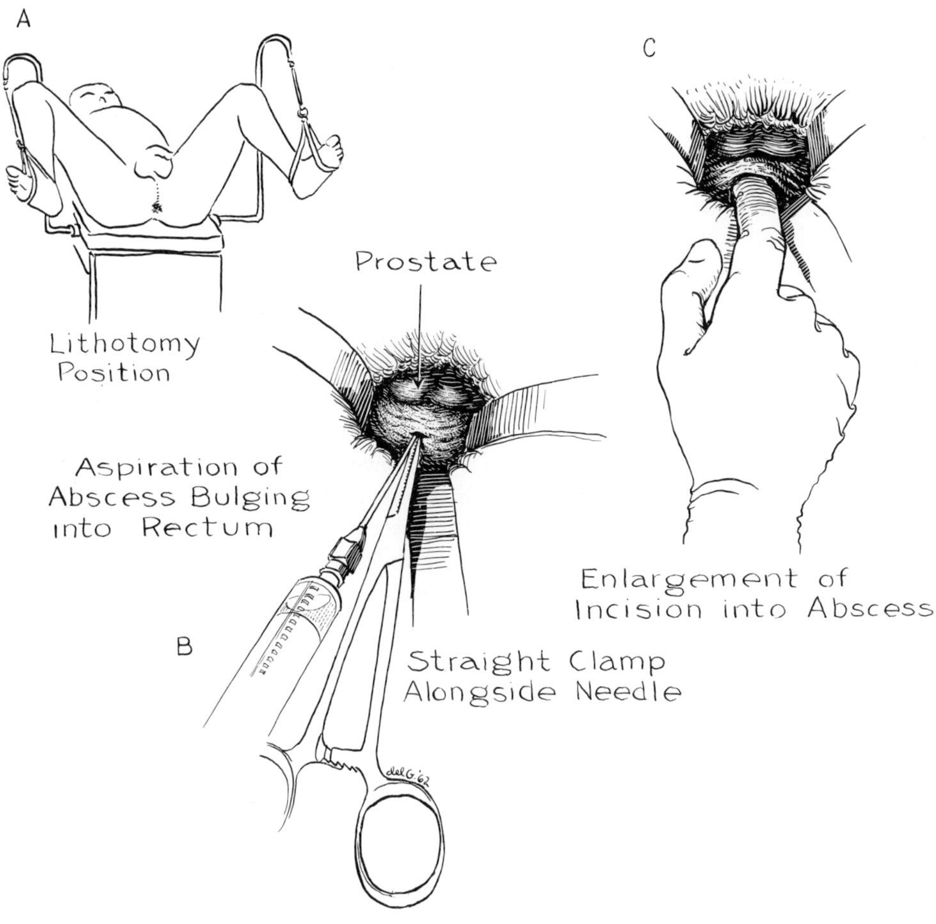

FIGURE 4. Pelvic abscess. (*A*) Position of the patient on the operating table. (*B*) Insertion of a clamp after a needle has been used to locate the abscess and has successfully aspirated purulent material. (*C*) Insertion of the operator's finger to enlarge the opening into the abscess cavity.

drainage it is usually found to be fluctuant on rectal examination, with a soft area near its center. A needle is inserted into this soft area. If the needle enters bowel, the rectal approach should be given up and the abscess approached and drained through the abdomen. However, if purulent material is aspirated, a clamp is inserted alongside the needle (Fig. 4B), the needle is removed, the blades of the clamp are spread, a finger is inserted between the blades of the clamp, the clamp is withdrawn, and gentle exploration and evacuation of the abscess cavity are accomplished (Fig. 4C). A large Penrose drain is inserted into the abscess cavity and fixed to the rectal wall with a catgut suture. This approach almost invariably results in cure of the abscess. In the female, on occasion, it may be preferable to drain a pelvic abscess through the vagina if the abscess seems to be pointed in that direction. The drain is usually evacuated, or is removed in a week or ten days. Care should be taken to assure obliteration of the cavity before the opening in the rectal wall seals.

Lesser Omental Cavity Abscesses

Abscesses in the lesser omental cavity need special mention since undiagnosed abscesses in this region have been occasionally found at autopsy. One should consider the possible presence of such an abscess if there are suggestive clinical findings following pancreatitis or the perforation of a gastric or duodenal ulcer.

The operative approach is through the gastrohepatic or the gastrocolic ligament, whichever appears more prominent over the abscess. Drainage should be established by the shortest feasible route from the abscess cavity, through a stab wound in the abdominal wall.

If an abscess secondary to pancreatitis has already taken the form of a pseudocyst, and a connection with a pancreatic duct seems probable, drainage into the stomach, duodenum, or jejunum by an anastomotic procedure is indicated if the wall of the pseudocyst is well established and of adequate thickness. The direction of drainage is discussed in Chapter 100. However, if the wall of the pseudocyst is not firm, fibrous, and of adequate thickness, it should not be anastomosed to a viscus, but should be treated as the usual abscess. It is opened, evacuated, and drained through a stab wound in the anterior abdominal wall. If an anastomosis is performed, using the fragile wall of such a pseudocyst, it will probably disrupt, and leakage of gastric or gastrointestinal secretions may produce dire results. If a connection is present or develops between a pseudocyst which has been drained through the abdominal wall, and a significant pancreatic duct, pancreatic secretions will usually continue to drain through the stab wound, and further surgery may be necessary to handle that problem.

Abscesses secondary to perforation of a gastric or duodenal ulcer are drained in the usual manner and other indicated surgery is accomplished.

Fistulas

Drainage of abscesses arising from either surgically or spontaneously perforated stomach or bowel may result in a fistula. But if drainage through such a fistula is adequate, and if the underlying viscus is relatively free of inflammatory disease, does not harbor a tumor, is not significantly obstructed distally, or does not hold a foreign body in its walls, the fistula will probably heal without further surgery. Also, the drainage tract itself must be free of foreign bodies. A fistula will not close readily if it is lined by a firm fibrous tissue wall, particularly if the tract is wide. In addition, if the mucosa of stomach or bowel reaches the skin level the fistula will probably not close spontaneously. Operative closure should be accomplished if nonoperative measures are unsuccessful after a reasonable period of time.

References

CRILE, G., JR. Peritonitis of appendiceal origin treated with massive doses of penicillin: report of 50 cases. *Surg., Gynec. and Obst.* 83:150, August 1946.

OCHSNER, A., and DEBAKEY, M. Subphrenic abscess—collective review and an analysis of 3,608 collected and personal cases. *Internat. Abstr. Surg.* 66:426, May 1938.

REDFERN, W. T., CLOSE, A. S., and ELLISON, E. H. Intra-abdominal abscess. A review of 100 consecutive patients. *Arch. Surg.* 85:278, August 1962.

XII. THE LIVER

72. *Liver Tumors*

THEODORE R. MILLER AND
GEORGE T. PACK

THE SURGICAL APPROACH to the treatment of liver tumors implies an intimate knowledge of the three intricate circulatory systems of the liver—the arterial, the portal venous, and the biliary—constituting an interlocking group of channels. The hazards of hemorrhage from the liver because of its fragility and vascularity make it necessary for the surgeon to be acquainted with the principles of hemostasis peculiar to this organ.

In the treatment of neoplasms of the liver one must be sure that they are localized and do not involve the hilar bile ducts or blood vessels. If metastatic cancer is localized to one lobe of the liver, some form of surgical resection should be attempted. Local excisions of benign tumors, such as hamartomas, embryomas, hemangiomas, and benign hepatomas, and of discrete metastatic cancers can be carried out with impunity if the surgeon has a thorough knowledge of the circulation and the methods of its control. For benign tumors occupying an entire lobe, and for cancers of the liver or gallbladder that offer some prospect of curability, a total lobectomy is indicated. Hepatic neoplasms, benign or malignant, primary or metastatic, if unilobular in distribution may be treated by local excision or by subtotal lobectomy. At times the complication of acute progressive hemorrhage from spontaneous or traumatic rupture of primary hepatomas or even metastatic cancers and injuries to the liver necessitates surgical intervention and excision of large sections of the liver.

Operative Technique

The first step in surgical treatment of liver tumors is abdominal exploration to obtain a reasonable assurance that the tumor is localized to the liver. The incision should be so planned that it may be extended into the chest to give more adequate exposure.

Enucleation or localized excision of tumors may be accomplished by the abdominal approach alone if the neoplasm is situated in the left lobe or is readily accessible in the right lobe; for example, along the inferior margin. Certain maneuvers are helpful in getting this exposure, such as elevation of the transverse bar or gallbladder rest to cause some dorsiflexion of the trunk at the hepatic level and to exaggerate the flare of the costal arch; transection, ligation, and gentle traction on the hepatic side of the round ligament in order to deliver the liver downward and forward; placement of warm laparotomy packs over the dome of the liver to increase the caudal displacement of the organ; severance of the triangular ligament; and the use of the reverse Trendelenburg position.

The abdominal incision may be vertical in the midline or right or left midrectus; or it may be obliquely situated across the epigastrium, extending upward toward the side of the lobe involved; or it may be parallel and subcostal from the xiphoid toward the end of the free ribs. Once the resectability of the neoplasm has been determined, the incision may be extended intercostally to enter the chest for additional exposure if a large excision is anticipated. The paracostal incision is enlarged by converting it into an inverted T with the upright limb extending across the costochondral margins. A right or left thoracoabdominal incision offers adequate exposure and control, and its adoption has made surgical treatment possible in many more patients with hepatic tumors.

At the time of the primary exploration, the surgeon should be prepared to remove the tumor or cancer by the method dictated by his experience and conscience, whether it be simple enucleation, partial hepatectomy, or total hepatic lobectomy.

Some slowly growing tumors such as cavernous angiomas or hamartomas, because of their weight, tend to extrude themselves from the liver and develop a long pedicle. Local enucleation of these tumors requires only control of the pedicle by interlocking sutures.

The use of the cautery in the past for control of hemorrhage was not particularly successful, although at times it may still be used with advantage. The difficulty lies in the fact that the coagulum and eschar tend to separate and produce delayed hemorrhage, biliary fistula, and liver abscess.

The conventional and present-day method of performing partial hepatectomy of the guillotine type and the local excision of liver tumors by sharp dissection with scalpel implies a hemostatic control. Encapsulated tumors such as hemangioma may be enucleated with the capsule intact without much bleeding, and the central vessels clamped and ligated. The removal of a small metastasis from one or both lobes may be carried out by using a hemostatic suture of the bootlace type. The sutures should be placed prior to the excision of the tumor, leaving a wide margin of normal tissue beyond the palpable margins of the neoplasm. A margin of about 1 cm. of normal liver tissue beyond the bootlace suture should be allowed, to prevent slipping of the ligature. After the segment has been isolated by the suture, the tumor can then be excised and the reduced bleeding controlled by packs, cautery, or individual ligation. The omentum can be used to cover the defects and also to increase the postoperative safety and help prevent delayed hemorrhage. Split-thickness grafts and free omental grafts as well as peritoneal grafts have been used. Foreign substances such as nylon, Oxycel, and Gelfoam are not particularly useful, because they tend to extrude and cause prolonged sinus formation.

While guillotine excision of segments of the liver and local excision and enucleation of liver tumors have their place in the management of these patients, controlled hepatic lobectomy (Fig. 1) is the only truly adequate surgical method of dealing with the problem of neoplasms in keeping with accepted principles of cancer extirpation. With adequate exposure, the liver hilum is approached and carefully dissected. The hepatic artery provides from 25 to 40 per cent of the blood supply of the liver. The remaining 60 to 75 per cent of the total blood supply to this organ is accounted for by the portal circulation. Control of the arterial and portal circulation to a segment of the liver, therefore, makes surgical excision of that portion of the liver less hazardous. Because of the great variability in the arterial supply of the liver, it is extremely important that the surgeon demonstrate the arterial supply to the portion of the liver which he wishes to preserve. On some occasions, this may take considerable time, but it must be carried out before any ligations are done, in order to avoid disaster.

In right hepatic lobectomy, the cystic duct is first ligated and then the right hepatic artery is dissected out and ligated. The right portal vein is relatively short and requires careful dissection in order that it be not traumatized before ligation. The right hepatic duct is carefully ligated after demonstration of the left duct.

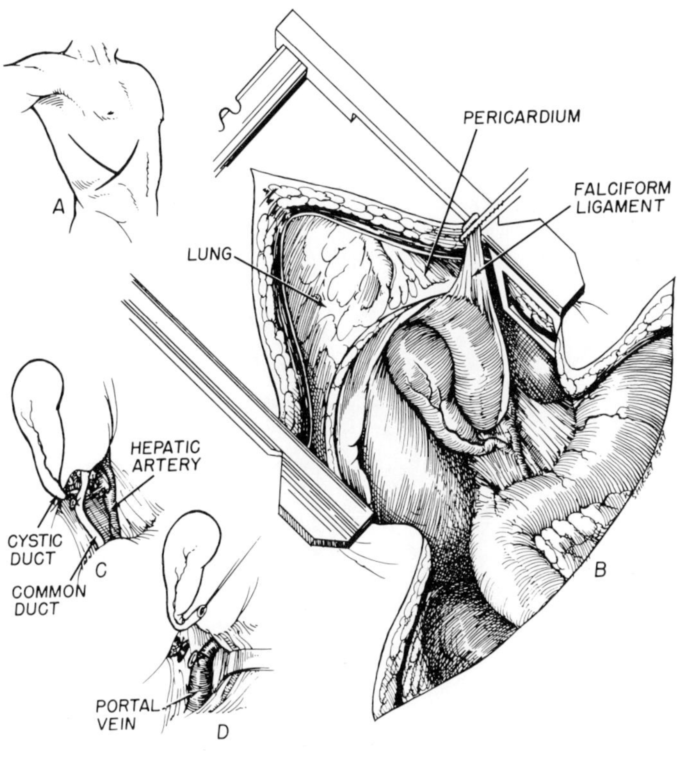

FIGURE 1. Technique of extended right hepatic lobectomy (right lobe plus medial segment of left lobe). (A) Incision. (*B*) Exposure. (C) Ligation and section of the cystic duct and right hepatic artery. (*D*) Ligation and section of the right portal vein.

The portion of the liver with impaired circulation is demarcated rapidly and easily seen. The inferior vena cava is then cleared, the liver is raised, and the individual hepatic veins are tied as they appear (Fig. 2). Care must be taken to avoid ligation of the hepatic veins from the left lobe of the liver in right hepatic lobectomy. This step may be tedious and fraught with some difficulty, as the vena cava may be kinked, causing a blockage of the return flow of blood to the heart, with immediate cardiac difficulty. When the control of the pedicle has been adequately carried out, this step of tying the individual hepatic veins may be omitted and simple guillotine amputation of the lobe done, using interlocking sutures of catgut to control the backflow from the hepatic veins. Finger fracture of the liver with individual ligation of the vessels as they are felt will also reduce the amount of hemorrhage at this stage. The falciform ligament may be brought down over the raw surface of the liver and sutured to the liver substance to lessen the seepage of bile and blood (Figs. 3 and 4). Nylon and other substances have been used, but tend to extrude and interfere with the convalescence.

It is important that the chest and the abdominal cavity be well drained. The intercostal tube should be left in place for a longer period of time than usual because of the possibility of bile seepage through the incision in the diaphragm.

Jaundice frequently appears postoperatively because of the increase in portal

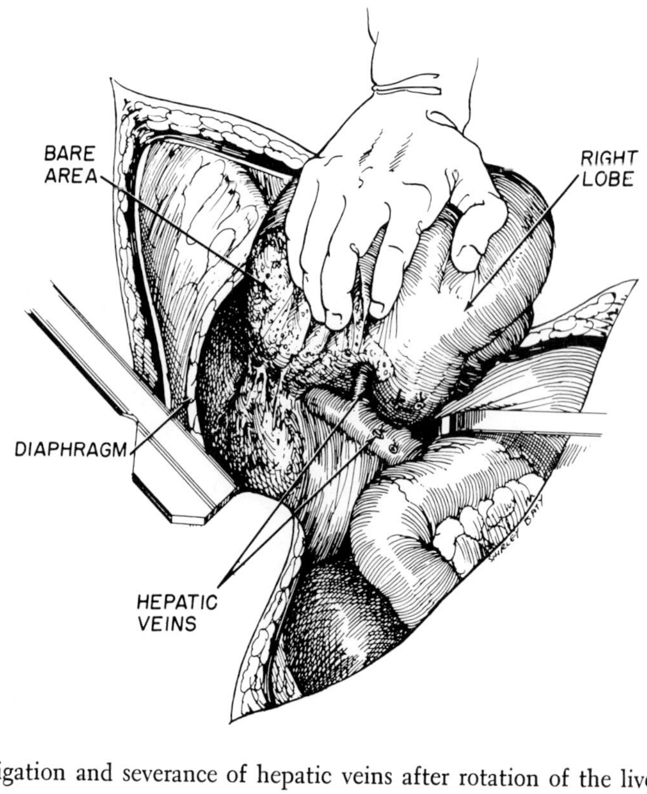

FIGURE 2. Ligation and severance of hepatic veins after rotation of the liver to the left.

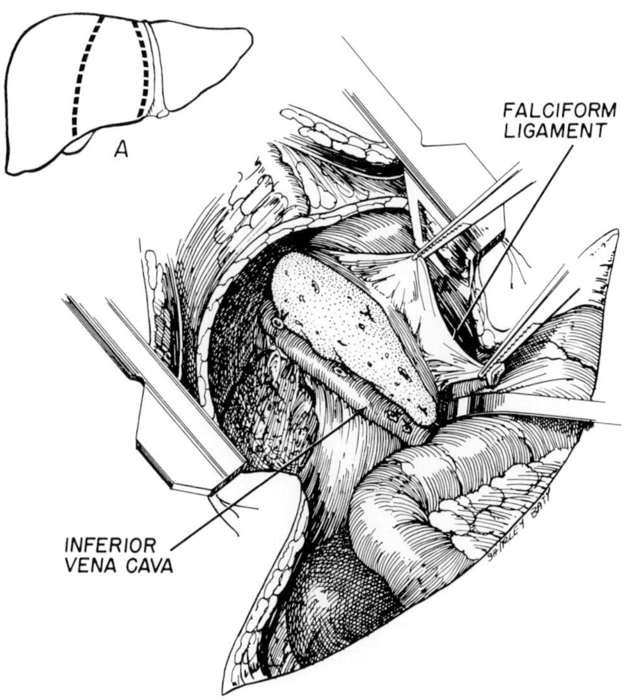

FIGURE 3. The right lobe and medial segment of the left lobe have been excised through the left segmental fissure.

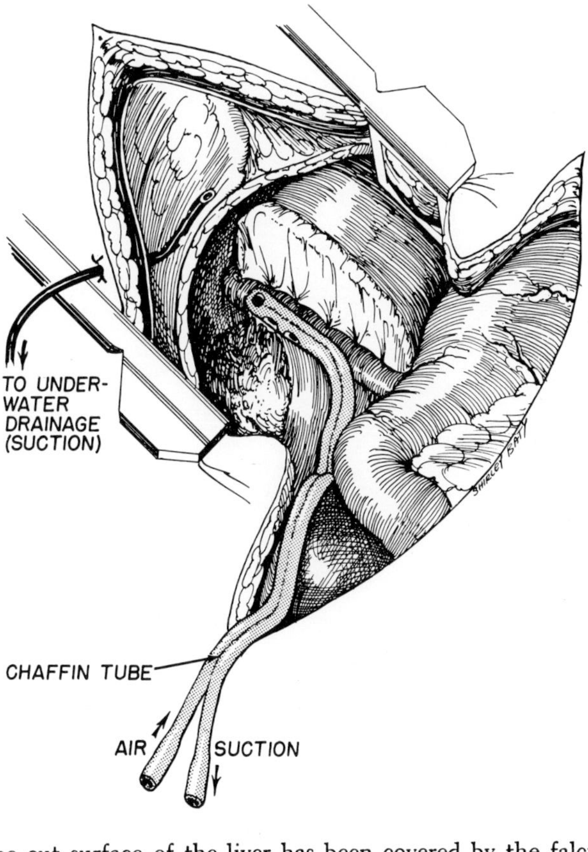

FIGURE 4. The cut surface of the liver has been covered by the falciform ligament to lessen seepage of blood and bile. Drains in position.

tension in the remaining portion of the liver, with concomitant compression of the biliary radicles. Because of the temporary disturbance of hepatic function, these patients require serum albumin, about 25 grams a day for the first four or five days postoperatively. Otherwise the patients experience edema and nutritional problems. Corticosteroids are useful in promoting liver regeneration.

References

Couinaud, C. Hépatectomies gauches lobaires et segmentaires. *J. Chir.* 68:697, November 1952.

Lortt-Jacob, J. L., and Robert, H. G. Hépatectomie droite réglée. *Presse méd.* 60:549, April 16, 1952.

Madden, J. L., and Lore, J. M. Surgical anatomy of the portal system. In *Surgical Forum,* 1951, American College of Surgeons. Philadelphia: W. B. Saunders, 1952.

Quattlebaum, J. K., and Quattlebaum, J. K., Jr. Technic of hepatic lobectomy. *Ann. Surg.* 149:648, May 1959.

Reifferscheid, M. *Chirurgie der Leber.* Stuttgart: Georg Thieme, 1957.

XIII. THE GALLBLADDER AND BILE DUCTS

73. Biliary Tract Surgery

FRANK GLENN AND
BJORN THORBJARNARSON

Cholecystectomy

Cholecystectomy for calculous disease is about the most common major operation at present. Since Langenbuch performed the first cholecystectomy in 1882 the indications for this operation have been better clarified and its beneficial effects more widely recognized. Also, more and more physicians realize that the silent or innocuous gallstone is a rarity and that preventive surgery, or the eradication of the calculous organ before severe symptoms set in, is more likely to give good immediate and long-term results than surgery performed in urgent situations.

The result is that larger numbers of patients are undergoing cholecystectomy, and also that a large proportion of these patients are receiving surgical treatment while they have minimal symptoms or disability from their calculous gallbladders. Surgeons feel justified in recommending removal of the calculous gallbladder in the presence of minimal or no symptoms because they know that the operation, when properly performed, carries minimal morbidity and mortality and in most cases permanently relieves the patient and eliminates the danger of later complications.

Every operation, however small and insignificant it may appear, entails some element of risk. Often the hazards are the same in a number of diverse operative procedures, but in addition to the common denominators there are important steps and precautions in the execution of the particular operation that demand special attention and care because they often determine its success or failure.

The most important aspect of cholecystectomy is to avoid injury to adjacent vital structures, or more specifically the common duct and the hepatic artery. Because of the common variations in the anatomical arrangement of vascular and ductal elements in the porta hepatis, it is impossible to know the location of these structures beforehand. We have gained the impression that damage to the common duct in particular seems to occur during what the surgeon describes as an "easy" cholecystectomy. Our approach to the problem therefore has been aimed at developing a routine procedure that eliminates as much as possible the chance of accidental injury to the common duct or right hepatic artery (Fig. 1), since dam-

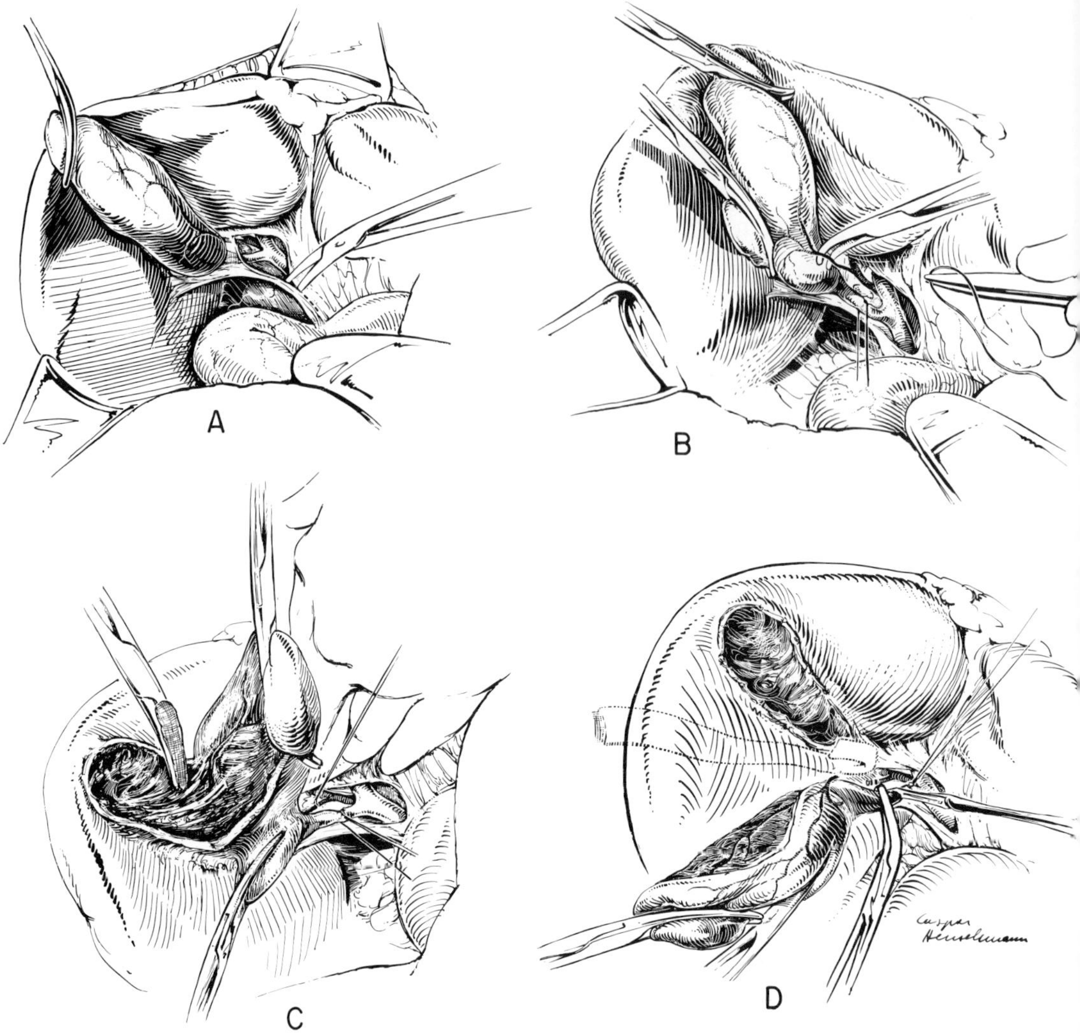

FIGURE 1. Cholecystectomy. (*A*) The peritoneum over Calot's triangle is incised and the cystic artery and duct are tentatively identified. (*B*) Ligatures of silk are looped around both artery and duct. (*C*) The gallbladder is removed from the fundus downward. (*D*) When the gallbladder is attached only by the cystic duct and artery, these structures are divided.

age to either one of these structures often leads to crippling complications that usually shorten the patient's life materially.

Prime requisites are adequate exposure and assistance. Unless the patient has a very narrow costal margin, we use a right subcostal incision curving from below the xiphoid process out into the right flank. After the porta hepatis has been exposed, the first assistant exerts a downward traction on the duodenum and pylorus of the stomach with his left hand. A clamp is placed on the fundus of the gallbladder and slight traction on the clamp outlines the peritoneal fold from the common duct out into the ampulla of the gallbladder. An incision is made in the peritoneum parallel to and just to the right of the estimated position of the common duct. Blunt dissection in this region with a Kuttner dissector and a long right-angle clamp exposes the junction of the cystic and hepatic ducts. The elements freed up during this maneuver are the lymphatics, autonomic nerves, and areolar fatty tissues. The cystic lymph node, a fairly constant finding in this area, sits on the ampulla of the gallbladder usually close to where the cystic artery divides into its branches. Once the cystic duct, or what is presumably the cystic duct, is exposed, a 3–0 silk thread is passed around the structure with the aid of the right-angle clamp. The ligature is pulled up lightly and an identifying clamp is applied to its ends.

Cephalad to the cystic duct the peritoneal incision is curved over the ampulla of the gallbladder, leaving a cuff at least 1 cm. wide attached to the liver. Dissection in this area is aimed at the cystic artery. Sometimes the right hepatic artery is found to buckle and courses in close approximation to the ampullary portion of the gallbladder. The size of the vessels encountered is of help in estimating whether one has found the cystic or the hepatic artery. When the cystic artery is identified, a thread of 3–0 silk is passed around it in the manner described for the duct.

The peritoneal incision is extended to the fundus of the gallbladder. A clamp can now be placed on the ampulla of the gallbladder and the organ shelled out of the capsule in the liver bed after the peritoneal covering of the undersurface of the gallbladder has been incised. Finally the gallbladder is hanging on the cystic duct and cystic artery. The cystic duct is now traced to its entrance into the common duct and ligated 0.5 cm. from this structure.

When the gallbladder is removed in this way, no major structures are divided until it has been definitely established that they enter the gallbladder alone. The ligature on the cystic artery also reduces the bleeding considerably during the removal of the gallbladder from the liver bed, and the ligature on the cystic duct prevents stones from escaping into the common duct. Should the ligatures be found not to be on the proper structure, they may be loosened and removed at the end of the procedure without having caused irreparable damage to the parts involved. Both the cystic artery and the cystic duct are secured with transfixion sutures of 3–0 silk in addition to the previously applied ligature, and a drain is always placed down to the foramen of Winslow.

Cholecystostomy

Cholecystostomy, or drainage and decompression of the gallbladder, is primarily useful in the treatment of certain aspects of acute cholecystitis. Although it is not a definitive attack upon the disease process, it may be a life-saving one. The decision for cholecystostomy in preference to cholecystectomy can be made before or during an operation for acute cholecystitis. Cholecystostomy should be decided upon as the treatment of choice when the general condition of the patient precludes the major intervention of a cholecystectomy. Cholecystostomy can also become the procedure of choice in planning an operation when adequate assistance or anesthesia for cholecystectomy cannot be secured.

The decision for cholecystostomy during an operation for acute cholecystitis depends on the gross appearance of the pathological changes. When gangrene and perforation with accompanying generalized peritonitis are present, simple drainage of the abdomen together with cholecystostomy is indicated. It is also the procedure of choice when extensive adhesions and inflammatory reaction preclude safe exposure and dissection of the structures in the hepatoduodenal ligament.

Cholecystostomy should place as small a burden on the patient as possible. Often local anesthesia may be successfully employed. Basically there are two types of cholecystostomy, one to be employed for the large and palpable gallbladder, the other to be resorted to when the organ is small or hidden under the liver so that its fundus cannot be brought into apposition to the parietal peritoneum. The latter is encountered in patients with long-standing biliary tract disease in which the gallbladder is contracted down about calculi.

The cholecystostomy for the large, palpable gallbladder (Fig. 2) is usually best performed through a short right upper rectus incision. The rectus muscle is separated in the direction of its fibers, and following this the peritoneum is opened. The fundus of the gallbladder is exposed but the surrounding areas are disturbed as little as possible. A purse-string suture of catgut is placed in the fundus of the gallbladder, and after a little nick has been made in the serosa with a knife, a trocar is inserted into the organ and all its liquid contents evacuated.

Following the emptying of the gallbladder the trocar is removed and a culture is taken from the inside of the organ. Stone forceps and scoops are used to evacuate all calculi. It is desirable to remove all the stones, and for this purpose the cholecystostomy may now be enlarged to give a direct view of the inside of the gallbladder. A Malecot catheter is next placed in the gallbladder. A size 16 to 18 French is usually sufficiently large. The purse-string suture is tied to hold the catheter in place. The circumference of the fundus around the point of exit of the catheter is sutured to the edges of the peritoneum and posterior rectus sheath. We usually use 00 silk for this unless there is frank purulent infection in the gallbladder. These sutures anchor the organ to the abdominal wall. The catheter emerges from a stab wound and the remainder of the wound is closed with similar interrupted sutures of silk. A Penrose drain is placed in the subcutanous tissues. The catheter is anchored to the skin with a silk suture that is tied around the catheter.

When the acutely involved gallbladder is small and deeply placed, as sometimes occurs in patients with acute obstructive cholangitis, a different approach has to be made (Fig. 3). Usually these gallbladders cannot be palpated. A larger exploring incision is needed, and this may be either of the subcostal or the right rectus type. The gallbladder is opened as previously described and emptied of its contents. Since it does not reach to the abdominal wall, the catheter is made to emerge through a stab wound in the most direct line to the fundus of the organ. In addition to the catheter, two cigarette drains should be placed alongside the gallbladder. These drains will serve if there is an escape of bile from around the catheter. The drains emerge through a stab wound separate from the one made for the catheter.

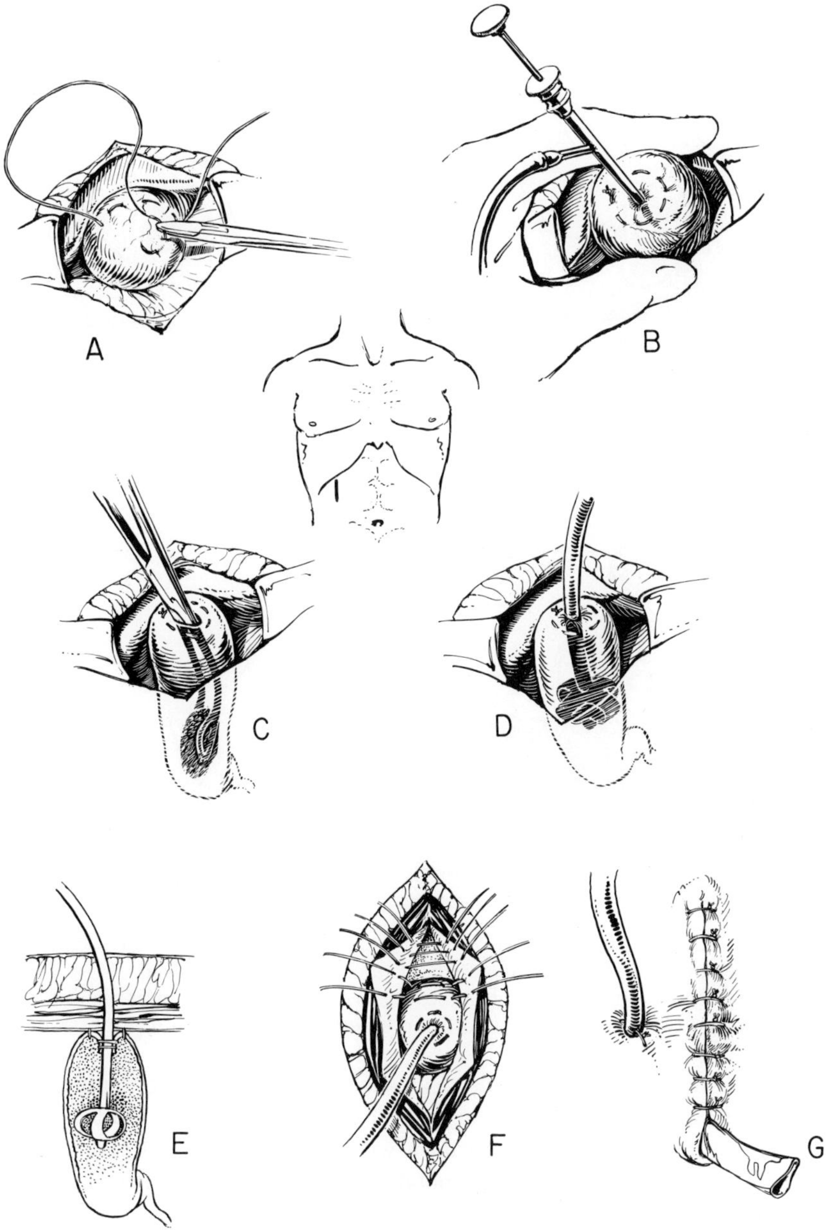

FIGURE 2. Cholecystostomy for a large gallbladder. (*A*) A purse-string suture is placed in the fundus of the gallbladder. (*B*) The gallbladder is decompressed by a trocar. (*C*) The stones are removed. (*D*) A Malecot catheter is in place. (*E and F*) The fundus of the gallbladder is sutured to the peritoneum and posterior rectus fascia. (*G*) The Malecot catheter emerges through a stab wound. A subcutaneous drain is in place.

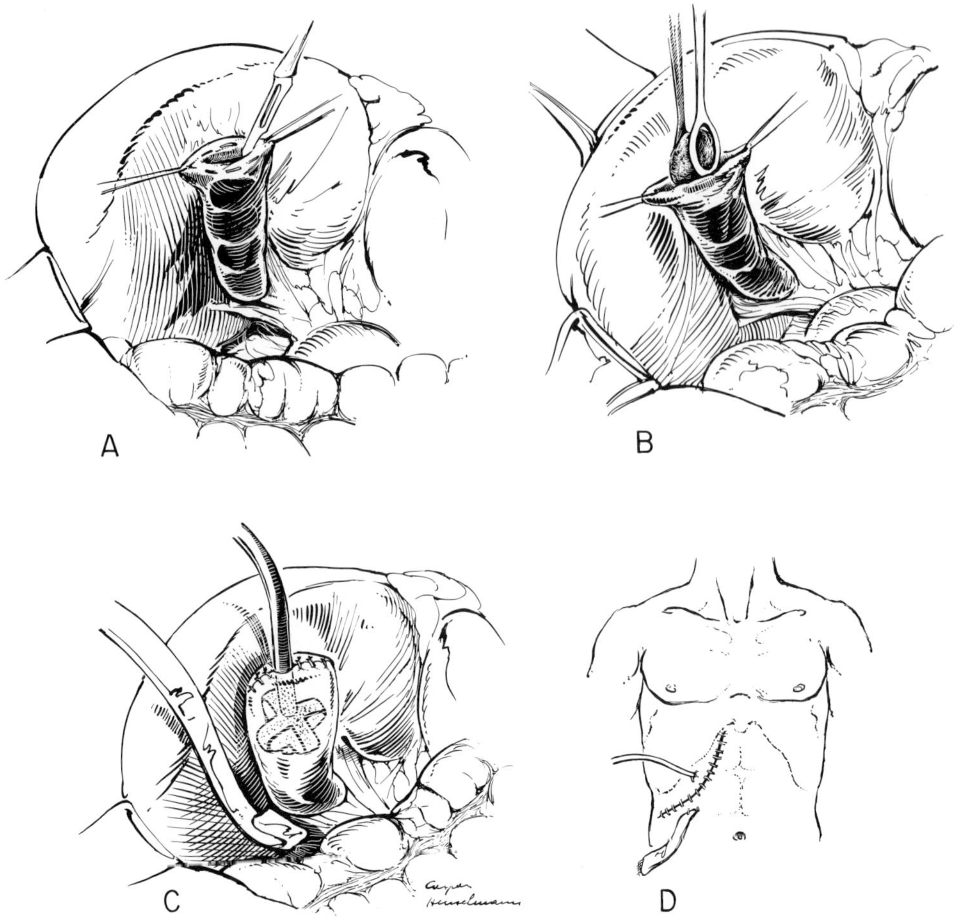

FIGURE 3. Cholecystostomy for a shrunken gallbladder. (*A*) The gallbladder is shrunken and deep under the liver. (*B*) The stones are removed. (*C*) The cholecystostomy is closed around a Malecot catheter. A cigarette drain is placed alongside the gallbladder. (*D*) The catheter and drain emerge through separate stab wounds.

The care of the cholecystostomy catheter is of considerable importance since, if it becomes blocked early in the postoperative course, leakage into free peritoneal cavity may be expected. Gentle irrigation with saline is quite permissible to insure patency. When the catheter is incorporated in the dressings, there is a tendency for it to kink at the level of the skin and thus become obstructed. We therefore make a point of preventing this occurrence. A gauze roll about 15 inches long is secured to the skin adjacent to the catheter, and the tube is brought over the roll to start the incline toward the drainage receptacle at the bedside. The tube is secured to the gauze roll and again to the skin outside the main dressings.

We feel that once the gallbladder has been drained in this way, it should later be removed as an elective procedure when circumstances allow. If this course is adopted, the cholecystostomy tube may be left in place until the second procedure is undertaken.

Drainage of the Common Duct

Following exploration of the common duct, drainage is essential. The passage of instruments through the sphincter of Oddi and removal of stones causes local damage with resultant swelling and impediment to the flow of bile into the duodenum. Without drainage, leakage of bile, subhepatic accumulations, and ascending cholangitis would be much more common than is necessary, and a catastrophe would result because overlooked stones happened to cause obstruction in the immediate postoperative period.

Common duct drainage can be accomplished by either a catheter or a T tube (Fig. 4). The catheter we usually insert through the cystic duct, the T tube through the choledochotomy. The size of the tube varies with the size of the duct. The tubes do not extend into the duodenum, and the upper limb of the T tube should be below the level of the bifurcation of the hepatic duct. The straight catheter through the cystic duct points distally and is secured in place with catgut ligatures around the stump of the duct.

Before placing a T tube, we usually make a notch where the limbs join together. This should not materially lessen the strength of the tube, and it makes removal easier. The choledochotomy is closed with interrupted sutures of 5–0 chromic catgut on an atraumatic needle. The catgut sutures go through all layers of the wall. This layer of closure is reinforced with interrupted sutures of silk which do not penetrate the lumen of the duct. The closure should be watertight. The common duct tubes are secured to the abdominal wall as described under Cholecystostomy.

The catheter or T tube remains in the duct for an average of 12 days. Prior to its removal a burette test is undertaken. The tube is attached to a burette which is by the bedside. Before the burette is attached to the tube it is filled with saline and a mark is made at the level of the fluid in the burette. The level of the fluid is watched for 12 hours and gives an indication of the pressure necessary to pass the sphincter of Oddi. The overflow outlet of the burette is located 15 cm. above the level of the common duct.

Following the burette test a cholangiogram is performed through the common duct tube. Before injection of the contrast material it is necessary to let all air bubbles out of the tube; otherwise the bubbles will show as radiolucent areas in the bile ducts. The contrast material should not be injected under pressure, but rather by gravity up to 30 to 40 cm. of water, since pain and febrile reaction may result.

Sometimes difficulties are encountered in visualizing the intrahepatic radicles of the bile ducts. This is usually caused by a patulous sphincter of Oddi which prevents adequate pressure from building up for filling of the smaller radicles. This obstacle may sometimes be overcome by tilting the x-ray table so that the patient assumes a Trendelenburg position. If this fails, an injection of morphine, 15 minutes before the examination, usually causes sufficient spasm at the lower end of the common duct to permit filling of the intrahepatic radicles. We usually

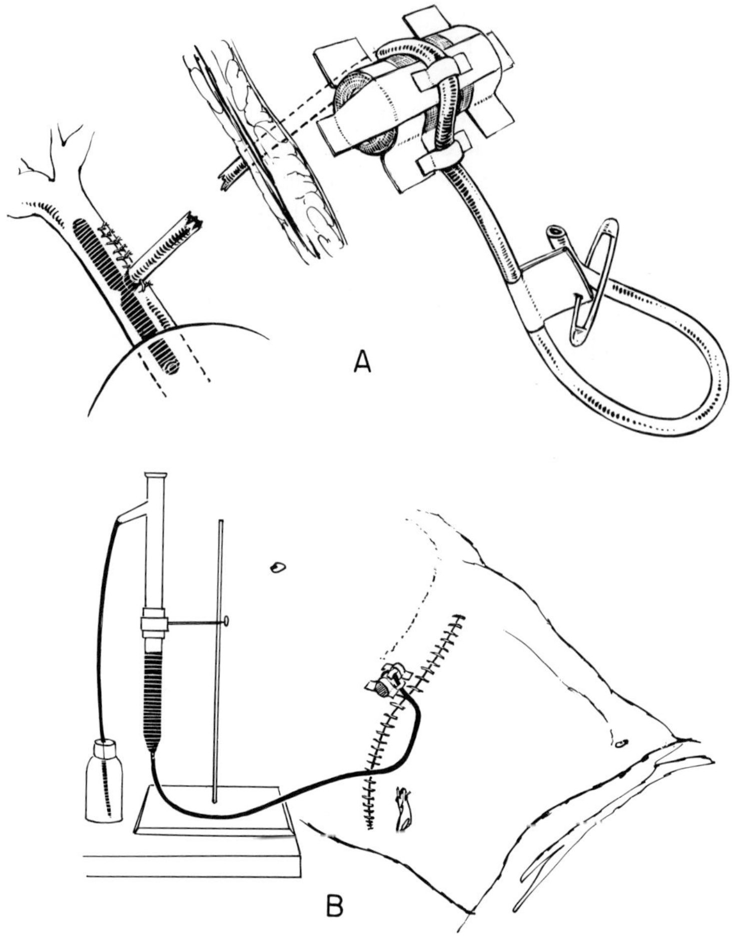

FIGURE 4. Drainage of the common duct. (*A*) The T tube inside the common duct and as it emerges through the abdominal wall. (*B*) The burette has been attached for determination of the intraductal pressure.

remove the common duct tubes 24 hours after the cholangiography. The delay is necessary because of the occasional febrile reaction following the procedure. This reaction may be due to mild cholangitis which subsides with continued drainage.

Surgical Relief of Obstruction to the Lower Common Duct

Long-standing biliary tract disease often afflicts the common duct. In addition to calculi in the duct, involvement of the head of the pancreas or simple fibrosis of the ductal wall may narrow the lumen and cause the tube to lose its resiliency and thus produce incomplete or complete obstruction. In the lower common duct this usually occurs at the sphincter of Oddi and causes gradual dilatation of the proximal duct. Occasionally the entire pancreatic portion of the duct is involved, as a rule in association with some degree of pancreatitis, and the dilatation of the common duct starts where the duct becomes visible above the level of the duodenum. Many etiological and pathological considerations are involved in the obstruction, and usually these patients have had previous and sometimes several operations for the relief of symptomatic biliary tract disease. The diagnosis at operation depends on demonstrating the proper level of the obstruction. Sometimes this can be done preoperatively by the use of intravenous cholangiography. In that case, the surgical problem is easier.

Fibrosis of the sphincter of Oddi causes uniform dilatation of the common duct. The pancreas usually is normal to inspection and palpation, and at least there is no narrowing of the intrapancreatic portion of the common duct. Exploration of the common duct through a choledochotomy allows passage of the exploring catheter or bougie down to the ampulla, where resistance is met. Often the smaller filamentous bougie may be passed and the sphincter gradually dilated.

Frequently duodenotomy reveals protrusion of the ampulla into the lumen, but the structure is fairly soft to palpation. Passage of a bougie from above through the sphincter under vision reveals the tight ring of fibrous tissue which blanches as the bougie is forced through. A cholangiogram reveals the dilatation of the duct and a smooth tapering at the level of the ampulla. The treatment here consists of a sphincterotomy or sphincteroplasty. The aim of the procedure is to widen permanently the entrance of the common duct into the duodenum without injury to the pancreatic duct, if this has a common channel with the bile duct (Fig. 5).

A grooved director is inserted into the ampulla from the duodenotomy. With the groove as a guide, two stay sutures are placed superiorly and slightly to the right. The sphincterotomy is now performed between these stay sutures. The fibrous tissues are completely divided and the incision is continued until the opening is of the same diameter as the duct at this level—or at least 1.5 cm. The duodenal and ampullary mucosa are approximated with interrupted sutures of 4–0 catgut. These sutures control any bleeding and tend to prevent the re-forming of the narrowed area. Bougies from the common duct side are inserted to demonstrate the wide patency of the ampulla. Before the mucosal sutures are placed, it is wise to try to demonstrate the pancreatic duct. If a common channel exists, a probe in the pancreatic duct prevents damage to this structure. The common duct is drained with a T tube that does not extend into the duodenum. This T tube is usually removed 12 days after surgery.

When pancreatitis or fibrosis of the common duct wall has caused narrowing or obstruction of the part of the common duct within the pancreas, the problem is different. Exploration of the duct through the routine choledochotomy and a duodenotomy reveals the long segment of the duct involved. Obviously a sphincterotomy will accomplish nothing for this patient since dilatation of the duct only starts at the upper border of the duodenum. In this situation we prefer to divide the common duct just above the retroduodenal area and perform a choledochojejunostomy Roux en Y (Fig. 6).

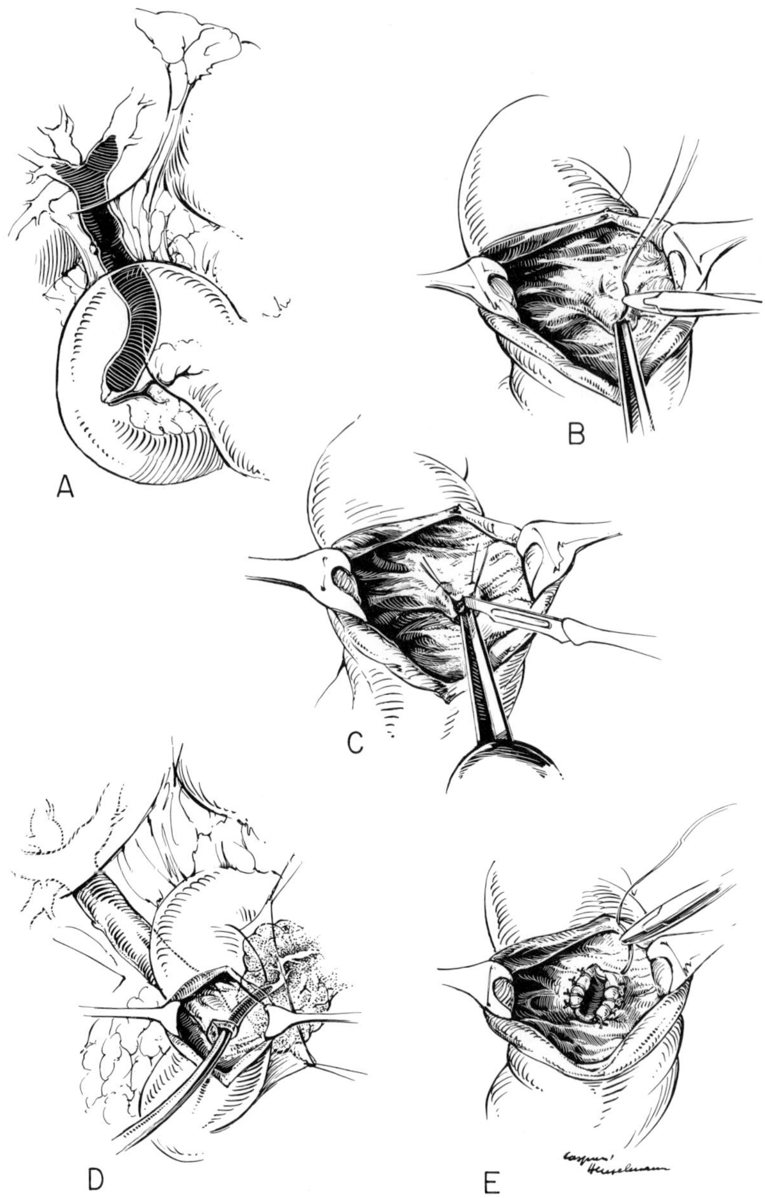

FIGURE 5. Sphincterotomy. (*A*) There is scarring and narrowing of the common duct outlet. (*B*) Stay sutures are placed using a grooved director. (*C*) The sphincter of Oddi is divided between the stay sutures. (*D*) A probe in the pancreatic duct avoids injury to it. (*E*) The common duct and duodenal mucosa are approximated with interrupted sutures of catgut.

After the common duct has been isolated and divided, the distal end is closed with interrupted sutures of fine silk. The Roux en Y loop is started sufficiently distal to the ligament of Treitz to permit the construction of a Roux en Y anastomosis

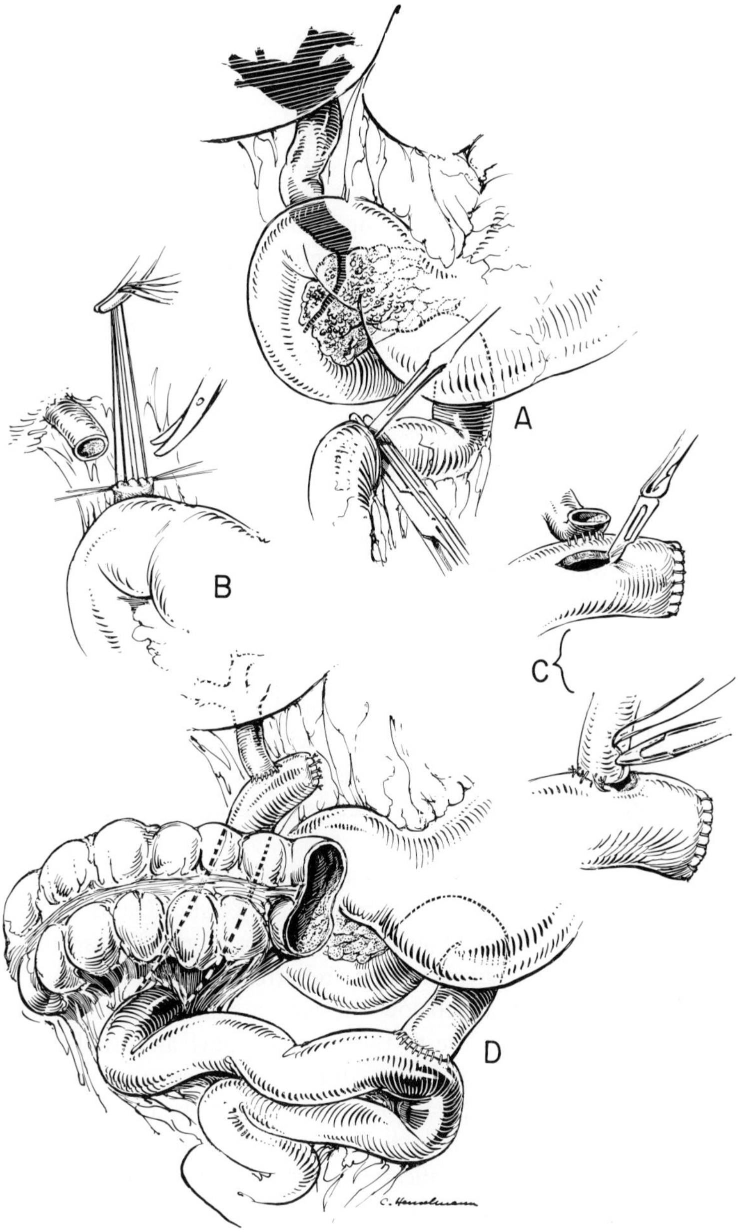

FIGURE 6. Choledochojejunostomy. (*A*) The narrowed intrapancreatic portion of the common duct is shown. The jejunum is being divided. (*B*) The common duct is divided just above the duodenal level. The lower end is closed. (*C*) The sutures are placed for the choledochojejunostomy. (*D*) The completed operation.

without tension, and is made almost 20 cm. long. The end of the vertical limb is closed with a continuous 3–0 catgut suture and then inverted with interrupted sutures of fine silk. The limb is now brought up through a rent in the transverse mesocolon and an end-to-side choledochojejunal anastomosis is performed. The anastomosis is on the antimesenteric border of the jejunum abut 5 cm. from the end. The anastomosis contains the full width of the common duct and is done in two layers. The posterior row of the superficial layer is placed before the jejunum is opened and consists of interrupted sutures of fine silk that do not penetrate the lumina. After this row has been placed the jejunum is opened and the deep layer of the posterior row placed, using 4–0 chromic catgut interrupted sutures. The anterior half of the anastomosis is then completed in a similar fashion. We usually leave a small caliber T tube in the common duct with the lower limb extending below the anastomosis. The tube is removed in 12 days.

Excision of a Cystic Duct Remnant

Excision of a cystic duct remnant is a secondary operation on the biliary tree. It includes the usual problems of handling adhesions and identification of structures in a previously operated area.

The preoperative diagnosis lies in the demonstration of the cystic duct stump by intravenous cholangiography. Thus the surgeon already has an idea of its location. We usually proceed from the common duct in identifying the cystic duct stump. When chronic infection is associated with this condition, there is usually extensive scarring and involvement of the surrounding structures which makes exact identification difficult, but it is necessary if untoward damage is to be avoided (Fig. 7).

By proceeding with the dissection up along the common duct, the stump can usually be identified without too much trouble, especially if it is of considerable size and contains bile or stones. The dissection is performed close to the organ, and the proximity of the right hepatic duct and artery is kept in mind. The wall of the common bile duct above and below the entrance of the cystic duct is clearly defined before it is ligated, as close to the common duct as feasible. Occasionally as the cystic duct is traced toward the common duct an abnormal insertion is found and the duct may curve posteriorly or anteriorly before entering the wall. Occasionally this abnormal insertion is the reason for the long stump, and its correction depends on proper identification of the insertion. Not infrequently the cystic duct is intramural in the common duct, with only a septum separating it from the main lumen. We do not remove the intramural portions of such ducts. Any stones present are removed through a choledochotomy. Once in a while excessive scarring completely obliterates landmarks, and identification of the cystic duct as a separate structure is impossible. In these cases we have opened the common duct and passed a probe from the inside into the structure and thus outlined its whereabouts. When probing from the inside does not reveal the entrance of the

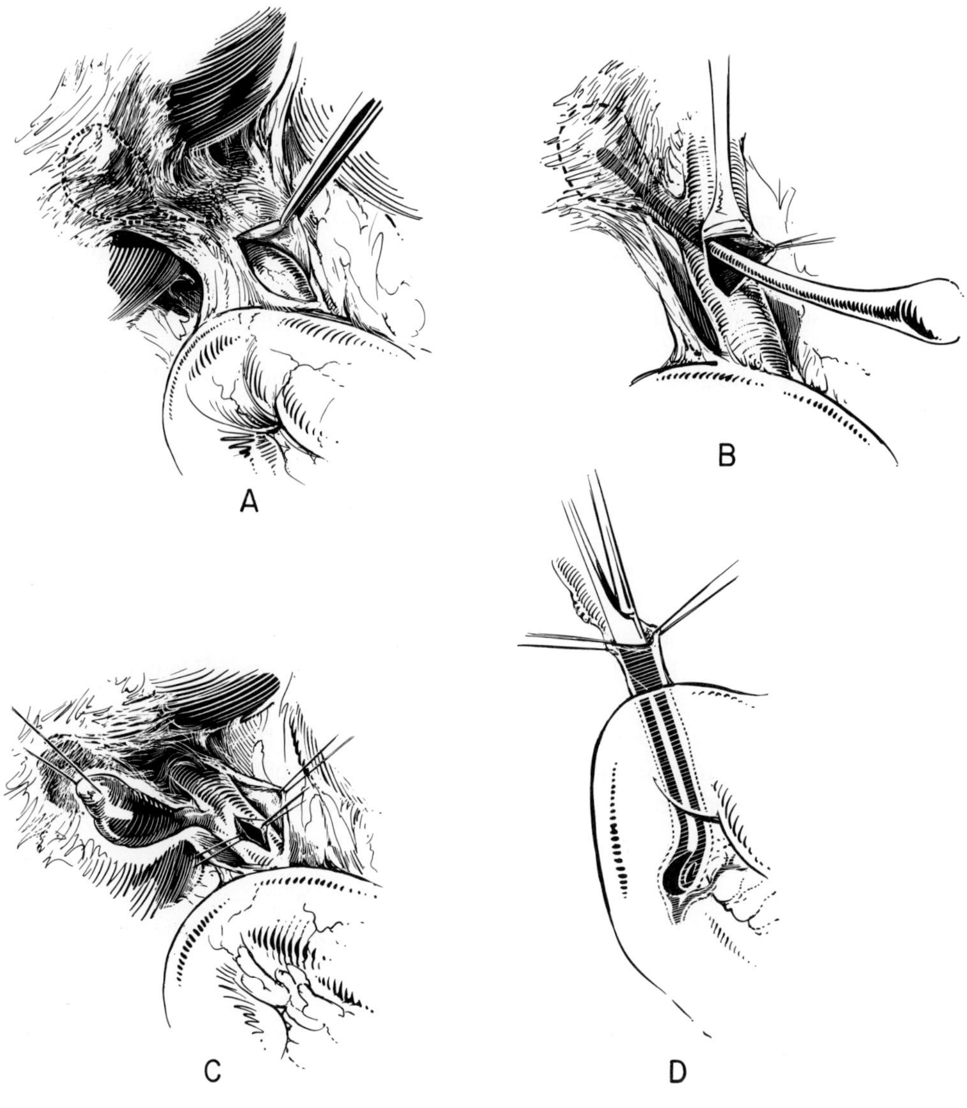

FIGURE 7. Removal of a cystic duct remnant. (*A*) The common duct is identified. (*B*) Sometimes probing from inside the common duct helps in identifying the cystic duct. (*C*) The cystic duct is dissected free until its junction with the common duct is clearly outlined. (*D*) Common duct stones are often associated with cystic duct remnants. Exploration of the duct follows.

cystic duct, an operative cholangiogram may do so. This is particularly helpful if an aberrant insertion is present.

We have the impression that common duct stones are a frequent companion of symptomatic cystic duct stumps. Consequently, exploration of the common duct for stones has become an integral part of our operations for removal of a cystic duct stump.

Choledochojejunostomy for Postoperative Stricture

When surgery is performed for the relief of postoperative bile duct stricture, the immediate results depend mainly on the operator's ability to re-establish continuity between the biliary and gastrointestinal tracts. The long-term success of the operation depends on how long the lumen of the anastomosis remains open, in the face of the known likelihood of secondary scarring at the site of such anastomoses.

We usually approach the severed common duct through a long right subcostal incision. The undersurface of the right lobe of the liver serves as a guide to the area of the gallbladder fossa, where the duodenum is usually found close to the liver surface. The angle between the hepatoduodenal ligament and the duodenum may often be recognized from the presence of a rather large lymph node. The duodenum is mobilized and swung over medially. This allows access to the retroduodenal part of the common duct. After the duodenum has been freed, the hepatic artery is identified by palpation, if possible. Only rarely can the bile duct be identified promptly in the dense scar tissues that characterize common duct injuries. Identification of suture material from previous procedures may help in locating the proximal end of the divided duct. Aspiration with a needle is also helpful in identifying the dilated duct and allows it to be carved out of the scar tissues.

Occasionally only a narrow area of stricture exists. In these cases we consider the optimal operation to be end-to-end anastomosis of the bile duct over a splinting T tube (Fig. 8). Identification of the lower end of the severed bile duct is facilitated

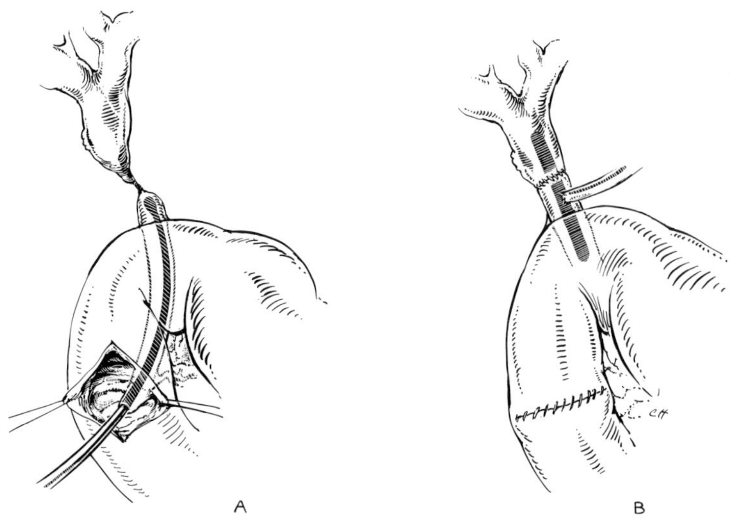

FIGURE 8. Choledochal anastomosis end-to-end for repair of stricture. The probe inserted in the distal common duct from the ampulla locates the blind end of the duct (*A*) and shows that an end-to-end anastomosis can be performed (*B*).

in these cases by doing a duodenotomy and passing a stiff silk woven bougie up the duct through the ampulla of Vater. Palpation of the bougie in the hepato-duodenal ligament then allows accurate localization of the severed end. When the distance between the two ends of the bile duct is too great for end-to-end anastomosis, we prefer to perform a choledochojejunostomy (Fig. 9).

Once the location of the proximal end of the duct is known, stay sutures are placed and a cuff is developed for anastomosis with the jejunum. A Roux en Y loop is prepared as described earlier, but the anastomosis is done end-to-end. The free end of the Roux loop is invaginated into itself by placing sutures of 3–0 silk through the wall of the bowel about 3 cm. from its end. These sutures are placed from the serosal surface through the wall. Once inside the lumen, the needle is brought to the outside through the wall close to its end. The needle then retraces its course to complete a mattress suture. Once four of these sutures have been placed, one in each quadrant, the bowel end is inverted by tying down all the threads. This maneuver creates a serosal surface for apposition to the end of the common duct, which then is invaginated and secured to the jejunum with interrupted sutures of silk. As a rule no catheter or tube is left in the common duct, but drains are placed down to the foramen of Winslow.

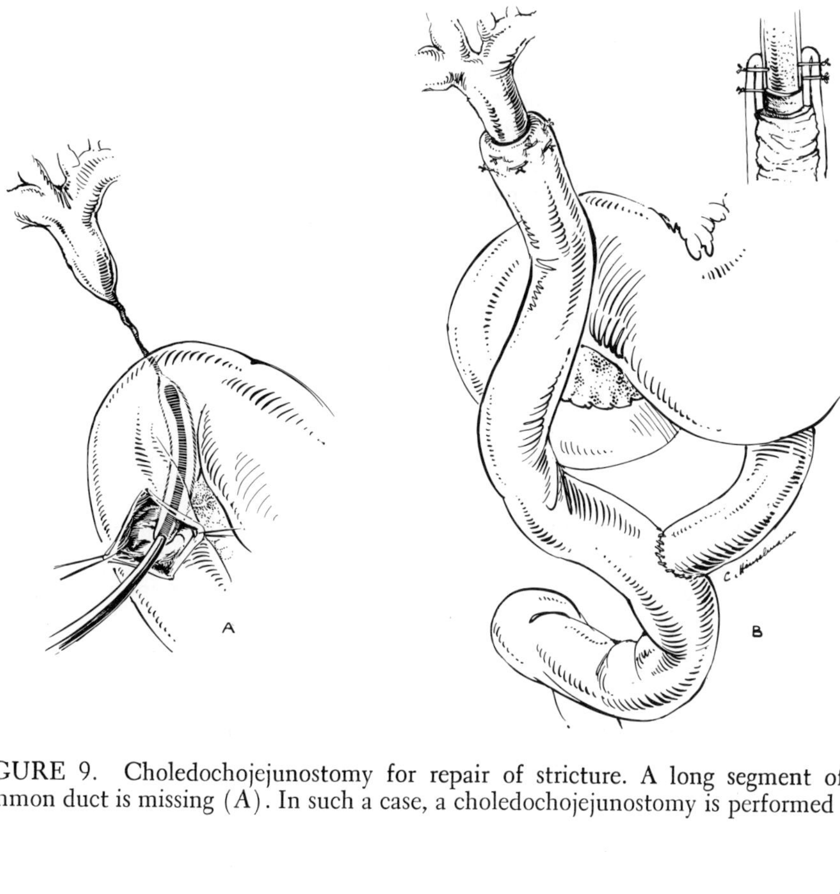

FIGURE 9. Choledochojejunostomy for repair of stricture. A long segment of the common duct is missing (*A*). In such a case, a choledochojejunostomy is performed (*B*).

Treatment of Intrahepatic Calculi

Intrahepatic calculi are rarely found in the United States and are usually the result of long-standing biliary tract disease associated with structural changes in the intrahepatic bile ducts. Primary intrahepatic calculi are commonly found in the Far East as a result of a fluke infestation, but in the United States, calculi in this location are almost always secondary to primary gallbladder disease.

The most common location of intrahepatic calculi in our experience is the left lobe of the liver. The stones are contained within a saccular or cisternal dilatation of the ducts; and although stones are usually also present in the distal common duct, the diameter of the intrahepatic cistern greatly exceeds the diameter of the extrahepatic ducts. Recognition of this condition at surgery may be difficult or easy, but proper assessment of it is essential for adequate treatment. At exploration in the most advanced cases the left lobe of the liver is small in size, with lack of substance to palpation. Areas of thinning and fibrosis may be seen on the surface, and correspond to the saccular dilatation of the duct. The stones may be easily palpable through the parenchyma. When there is less involvement of the liver this condition may be recognized only during common duct exploration. The left hepatic duct is found to be filled with stones, and difficulty is experienced in removing the calcareous material, since more and more keeps appearing as the exploration proceeds. The true condition of the ductal system in this case becomes apparent only after prolonged exploration. The problems to be overcome during surgery are twofold: first, to remove all the stones already present; and second, to try to reduce the size of the cistern so that stasis, infection, and subsequent reformation of stones are less likely to occur. The procedure described here hardly applies when most of the liver parenchyma has been destroyed; in such cases, removal of the lobe is the only effective therapy.

When intrahepatic calculi are found or strongly suspected at surgery, an operative cholangiogram is performed through a catheter inside the common duct. We usually use 30 per cent Urokon, which is instilled under gravity. To assist the filling of the intrahepatic radicles, the table is tilted or the common duct is compressed distal to the catheter. The cholangiogram often shows the exact location and number of stones in the intrahepatic cistern. A choledochotomy is then performed, long enough to admit a finger for exploration. The choledochotomy should reach close to the confluence of the hepatic ducts (Fig. 10). During the removal of the stones and afterward, palpation inside the duct helps in locating elusive concretions. Thorough irrigation with saline is carried out. During the palpation of the inside of the duct, it should be borne in mind that occasionally carcinoma may have developed, and should be differentiated from inflammatory changes. If difficulties are encountered in removing all the stones through the common duct, an incision is made in the surface of the liver. The most suitable area is chosen by palpation of an instrument inside the duct through the substance of the liver. By working through both openings it should be possible to remove all the stones present. Following the exploration a T tube is placed in the common duct and a mushroom

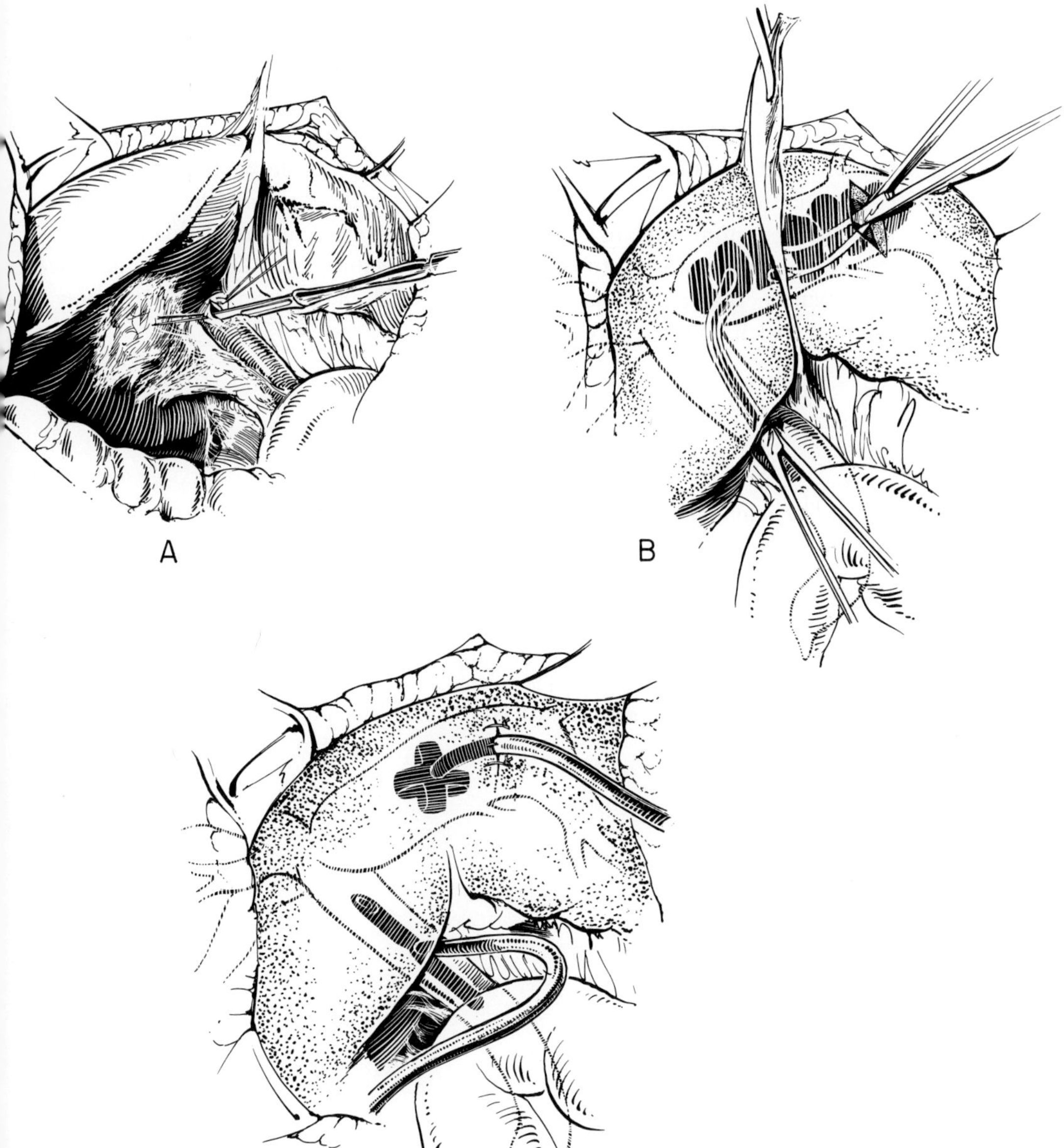

FIGURE 10. Intrahepatic stones. (*A*) The scarred and shrunken appearance of the left lobe of the liver is apparent. The choledochotomy is in the common hepatic duct. (*B*) An incision has been made through the dome of the liver, and stones are being removed from both directions. (*C*) Drainage is established both through the common duct and by a Malecot catheter through the substance of the liver.

catheter is placed through the incision in the liver, into the duct. The liver substance is closed about the catheter with mattress sutures of catgut. The size of the mushroom catheter varies with the size of the dilated intrahepatic duct.

We hope that postoperatively the intrahepatic ductal system will return to more normal size, and have actually seen this happen to some degree. We remove the common duct T tube in approximately 12 days, but leave the mushroom catheter in place much longer, or as long as we see decrease in the size of the ducts as estimated from cholangiograms. When there is continued dilatation of the ducts and re-formation of stones after this procedure and the process is unilateral, we believe that a hepatic lobectomy should be undertaken as the only procedure left which could relieve the patient.

References

GLENN, F. The importance of technique in cholecystectomy. *Surg., Gynec. and Obst.* 101:201, August 1955.

GLENN, F. The management of common duct drainage. *Surg., Gynec. and Obst.* 105:238, August 1957.

GLENN, F., and MOODY, F. G. Intrahepatic calculi. *Ann. Surg.* 153:711, May 1961.

GLENN, F., and WHITSELL, J. C., II. The surgical treatment of cystic duct remnants. *Surg., Gynec. and Obst.* 113:711, December 1961.

GLENN, F. *Atlas of Biliary Tract Surgery.* New York: Macmillan, 1963.

74. *Cholecystectomy, Common Duct Exploration, and Choledochoduodenostomy*

ALFRED HURWITZ

Cholecystectomy

Good lighting, proper exposure, and an adequate incision are essential to the conduct of a safe operation. An x-ray film is placed in the Bucky frame under all patients undergoing biliary tract surgery, so that a film may be obtained at the time of operation if indicated. It is reassuring for the surgeon to have this additional diagnostic procedure at his disposal, because it may be of inestimable help in the diagnosis of anomalies and in the identification of stones in the common or hepatic ducts.

Technique

After the peritoneum has been opened, a careful exploration of the organs within the peritoneal cavity is performed. Many surgeons do not take the few minutes necessary for the execution of this examination and, as a result, miss undiagnosed lesions which often are of more serious import to the patient than the diseased gallbladder.

To facilitate dissection and to avoid rupture, the tense gallbladder should be emptied of its contents by aspiration. The gallbladder can then be clamped with ring clamps at its fundus and at Hartmann's pouch. Traction on the latter clamp straightens out the cystic duct, which can then be more readily delineated. A Kocher maneuver is carried out to free the duodenum so that it can be retracted to the left and a greater length of the common bile duct exposed. Invariably the telltale common duct lymph node which is situated just lateral to the duodenum and inferior to the common duct can be seen. It is a useful landmark since the common duct invariably lies cephalad to it.

EXPOSURE AND LIGATION OF THE CYSTIC DUCT AND CYSTIC ARTERY. The peritoneal covering over the cystic duct is opened and the dissection proceeds distally to expose the common duct. Painstaking palpation of the cystic and common ducts is performed at this time in an attempt to locate stones or tumor. A ligature is then placed around the cystic duct and the duct is retracted to the left.

The cystic artery can be visualized next and the peritoneal covering stripped carefully away from its wall. It usually divides into anterior and posterior branches which may be ligated separately if they are elongated. In most instances, the main cystic artery can be easily visualized by gentle sharp and blunt dissection, and ligatures of 00 silk placed around it (Fig. 1). Before these ligatures are tied, the surgeon must be sure that the vessel is the cystic and not the hepatic artery. Distinguishing features of the cystic artery are its relatively small diameter (less than 1 to 2 mm.) and its course, which is usually perpendicular to the gallbladder wall and *terminates* as an *end* artery in the wall of the gallbladder. If the artery is larger than 2 mm. and if it cannot be demonstrated to enter the gallbladder wall, it is probably the hepatic artery and should be spared. The cystic artery is tied in continuity with silk ligatures and divided. This vessel should not be divided between hemostats, because of the danger of dislodging the hemostats and also because the tie cannot be placed as accurately behind the bulky hemostat.

Often a small artery enters the cystic duct just proximal to its junction with the common duct. This vessel, which is less than 1 mm. in diameter, should be ligated with 3–0 silk ligatures and then sectioned between them.

At this point in the operation, the cystic and common ducts should be palpated again for the presence of calculi. The diameters of both ducts are measured with a specially designed caliper. If the cystic duct is larger than 3 mm. and the common duct larger than 12 mm., we consider these ducts to be abnormally large and usually explore the common duct under these circumstances.

The cystic, common hepatic, and common bile ducts should be carefully delineated. If all three ducts are clearly visualized, the chance of damaging the

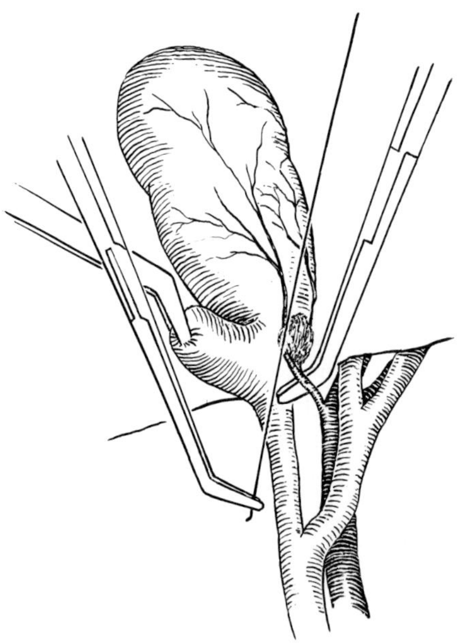

FIGURE 1. Method of ligating the cystic artery in continuity as it enters the gallbladder under a small lymph node. The silk ligature around the cystic duct is not shown.

common or hepatic duct is extremely remote. The ligature around the cystic duct can now be tied just below the junction of the cystic duct and the gallbladder to prevent the descent of stones from the gallbladder into the cystic duct (Fig. 2). Another ligature is placed loosely around the duct, the duct is opened along its anterior wall, and a ureteral catheter, usually a No. 5, is inserted into the cystic duct and passed into the common duct and finally into the duodenum. This maneuver assures patency of the cystic duct and the ampulla of Vater and also enables the surgeon to palpate stones along the catheter. The ureteral catheter is withdrawn to the junction of the cystic and common ducts and 8 to 10 cc. of Hypaque injected. After the x-ray film has been taken and read, the catheter is removed and the cystic duct ligated *in continuity* and divided. The duct is ligated about 5 mm. proximal to its junction with the common duct. If it is ligated flush with the duct, stenosis may ensue. Of course, if too long a stump is left, the patient may subsequently develop symptoms secondary to stones or inflammation in the long cystic duct remnant.

In the extirpation of the acutely inflamed gallbladder, it is often safer to remove the gallbladder from the fundus downward and to secure the cystic artery as it passes into the wall of the gallbladder. Under such circumstances, it may be too difficult and dangerous to attempt delineation of the common duct. The cystic duct should be ligated close to the junction to the gallbladder so that the risk of damaging a markedly inflamed and poorly discernible common duct will be reduced.

Removal of the Gallbladder. Saline is injected under the peritoneal layer that covers the gallbladder, which can then be peeled from the liver bed with greater ease and less bleeding. The peritoneum is opened and the flaps dissected away from the gallbladder. Small blood vessels and fine bile ducts can be seen emerging from the liver bed and entering the gallbladder wall. These structures are clamped, cut, and tied with fine silk sutures (Fig. 3). By employing this step,

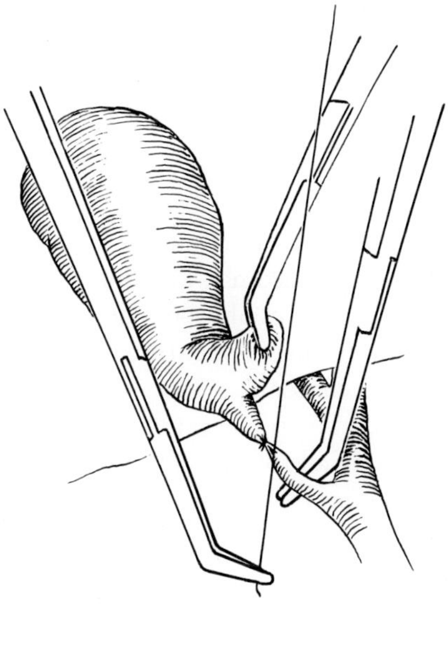

FIGURE 2. Ligation of the cystic duct in continuity. The final ligature is placed about 5 mm. from the common duct.

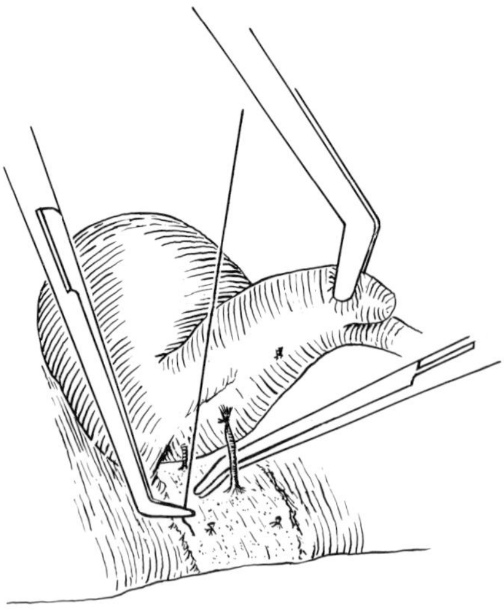

FIGURE 3. Ligation of the small bile ducts and blood vessels which emerge from the liver bed to enter the wall of the gallbladder.

postoperative leakage of bile and blood can be diminished and in most cases eliminated. The peritoneal flaps are resutured with continuous 3–0 chromic catgut.

The right upper quadrant is irrigated with large amounts of saline and aspirated completely. This maneuver enables the surgeon to remove any bile or exudate that might have been spilled during the operation. It also assures him, if the saline remains colorless, that hemostasis has been complete.

Common Duct Exploration

The indications for common duct exploration are: (1) palpable stone in the common duct; (2) duct diameter larger than 12 mm.; (3) jaundice; (4) evidence of stones in the common duct by operative cholangiogram; (5) cystic duct larger than 3 mm.; (6) repetitive attacks of biliary colic, especially with pain referred to the left hypochondrium.

Technique

Small blood vessels coursing transversely across the common duct should be transfixed before the duct is opened, to prevent troublesome bleeding. The duct is first aspirated with a 20 gauge needle, and the recovery of bile establishes the identity of the duct. On rare occasions an anomalous portal vein may be confused with the common duct until aspiration reveals the nature of its contents.

The duct is opened in a longitudinal direction for 1.5 to 2 cm. Obvious stones are removed in both directions by the gentle use of Randall forceps. The cystic duct should be probed from within the lumen of the common duct to prove the presence or absence of stones in the stump. No metallic instrument is employed to traverse the sphincter of Oddi, because of the danger of creating a false passage at the

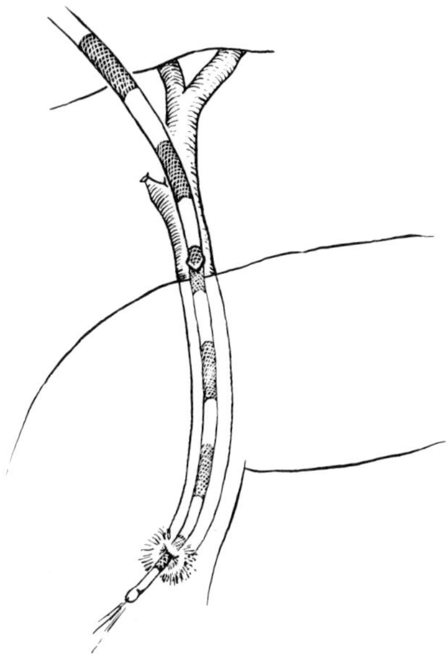

FIGURE 4. Insertion of a ureteral catheter through the ampulla of Vater.

lower end of the duct which might initiate acute pancreatitis or subsequently cause fibrosis and stricture in the lower end of the common bile duct. I employ a ureteral cathether, usually size 7 or 9, and pass it gently through the ampulla of Vater into the duodenum (Fig. 4). The catheter is irrigated as it is slowly withdrawn, to wash out additional stones. The hepatic ducts are irrigated through a conventional rubber catheter. After the patency of the lower end of the duct has been demonstrated by the passage of the ureteral catheter, a No. 8 Foley bag (pediatric) catheter is inserted into the lower portion of the duct and the bag inflated just enough to prevent egress of saline from around the balloon (Fig. 5).

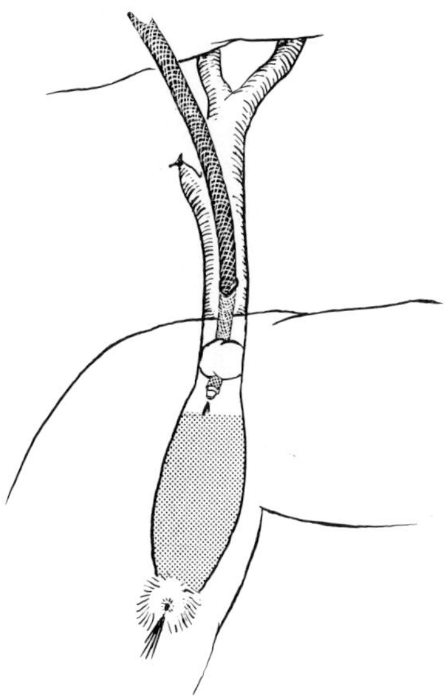

FIGURE 5. Lavage of the lower end of the duct after dilatation, through a No. 8 Foley (pediatric) catheter. Through this same catheter x-ray visualization can be obtained.

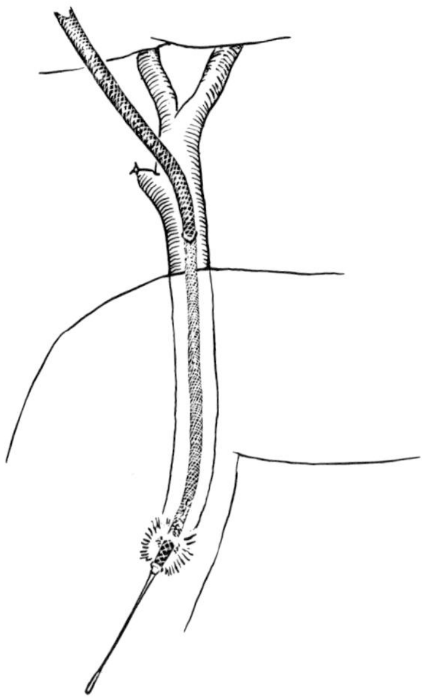

FIGURE 6. If the ureteral catheter does not traverse the ampulla of Vater, a filiform and follower are employed.

The lower end of the duct is flushed with copious amounts of saline. This maneuver enables the surgeon to wash detritus and small calculi into the duodenum. In one instance, I encountered difficulty in pushing the saline into the duodenum despite the fact that a ureteral catheter had been previously passed into the duodenum. Re-exploration of the duct revealed an 8 mm. calculus which had been overlooked. If the ureteral catheter does not pass through the ampulla of Vater, a filiform and follower are used. They may also be employed to dilate gently the sphincter of Oddi (Fig. 6). I have employed this method after observing how successful urologists are in dilating strictures of the urethra with minimal trauma.

A T tube is inserted into the common duct and the duct closed with interrupted 3–0 catgut sutures in a watertight fashion. A T tube that is smaller than the lumen of the duct is employed. I excise its entire posterior wall so that it can be removed in the postoperative period with less trauma. I have not closed the duct primarily because leakage of bile might occur if the sphincter of Oddi was spastic or a calculus was left behind in the common duct. Moreover, one may be able to flush small stones into the duodenum by injecting saline through the T tube in the postoperative period. In these instances repetitive choledochograms are of inestimable value.

Summary of Recommendations for Avoiding Pitfalls in Biliary Tract Surgery

1. Adequate incision.
2. Good lighting.
3. Good exposure.

4. Delineate all three ducts—cystic, common hepatic, and common bile—before ligating the cystic duct.

5. Make sure that the cystic artery is of appropriate size and terminates in the gallbladder wall as an end artery.

6. Ligate the cystic duct about 3 to 5 mm. from its junction with the common duct or at its junction with the gallbladder when the common duct cannot be clearly delineated.

7. Ligate all blood vessels and bile ducts traversing the liver bed during the stripping of the gallbladder from its bed.

8. Aspirate the common bile duct before opening it.

9. Use stone forceps gently.

10. Traverse the ampulla of Vater with a ureteral catheter.

11. Dilate the lower end of the duct with a filiform and graduated followers.

12. Irrigate the lower end of the common duct through a pediatric Foley catheter.

13. Employ operative cholangiograms.

Choledochoduodenostomy

Stenosis of the terminal end of the common bile duct is a frequent finding in chronic disease of the biliary tract. The pathogenesis of this condition is not clear and many explanations have been offered. In chronic cholecystitis and cholelithiasis, stenosis of the common duct may be secondary to the chronic inflammatory process involving the biliary tract. In those cases in which there are stones in the common duct or a history of previous common duct exploration, trauma may also be a contributing factor. Various theories have been advanced to explain the development of stenosis of the terminal portion of the common duct in the absence of biliary calculi or of previous exploration of the duct. Hypertrophy and stenosis of the sphincter could be part of the general thickening of the common duct which occurs in chronic cholangitis. It has also been suggested that the presence of smooth muscle and nerve fibers may, under proper conditions of hypertrophy and stimulation, make the common bile ducts capable of dynamic independent activity. Advocates of this theory believe that the symptoms which occur after cholecystectomy may be related to functional spastic phenomena in the extraduodenal common bile duct itself, as well as in the sphincter of Oddi. In the experimental animal, bile stasis which resulted from the narrowing of the terminal portion of the common duct favored the formation of stones.

The surgical objective in the treatment of stenosis of the terminal portion of the common duct is to re-establish the free flow of bile into the gastrointestinal tract. Choledochoduodenostomy is our recommended procedure for most of these cases. Other operative procedures that have been employed have failed in a great number of cases or have been associated with a high incidence of complications. Included in these operations are dilatation with Bakes dilators and sphincterotomy. The latter procedure has been modified so that both the sphincter of Oddi and the choledochal muscle are divided. Under these circumstances, sphincteroplasty ceases to be a simple procedure and becomes a rather extensive and hazardous operation.

It is our opinion that exploration of the common duct and dilatation of its sphincter by the use of metallic instruments may be followed by iatrogenic complications. A false passageway may be created during this manipulation, especially if any degree of force is used. There is also the danger of producing postoperative pancreatitis and stricture formation. Finally, the improvement obtained by dilating the narrow terminal duct and sphincter may be only temporary. We also consider it impractical to attempt to drain a large and dilated duct through a relatively small opening. We have therefore abandoned the use of metal dilators and are employing ureteral catheters and also urologic filiforms and followers during common duct exploration since they are less traumatic. When an absolute or relative narrowing of the lower end of the common bile duct is found at operation, we believe that a bypass operation should be performed. This situation would be comparable to the slow flow that occurs when fluid, especially if it is viscid, drains through a narrow outlet from a wide reservoir.

Technique

Our technique of choledochoduodenostomy is easy to perform. The duodenum is mobilized by the Kocher maneuver. An incision is then made in the lower part of the common duct and the duct is explored. If it is decided that a choledochoduo-

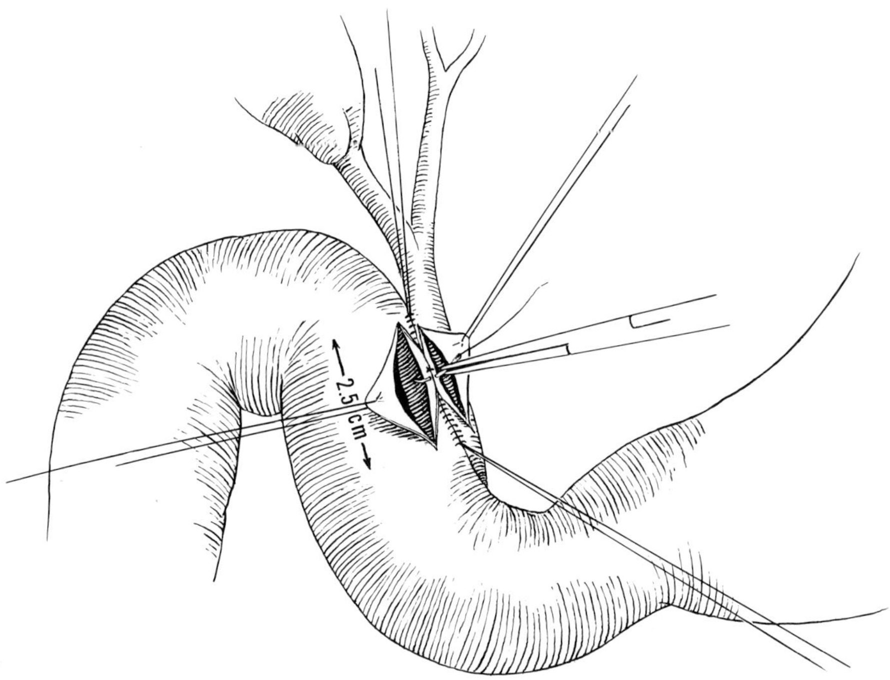

FIGURE 7. Side-to-side anastomosis of the common bile duct to the duodenum. Note the obliquity of the incision in the common bile duct.

denostomy is indicated, the incision is enlarged to about 2.5 cm. or more. A side-to-side anastomosis is then performed between the duct and the duodenum, using an inner layer of interrupted 3–0 chromic catgut and an outer layer of interrupted 3–0 silk sutures (Fig. 7). When completed, the stoma should measure 2.5 cm.

Comments

In one case we decided to perform this operation although stenosis was not demonstrated. Since this was the patient's third operation and her second common duct exploration, choledochoduodenostomy appeared to be the procedure most likely to insure permanent relief. In our cases this operative procedure has not presented any unusual technical problems and has been followed by an uneventful postoperative course. We have been especially impressed with the fact that our patients have remained asymptomatic. We attribute the good results to the fact that in each case the stoma between the common duct and the duodenum was large enough (2.5 cm. or more) to insure its patency. It is possible that sphincteroplasty would be equally effective, but this procedure is more difficult to perform and may be followed by a higher incidence of complications. The length of the follow-up in our cases has varied from six months to eight years. These studies have shown that the patients have remained well and presented no evidence of recurrent biliary disease. Our experience, together with that of an increasing number of other surgeons, makes us feel that side-to-side choledochoduodenostomy is an efficacious and safe operation.

References

COLE, W. H. *Operative Technic in General Surgery*. New York: Appleton-Century-Crofts, 1949. P. 543.

IMAMOGLU, K., PERRY, J. F., JR., and WANGENSTEEN, O. H. Experimental production of gallstones by incomplete stricture of the terminal common bile duct. *Surgery* 42:623, October 1957.

ISZAK, F. C., and STEIGER, Y. Post-cholecystectomy syndrome: its prevention and treatment by choledochoduodenostomy. *J. Internat. Coll. Surgeons* 300:802, December 1958.

LAHEY, F. H. The surgical exposure of the gallbladder and bile ducts. *Surg., Gynec. and Obst.* 75:1, July 1942.

SCHWARTZ, F., BENSHIMOL, A., and HURWITZ, A. Choledochoduodenostomy in the treatment of stenosis of the lower portion of the common bile duct. *Surgery* 46: 1020, December 1959.

75. *Reconstruction of the Common Bile Duct*

HAROLD A. ZINTEL

RECONSTRUCTION of the common bile duct is one of the most difficult problems with which the surgeon is confronted and one of the most difficult in which to obtain a permanent and satisfactory result. It will frequently tax to the utmost the ability, equipment, and experience of a surgeon and his operating team.

Almost all common duct strictures follow cholecystectomy or other biliary tract surgery. Occasionally strictures are produced in the course of operation on the stomach or duodenum. According to the literature, 85 to 99.9 per cent of the cases represent true surgical complications. The remaining strictures are caused by inflammation or tumor. Common duct strictures result when the surgeon does not adequately expose or understand the anatomical details of the operative area, or when there has been massive, or at least excessive, bleeding. Many of these patients have been operated upon several times, and an occasional patient has had seven or eight previous operations. With each operation, the scar tissue in the region of the hepatoduodenal ligament and the inferior surface of the liver increases. Usually there is also some additional loss of bile duct substance. The report, from one or several surgeons, that no extrahepatic ductal structures exist does not necessarily mean that another surgeon cannot find duct remnants with which to make a satisfactory repair.

With biliary obstruction, there is increasing liver damage, associated with dilatation of the intrahepatic biliary duct tree—the so-called hydrops of the liver. Persistent, very deep jaundice, associated with ascites, usually indicates severe liver damage and is ordinarily a contraindication to operation.

The major portion of the abdominal dissection, from the inferior edge of the anterior surface of the liver to the hepatoduodenal area, may be through one solid mass of dense scar tissue. The duodenum is frequently pulled upward into the cleft between the caudate lobe, the caudate process, and the inferior surface of the medial segment of the right lobe of the liver. Thus, a small portion of the duodenal loop may appear to be posterior to the inferior surface of the liver. The operative field is usually bloody. Much time must be spent in providing an adequate approach to and exposure of the area for reconstruction. If there is one step that is more critical than any other in the operation for common duct reconstruction, it is the adequate exposing and identifying of all structures in and surrounding the hepatoduodenal area. Under the best of circumstances there never seems to be too much room in which to readily make an anastomosis close to the liver surface. All too frequently the completed anastomosis is not as neat as one would like to have it. Only 25 per cent of patients present what can be referred to as normal anatomy of the bile ducts and the cystic and hepatic arteries (Michels, 1953). The surgeon must be equipped to recognize and deal with any of these ductal and vascular abnormalities as they are exposed in the scar tissue.

Technique

The surgeon's frame of mind is highly important. He must be prepared to spend as much time as is necessary to perform a satisfactory operation. The endeavor should be the only operative procedure scheduled for the surgeon that day. He must also keep in mind that each unsuccessful attempt at common duct reconstruction reduces the patient's chances of ever having a successful reconstruction.

The operation requires wide exposure by a very long abdominal incision and by a very adequate separation of the structures in the right upper quadrant along the plane of the inferior surface of the liver. In few operations is it so important to have adequate relaxation, a dry field, and good illumination.

The object of the operation is to obtain an adequate mucosa-to-mucosa suture of the upper and lower bile duct remnants with an intact sphincter of Oddi. The proximal portion of the biliary tree must be located first. Without the proximal portion of the ductal system—the common hepatic or the right and left hepatic ducts—an entirely satisfactory procedure cannot be accomplished.

The incision of choice is a liberal right subcostal incision. It is made parallel to and 1.5 cm. below the right costal margin, dividing the right rectus muscle and curving to cross the medial part of the left rectus muscle. The left rectus can then easily be divided later, if necessary. The subcostal incision should lie immediately over the plane of the inferior surface of the liver. This is the plane of major dissection necessary to free all the structures of the right upper quadrant and to expose the inferior surface of the liver leading to the hepatoduodenal ligament and its contained structures. Frequently, previous scars and drainage tracts will alter one's choice of incision. When a fistulous tract is present or a T tube has been left in place, the tissue surrounding the tract or a tube is excised from the abdominal wall. This is done either as part of the initial incision or as a separate incision.

The surgeon who finds no adhesions or only a very few flimsy ones on his way to the hepatoduodenal ligament is most fortunate. When no free peritoneal cavity is encountered and the structures in this area are adherent, the first step is to find the inferior edge of the anterior surface of the liver by entering the space between the anterior surface of the liver and the undersurface of the abdominal wall (Fig. 1). Once the anterior surface of the liver tissue has been exposed, it is easy to locate the liver edge. The dissection is carried to Morison's pouch and the area of the hepatoduodenal ligament posteriorly, and from the midline to the right lateral abdominal wall. The ligament teres is partially or completely divided. The

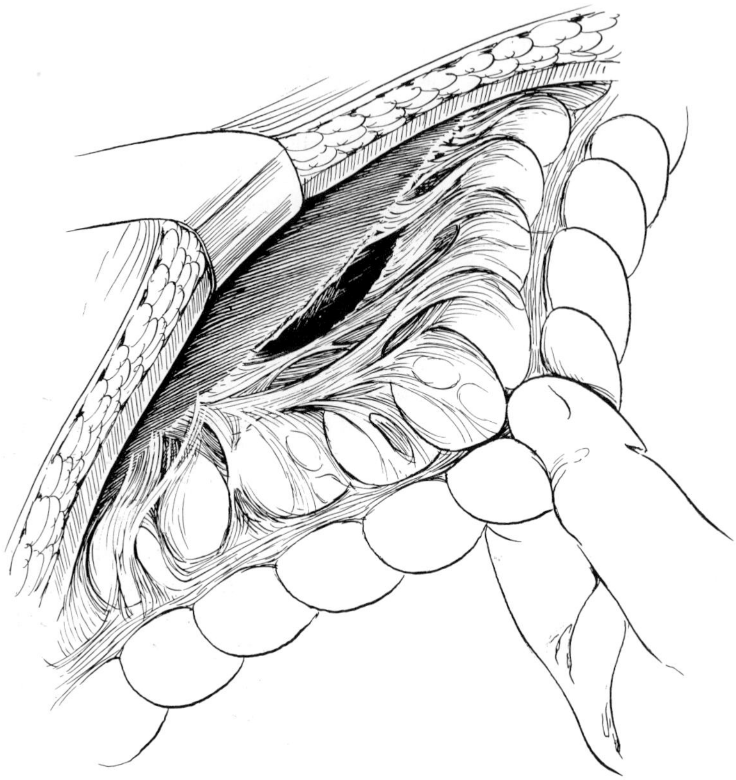

FIGURE 1. A subcostal incision is usually in the plane of major dissection in common duct reconstruction operations. In the presence of excessive scarring and adhesions the inferior edge of the anterior surface of the liver is readily found by separating the abdominal wall from the anterior surface of the liver.

colon is detached completely from the right lobe of the liver. The distal portion of the stomach and the duodenum are freed from the undersurface of the liver. When the scar tissue is thick, this can be a most tedious dissection. If an error is made in attempting to follow this cleavage line, one should cut into the substance of the liver rather than into the bowel.

The assistant constantly removes the blood—sometimes with each scalpel stroke. A tonsil suction tip or a slightly smaller tip is used. It is good to have available several such suction tips, and an extra suction tube to connect to the suction apparatus. If oozing becomes too profuse, apply Gelfoam and an abdominal pad, and hold it firmly in place with a retractor. Meanwhile continue the dissection elsewhere. There is much to be done.

As one approaches the general area of the gastrohepatic ligament, one should palpate frequently for an anomalous hepatic artery or its right and left branches. It should be remembered that the scar tissue may not only have pulled the hepatoduodenal ligament content and the duodenum up toward the posterior surface of the liver, but it can also have pulled these structures anteriorly. Unless one is thinking of these possibilities, one might accidentally enter the common duct, the hepatic artery, or even the portal vein. Furthermore, the liver of these patients is enlarged—bulging, so to speak. The entire intrahepatic biliary duct tree may be markedly distended and may contain several ounces of bile—hydrops.

The next step before entering the scar tissue in the hepatoduodenal ligament area is to expose and identify the anterior surface of the first and second portions of the duodenal loop. Then the pyloric area and several centimeters of the anterior surface of the stomach are exposed. The pyloric ring can usually be identified by locating the transverse vein of Mayo along its anterior surface and also by palpating the increased substance—muscle—of the pyloric ring itself. The duodenal loop is then mobilized by the Kocher maneuver. Scar tissue of previous operative procedures is rarely found along the lower part of the second and third portions of the duodenum or behind the head of the pancreas. Thus, this maneuver usually is carried out easily. The duodenal loop and the pancreatic head are mobilized to the point where one can readily visualize most of the posterior surface of the head of the pancreas. One should then take a minute or two of extra time to expose and positively identify the anterior surface of the inferior vena cava if it is not already evident. Thus far, the exposure in the abdomen has included separation and identification of all structures in the right upper quadrant. The hepatoduodenal ligament has been approached anteriorly, posteriorly, and laterally by wide separation of the structures.

Deaver retractors 1 or 2 inches wide, with pistol-grip handles, will be found most useful in this operation. The regular, medium, and deep types should always be on hand. Occasionally in an extremely obese individual the deep, deep Deaver retractors will prove to be most useful. They have a total depth of 9 inches from the highest point on the blade to the tip when the handle is held horizontally. With the aid of wide retractors over abdominal pads, the inferior surface of the liver in the general area of the hepatoduodenal ligament is lifted upward or cephalad and toward the patient's right side. Similarly, a retractor is used to retract the mobilized loop of the duodenum and the head of the pancreas caudad and toward the patient's left side. Such contralateral retraction tends to put the hepatoduodenal ligament on a stretch and to open up the foramen of Winslow, the entrance to the lesser peritoneal cavity. If the foramen of Winslow is not patent, an attempt should be made to separate the structures of this area to allow insertion of a finger into the foramen. Then it will be possible in a moment to control severe arterial hemorrhage by thumb and finger compression of the hepatic artery in the hepatoduodenal ligament. The hepatic artery should be located by palpation or by exposure of a short segment. In most patients the hepatic artery will parallel the course of the common duct a little medially and slightly posterior to the duct. Occasionally I find it helpful to locate the portal vein. It can usually be found by following the anterosuperior surface of the first portion of the duodenum, just distal to the pyloric ring. Just posterior to this area the superior edge of the pancreas is separated from the hepatoduodenal ligament. The portal vein will be found in this area, as it emerges from the cleft between the uncinate process and the neck of the pancreas. Fortunately this area usually is not bound in dense scar tissue.

Once the hepatoduodenal ligament area has been cleared, wide exposure obtained, and all surrounding structures identified—including those that might give rise to serious trouble—one can begin the search for the ends of the duct. If one has a fistulous tract or a T tube to follow to the proximal portion of the extrahepatic biliary duct, half—and the most important part—of the battle is won. One must proceed most cautiously because of the very dense scar tissue. Usually progress can be made only by sharp dissection, and frequently only by knife dissection. A No. 26 hypodermic needle ¾ or 1 inch long, on a 5 or 10 cc. syringe, is used to probe the scarred tissue in the search for bile in a patent proximal bile duct remnant (Fig. 2). One should insert the needle very slowly. As the needle is inserted and then withdrawn from the tissues, gentle aspiration is used. Since, occasionally, only a fraction of a drop of bile may be obtained, it is helpful to expel the contents of the syringe or needle onto the surface of a clean white towel or abdominal pad. The yellow color of bile is most easily seen on a white background. Frequently the aspirated material is mixed with blood. One may not be able to aspirate additional bile from the same segment of the duct or a fistulous tract. A small contracted bile duct segment or a small fistulous tract containing bile must connect with a normal-sized or bulbous proximal end of the duct. If such a tract is found, one need only follow the tract to the undamaged portion of the bile duct.

When no bile is obtained in the proximal hepatoduodenal ligament area the needle must be inserted into the hilum of the liver. If bile is obtained the needle should be left in place or the position of the needle should be noted carefully. It may be most difficult to find again. Once bile has been obtained in the hilum of the liver, an attempt is made to find the distal end of the proximal duct by serial needle aspirations along its suspected course. Only the amount of proximal duct necessary to allow placement of one row of fine sutures is separated from the surrounding tissue. More extensive separation might jeopardize the blood supply and lead to necrosis of that segment of the duct. When no duct protrudes from the undersurface of the liver, it becomes necessary to dissect into the liver. A No. 15 scalpel blade is inserted into the scar tissue and liver substance along the hypodermic needle. The opening is gradually enlarged to the maximum diameter of the distal end of the duct. By means of Bakes dilators (3 or 4 mm.) one can determine

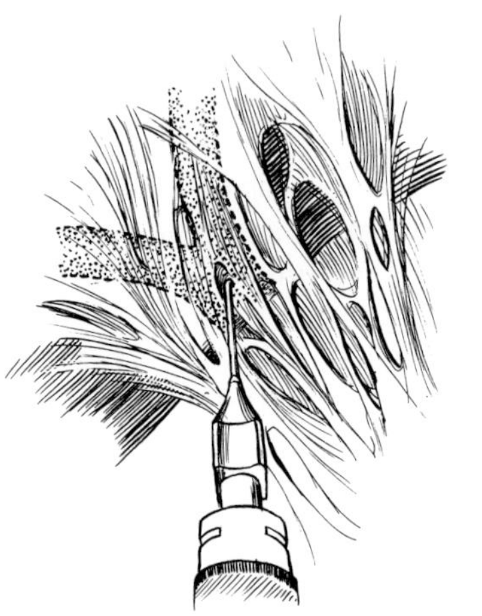

FIGURE 2. A hypodermic needle is inserted into the scarred hepatoduodenal ligament—and when necessary into the base of the liver—in search of bile in a bile duct.

whether an entrance has been gained into the common hepatic or the right or left duct. If necessary, a portion of the liver substance is removed around the ductal system (Fig. 3). A Bovie or cutting edge loop may be useful. Oozing from the cut liver surface will usually respond satisfactorily to compression through an abdominal pad over a piece of Gelfoam. Occasionally it is necessary to place a mattress suture of chromic 00 catgut in the liver substance around the bleeding point. Such suture ligatures should be placed and tied very gingerly since one can easily cut through liver substance with very little tension. One must always remember it takes *very* little tension to provide sufficient pressure to occlude a rather small artery or vein. It is helpful for anyone who undertakes this operation to investigate the anatomy of the bile ducts and the blood vessels within the liver, as described by Goldsmith and Woodburne (1957).

Once one has found the proximal end to the biliary tree and separated a sufficient amount of duct to allow suturing of its cuff, attention is turned to the problem of finding the distal common duct. One should explore not only along the hepatoduodenal ligament, but also along the posterior surface of the superior and right lateral borders of the pancreas just below the surface of the second portion of the duodenum. The common duct in the region of the head of the pancreas may assume several positions. It may enter into and be completely buried in pancreatic tissue. It may be on the posterolateral surface of the pancreas or may lie in a groove of pancreatic tissue before becoming buried in pancreatic tissue.

I do not dissect into the lateral and into the under surface of the pancreatic head in an attempt to locate the distal common duct, as recommended by Lahey (1950). If the duct cannot be found on the posterolateral surface of the duodenal loop or on the posterolateral surface of the edge of the pancreas, I resort to a duodenotomy. In my opinion, a properly done duodenotomy is a far safer and more direct approach to the problem (Fig. 4). The duodenum is opened longitudinally along the anterolateral surface from the midpoint of the second portion to the beginning of the third portion. The duodenal loop is rotated anteriorly so that the lateral wall of the duodenum can be more readily inspected. Such an approach makes it much easier to find the very small papilla because, with the duodenum rotated, the surgeon should be looking directly at the papilla. The cut intestinal wall edges are held apart by means of Allis or Babcock clamps.

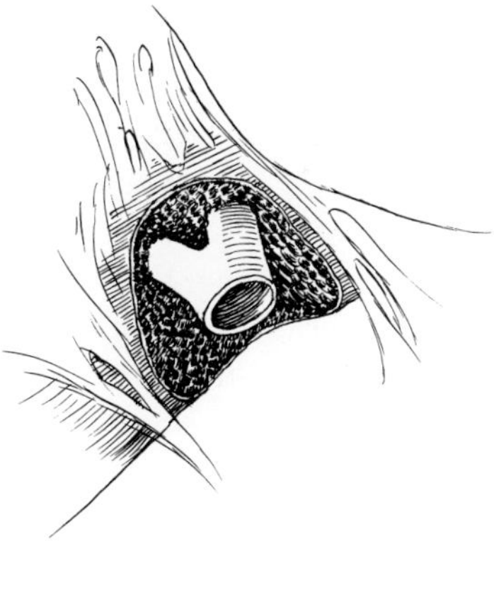

FIGURE 3. No duct protrudes beyond the inferior surface of the liver. A wedge of liver tissue has been removed to allow placement of sutures in the proximal common hepatic duct.

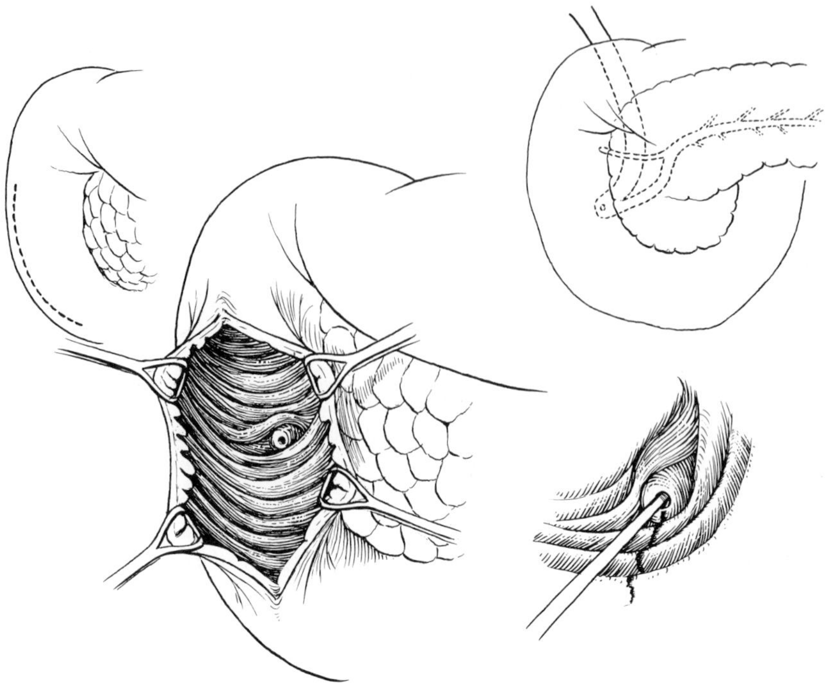

FIGURE 4. Upper right diagram shows the usual relationship of the ducts in the head of the pancreas. Upper left diagram shows the location of the duodenotomy incision. The duodenal loop and head of the pancreas are rotated forward so that one can look directly toward the papilla in the opened duodenum. The lower right diagram is an enlarged version of the placement of a probe through the ostium of the papilla of the duct of Wirsung.

A diligent search is made for the papilla of Vater. Usually Roux or vein retractors are necessary to scrutinize adequately the recesses between the heavy transverse mucosal folds. The blunt end of the scalpel handle is useful in visualizing both sides of the folds. The papilla is usually 2 to 3 mm. in diameter and projects 2 to 3 mm. into the duodenum. The orifice in the papilla is not always apparent, but by gentle probing with a wire probe or with lacrimal dilators, one can usually gain entrance into the orifice and demonstrate both the main pancreatic duct and the common bile duct. Frequently a wire probe can be passed through one-half to three-quarters of the entire length of the pancreatic gland. Occasionally, when there is doubt about whether or not the papilla has been seen, pressure over the portion of the stomach that overlies the pancreas and gentle milking of the pancreas from its tail toward the head will produce a drop or two of water-clear, slightly viscous pancreatic fluid from the papilla. It is possible that the papilla of the accessory duct may be found. However, in most instances the accessory duct does not communicate with the main pancreatic duct in the adult.

Only rarely is it possible to introduce a No. 3 Bakes dilator into the lower common bile duct through the papilla. Ordinarily, one must first insert a wire probe and with a No. 15 scalpel blade do a minimal sphincterotomy. Usually this means cutting the cephalad side of the ampulla and part of the sphincter for a distance of 2 to 3 mm. Rarely is it necessary to extend the incision more than 5 or 6 mm. With a small Bakes dilator in the ampulla of the common bile duct, one can readily determine the position of the proximal end of the distal duct remnant. Usually it will be found protruding beyond surrounding pancreatic tissue. If it is necessary to enter pancreatic tissue, the dissection can be done with much less disturbance of pancreatic acini and ducts than by a blind search for the duct without a duodenotomy and without the aid of a probe in the duct.

Finally, one must decide on the kind of reconstruction procedure. This is largely determined by how successful one has been in finding the ductal remnants. Where adequate lengths of remaining hepatic and common bile duct are found, end-to-end anastomosis with interrupted sutures of 4–0 silk will suffice. This is easiest done if one begins the approximation with a suture at the posteromedial aspect of the ends of the ducts, leaving all sutures long so that they can be used as rotators to bring relatively inaccessible parts of the anastomotic site into view

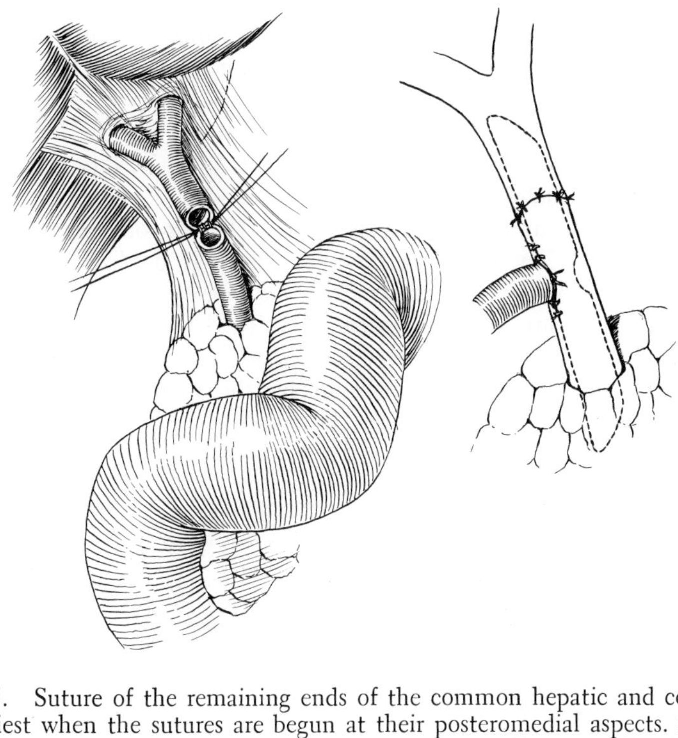

FIGURE 5. Suture of the remaining ends of the common hepatic and common bile ducts is easiest when the sutures are begun at their posteromedial aspects. Suture ends are left long to facilitate placement of subsequent sutures. The suture line is completed over a T tube which is exteriorized through a separate opening in the duct. The sutures immediately beside the T tube are of 00 chromic catgut. The corresponding knots are tied to the corresponding ends of the suture on the other side of the tube to form a temporary restraining bridle. A notch is cut in the T tube opposite the stem of the T to facilitate eventual removal of the tube.

(Fig. 5). Because of the previous mobilization of the duodenal loop, approximation usually is easily achieved. It is best to use atraumatic or swaged sutures on three-eighths inch round needles. Quite frequently one has only limited space in which to maneuver the needle; therefore, smaller-sized needles are very useful. A T tube is inserted to serve as a stent as suturing progresses. The T tube is always inserted through a separate opening. I much prefer to use a double-bridle stitch of chromic 3–0 catgut in the duct wall to keep the T tube from sliding out of place before the operation has been completed, and also to help keep it in place during the first few days of the postoperative period.

If only the right and left hepatic ducts remain, a small V can be cut between the adjacent walls and the cut edges sutured together with interrupted sutures (Fig. 6) as described by Lahey. Thus the two hepatic ducts are joined to form a single opening. When an anastomosis is made at or very close to the junction of the right and left hepatic ducts, a Lahey T tube is used. This is a T tube one limb of which divides into two shorter tubes to fit the right and left hepatic ducts.

Frequently the distal segment of the common duct will be found to be quite small. However, it should be remembered that a duct that will admit a 3 mm. Bakes dilator ordinarily will allow an adequate flow of bile in a normal individual.

When the distal common duct cannot be found, a hepatoduodenostomy, a hepatojejunostomy with a jejunojejunostomy, or a Roux en Y procedure is done. I prefer a Roux en Y procedure because one can be assured of a more satisfactory anastomosis than can be obtained with the duodenum or with a loop of jejunum. This is especially true if the anastomosis is made at or near the liver surface. Frequently the hepatic bile duct is enlarged to a size of 1.25 to 1.5 cm. and the anastomosis may be made end-to-end with only moderate puckering of the jejunal end (Fig. 7). As in an intestinal anastomosis, the mucous membrane must be completely inverted. To do this a Connell suture is used. The sutures in the jejunum are placed 3 to 5 mm. away from the cut end of the jejunum and are spaced 3 to 5 mm. apart, while the suture bites in the bile duct are much smaller and are placed closer together. Silk 4–0 sutures are used. If the caliber of the proximal portion of the duct is rather small, or only the openings of the right and left

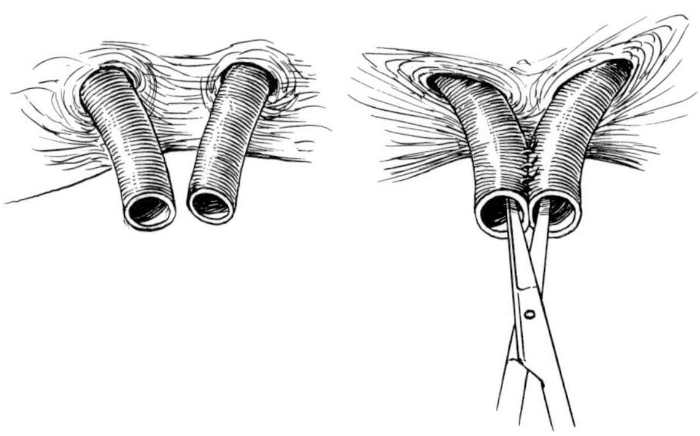

FIGURE 6. The maneuver, described by Lahey, converting the right and left hepatic bile ducts into a single tube or a reconstructed proximal common hepatic duct.

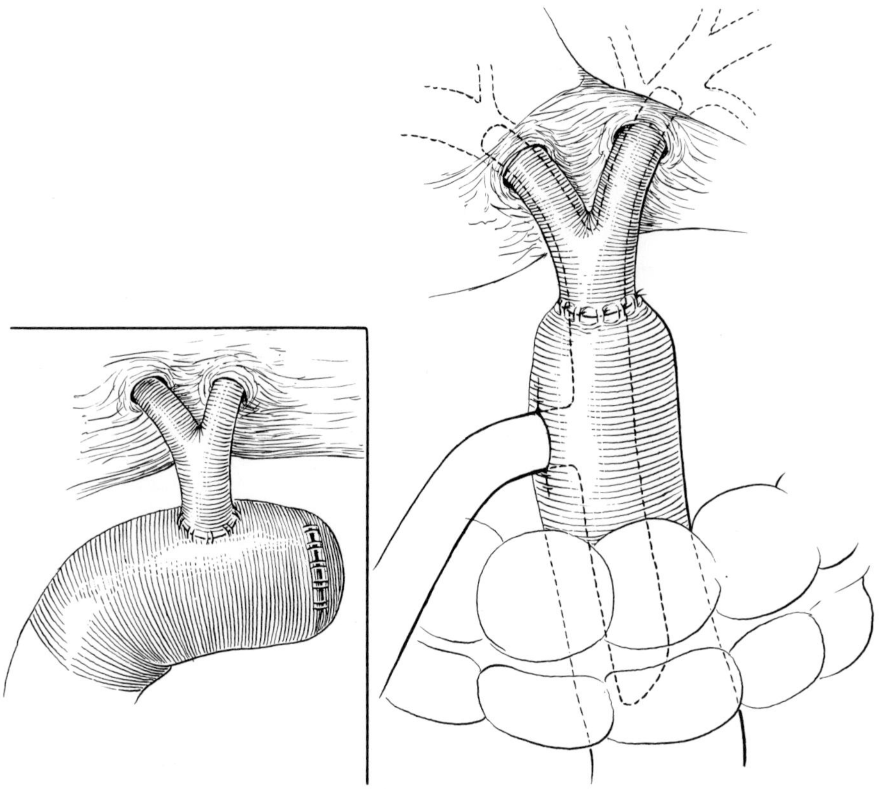

FIGURE 7. If the remaining common hepatic duct is large, an end-to-end anastomosis to the cut end of the jejunum is rather easily accomplished. A T tube, a T tube split by a scissors cut, or a Lahey T tube (shown) is used as a splint. If the common hepatic duct is small, the end of the jejunum is closed and the bile duct anastomosis is made end-to-side.

hepatic duct remain, one can close the open end of the jejunal limb and anastomose the single hepatic duct or the right and left ducts to the side of the jejunum, as the case may be. To do this adequately, it may be necessary to place all sutures first and then draw them up and tie them one by one.

If the patient's condition is not satisfactory during the operation, and the hepatic duct or hepatic ducts have been found, a catheter can be inserted into the duct to form a fistulous drainage tract through the abdominal wall. At a subsequent operation, one may find that the hydrops of the liver has disappeared and the bulk of the liver decreased in size to the point that the operation is facilitated.

When one finds that a small portion of the bile duct has been destroyed, as when a clamp has been placed partially, but not completely, across the duct, I am convinced that one should not attempt to do a Heineke-Mikulicz plastic procedure. In this procedure the scar tissue is excised by a vertical elliptical incision, which is closed transversely. I believe it is much more satisfactory to excise a segment completely and rejoin the cut ends.

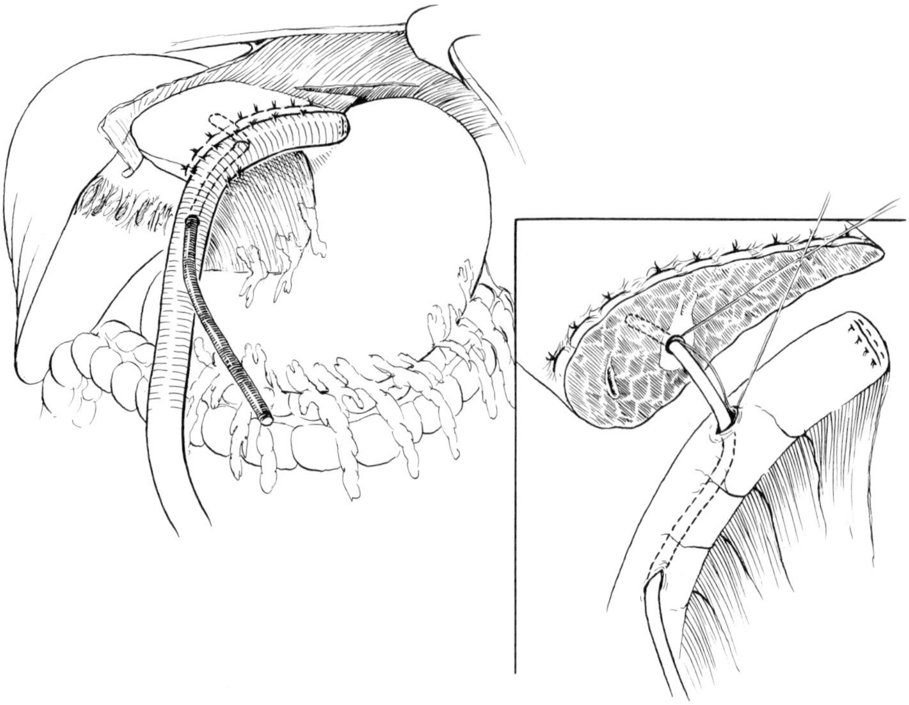

FIGURE 8. When the common hepatic or right and left hepatic bile ducts cannot be found the Longmire procedure is used. A sufficient portion of the left lobe of the liver is amputated to find and expose a sizable portion of a main duct of the lobe. The cut end of the duct is sutured to the jejunum by an end-to-side anastomosis over a T tube or a catheter (shown). The capsule of the liver is then sutured to the serosa of the jejunum.

As a last resort, the procedure suggested by Longmire can be used (Fig. 8). The left lobe of the liver can be partially amputated to obtain access to a bile duct of a size large enough to permit bile flow. The duct then can be anastomosed to a small opening in the mucous membrane of the duodenum over a T tube or a catheter with side holes to allow bile drainage into the duodenum.

The length of time that should elapse before removal of the T tube is always a debatable question. If one fortunately should find no scarring except at the point of obstruction, then one would be perfectly justified in removing the tube after a satisfactory cholangiogram report at 7 to 10 days postoperatively. In almost all instances when scar tissue is present the T tube must be left in place at least six months and preferably one year. In one instance, when very extensive and thick scar tissue was present, I left the tube in until the rubber began to decompose, at about two years. My thought was that the patient had been getting on perfectly well with the tube, and I was not absolutely sure that she would do well without it. All patients who have tubes in place for more than several weeks are instructed to irrigate the tube with 5 to 10 ml. of physiological saline solution every second day, without fail.

References

Goldsmith, N. A., and Woodburne, R. T. The surgical anatomy pertaining to liver resection. *Surg., Gynec. and Obst.* 105:310, September 1957.

Lahey, F. H., and Pyrtek, L. J. Experience with the operative management of 280 strictures of the bile ducts. *Surg., Gynec. and Obst.* 91:25, July 1950.

Michels, N. A. Variational anatomy of the hepatic, cystic, and retroduodenal arteries: a statistical analysis of their origin, distribution, and relations to the biliary ducts in two hundred bodies. *Arch. Surg.* 66:20, January 1953.

XIV. THE STOMACH AND DUODENUM

76. Gastric Vagotomy in the Treatment of Duodenal Ulcer

LESTER R. DRAGSTEDT

THE EMPLOYMENT of gastric vagotomy in the treatment of duodenal ulcer is based upon the concept that the cause of this disease is a hypersecretion of gastric juice of nervous or vagus origin. It is imperative to make certain that a pathological hypersecretion of gastric juice of nervous origin actually exists in the patient before the operation is undertaken. This can be easily done. With few exceptions, the secretion of gastric juice in the fasting empty stomach, as at night, is chiefly of nervous origin, and a comparison of the acid output in a measured period of time with that secured from normal individuals under the same circumstances provides an index of the pathological hyperactivity of the vagus nerves. If this determination is made by means of an intragastric nasal tube of the Levin type, the tube should be left in place for the operative procedure.

Technique of Gastric Vagotomy

The anesthesia should provide good relaxation and the choice is best left to a skilled anesthetist. Continuous spinal anesthesia is satisfactory if well given, but I have abandoned it because of the frequency of postanesthetic headache. Ethylene induction with ether as the major anesthetic agent has usually been my choice, at times supplemented with curare or a similar drug for greater relaxation.

I have usually employed a midline incision extending from the xyphoid cartilage to the umbilicus. The incision should be adequate for the purpose. The stomach and duodenum are examined carefully, to determine the presence and extent of pathology in the duodenum and also the possible presence of a secondary peptic ulcer in the stomach. Examinations of the gallbladder and other abdominal organs follow in orderly sequence. If no forbidding pathology is encountered, division of the vagus nerve supply to the stomach is carried out. Two assistants are usually required, and each rib margin is elevated with a broad abdominal retractor. The omentum is gently pushed to the left and held out of the way by a large abdominal pad in the left gutter. Occasionally the omentum is attached to the spleen, and great care must be observed lest in pulling the omentum away from the spleen persistent bleeding, even requiring splenectomy, be produced.

With the upper part of the stomach cleared, the surgeon grasps the left lobe of the liver and exerts downward traction to expose the triangular ligament. It is convenient to have the first assistant divide this ligament while the surgeon exerts traction to keep it clearly in view. The ligament should be divided close to the liver to avoid the possibility of cutting one of the diaphragmatic veins. Division of the ligament is continued until the liver is freed past the esophagus and can be retracted well to the right (Fig. 1A). The margin of the ligament often bleeds a little and usually requires a clamp and ligature. The left lobe of the liver is now protected with a warm gauze pack and retracted to the right, using a spring retractor of the type frequently used in gallbladder surgery.

The surgeon next palpates the abdominal esophagus and identifies its center portion by means of the Levin tube, which extends into the stomach. With the index finger of his right hand on the Levin tube in the esophagus, he picks up the diaphragm with a rat-tooth forceps and makes a short transverse incision in the diaphragm about 2 cm. above the hiatus and approximately midway between the hiatus and the left inferior phrenic vein. This incision is conveniently made with a large pair of scissors of the type commonly employed for abdominoperineal resection of the rectum. After the short incision in the diaphragm has been made, the point of the scissors is introduced into the mediastinum, the scissors are opened, and the incision is extended for a distance of about 4 cm. This blunt opening of the diaphragm minimizes bleeding. The surgeon then introduces his index finger into the mediastinum and gently separates the wall of the esophagus and the vagi from neighboring tissues (Fig. 1B). Following this, two fingers are introduced into the mediastinum and gently passed around the esophagus, picking up all the vagus branches with the esophagus and pulling it downward through the opening in the diaphragm into the abdomen. *This maneuver is most important in that, more than anything else, it probably insures the completeness of the vagotomy.* In executing it, the surgeon must take special care not to insinuate his fingers between the large posterior vagus trunk and the esophagus and thus displace the right vagus nerve and leave it undivided. To make certain that all vagus fibers are included in the surgeon's grasp, sweeping movements within the mediastinum are made with the fingers, care being taken, however, not to perforate the pleura.

When the esophagus has been pulled downward into the abdominal cavity, the posterior vagus trunk is felt as a large cord behind the esophagus and can be gently separated by manual dissection. This procedure often includes not only the right or posterior vagus nerve, but sometimes additional branches along the posterior esophagus. With the vagus trunk held in the fingers, a Harrington clamp or similar long hemostat is placed across the right vagus at its superior margin. Previous cocainization of the nerve trunk is not necessary. The vagus trunk is now divided and a similar hemostat is placed across its distal margin. From 2 to 3 cm. of the trunk is resected and the proximal and distal ends are tied off with silk or linen ligatures. After this has been accomplished, the fingers of the right hand are again placed around the esophagus retracting it into the abdomen.

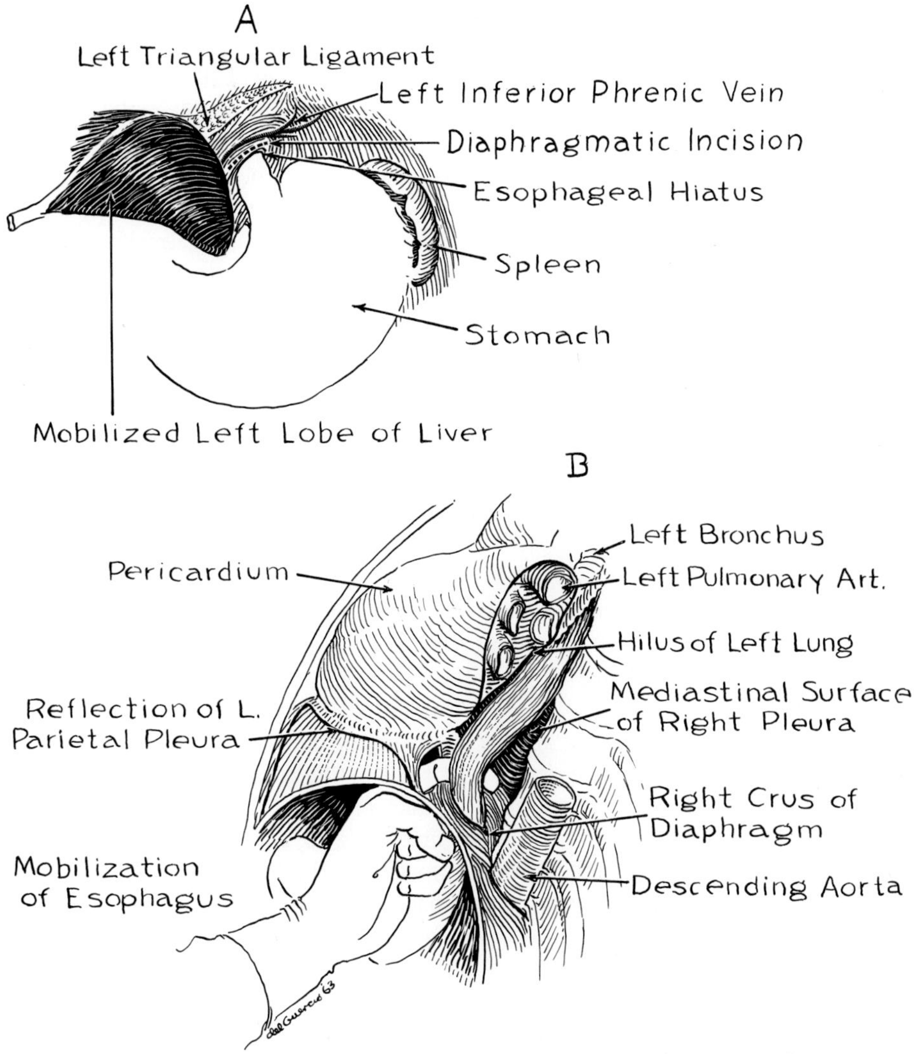

FIGURE 1. (A) The triangular ligament has been sectioned and the left lobe of the liver retracted, exposing the esophageal hiatus area. The planned diaphragmatic incision is shown as a dashed line. (*B*) Mobilization of the esophagus and vagus nerves by finger dissection through the diaphragmatic incision. The esophagus and the vagus nerves are then delivered into the abdomen.

The anterior vagus nerve and its branches are seen on the anterior wall of the esophagus or their location is indicated by a longitudinal groove. Again it is my practice to separate the anterior nerves from the esophagus by manual dissection and to excise a segment, tying off the proximal and distal ends as was done with the right vagus. After this has been accomplished, the fingers of the left hand are passed around the esophagus and it will now be found that it comes much more readily into the abdomen.

With a blunt tissue forceps, the surgeon picks off all strands of fascia or nerve fibers that can be seen or felt for a distance of 2 inches along the lower esophagus. The esophagus is rotated to facilitate clearing the posterior wall of any structure that might be a nerve fiber. Small blood vessels are frequently torn in this process, but bleeding usually stops almost immediately. Occasionally an inelastic fiber is felt within the longitudinal musculature and must be pried out and divided. When the procedure is completed, the bare longitudinal musculature of the esophagus is cleanly in view and no inelastic material is felt on palpation. By traction on the esophagus it can be determined that no vagus fibers extending to the lesser curvature of the stomach have remained undivided. After careful hemostasis, the esophagus is allowed to fall back into the mediastinum and the incision in the diaphragm is closed with three interrupted catgut sutures. The left lobe of the liver is allowed to fall back in place but no attempt is made to suture the ligament.

Drainage and Decompression

After the vagotomy has been completed, some type of drainage procedure must be carried out or the antrum resected. A pyloroplasty of the type described by Weinberg is now done, or if the findings are not favorable for this procedure, a gastroenterostomy of small size is established between the antrum of the stomach and the jejunum.

The most frequent cause of recurrent ulceration after a vagotomy and drainage procedure, in my experience, is stasis of food in the stomach. There is satisfactory evidence to indicate that prolonged contact of food with the antrum mucosa leads to continued elaboration of gastrin and thus to continued stimulation of gastric secretion. Ultimately, the buffering capacity of the food is overcome and the acidity of the gastric content begins to approach that of pure gastric juice. Stasis of food in the stomach appears not to be ulcerogenic if the antrum has previously been removed, and there is no doubt that gastric vagotomy combined with antrum resection provides the duodenal ulcer patient with his best chance to remain free of recurrent ulceration. The price for this insurance, however, is an immediate mortality which is four to eight times greater than that following gastroenterostomy or pyloroplasty. The dumping syndrome is likewise more frequent and more severe and the subsequent nutritional impairment somewhat greater. If the duodenal ulcer is large and extends to the vicinity of the common bile duct or the pancreatic ducts and if there is an inflammatory reaction with hyperemia and edema of neighboring structures and as a result closure of the duodenal stump appears hazardous, resection of the antrum had better be abandoned in favor of a posterior gastroenterostomy.

If the duodenum is markedly deformed and narrowed by scar tissue, probably a contemplated pyloroplasty should also give way to a posterior gastroenterostomy. It is not certain at present whether pyloroplasty or gastroenterostomy is the better drainage procedure. Pyloroplasty is more physiological in that it diverts the gastric content into the duodenum, which is the normal route, rather than into the jejunum, which is less prepared to receive the hypertonic gastric chyme. Recurrence of ulceration after vagotomy and pyloroplasty appears to be as low as after vagotomy and gastroenterostomy, or even lower. There is not yet sufficient evidence, however, to state that pyloroplasty provides as good drainage of the vagotomized stomach as may be secured by a gastroenterostomy with the stoma near the pylorus.

It was my custom in my early experience to decompress the stomach after operation with the indwelling nasal gastric tube that had been introduced before the operation for preliminary determinations of the nocturnal secretion. However, in recent years it has become my practice to decompress the stomach after vagotomy by means of a gastrostomy using a Foley bag and catheter. The Foley bag is inserted into the body of the stomach along the greater curvature with two infolding catgut sutures. The catheter is wrapped with omentum and led through a stab wound to the left of the incision and immediately beneath the costal margin. Complete decompression of the stomach is secured by continuous suction applied to this tube for five days after the operation. During this time, the patient is given 3000 cc. of physiological salt solution intravenously each 24 hours. The 12-hour night secretion is collected in the usual way and the acid output determined. In the usual case, the output of acid is less than 10 mEq. in a 12-hour period. If values of more than 20 mEq. are repeatedly found, it is probable that all the vagus fibers have not been divided or that an Ellison-Zollinger tumor is present. On the sixth postoperative day, the patient is permitted small amounts of liquid and this feeding is gradually increased by the addition of semisolid food. Satisfactory emptying of the stomach is determined by aspiration on the gastrostomy tube in the evening. A final determination of the night secretion is made on the eleventh postoperative day and the tube removed.

The patient is brought back for subsequent measurements of the nocturnal gastric secretion at intervals of six months, one year, and two years. If the fasting nocturnal gastric secretion still remains below 20 mEq. and if x-ray examination shows no stasis in the antrum, the patient will probably remain free of recurrent ulceration.

References

Dragstedt, L. R. The pathogenesis of duodenal ulcer. *Arch. Surg.* 44:438, March 1942.

Dragstedt, L. R., and Owens, F. M., Jr. Supra-diaphragmatic section of the vagus nerves in the treatment of duodenal ulcer. *Proc. Soc. Exper. Biol. and Med.* 53:152, June 1943.

Dragstedt, L. R. Is gastric ulcer due to hyperfunction or dysfunction of the gastric antrum? *Surg., Gynec. and Obst.* 97:517, October 1953.

Holt, R. L., and Robinson, A. F. The treatment of duodenal ulcer by vagotomy and gastrojejunostomy. *Brit. J. Surg.* 42:2, March 1955.

Palumbo, L. T., Sharpe, W. S., Lulu, D. J., Bloom, M. H., and Porter, H. R. Results in 300 cases of antrectomy with bilateral vagectomy for chronic duodenal ulcer. *Surgery* 51:289, March 1962.

77. *Transabdominal Vagus Transection*

STANLEY O. HOERR

A VERY SATISFACTORY INCISION for transabdominal vagus transection is the midline incision depicted in Figure 1. It is important to extend this incision as high as possible along the left side of the xiphoid, and it may be swung to the left of the umbilicus for added length. It is usually not necessary to excise any of the xiphoid. Surgeons closing abdominal incisions with catgut or silk may prefer to create two fascial layers by cutting through the anterior fascia over the left rectus muscle, retracting the muscle to the left and then cutting through the posterior rectus sheath. If the abdominal wall is cut directly in the midline between the rectus muscles, a closure with interrupted sutures of No. 30 stainless steel wire through fascia, muscle, and peritoneum in one layer is very satisfactory.

The Balfour self-retaining retractor shown in Figure 2 may be used to hold the wound open. After the retractor has been placed it occasionally becomes clear that the incision can be lengthened upward to advantage either in skin or fascia or in all layers.

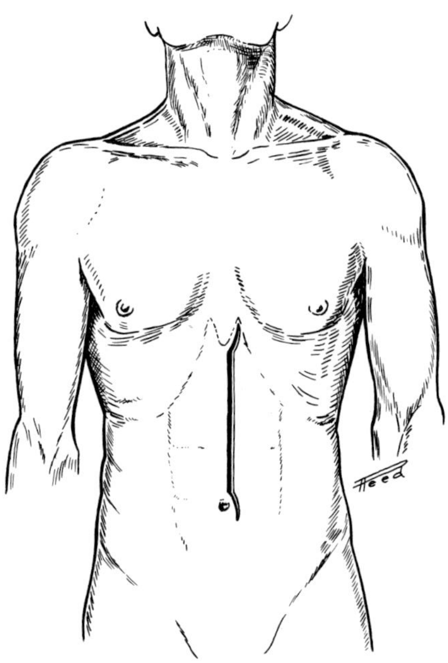

FIGURE 1. A midline incision useful for transabdominal vagus transection. It may be swung to the left of the umbilicus for added length.

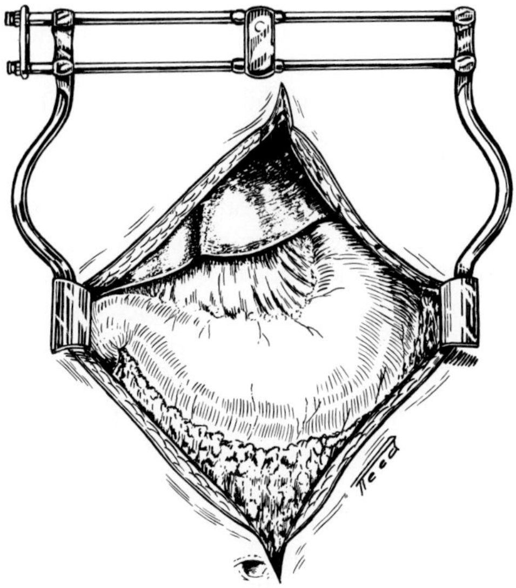

FIGURE 2. The Balfour self-retaining retractor, so useful for pelvic work, is shown positioned here. The arm of the retractor used for vertical retraction in pelvic work is not needed.

Very few special instruments (Fig. 3) are needed: a malleable ribbon retractor of suitable width, long nerve hooks, a little instrument which can be used for stripping the nerve, a long Moynihan right-angle clamp, a long curved Kelly clamp, and extra-long scissors.

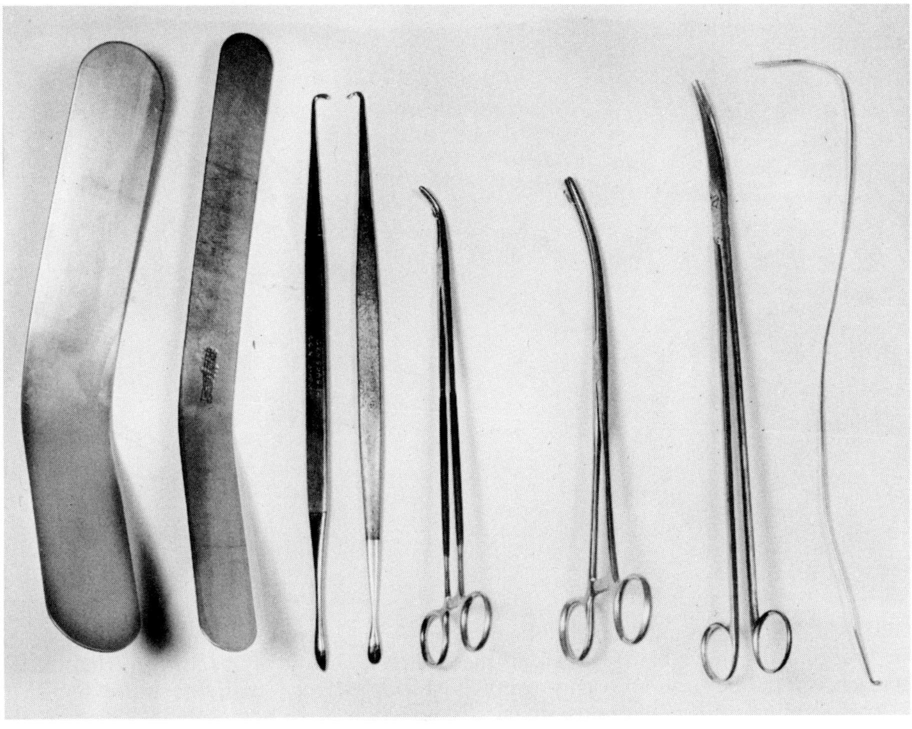

FIGURE 3. *Left to right*, two malleable retractors, two nerve hooks, extra-long Moynihan clamp, extra-long Kelly clamp, extra-long scissors, nerve stripper.

The malleable ribbon retractor, bent at the appropriate spot, is placed under the left lobe of the liver and judiciously retracted cephalad. This maneuver exposes the area near the hiatus, where the vagus nerves are to be mobilized (Fig. 4A). It is hardly ever necessary to divide the left triangular ligament if this technique is utilized. There is usually an avascular area 1 to 1½ inches long, just below the hiatus, and it is in this area that the nerve hook is used, to tear through the thin layer of peritoneum and pick up the vagus nerves. The surgeon grasps the stomach with his right hand through a gauze pack or sponge and retracts it strongly toward the left great toe of the patient, while feeling with his left index finger over the region of the esophagus. With this technique the vagus nerve stands out like a violin string and is easily palpated. With his finger on the nerve and the stomach on the stretch, the surgeon transfers the stomach to his first assistant. In Figure 4B the nerve has been picked up with a nerve hook and freed for a little distance from adventitious tissue with a second nerve hook. The nerve may then be divided by placing the specially long Moynihan clamp and then a specially long curved clamp to facilitate cutting between the two clamps (Fig. 5).

Usually it is not necessary to ligate the cut nerve ends, but occasionally a small vessel may accompany the nerve, particularly the posterior vagus. If doubt exists, it is easier to ligate than to cope with bleeding after the clamp has been removed.

The right or posterior vagus is palpated in a similar way (Fig. 6). This nerve trunk may lie a centimeter or more posterior to the esophagus when it is placed

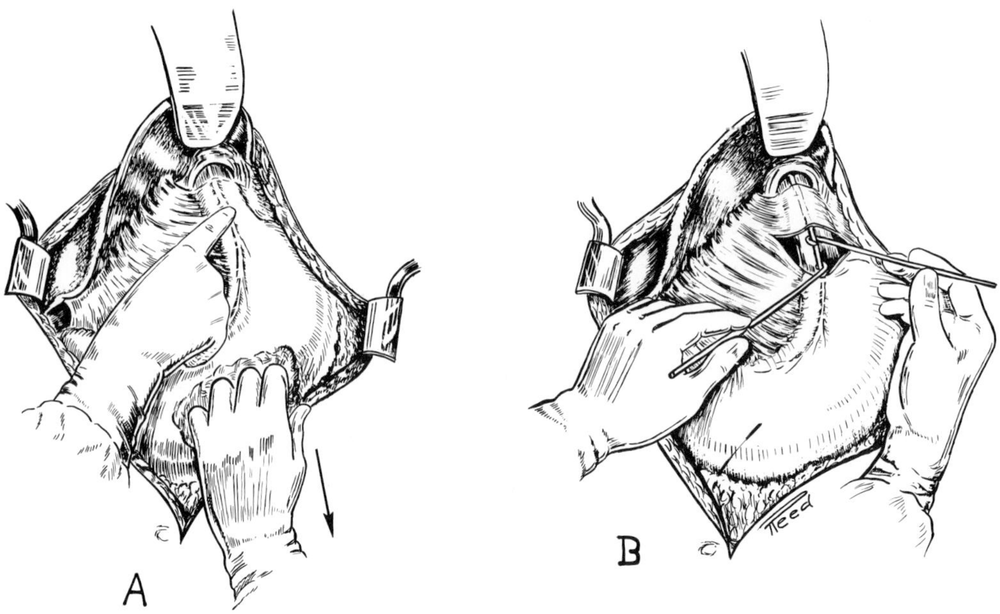

FIGURE 4. (A) A malleable ribbon retractor is shown elevating the left lobe of the liver and the nerve being placed on the stretch by cautious but firm traction on the stomach. (*B*) The anterior vagus trunk is shown elevated with the nerve hook. Its relative position at the hiatus is shown through the artist's "peephole," next to the retractor. (The nerve will normally not be seen at that level.)

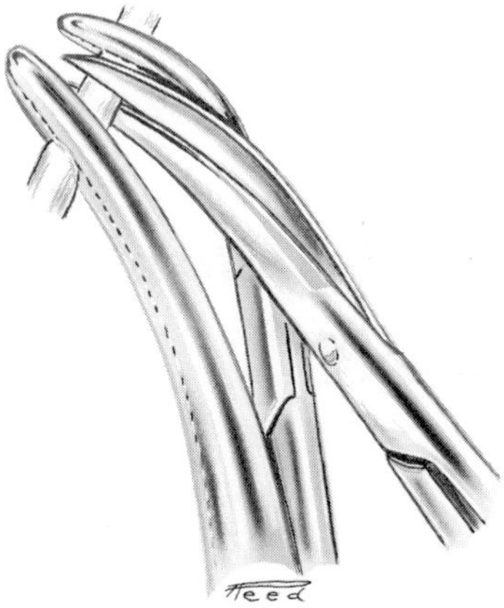

FIGURE 5. The difference in shape of the long Moynihan clamp and the long curved clamp facilitates cutting the nerve between the clamps.

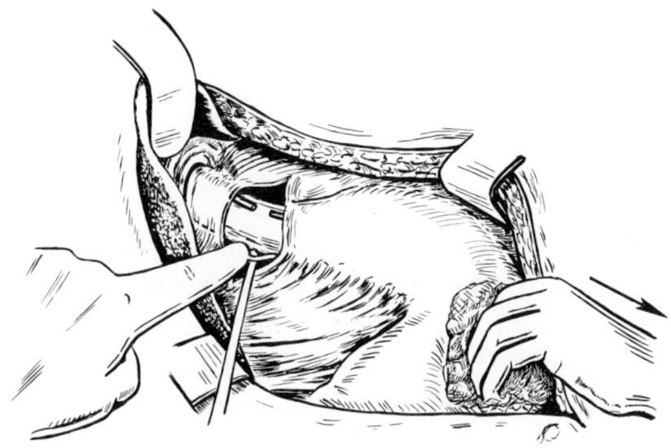

FIGURE 6. The posterior vagal trunk is shown exposed. With traction on the stomach it often lies a centimeter or more posterior to the esophagus.

on the stretch, and characteristically it crosses at a slight angle from right to left as it courses downward over the aorta.

The final maneuver is accomplished when a finger of the left hand (forefinger or middle finger) is carefully worked about the esophagus posteriorly until the esophagus is completely encircled. The surface of the esophagus is then examined for additional fibers, and a nerve hook used to rupture any suspicious ones that might be there.

78. *Selective Gastric Vagotomy, Hemigastrectomy, and Gastroduodenostomy: The "Revised Combined Operation"*

HENRY N. HARKINS AND
CHARLES A. GRIFFITH

WE PERFORM selective gastric vagotomy, hemigastrectomy, and gastroduodenostomy upon the majority of patients with duodenal ulcer who present the surgical indications of intractability or obstruction. We also perform this operation upon carefully selected patients with bleeding or perforated duodenal ulcer, but we usually perform less complicated and time-consuming procedures in such emergent circumstances. Furthermore, we have utilized this operation as described herein for a few selected cases of peptic esophagitis as an acid pepsin reducing and gastric drainage operation.

We have described in previous publications our experience with the "combined operation" of conventional total abdominal vagotomy, hemigastrectomy, and gastroduodenostomy. This clinical combination was the direct outgrowth of our previous animal experiments. Now that we have adopted clinical selective gastric vagotomy, we refer to the procedure as the "revised combined operation."

In the following account of our current technique, these three steps of selective gastric vagotomy, hemigastrectomy, and gastroduodenostomy are serially described. We believe that each of them contributes individually and in combination to the overall success of the "revised combined operation."

Selective Gastric Vagotomy

We are convinced from our recent experimental studies and our clinical observations, plus the observations of others (Jackson, 1948, 1960; Franksson, 1948; Burge et al., 1961), that many undesirable symptoms and sequelae of conventional total (truncal) abdominal vagotomy are due to vagal denervation of the biliary tract, pancreas, and bowel. In confining vagal denervation to the stomach with

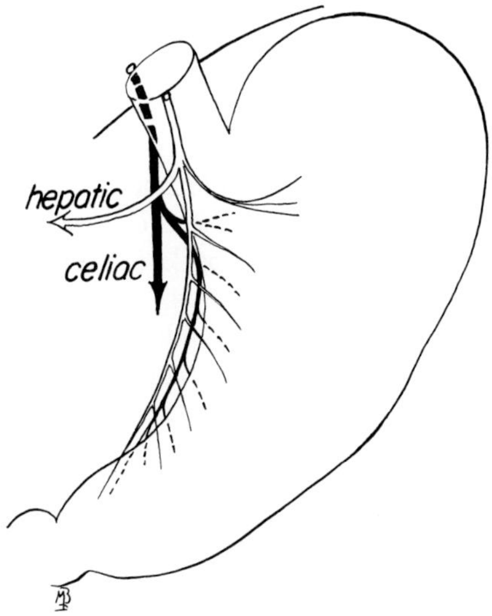

FIGURE 1. Anatomical arrangement of the anterior and posterior vagi. The anterior vagal trunk (hollow lines) divides into hepatic and anterior gastric branches of relatively equal size. The posterior trunk (dashed and solid lines) divides into a large celiac branch and a posterior gastric branch. Selective gastric vagotomy entails transecting the gastric branches and sparing the hepatic and celiac branches. The hepatic branch runs across the lesser omentum to the hepatic plexus which enmeshes the hepatic ducts and arteries. The celiac branch runs to the celiac plexus, from which its fibers reach the bowel with sympathetic fibers via the superior mesenteric artery and its branches. Exact vagal pathways to the pancreas and biliary tract have not been determined, but most evidence indicates that the hepatic and celiac branches both send fibers to these viscera. The stomach receives all its vagal innervation along the lesser curvature by individual terminal gastric branches from the vagal trunks and their primary gastric divisions. Each of these branches innervates its own localized segment of stomach. None is capable of triggering the entire glandular apparatus. Thus the physiological result of vagotomy does not obey the "all or none" phenomenon.

selective gastric vagotomy (Fig. 1) we have minimized these undesirable symptoms and sequelae in our patients. Furthermore, our experience with the selective technique has demonstrated to us repeatedly that the anatomical accuracy of the dissection required to perform selective gastric vagotomy assures complete vagotomy of the stomach. In contrast, our experience with more conventional techniques often failed to afford us anatomical proof that our vagotomy was complete.

Technique

In performing a complete gastric vagotomy, one must first meet the prime requisite of adequate access to the undersurface of the diaphragm. Poor surgical exposure not only subjects the patient to the hazards of unrecognized injury to the pleura, esophagus, spleen, vasa brevia, and esophageal vessels, but also thwarts the accomplishment of a complete gastric vagotomy. Although conventional midline and transverse incisions usually suffice, these incisions sometimes fail to afford adequate exposure in obese or muscular deep-chested patients, particularly when anesthetic relaxation and surgical assistance are less than optimum. Under these circumstances, we remove the xiphoid to increase exposure of a vertical incision. In patients of particularly difficult body habitus, the incision of Ross (1950) offers superb exposure.

Two other details of technique provide good exposure of the esophageal hiatus. (1) Care is taken not to injure the spleen or vasa brevia; the gastric fundus and spleen are cleared from the field with a pack. (2) The left hepatic lobe is held forward with a retractor designed by Weinberg especially for this purpose. This retractor has a long and wide blade with rounded edges that do not lacerate the liver. We do not routinely divide the left triangular ligament of the liver, but when we do, we do not cut it too close to the liver because of the danger of opening small outcroppings of bile canaliculi. Finally, if the ligament is cut, the left lobe must be inspected at the end of the operation to be sure it is no longer kinked on itself.

The key technical feature in the performance of selective vagotomy involves identifying the hepatic, celiac, and gastric vagal branches in their *constant* peripheral positions, and then tracing them centrally to their origins from the vagal trunks. The key to identifying the anterior vagal trunk and its hepatic and gastric branches is downward traction on the stomach. A portion of the greater curvature is freed of omentum to permit secure manual purchase on the stomach. Traction on the stomach stretches out the lesser omentum and *always* brings the hepatic branch into view. This branch is sometimes single but usually consists of three or four closely approximated parallel fibers. When present, the accessory left hepatic artery arising from the left gastric artery runs alongside the hepatic vagal branch in the lesser omentum to the porta hepatis. In thin patients the anterior gastric branch is seen in its constant position beneath the anterior peritoneal layer of the lesser omentum adjacent to the cardia and lesser curvature. One or more of its larger proximal terminal gastric branches are usually also visible. If fat hides these gastric branches in the obese patient, they can always be palpated as taut cords when they are tensed by traction on the stomach. Dissection of the gastric branches and anterior vagal trunk for selective anterior vagotomy is illustrated in Figures 2 and 3.

The posterior vagal trunk actually continues as the large celiac branch to the celiac plexus. Application of this fact is the key to foolproof identification of the posterior trunk. When conventional truncal vagotomy is performed, the operation is often incomplete; and in the incomplete operations, in most instances it is the posterior trunk which is not completely sectioned. Usually the celiac branch runs alongside the left gastric artery in the gastropancreatic peritoneal fold, but occasionally it runs closely applied to the right diaphragmatic crus and aorta. Accordingly, with traction on the stomach, the posterior trunk or its celiac continuation can always be located by palpation with a finger directed either alongside the right posterior surface of the distal esophagus and cardia or against the right crus. Dissection of the posterior vagal trunk for selective posterior vagotomy is illustrated in Figure 4.

With both vagal trunks dissected to the hiatus, and all gastric branches tran-

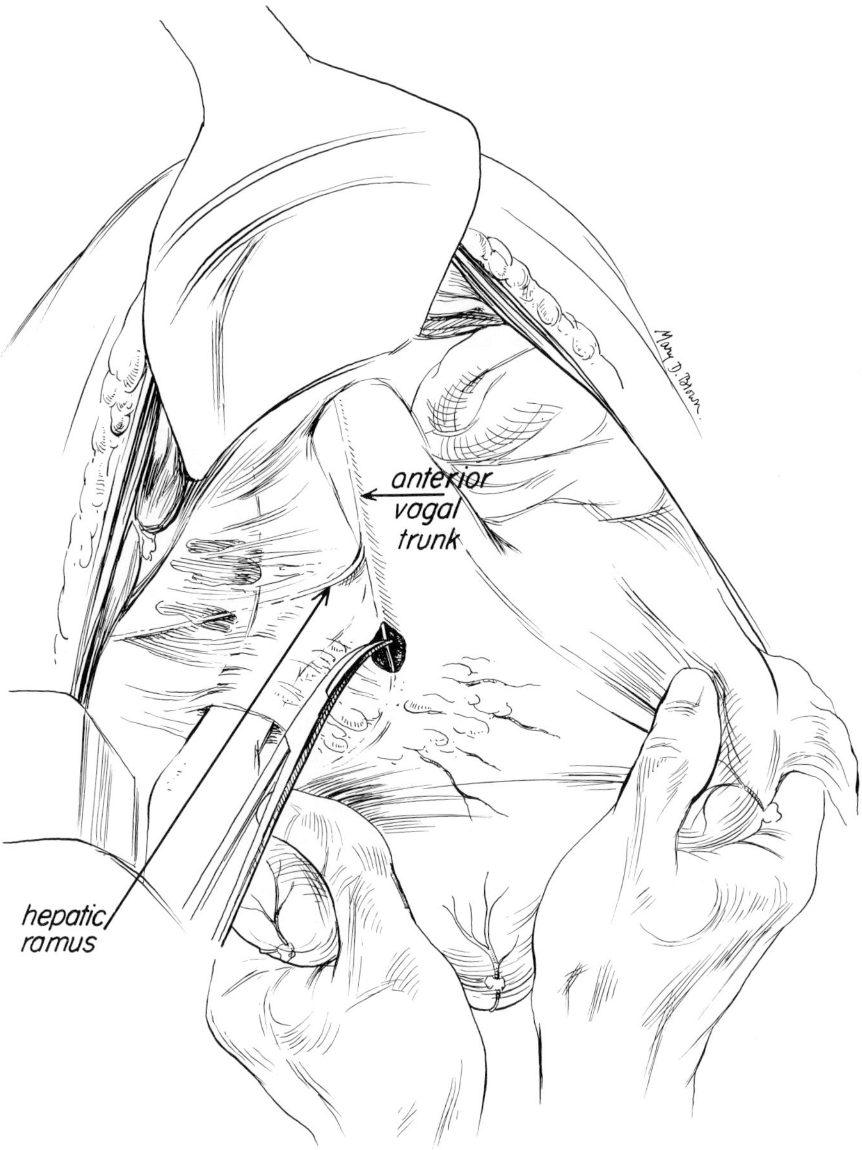

FIGURE 2. Traction exposure of the anterior vagal trunk including the large extragastric hepatic ramus and anterior gastric ramus. The main gastric division ("anterior gastric nerve of Laterjet") of the anterior vagal trunk that descends along the lesser curvature, or one of its large proximal terminal gastric branches, has been exposed in the lesser omentum and grasped with a clamp. Downward traction on this clamp tenses the anterior vagal trunk and enables foolproof identification by palpation as a taut cord up to the hiatus. A finger inserted into the lesser space through an avascular opening in the lesser omentum supplements this identification by palpation from behind. The origin of the hepatic branch is also identified by inspection or palpation. Note the midline incision, Weinberg retractor, downward traction of the stomach, and packing away of the fundus and spleen.

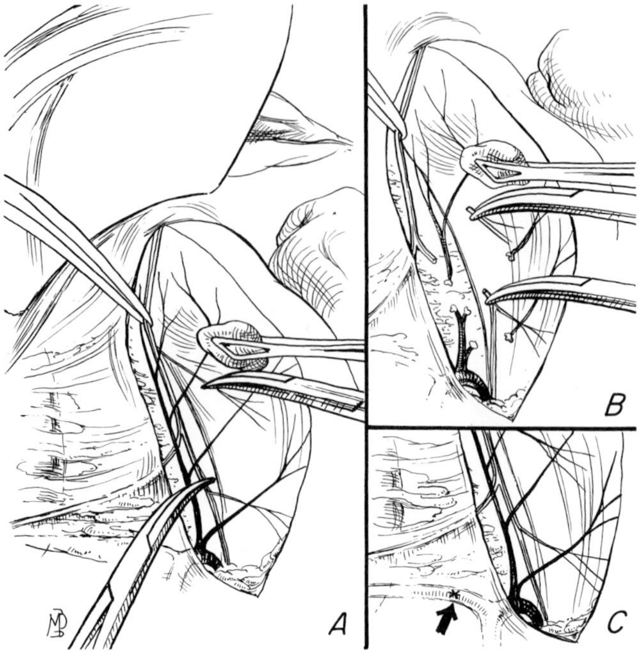

FIGURE 3. Technique of anterior selective vagotomy. (A) The peritoneum to the left of the anterior vagal trunk has been incised up to the hiatus, and the anterior vagal trunk freed from its bed and encircled with a Penrose drain. (*B*) Anterior selective vagotomy is performed by transecting the gastric division below the origin of the hepatic branch, and transecting all individual terminal gastric branches from the vagal trunk. This technique entails ligating and transecting esophageal vessels from the left gastric artery in order to separate the vagal trunk and hepatic branch completely from the esophagus and lesser curvature. (*C*) Accessory left hepatic artery from left gastric artery (* and arrow). This anomaly occurs in 10 to 18 per cent of cases.

sected below the hiatus, the only gastric vagal fibers that can possibly remain are individual terminal gastric branches that uncommonly arise from the vagal trunks or esophageal plexus above the hiatus. If present, these branches always lie to the left of the vagal trunks and run in the same fascial plane as the vagal trunks. This fascial plane is entered by insinuating a finger between the esophagus and the vagal trunks up into the mediastinum. Small branches that by palpation plunge into the esophagus innervate only the esophagus. These branches are therefore left intact in order to prevent postoperative dysphagia. But small branches that can be lifted off the esophagus and traced to the stomach are transected.

Missing one or two of these small branches may prove to be insignificant, for they each innervate only a small area of mucosa, and therefore cause only a small secretory response to insulin. But missing a main trunk results in persistence of a large secretory response that can cause recurrent ulcer. The selective technique guarantees elimination of a large secretory response by guaranteeing foolproof identification of both vagal trunks on an accurate anatomical basis. However, our goal is complete gastric vagotomy, and we therefore carefully search for and find

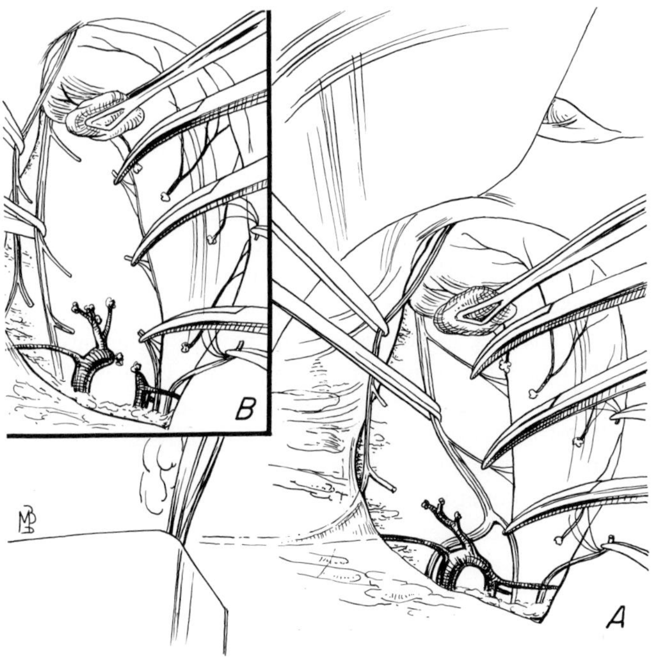

FIGURE 4. Technique of posterior selective vagotomy. (A) The posterior vagal trunk has been dissected up to the hiatus and encircled with a Penrose drain. Palpating or visualizing its continuation to the celiac plexus verifies identification of the posterior trunk. (*B*) All gastric vagal fibers are transected below the hiatus. The posterior trunk is completely separated from the esophagus and lesser curvature by ligating and transecting esophageal vessels. The left gastric artery is transected just distal to its hairpin turn adjacent to the lesser curvature. The level of gastric resection on the lesser curvature is at or just proximal to this point. The operative field now reveals intact anterior and posterior vagal trunks and their hepatic and celiac branches. The cardia and proximal lesser curvature are free of all omental attachments and nerves and vessels. This devascularization does not threaten viability of the gastric remnant, which receives adequate circulation via the vasa brevia and left gastroepiploic vessels.

small gastric branches that occasionally originate above the hiatus and may provide a source of vagal reinnervation of the stomach by sprouting. We believe that with the technique of selective gastric vagotomy we use, there is definitely less chance of an incomplete gastric vagotomy than with the standard truncal or total abdominal vagotomy. In addition, the selective technique does not unnecessarily vagotomize the other important organs in the abdomen, as discussed above.

Hemigastrectomy

Initial studies by Farmer and his co-workers in 1951 showed that vagotomy plus hemigastrectomy reduces gastric acidity more effectively than any other procedure. The clinical significance of this finding is the fact that vagotomy plus hemigastrectomy enjoys the lowest rate of recurrent ulcer of all procedures. Hemigastrectomy supplements an incomplete vagotomy, and vagotomy supplements inadequate resection.

The purpose of our "hemigastrectomy" is to perform a complete "antrectomy." We realize that the *average* antrum (i.e. the area of the pyloric glands) *usually* comprises no more than 25 per cent of the area of the stomach. However, as has been pointed out by Oi (1962) and will be discussed later in this chapter, this extent has considerable variations. Hence, to insure a complete antrectomy we perform a hemigastrectomy. Furthermore, as is also pointed out later, we take cognizance of the usual shape of the antrum as well as its overall size.

Since adopting selective gastric vagotomy, we are certain we have lowered, if not eliminated, our incidence of incomplete vagotomy. In view of this fact, plus the fact that with only a drainage procedure the incidence of recurrent ulcer is negligible when vagotomy is complete, we have carefully evaluated the controversy of hemigastrectomy versus pyloroplasty. Although we are becoming more impressed with the merits of pyloroplasty with suture ligation in the presence of massive hemorrhage from duodenal ulcer, and pyloroplasty after excision of *chronic* duodenal ulcer with acute perforation (simple closure of the *acute* duodenal ulcer with perforation), we still prefer hemigastrectomy for intractable and obstructing duodenal ulcer, for the following reasons.

1. Hemigastrectomy prevents the development of a flaccid dilated gastric sac and eliminates the symptoms and complications (recurrent ulcer) of gastric stasis more effectively and more consistently than pyloroplasty or gastrojejunostomy. This advantage is particularly manifest in patients with fishhook stomachs. Furthermore, the amount of stomach removed by hemigastrectomy does not embarrass the function of the stomach as a reservoir and does not appreciably increase the incidence or severity of dumping.

2. Vagotomy continues to receive criticism because of failure due to subsequent vagal reinnervation of the stomach. However, hemigastrectomy by a high resection of the lesser curvature (Schoemaker-like line of resection as opposed to Polya or Hofmeister) eliminates the possibility of vagal reinnervation by removing the distal vagal fibers on the stomach. Vagal reinnervation cannot occur if the distal nerve sheaths are not accessible to proximal regenerating or sprouting vagal fibers.

3. Vagotomy has been criticized because of the possibility of residual parasympathetic innervation by extravagal parasympathetic fibers carried to the stomach by sympathetic nerves. We doubt the validity of this criticism. Nevertheless, extravagal parasympathetic fibers may exist in the splanchnic nerves as the result of either (1) communications between the vagus nerves and sympathetic chains in the neck and thorax, or (2) separate origins of parasympathetic fibers in dorsal thoracic nerve roots (Kure, 1931). However, hemigastrectomy removes these extravagal parasympathetics because they reach only the antrum and not the acid-pepsin secreting corpus and fundus. The gastric remnant following hemigastrectomy is actually a liberal, permanent, well-drained Heidenhain pouch in continuity. This pouch neither ulcerates itself nor causes stomal ulcer.

Technique

To insure complete excision of the antrum, we must heed the distal and proximal extents of the antrum, which cannot be determined by gross external examination. The vast majority of duodenal ulcers occur at or just a centimeter or two beyond the *mucosal* gastroduodenal boundary. This boundary usually lies within the pyloric sphincter, but may occur either immediately proximal or distal to it. Accordingly, leaving a duodenal ulcer in situ means leaving some antrum in those patients whose duodenal ulcer is at a mucosal gastroduodenal boundary *distal* to the pylorus. We therefore remove the ulcer by the technique described by Strauss (1951), who has taught us how to remove a posterior penetrating ulcer quickly, safely, and easily (Fig. 5). We attach tremendous importance to the Strauss maneuver, which in

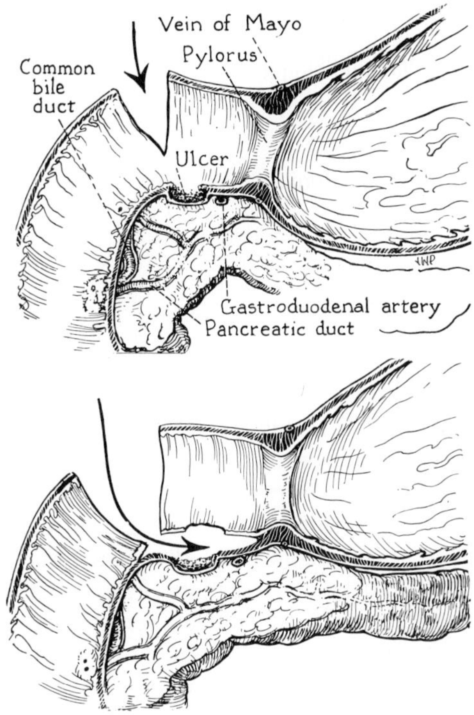

FIGURE 5. Strauss maneuver. The anterior wall of the duodenum is opened just distal to the ulcer. The mucosa of the posterior wall is incised just distal to the ulcer, and then the proximal mucosa is peeled off scar tissue and thickened pancreatic capsule in a distal-to-proximal direction, leaving the ulcer bed in situ. When the ulcer has not penetrated into the pancreas, but the duodenum is merely adherent to the pancreas, the posterior mucosa and duodenal muscularis are peeled from the pancreas. This technique eliminates the tedious and bloody dissection of conventional techniques that remove the duodenum from the pancreas in the proximal-to-distal direction in an attempt to avoid entering the duodenal lumen. Performing the Kocher maneuver first (Fig. 8) facilitates transection of the duodenum by the Strauss maneuver. (From Harkins, H. N., and Nyhus, L. M., *Surgery of the Stomach and Duodenum*. Boston: Little Brown, 1962. P. 690.)

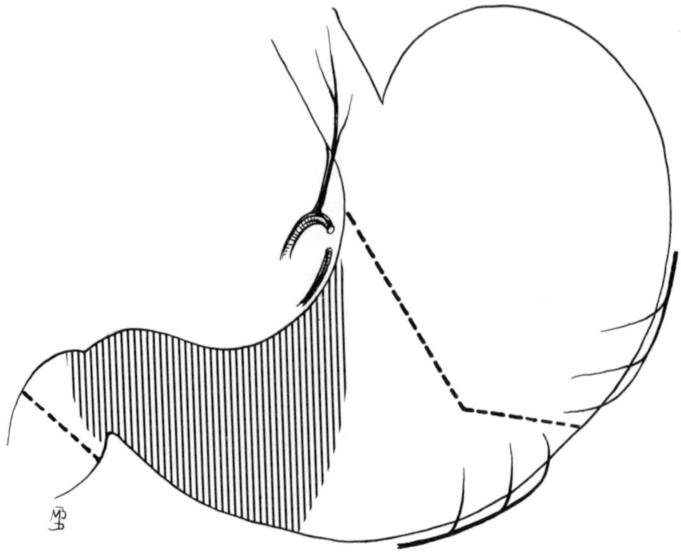

FIGURE 6. Transection of the stomach and of the duodenum for hemigastrectomy. The greater curvature is transected where the right and left gastroepiploic vessels anastomose. The line of resection is then angled up to the lesser curvature at or above the level of the hairpin turn of the left gastric artery (or where this artery bifurcates into its ascending esophageal and descending gastric branches). This level is often within two or three centimeters (or less) of the esophagus. This resection averages approximately 50 per cent, and always removes the antrum (*shaded area*) plus a small cuff of the acid-pepsin secreting glands.

our hands has made the previously difficult duodenum easy. Only rarely will this technique fail to permit safe removal of the ulcer.

The proximal extent of the antrum varies, but usually the antrum extends much higher on the lesser curvature than on the greater curvature. We therefore resect the lesser curvature much higher than the greater curvature. Vascular landmarks (Payne, 1962) guide our line of resection (Figs. 6 and 7).

We use the von Petz clamp to control hemorrhage and close the lesser curvature portion of the gastric remnant. But this clamp is expensive and not generally available. If a Payr clamp is used, we remove it carefully in an attempt to keep the opposed crushed edges together. The crushed edges are then grasped with many Allis clamps and oversewn with catgut for hemostasis. On some occasions we individually clamp and ligate the vessels of the submucosal plexus by a technique described in the next section. But this method is time-consuming. Banzet's noncrushing clamp, or Rienhoff's modification of it,* is an excellent instrument to control hemostasis and hold the stomach for its suturing.

We bury the von Petz clips or the catgut suture with a row of interrupted silk sutures in the seromuscular layer. These sutures are carried on up the remaining two or three centimeters of lesser curvature to the cardia in order to bury any distal vagal fibers and make them inaccessible to proximal sprouting fibers.

* Made by Pilling & Son, Company, Philadelphia, Pennsylvania.

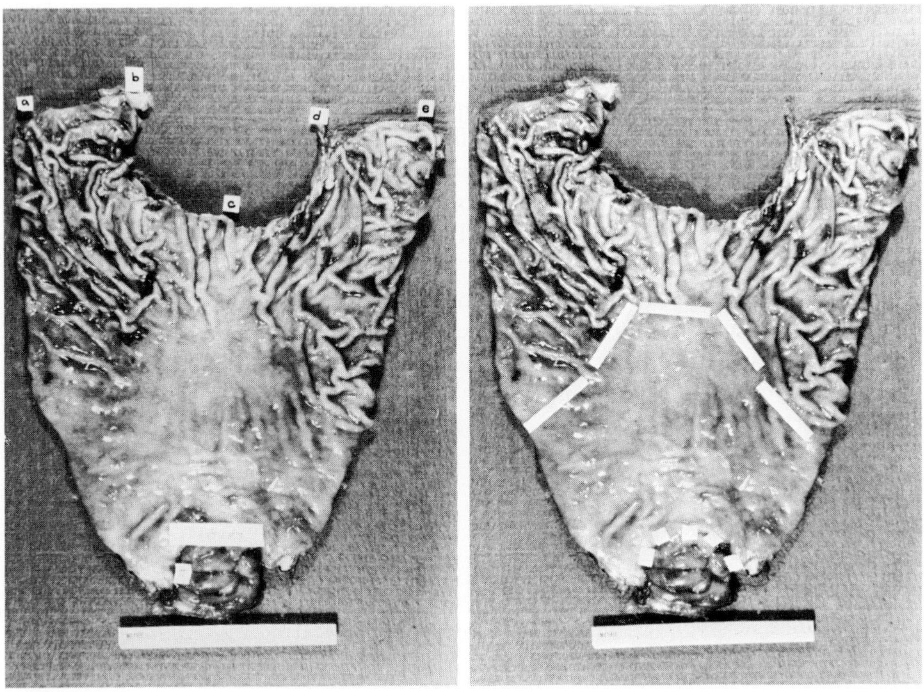

A B

FIGURE 7. Typical specimen excised according to the line of resection in Figure 6 and showing the extent of the antrum. (*A*) The boundary between the acid-pepsin secreting glands of the corpus above and pyloric glands of the antrum below occurs where the rugal folds flatten out distally. Sections taken in the longitudinal axis through this landmark reveal that the microscopic border between corpus and antrum is usually less than one centimeter wide. The specimen has been opened along the greater curvature and is seen on its mucosal surface. The five markers at the top of the figure represent (*a*) the greater curvature, (*b*) the angle of junction on the anterior wall of the horizontal section and ascending (Schoemaker) section, (*c*) the lesser curvature, (*d*) the angle as in *b* on the posterior wall, and (*e*) the greater curvature. (*B*) The white rectangles in the middle of the specimen further identify the boundary between the corpus above and the antrum below. The smaller white squares at the bottom outline the pylorus. A cuff of duodenum below this has been resected as is usual by our technique.

If the esophageal hiatus is lax, the crura posterior to the esophagus are approximated with one or two sutures. In addition, we fix the esophagus and cardia to the right crus with three or four silk sutures to prevent hiatus hernia.

Gastroduodenostomy

We perform gastroduodenostomy because, in our experience with gastric resection, our rate of recurrent ulcer was lower with the Billroth I than with the Billroth II. Certain authors have reported a higher incidence of stomal ulceration following resection with restoration of continuity *ad modum* Billroth I as opposed to Billroth II. However, we are convinced that a number of technical factors (some of these are discussed below) explain the difference. Of these factors, we believe that relative extent of resection is the most important. We know of no published report of a high incidence of stomal ulceration following the Billroth I technique of subtotal gastrectomy in which a *quantitation of the extent of resection is recorded.* Since the present chapter does not recommend the Billroth I—or II—operation without vagotomy for duodenal ulcer, this matter is largely academic, but we believe it is pertinent to our discussion because we do incorporate this type of anastomosis as one of the three ingredients in our combined operations.

Furthermore, we have found that gastroduodenostomy can be performed more easily and quickly than gastrojejunostomy. Lastly, gastroduodenostomy eliminates the complications of gastrojejunostomy. We are convinced that the following technical details account for our success with gastroduodenostomy.

Technique

Performing the Kocher maneuver (Fig. 8) affords two advantages. First, in the initial stages of the operation, mobilizing the duodenum and bringing it into the wound makes a much easier and quicker task of ligating the right gastric and gastroepiploic vessels and transecting the duodenum. Second, the Kocher maneuver allows the gastroduodenostomy to lie comfortably without tension near the midline or often to the *left* of the midline.

In transecting the duodenum by the Strauss maneuver distal to a posterior ulcer penetrating the pancreas, the gastroduodenal artery, or its superior pancreaticoduodenal branch, is usually exposed in its course between the duodenum and the head of the pancreas. This landmark signifies that the accessory duct of Santorini, if present, is not too far beyond. We therefore do not dissect the posterior wall of the duodenum distal to the ulcer in the pancreas. If the ulcer is anterior, we still remove the proximal duodenum as far as the head of the pancreas so that the anastomosis is close to the outlets of neutralizing pancreatic juice and bile. This technical detail may be quite important in view of the experimental work of Salmon and his coworkers in 1959, who suggested that gastroduodenostomy spatially removed from the minor and major duodenal papillae may not allow adequate buffering of gastric content in between the stoma and duodenal papillae. We also consider important the fact that the gastroduodenostomy is constructed in the area of maximum concentration of Brunner's glands, which secrete mucus that accounts for an intrinsic greater resistance of the duodenum than of the jejunum to ulcer.

We perform the anastomosis by a meticulous open technique learned from Banzet (1952). Surgically considered, the stomach and duodenum (and the esophagus, small intestine, colon, and rectum) have two distinct layers, an outer muscular and an inner mucosal. In preparing for anastomosis, the muscle is cut cleanly with a knife as a single avascular layer. The muscle retracts and exposes the submucosal vessels, which are next individually clamped, cut, and ligated. The submucosa and mucosa are then incised as the second layer. Anatomical anas-

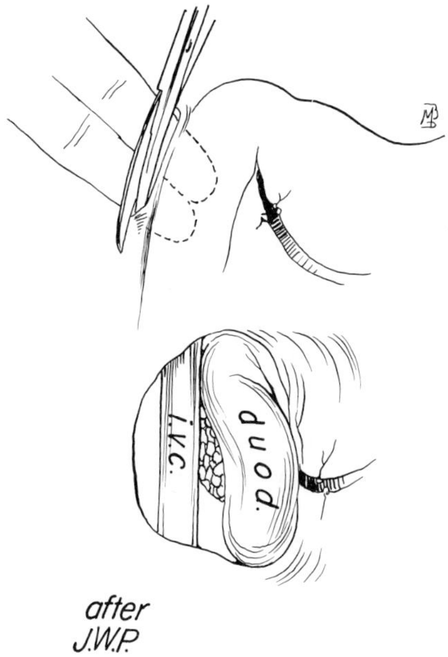

FIGURE 8. Kocher maneuver. This important maneuver restores embryological mobility of the duodenum and head of the pancreas, which it sweeps off the retroperitoneal areolar tissue medially to the midline. The inferior vena cava is always completely exposed, and sometimes the right aspect of the aorta. This technique often requires separating the duodenum from the hepatic flexure of the colon. In many instances, the anterior fold of the hepatoduodenal ligament, which contains the right gastric and supraduodenal vessels, is foreshortened and indurated by periduodenal inflammation, and adherent to the posterior fold of hepatoduodenal ligament containing the common duct, hepatic artery, and portal vein. In addition to ligating and transecting the right gastric and supraduodenal vessels, the anterior fold of hepatoduodenal ligament must be completely transected and peeled from the posterior fold in order to swing the duodenum medially for proper gastroduodenostomy without tension.

tomosis is performed with running 3–0 or 4–0 chromic catgut *to the mucosal* layers only. Interrupted 4–0 silk sutures unite the muscle layers *end-on with no inversion.* In instances of penetrating posterior ulcer, the posterior row of sutures is taken through the fibrous ulcer bed and pancreatic capsule. The stoma always admits the thumb tip with ease.

Since our adoption of this technique of anastomosis, our incidence of stomal obstruction has been negligible. We have never had to use any medications such as Urecholine to stimulate gastric contraction and promote gastric emptying. We do not perform the anastomosis with the idea of deliberately constructing a small stoma to prevent dumping. Dumping occurs in a few of our patients, but its severity and incidence are minimal compared with previous experience with both Billroth I and II "subtotal" gastric resections.

To sum up, proper performance of the Strauss maneuver, the Kocher maneuver, and the Banzet suture technique results in a stoma that is (1) close to the outlets of pancreatic juice and bile, (2) in the area of maximum concentration of Brunner's glands, (3) of ample circumference and not obstructing, and (4) under no tension. We consider these four points to be absolute requirements of gastroduodenostomy. Failure to meet these requirements may result in recurrent ulcers, many of which are not stomal ulcers in the true sense, but are gastric ulcers secondary to partial obstruction by a constricting anastomosis under tension. If recurrent ulcer results from incorrect application of the Billroth I technique, the patient would have been better served by a gastrojejunostomy.

Summary

Our current operation of choice for duodenal ulcer is the "revised combined" procedure of selective gastric vagotomy, hemigastrectomy, and gastroduodenostomy. Each of these three steps was investigated in our experimental laboratories prior to clinical application. From this experience we believe that each has its own merits, and that each supplements the other.

By *selective gastric vagotomy,* we eliminate the cephalic or nervous phase of gastric secretion. This technique provides us maximum anatomical assurance at the time of operation that vagotomy of the stomach is complete. At the same time, this technique also avoids undesirable sequelae of vagotomy of other abdominal viscera.

By *hemigastrectomy* we accomplish a complete antrectomy and eliminate the gastric or hormonal phase of gastric secretion. Our technique of hemigastrectomy provides us anatomical assurance of complete excision of the gastrin-secreting pyloric glands plus a small cuff of acid-pepsin secreting gastric glands.

By *gastroduodenostomy* we restore normal gastroduodenal continuity with its attendant physiological and technical advantages.

Our results to date with the "revised combined operation" described in this chapter satisfy us that this operation, particularly for duodenal ulcer, provides maximum protection against recurrent ulcer and minimizes undesirable secondary sequelae.

References

Burge, H. W., Rizk, A. R., Tompkin, A. M. B., Barth, C. E., Hutchinson, J. S. E., Longbeach, C. J., McLennan, I., and Miln, D. C. Selective vagotomy in the prevention of post-vagotomy diarrhea. *Lancet* 2:897, October 21, 1961.

Franksson, C. Selective abdominal vagotomy. *Acta chir. scandinav.* 96:409, April 30, 1948; *Nord. med.* 39:1473, 1948 (discussion of paper presented at meeting of Svensk kirurgisk förening, October 24, 1947).

Franksson, C. Personal communication, 1960.

Griffith, C. A. Selective gastric vagotomy. In Harkins, H. N., and Nyhus, L. M., *Surgery of the Stomach and Duodenum.* Boston: Little, Brown, 1962. Ch. 10B7.

Harkins, H. N., and Nyhus, L. M. Personal operative technique for the surgical treatment of duodenal ulcer. In *Surgery of the Stomach and Duodenum.* Boston: Little, Brown, 1962. Appendix A.

Jackson, R. G. Anatomic study of the vagus nerves, with a technique of transabdominal selective vagus resection. *Arch. Surg.* 57:333, August 1948.

Jackson, R. G. Personal communication, 1960.

79. *Billroth I Operation*

NORMAN C. TANNER

THE BILLROTH I OPERATION, also known as the Rydygier or Péan operation, entails a reconstruction by gastroduodenal anastomosis, following resection of part of the stomach and duodenum ("lower partial gastrectomy"). In this reconstruction, part or all of the cut end of the stomach is used to form the stoma. It is usually joined to the divided end of the duodenum; however, the duodenum may be closed and the gastric remnant anastomosed to the side or anterior wall of the duodenum. (This variant is most commonly employed in converting a gastrojejunal —Polya, Reichel, Billroth II—gastrectomy into a Billroth I form.)

This method of reconstruction may be used following the resection of a gastric, duodenal, or stomal ulcer, or of a simple or malignant tumor, or following gastrectomy for a nonmalignant lesion of the stomach, e.g. tuberculosis or corrosive stricture.

In considering the desirability or the inexpediency of using this reconstruction, we must review its physiological effects and clinical results as compared with those of the alternative procedure, the Billroth II or Polya operation.

Physiological Effects and Clinical Results of the Billroth I Operation

It is self-evident that the Billroth I operation simulates the normal anatomy and interferes less with the normal physiology than does the Billroth II operation. The food and gastric chyme meet the biliary, duodenal, and pancreatic juices immediately after leaving the stomach, as is normally the case. There is no long side loop with potentialities for producing "blind loop" effects as in the Billroth II. Gastric emptying is usually a little slower than in the Billroth II. However, let there be no mistake: although a Billroth I operation on its completion closely resembles a normal stomach of reduced dimensions, its physiology is much disturbed. The gastric antrum with its internal and external secretion is gone. The pylorus and the control of gastric emptying are gone. All forms of gastrectomy lead to a diminished digestive efficiency and increased excretion of fat, iron, and other foodstuffs. After all, in ulcer cases, one of the objects of the operation is to reduce the digestive efficiency in order to mitigate the recurrent autodigestion of the ulcer site.

This changed physiology is reflected in the clinical results of the Billroth I operation. Early postcibal or "dumping" symptoms of "fullness," palpitations, sweating, heat, or fatigue may be experienced. Later postcibal effects, similar to the symptoms of hypoglycemia, may be noted. Indeed, these are no less common than after the Billroth II operation. The incidence of these effects was compared in a late follow-up of 600 of my gastrectomy cases. From that study alone it appeared that early postcibal symptoms were a more severe problem after Billroth I than after Billroth II. There are other considerations, however.

The first is that in the majority of cases early postcibal symptoms are only a temporary disability, occurring in the early months after any form of gastrectomy. Though frequent, they tend to become less severe after the Billroth I procedure. The second consideration is that the most troublesome postcibal symptom is bilious vomiting and this is much more rare and much less severe after the Billroth I operation. Another point is that the ability to take certain foodstuffs, notably milk and eggs, is interfered with least of all by the Billroth I procedure, although the patient may complain that his taste for these articles is reduced by either kind of gastrectomy or, alternatively, that if he does take them he suffers discomfort and the milk or egg "will not digest."

As a result of the inability to take egg and milk, together with the increased excretion of undigested foodstuff, the patient may lose weight. The greatest factor in producing weight loss, however, is the degree of discomfort, particularly bloating, nausea, or bilious vomiting, which may occur after meals. This weight loss is less marked after the Billroth I operation than after the Billroth II.

After gastrectomy there is at times intermittent postprandial diarrhea, usually of a mild nature, which may continue for several years. This is less common with the gastroduodenal anastomosis.

The incidence of postoperative peptic ulceration differs according to the type of gastrectomy as well as according to the condition for which it was performed. After the Billroth I operation, stomal ulceration is commoner than after the Billroth II. This is probably the penalty of reproducing a too near to normal physiology. Even pure duodenal ulceration may occur, or recur, after Billroth I, though this is of the greatest rarity, if it occurs at all, after the Polya operation. True *gastric* ulceration may occur after the Billroth I operation, and this is something which I believe never occurs after the Billroth II operation, despite the fact that radiologists occasionally report it.

Technical Considerations

The Billroth I operation, the first form of gastrectomy to be carried out successfully, is simpler in design than the Billroth II reconstruction, and in most cases is a simpler procedure to perform. Approximation of the two cut surfaces is nearly always possible without difficulty. Indeed, it is possible in many cases to remove the whole stomach and make an esophagoduodenal anastomosis, although this does not produce a very satisfactory clinical result, because of the bilious regurgitation which occurs freely into the gullet after removal of the cardia mechanism. Technical difficulties may arise, however, in dealing with certain pathological conditions, which make the Billroth I operation less expedient, though rarely impossible.

Gastric Ulcer

Almost all forms of gastric ulcer, even those close to the cardia or those on the posterior gastric wall, may be dealt with by appropriate modification of the Billroth I operation.

Duodenal Ulcer

With mild duodenal ulceration or scarring confined to the proximal part of the bulb, the Billroth I operation can be combined with resection of the ulcer without technical difficulty. Because of the greater risk of stomal ulceration, there is much to be said for adding a vagotomy in such cases. Although this slightly increases the surgical risk and adds the chance of postvagotomy complications, these risks and side effects are not severe in practice. If a vagotomy is added, there is the advantage that a lower gastrectomy, as little as a 25 to 35 per cent resection, may be needed.

With penetrating postbulbar or distal bulbar ulceration, considerably more difficult duodenal dissection is required in order to obtain sufficient healthy duodenum for safe approximation to the stomach. In such cases the advantages of the Billroth I over the operation of closing the duodenum and performing a gastrojejunal anastomosis are not so great as to justify the greater technical demands and the increased risk of stomal ulceration. Resection of the rare ulcer of the second part of the duodenum is hazardous and unjustifiable, and the Billroth I operation should be regarded as the least desirable operation for such ulcers.

Gastric Tumors

If partial gastrectomy is required for the removal of a simple gastric tumor, the Billroth I operation is usually the best reconstruction to follow it.

For malignant tumors of the lower stomach, the subpyloric and suprapyloric lymph nodes must be carefully removed. This involves removal of the attendant blood vessels; hence, the devascularized first part of the duodenum should also be removed for safety. This renders gastroduodenal anastomosis less satisfactory than careful closure of the duodenal stump followed by high gastrojejunal anastomosis. In addition, recurrent tumor is prone to occur in the region of the pancreatic head and it may invade a gastroduodenal stoma and cause late recurrent obstruction, an event which reduces the palliative value of the Billroth I gastrectomy for cancer.

For cancer of the midstomach, a total gastrectomy is usually required and, as already indicated, esophagoduodenal anastomosis is possible but often an unhappy one for the patient's comfort.

In cases of upper gastric cancer a length of esophagus should be excised. For this reason the Billroth I operation is not feasible.

Indications for the Billroth I Operation

Bearing in mind these physiological, clinical, and technical considerations, we can summarize, though rather dogmatically, as follows:

The Billroth I operation is satisfactory for almost all forms of gastric ulcer, both technically and on account of the lessened risk of stomal ulceration after gastric ulcer resection.

The Billroth I operation may be used in cases of mild ulceration or scarring of the proximal duodenum. Because of the higher risk of stomal ulceration attendant on the Billroth I operation and on operations for duodenal ulceration, such resection must be high in the stomach *or* combined with a vagotomy. The Billroth I operation is not the best procedure in cases of severe distal bulbar or postbulbar ulceration and is absolutely contraindicated in ulcer of the second or descending part of the duodenum.

The Billroth I operation may be used for postgastrojejunostomy stomal ulceration provided that the duodenal scarring is slight, but it entails a higher risk of further stomal ulceration than does the Billroth II operation unless a vagotomy is added.

Because acutely perforated gastric or duodenal ulcers are often associated with anterior rather than posterior lesions, and because the most simple and expeditious operation is called for in such cases, a Billroth I operation is usually satisfactory if gastrectomy is judged to be desirable. This is not the case, however, if a difficult duodenal stump is encountered.

The most expeditious and usually the best operation for bleeding gastric ulcer is the Billroth I operation. For bleeding duodenal ulcer the Billroth II is usually the better procedure.

The Billroth I operation is satisfactory for most simple tumors of the stomach.

The Billroth I operation is but rarely indicated for malignant gastric lesions. It may occasionally be indicated for restricted lesions of the lower greater curvature, for ulcer cancers with local invasion only, and for certain leiomyosarcomas, particularly in poor risk or aged patients.

The Billroth I operation is the most satisfactory procedure in certain nonulcerative conditions, e.g. inflammatory lesions, strictures, or rarely for severe acute or recurrent volvulus.

Technique

The Approach

The Billroth I operation can be carried out through any of the standard upper abdominal incisions. If the patient is having his second or third upper abdominal operation, it is desirable, whenever possible, to use one of the old scars again, although in such a case a direct incision through all layers, rather than a muscle-displacing one, should be used. To make the successive incisions in different parts of the upper abdomen increases the extent of peritoneal adhesion and thereby the difficulty of subsequent surgery, and is a most depressing sight for the patient.

A left or right paramedian or median epigastric incision is satisfactory and is the most commonly used. In subjects with a wide subcostal angle, a high transverse incision gives good access and leaves a strong scar.

Occasionally, if there is a high ulcer in an obese patient with a wide subcostal angle, an upward extension from the middle of a transverse incision, making it T-shaped, and temporary suturing of the two right-angled flaps so produced onto the chest wall will give excellent visualization of the stomach and the upper abdominal viscera.

Further help toward visualizing and mobilizing a high ulcer may be obtained by dividing the avascular left triangular ligament of the liver, and then with a retractor drawing the left lobe of the liver downward to the right. More light can be directed to the cardia region by removing the xiphoid process after dividing the costoxiphoid ligaments and the diaphragmatic slips running to it.

Preliminary Exploration

Before any step is taken to mobilize the stomach, careful palpation and, where possible, inspection of the other abdominal viscera are carried out. It will be disconcerting to remove part of the stomach, even though it contains an ulcer, only to discover a neoplasm of the pancreas, colon, or kidney. The state of the esophageal hiatus in the diaphragm is estimated, and palpation of the gallbladder and bile ducts must be included in this examination.

The gastric condition must then be examined in detail and the extent of the operation planned. One must be certain that there is no posterior duodenal ulcer beyond the level of the proposed duodenal transection and that the distal duodenum is unobstructed and free of tumor. The fundus and parts of the stomach to be retained must be confirmed to be free of ulcer, scar, or tumor. Sometimes the ulcer or scar will be found to involve the posterior wall rather than the lesser curvature, or the upper margin of the ulcer may be as high as the cardiac orifice. Either of these variants can be dealt with by a Billroth I resection.

In many cases, particularly of duodenal or marginal ulceration, it will be decided to add a vagotomy to a Billroth I gastrectomy. My practice at present is to use a selective vagotomy, preserving both the hepatic and the celiac nerves. If this procedure is to be employed, it is desirable to carry out the vagotomy and repair the phrenoesophageal ligaments before proceeding to the partial gastrectomy.

Mobilization of the Stomach and Duodenum

The first stage of the operation is to free the part to be removed, together with the adjacent duodenum and stomach. The greater omentum and middle transverse colon are drawn out of the incision. An opening is made into the lesser sac wall to the left of the gastrocolic ligament. The gastrocolic ligament is divided from left to right by underrunning the epiploic branches of the gastroepiploic vascular arch one by one and dividing them between ligatures. In a slim subject the vessels are clearly seen; in the obese a finger must palpate the colon to prevent accidental ligation of part of its wall. Toward the right half of the gastrocolic ligament it will be found that there are adhesions between the mesocolon and the posterior wall of the pyloric antrum, in such a way that the middle colic artery and the right gastroepiploic vessels come into very close apposition (Fig. 1). These adhesions can be separated in an avascular plane, and the two vessels widely separated, by gently brushing them downward from behind the lesser curvature of the antrum. When they are well separated, the ligation and division of the gastrocolic ligament can be continued to the right until the inferior surface of the duodenum is met.

The right gastroepiploic artery and vein, usually accompanied by lymph nodes of variable size, will be found coming forward from behind the duodenum and must be carefully isolated, ligatured, and divided. If the duodenum is healthy and there is no real evidence of malignancy, the division should be about 1.5 cm. to the right of the pylorus, leaving good branches intact to supply the duodenum.

Having thus cleared the greater curvature of the stomach and the inferior border of the duodenum, one turns to the superior lesser curvature.

A finger is passed up behind the antrum and is easily thrust through an avascular part of the tenuous hepatogastric ligament. The stomach is drawn to the left

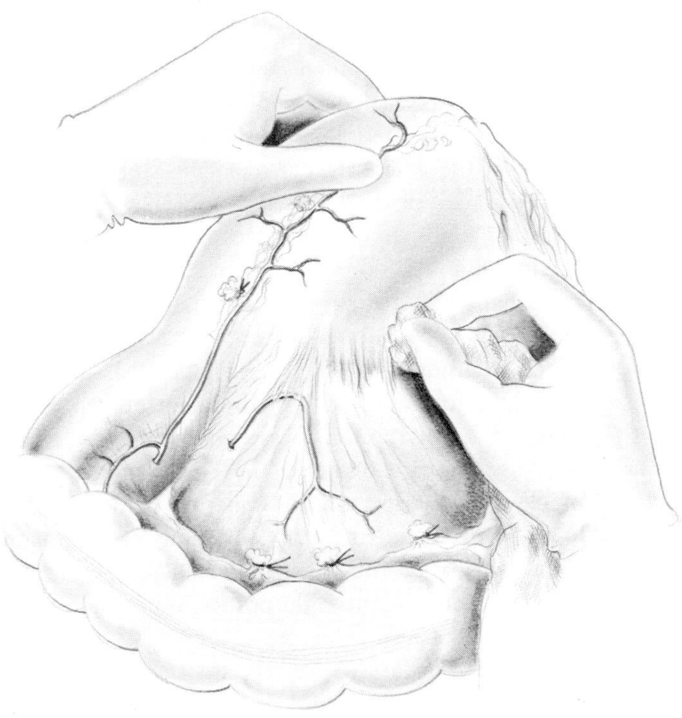

FIGURE 1. The mesocolon and posterior antral wall are usually lightly adherent; consequently the right gastroepiploic and middle colic vessels are in close proximity. These adhesions can be separated easily with a gauze swab.

and the superior border of the duodenum is outlined with a scalpel, to demonstrate the line of division between it and the hepatogastric ligament. The part of the hepatogastric ligament lying between the superior border of the duodenum and the opening made in the ligament will be seen to contain the right gastric vessel or vessels. These are carefully ligatured and divided about 1.5 cm. to the right of the pylorus. Fine adhesions between the proximal duodenum and the adjacent pancreas are separated by blunt dissection, in order to mobilize the posterior duodenal wall. If a duodenal ulcer or scar is present, it will be necessary to free the duodenum for at least 1.5 cm. beyond the ulcer or scar.

It is convenient to transect the duodenum at this stage. If the duodenum is healthy and there is no suggestion of gastric malignancy, it is well to preserve as much of it as possible. The duodenum is clamped with two fine clamps close to the pylorus and divided between the clamps. I use the fine crushing clamps designed by Lang Stevenson for this purpose.

The stomach is now drawn forward out of the wound and then to the left over the costal margin. After freeing some avascular adhesions normally encountered between the pancreas and the posterior wall of the upper stomach, and putting a retractor under the liver to draw it upward, a good view is obtained of the undivided part of the hepatogastric ligament, and also of the ligament passing from the upper border of the pancreas to the lesser curvature of the stomach, which contains the left gastric artery and vein, the celiac branch of the vagus nerve, and lymphatics. It is now important to palpate and inspect the hepatogastric ligaments carefully, for at times a large hepatic branch may pass upward from the left gastric artery and arch under the hepatogastric ligament to enter the liver. This branch, if found, usually supplies part of the left lobe of the liver, but occasionally supplies the whole left lobe or even the whole liver ("replacing common hepatic artery"). In other instances a large branch of the left gastric vein may leave the stomach and enter the liver by a similar route. If no major vessel is present, the hepatogastric ligament is divided, tying off any minor vessel encountered. If an artery of appreciable size is found it is usually wise to spare it, though accessory left hepatic vessels may be sacrificed, particularly in carcinoma cases.

The next step is the division of the left gastric vessels. In simple ulcer cases it is not necessary to make a formal ligature of the main branch of the left gastric artery above the point of its division into ascending and descending branches. Indeed, this carries a disadvantage, because the celiac branch of the posterior vagus nerve runs in close apposition to the superior border of the left gastric artery and is very likely to be included in high divisions of the main artery. This is undesirable, because division of the celiac nerve increases the possibility that the patient may develop certain disagreeable postvagotomy side effects, e.g. postoperative distention or, later, diarrhea.

In the average case the left gastric vessels are transected at their point of branching. At this level the lesser curvature of the stomach is defined by palpation between finger and thumb, and a slim nontoothed dissecting forceps is passed between the muscle of the lesser curvature on the one hand and the fatty and vascular tissue on the other. An aneurysm needle carrying a stout ligature (e.g. No. 60 or No. 40 linen) is passed through and round the left gastric vessels and they are firmly ligatured and divided between clamps; then second ligatures are applied.

This usually leaves the stomach freed above the level of disease or desired transection, although in certain cases further mobilization of the lesser curvature will be required. To effect this, the muscle of the lesser curvature is exposed by upward traction on the upper divided part of the left gastric vessels; then by tying and dividing any small vessels as they enter the lesser curvature, eventually the desired length of lesser curvature is freed. The mobilization may even be continued to the level of the esophagus in this way.

In most cases it will be necessary to dissect higher up the greater curvature of the stomach than the gastroepiploic arch. In all but the most obese patients, this is best done by ligature and division from the lesser sac side, for the vessels running in the gastrosplenic omentum are most evident from its posterior surface. The colon is withdrawn from the wound, and the assistant draws it downward and to the right with his left hand. A retractor is placed under the upper part of the left wound edge, and light is directed to the gastrosplenic omentum, so that when the operator draws the stomach to the right and forward, and looks into the lesser sac, the left gastroepiploic vessels and the vasa brevia are clearly transilluminated. It is helpful if at this stage the anesthetist can empty the stomach completely, or the surgeon can manipulate the contents of the stomach into the pyloric end, since this makes the upper stomach much easier to manipulate. It is now easy to individually clamp, divide, and ligature these vessels. A Moynihan cholecystectomy forceps or similar curved long artery forceps is useful for this.

In slim patients with lax ligaments it is so easy to divide the vasa brevia by this means that there is even a risk that the surgeon may divide more vessels and so resect more stomach than he intends or had thought necessary. The mere fact that it is easy to make a very high resection is not really an indication for resecting higher, but rather the reverse, for the "easy case" is the thin patient who needs as much stomach as can reasonably be left to him. "Be kind to the patient who is kind to you."

If a very limited partial gastrectomy is intended, as may be the case when a coincident vagotomy is performed, then neither the left gastroepiploic artery nor any of the vasa brevia need be divided.

The Resection

The extent and pattern of the resection are now finally decided. My routine for performing it is as follows.

The mobile stomach, emptied of its contents, is lifted upward. A point on the greater curvature is chosen which is to be the level of the transection. *This need not be above the ulcer level,* but may be below it, provided that the ulcer is on or near the lesser curvature. A strong but slim crushing clamp is placed across the greater curvature half of the stomach diameter at this level and closed. This is to be the part of the stomach used in the new stoma. It will be noted that the width of the stomach clamped is *not* necessarily related to the diameter of the duodenum, but is always one-half of the gastric diameter. This diameter is usually a little, sometimes considerably, wider than the duodenum. A noncrushing clamp is put across the whole gastric diameter to prevent spilling from the distal stomach, and the greater curvature half of the stomach is transected just distal to the crushing clamp (Fig. 2). The lesser curvature half of the stomach is now clamped. If the ulcer is low, a straight Payr clamp may be used, continuing in the same transverse direction as the clamp already on the greater curvature. If, however, the ulcer is higher than the level of the greater curvature transection, strong curved crushing clamps, e.g. Parker-Kerr clamps, may be put on to arch well over the ulcer to the lesser curvature. The stomach is sectioned between them (Fig. 3).

The lesser curvature part of the stomach is now closed with a running continuous stitch of 00 chromic catgut placed over the clamp rather slackly. The clamp is withdrawn and the suture then tightened. A second continuous Lembert suture is placed over this, using the same suture material.

This leaves a structure superficially resembling a small stomach, held at its distal end in a clamp, ready for anastomosis to the duodenum.

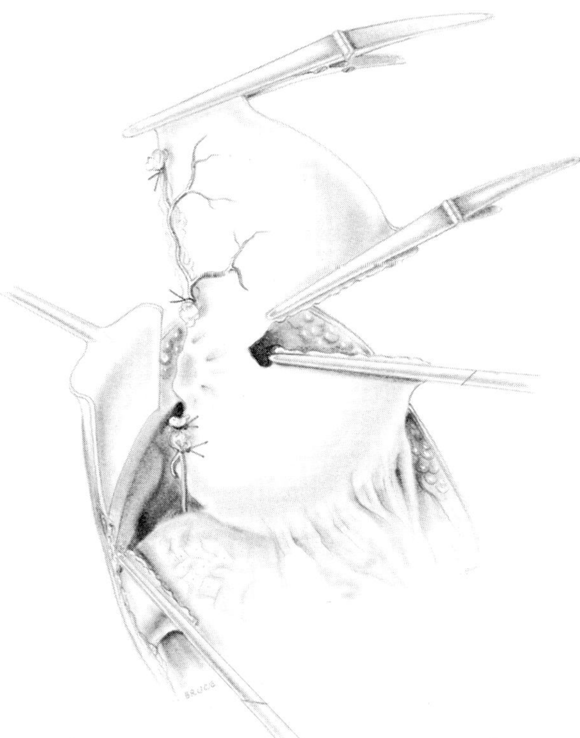

FIGURE 2. The stomach is lifted up and two strong, slim clamps are placed across the greater curvature half of the stomach at the desired level of transection (which may be below the ulcer level). The greater curvature half of the stomach is divided between them.

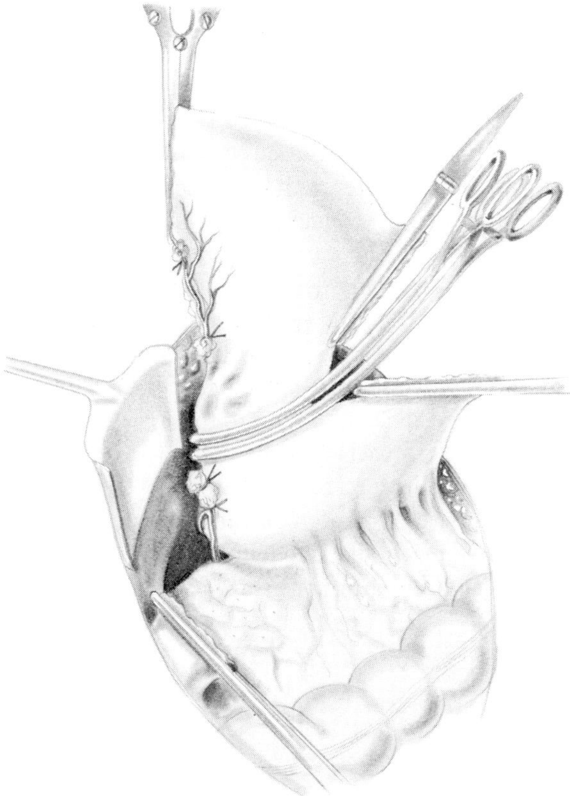

FIGURE 3. A pair of Parker-Kerr or similar curved crushing clamps are made to arch above the ulcer level, and the stomach is divided between them.

The Anastomosis

It will usually be found that the duodenal and gastric cut ends can be approximated with ease, even after a high resection. If there is any suspicion of tension, the duodenum, and even the head of the pancreas, may be mobilized after incising the peritoneal fold to the right of the descending duodenal limb, together, of course, with the cholecyst-duodenal fold and any adventitious adhesions. By this means, and if necessary by mobilizing the third part of the duodenum, the cut end of duodenum can be brought to the level of the esophagus. It is better not to overmobilize the gastric remnant—in the first place for fear of endangering its blood supply, though this is usually more than ample, and in the second place to prevent pulling the fundus downward and so flattening the esophagogastric angle.

There are many satisfactory methods of uniting the duodenum and stomach. I find a two-layer anastomosis, using continuous 00 chromic catgut on an atraumatic needle and carried out as follows, to be absolutely leakproof and hemostatic. The first suture, starting at the greater curvature side of the stomach and ending at the suture line on the new "lesser curvature," is placed very loosely between the posterior walls of the stomach and duodenum, running downward on the gastric side, upward on the duodenal side, rather like the progress of a corkscrew or the movement of a spirochete. The final stitch on the gastric side passes through *both* edges of the suture line on the lesser curvature side of the stomach (Fig. 4). This is passed loosely because of the disparity in size of the two cut ends. The loose stitching enables the operator to see each stitch clearly and place it exactly to compensate for the differing diameter; naturally the stitches are closer together on the narrower organ. Any excess of stomach or duodenum projecting beyond the clamps is excised and the clamp on the narrower structure, usually the duodenum, is removed. The loose suture is tightened stitch by stitch and the remaining clamp is removed. The contents of the stomach and duodenum are aspirated. The suture line is controlled by having the assistant hold the ends of catgut uniting the posterior surfaces. Any spouting vessel may be caught and tied; minor oozing will be adequately controlled by the "all-coats" layers to follow.

With the cut ends of the stomach and duodenum steadied by the assistant, and the anterior walls held by Allis forceps, the "all-coats" suture is inserted, starting at the greater curvature, with a simple continuous suture, which is continued all round the open ends of stomach and duodenum to meet the first stitch again. On the anterior wall also, a simple continuous suture is used, rather than a Connell

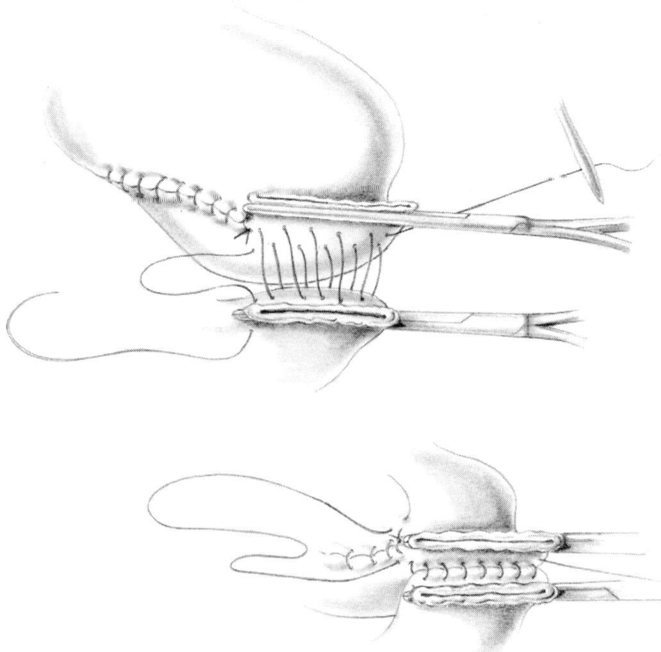

FIGURE 4. After closure of the lesser curvature half of the stomach with two layers of fine catgut the gastroduodenal anastomosis is commenced. A slack continuous suture is passed between the seromuscularis of the stomach and that of the duodenum, and then tightened. This Lembert layer should be made to bury the lower end of the united lesser curvature—the "critical angle."

stitch, as this is more hemostatic, but as each suture is tightened, the mucosa is inverted into the stomach. These sutures must be closely placed and not take too big bites of tissue, or the suture line will be narrowed and postoperative delay in emptying will result. Chromic catgut, size 00, is used for these layers (Fig. 5).

The Lembert suture from the posterior wall is now continued round the anterior wall and tied when the beginning of the suture is met. Next a reinforcing stitch is placed on the lesser curvature side of the anastomosis, taking bites of the anterior and posterior parts of the stomach and the adjacent duodenum. To complete the anastomosis, two or three stitches are placed between the remnants of hepatogastric ligament adjacent to the right gastric pedicle and the sutured lesser curvature half of the stomach. These reinforce the closure of the cut end of the stomach and help to prevent any tension arising in the suture line in the postoperative period.

Special Difficulties Encountered

THE NARROW DUODENUM. Sometimes the duodenum is extremely narrow. This is especially troublesome when the operation is being performed in a patient with stenotic scarring of the duodenum, even though one transects well beyond the fibrous tissue. In such a case the anastomosis is commenced as already stated, making the posterior Lembert and the posterior all-coats sutures but, of course, taking much wider bites of stomach than of duodenum. Before commencing the anterior suture line, an incision is made with scissors into the anterior wall of the duodenum, starting at the cut end of the duodenum (Fig. 5). This greatly increases the length of the anterior suture line. In addition, when the anterior line has been completed, the full suture line is elliptical. Consequently the anterior and posterior

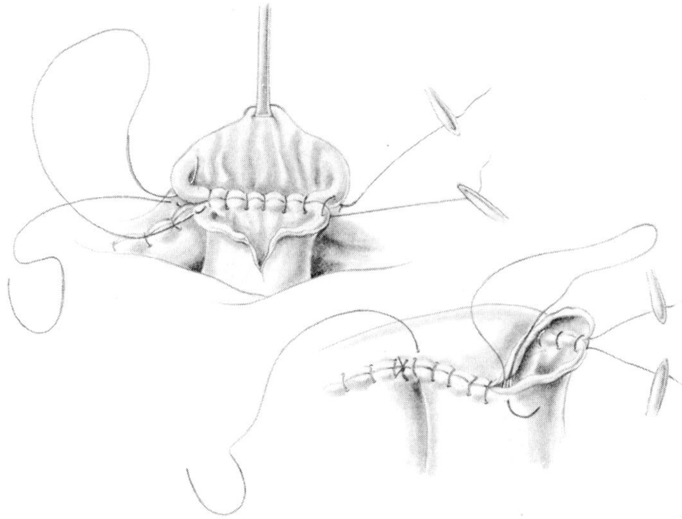

FIGURE 5. The "all-coats" layer of the gastroduodenal anastomosis. In this case the duodenal lumen has been enlarged by making a small incision in the middle of its anterior wall.

suture lines are not in contact. This is an aid to gastric evacuation, for no matter how edematous or bruised the suture line may be, it will not be encircling at any one level. Delayed emptying of the stomach is most unusual after this variation of the operation.

Penetrating Gastric Ulcer. Not infrequently it will be found that the gastric ulcer is penetrating a neighboring organ, most often the pancreas. On elevating the stomach after division of the duodenum, broad adhesions are seen uniting the stomach to the pancreas at the site of penetration. The main thing to bear in mind is that the pancreas is ulcerated only because it is in contact with gastric juice; its surface is covered with healthy granulations and there is no need—indeed, it is extremely dangerous—to remove or shave off any part of the pancreas. Even diathermy of the base of such an ulcer may open a pancreatic duct and lead to a pancreatic fistula.

The best technique is to "pinch off" the stomach from the pancreas. To effect this, the flimsier adhesions around the penetrated part are freed as much as possible, particularly proximal to the ulcer. A gauze pack is placed round the site to prevent diffuse soiling with gastric content. The edges of the ulcer are then squeezed between thumb and forefinger from one side to the other, and in most cases the stomach will separate bloodlessly from the pancreas, exactly in the line in which they had adhered. As soon as separation commences, a "sucker" is introduced into the stomach and it is emptied.

In occasional cases pressure or pinching of this sort will not completely separate the two organs because of more extensive fibrosis uniting them. Rather than use extreme pressure or risk tearing one of the viscera, it is better to separate them, or complete the separation, by means of a scalpel. In doing this the line of incision should never encroach on pancreatic tissue. Not the least harm is done if a circle of seromuscularis of stomach remains round the pancreatic crater, but a pancreatic fistula may occur if a ring of pancreas is cut off and left attached to the part of the stomach to be removed.

When the two are separated a wide perforation will usually be left in the stomach. This may be temporarily closed with a coarse line of suture, after which the gastrectomy proceeds as already indicated.

High Gastric Ulcer. The ulcer may be at any height; its upper margin may even involve the esophagus. So long as not more than half of the esophageal circumference is involved in the ulceration, and so long as the ulceration is innocent, it is never necessary to carry out total resection for high gastric ulcer. The operation must be varied as follows.

In the preliminary mobilization of the lesser curvature, in order to free the stomach more thoroughly, the main trunk of the left gastric artery and vein may be divided, even though this may sacrifice the celiac nerve too. To free the stomach above the ulcer level, it may be necessary to divide the peritoneum and phrenoesophageal ligaments around the cardia and mobilize the lower few centimeters of esophagus, though the inferior thoracic artery to the esophagus should not be divided. At a point opposite healthy stomach just above the ulcer level, the fatty, lymphatic, fibrous, and vascular tissue surrounding the ascending branch of the left gastric artery is defined, separated from the musculature of the lesser curvature of the stomach, ligatured, and divided. Sometimes this point is at the esophageal rather than the gastric level.

In other cases it may be simpler to divide the left gastric artery at a low level and distal to the ulcer, as previously described, and then slowly and carefully dissect the tissues of the lesser curvature of stomach from the fatty tissues surrounding the ascending branch of the left gastric artery. Paired vessels enter the anterior and posterior parts of the lesser curvature of the stomach, with occasional branches entering the middle of the lesser curvature. These must all be individually ligatured and divided. By this means the dissection can ascend as high as the gullet. This is also the best way of dealing with the situation when it is particularly important to spare the main branch of the left gastric artery because it gives origin to a left or main hepatic artery.

Attention is now turned to the greater curvature. Here the clamp is placed across the greater curvature half of the stomach as previously described. One should remember that *this may well be below the level of the ulcer*. To remove the ulcer, the Pauchet maneuver is used, excising a tongue-shaped piece of lesser curvature containing the ulcer. This may in many cases be effected by passing a curved Parker-Kerr crushing clamp across the lesser curvature and upward to encircle the ulcer, after which the clamped part is sutured as previously described.

In many cases the use of a clamp is impracticable because of the danger of occluding the gullet. Instead, the segment of lesser curvature containing the ulcer is removed with scissors. It is best to incise about 2 to 3 cm. at a time, stitching up the lesser curvature as one goes (Fig. 6). The upper part of the incision may enter and remove a segment of esophagus. This is safe so long as about one-half of the esophageal circumference remains, although in such cases it is wise to have a stomach tube in the gullet during the stitching.

The lesser curvature having been closed by one of these methods, the further progress of the operation may, in most cases, continue as previously described, by inserting a second row of Lembert suture and then completing the gastroduodenal anastomosis. If, however, the esophagus has been encroached upon by this all-coats suture, it will be impracticable to invert it now by a second (Lembert) layer, and too hazardous to trust to a single row of suture. In such cases, therefore, it is my practice to abandon any thought of the Billroth I repair. Instead a loop of jejunum is brought up and sutured from the greater curvature of the stomach, up behind the sutured lesser curvature, to the esophagus. The loop of jejunum is then attached first above and next in front of the sutured lesser curvature. Opposite the greater curvature half of the stomach, the jejunum is opened and an anastomosis is made between the stomach and the jejunum (Fig. 7). By this means, instead of putting a Lembert layer in the sutured lesser curvature half of the stomach and adjacent esophagus, a "graft" of healthy jejunum is securely placed over it. In many experiences of this modification it has never leaked or given rise to any complication. This method has been successfully used even in patients admitted with severe dysphagia and a dilated esophagus due to esophagogastric ulceration. Temporary dysphagia, particularly for solids, may be present for a few weeks after such an operation, but this gradually disappears entirely.

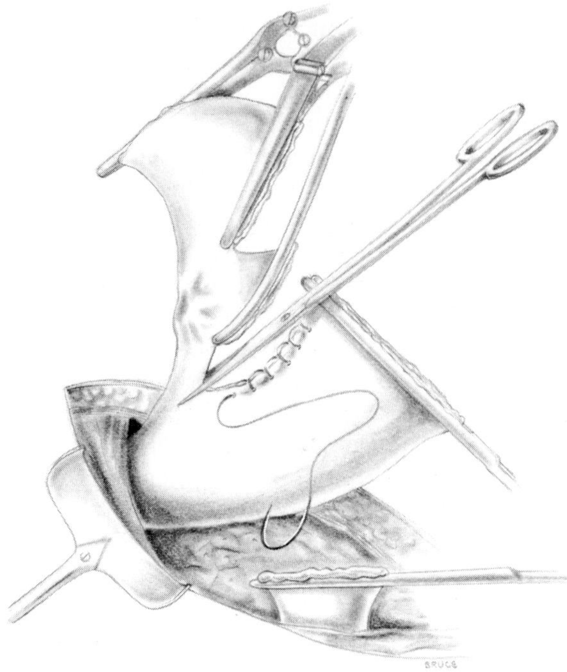

FIGURE 6. The very high gastric ulcer. In this case the ulcer is too high, too indurated, or too near the esophagus to use curved crushing clamps. The incision is made with scissors, suturing as one proceeds. A clamp may be placed part way on the part to be removed.

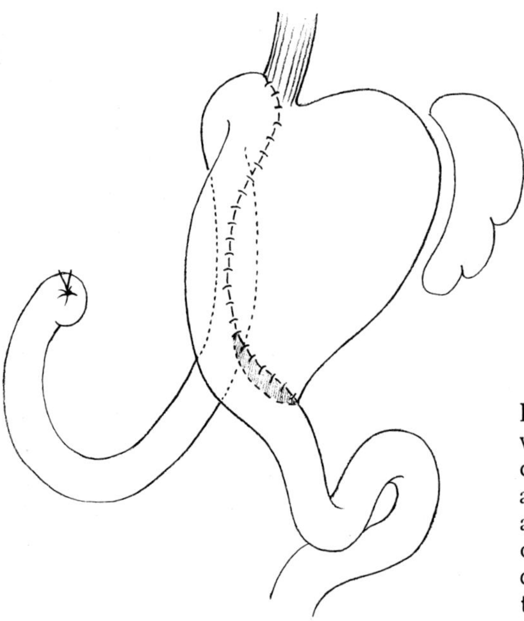

FIGURE 7. Juxtaesophageal ulcer with excision of part of the esophageal diameter. The new lesser curvature and esophagus are closed in one layer, and then the afferent jejunal loop is drawn up and sutured over the lesser curvature and esophagus to reinforce them.

Gastrectomy Below the Ulcer. Is there a place for this modification? If a healed high gastric scar is present in an obese or poor risk subject, it is occasionally possible to carry out gastrectomy below the ulcer, and I have done so, with good immediate and late results; but because gastric ulcer may develop or recur after the Billroth I operation, the Billroth II modification was and should be always used in such cases.

Posterior Gastric Ulcer. In a review of gastric ulcers in 1953, I found a high percentage (44.2 per cent in women, 29.3 per cent in men) to be on the posterior wall of the stomach, rather high up, particularly in women. For this contingency I have used what I call the "Rotation Billroth I," in which the gastric stump is mainly fashioned from the *anterior* wall of the stomach and a tongue-shaped part of the posterior wall is removed. This may be effected most simply by the following means.

The stomach is well mobilized, particularly on the lesser curvature, to above the ulcer level. The ulcer is then grasped with the left hand and the stomach rotated in a clockwise direction. To form the new stoma, the fine crushing clamp is placed across half the gastric diameter; but being placed opposite the ulcer, it takes mainly anterior wall (Fig. 8). Half the stomach having been thus transected,

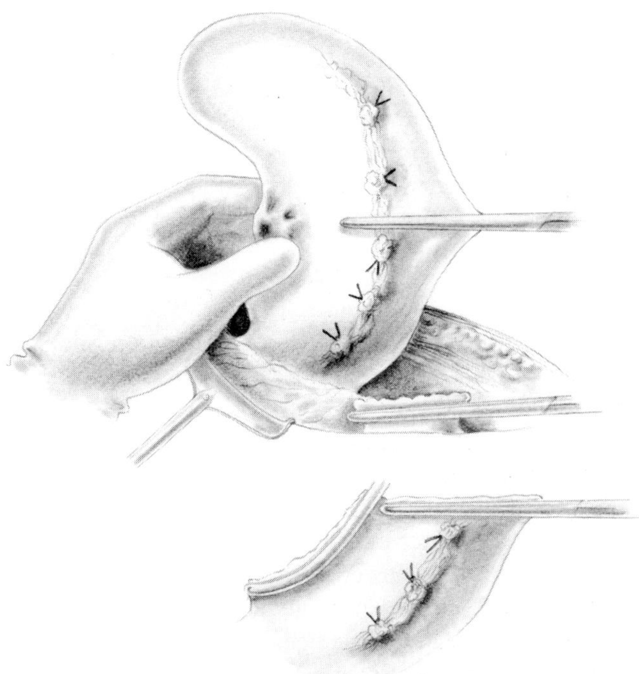

FIGURE 8. Rotation gastrectomy for ulcer high on the posterior wall of the stomach. The stomach is rotated; the ulcer is held in the left fingers and the clamp placed halfway across the stomach opposite the ulcer, i.e., mainly on the anterior wall of the stomach. After division of the stomach beyond the clamp, a second curved crushing (Parker-Kerr) clamp is made to encircle the ulcer, and the stomach beyond is removed.

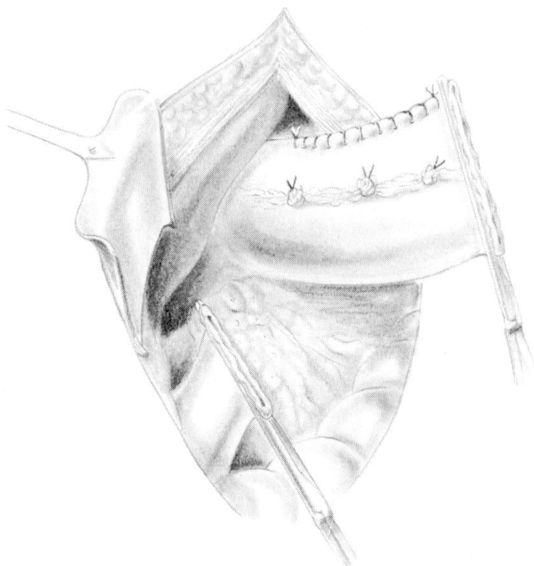

FIGURE 9. Rotation gastrectomy. The posterior wall of the stomach is closed and the stomach stump and duodenum are ready for anastomosis in the usual way.

a curved crushing (Parker-Kerr) clamp is placed so as to surround the ulcer, which is still held between thumb and finger, and the segment enclosed in the clamp is removed, thus excising part of the posterior wall (Fig. 9). The operation is completed precisely as described before. The fact that anterior wall only is united to the duodenum does not distort it at all; indeed, it appears to lie more satisfactorily than it does when the greater curvature half of the stomach is used.

Final Inspection

At the end of any gastrectomy, a methodical inspection should be made. My routine is to examine, visually, first the spleen, to make sure there is no tear; then the lesser sac, to exclude bleeding from vasa brevia; next the left gastric pedicle and the right gastric and right gastroepiploic pedicles. Then the greater omentum and colon are withdrawn from the wound. The inspection is continued to insure that the epiploic ties are secure, the mesocolon intact, the colon of good color and viable. The devascularized greater omentum may have some venous congestion but usually appears quite viable. If, however, the greater omentum or part of it is of poor color *and* obese, the affected part should be removed, because fat necrosis of the greater omentum can lead to prolonged suppuration.

One must also make sure that there is no tension on the suture lines. If there is any tension, it is relieved by a little further mobilization of the duodenum or head of the pancreas. Any collection of blood is carefully aspirated.

Finally, all being well, the greater omentum is rotated up to lie over the stomach and duodenum and below the liver. The wound is then closed.

Complications Peculiar to the Billroth I Operation

It is often found that the normal temporary postoperative delay in gastric emptying is a little more prolonged after the Billroth I than after gastrojejunal anastomosis. There should not be a pronounced difference, however. If the surgeon finds that his patients are slow in starting evacuation, he should attend to the points mentioned as aids to a satisfactory result: namely, the use of small, frequent stitches round the anastomosis; the use of half the gastric diameter; and, if necessary, the use of a small anterior incision to widen the duodenum and gain an elliptical stoma.

One might expect jaundice or pancreatic difficulties to follow wide mobilization of the pancreatic head. I have seen a transient jaundice on one occasion only.

Necrosis of the suture line has been reported. To prevent it, it is important to retain right and left gastroepiploic branches, close to the suture line, to the duodenum and stomach respectively.

References

Michels, N. A. *Blood Supply and Anatomy of the Upper Abdominal Organs with a Descriptive Atlas.* Philadelphia: J. B. Lippincott, 1955.

Moore, H. G., and Harkins, H. N. *The Billroth I Operation.* Boston: Little, Brown, 1953.

Swynnerton, B. F., and Tanner, N. C. Chronic gastric ulcer: a comparison between a gastroscopically controlled series treated medically and a series treated by surgery. *Brit. M. J.* 2:841, October 17, 1953.

Tanner, N. C. Non-malignant affections of the upper stomach. *Ann. Roy. Coll. Surgeons England* 10:45, January 1952.

Tanner, N. C. Surgery of peptic ulceration and its complications. *Postgrad. M. J.* 30:448, September 1954.

80. *Billroth II Operation*

PIETRO VALDONI

SURGERY for gastric and duodenal ulcer usually follows a long period of difficulty. By creating a new pathophysiological gastric state, it may initiate a series of problems that result from resection of the stomach. Therefore, surgery should aim to assure not only anatomical healing but also a proper functional result. Vagotomy, which is considered by most surgeons as a necessary adjunct to gastric resection for the treatment of duodenal ulcer, is discussed in other chapters.

Before describing the technique of gastric resection that I use for gastric and duodenal ulcer disease, I must emphasize certain points. The first pertains to indications for operation. Candidates include patients with verified complications of the ulcer, such as hemorrhage, penetration, perforation, or obstruction; those in whom pain has been severe; and those in whom medical and dietary measures, although diligently applied, have not brought about relief of the symptomatology. Regardless of symptomatology, another indication for radical surgery in gastric ulcer is the need to exclude malignant disease.

The technique that I shall describe is one that I have used for twenty years without major modifications. I performed my first operation for duodenal ulcer in 1926 and have employed techniques of gastric surgery varying from the simplest to the most radical. Many of these techniques are now primarily of historical significance. The successive modifications I have employed have been influenced by postoperative studies of my patients, with the intent to select those techniques which are associated with the lowest mortality, the best postoperative course, and the most satisfactory functional results.

I have followed, by personally examining them, 286 patients operated on in a five-year period. There were 23 women and 263 men. Forty-two patients had a gastric and 234 a duodenal ulcer. Ten had both gastric and duodenal ulcers. In 14 patients an afferent loop syndrome was noted after surgery. This is characterized by the projectile vomiting of bile and is accompanied by repeated nausea and a sensation of heaviness in the right hypochondrium, especially in connection with meals. We have not observed any patient with the small-pouch syndrome. In 15 cases we observed an early postprandial syndrome that disappeared within a period of six months. In 12 cases a late postprandial syndrome developed. Loss of weight from the presurgical levels was noted in 19 per cent and an increase in weight was noted in 50 per cent of cases. There were no cases of anemia, and work capacity either was increased or remained unchanged.

Technique

The operation is performed under general anesthesia. Immediately before surgery a nasogastric tube is introduced to maintain decompression.

The Incision

I have always used a midline incision, extending it below the umbilicus in obese patients. I believe major problems can arise from an inadequate incision and that no harm follows the use of an ample incision provided the closure, at the completion of the operation, is performed with particular care.

The Extent of Resection

The exact extent of the resection cannot be readily estimated. In ulcer patients the stomach size varies greatly, especially when there is a coexisting functional or organic stenosis which selectively increases the size of the antrum. The important point is not how much stomach to resect, but what portion of the stomach to leave. To establish the proper limits of resection I regularly identify two anatomical guideposts, one on the greater and the other on the lesser curvature, and precisely mark them with Allis clamps. The guide on the greater curvature is the spot at which the

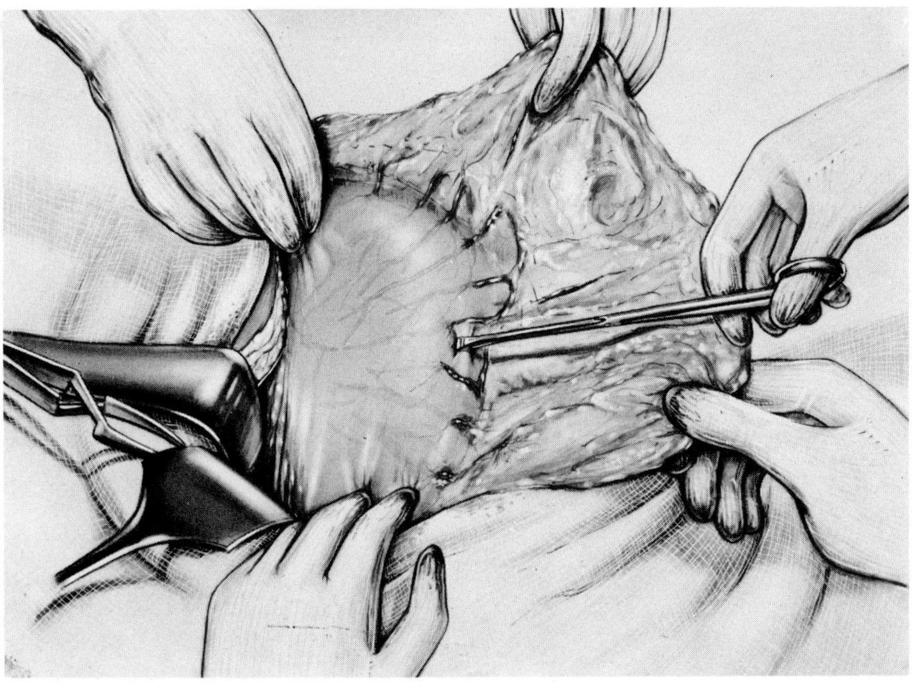

FIGURE 1. An Allis clamp fixes the point of resection on the greater curvature where the branches of the right gastroepiploic join with those of the left gastroepiploic artery.

branches from the right gastroepiploic unite with those arising from the left gastroepiploic artery (Fig. 1). On the lesser curvature, I identify the left gastric artery after I have transected the gastrohepatic ligament. The artery divides into two branches near the lesser curvature, one ascending and the other descending. I transect the descending branch close to the lesser curvature immediately after I have identified its origin (Figs. 2 and 3). An important advantage of this line of resection is that one obtains a line of anastomosis that runs obliquely in an almost vertical direction. This assures that the point of emptying of the stomach will be at the most dependent portion.

It is essential not to use gastric clamps. There is no justification for the use of these clamps to avoid contamination of the operative field, because the stomach is essentially empty at the time of the operation. Furthermore, their use precludes complete hemostasis of the submucosal vessels. Also, if the pressure of a gastric clamp is excessive, it can easily produce a traumatic tear of the gastric mucosa, and may thereby cause operative complications such as hemorrhage from the lacerated vessels, or infection in the submucosa.

The Gastric Pouch

Another important feature of our technique is the sectioning of the vasa brevia, leaving only the upper two vessels intact. The separation of the major portion of the greater curvature from the spleen frees the gastric pouch from its attachment to that organ and renders it fully mobile (Fig. 4). I consider that this maneuver accounts

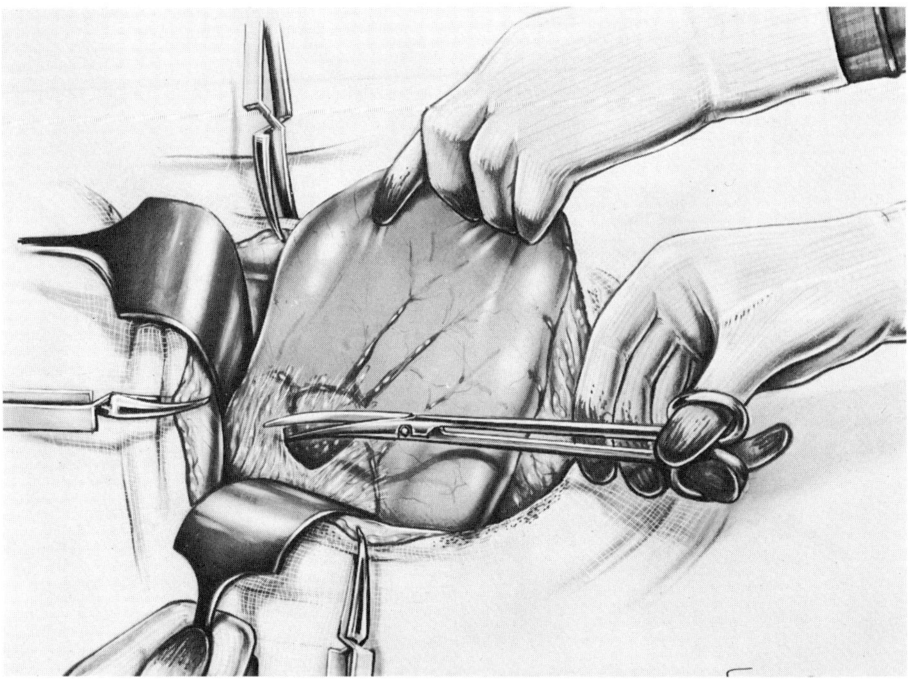

FIGURE 2. The gastrohepatic ligament is transected in order to expose the trunk of the left gastric artery and its ascending and descending rami.

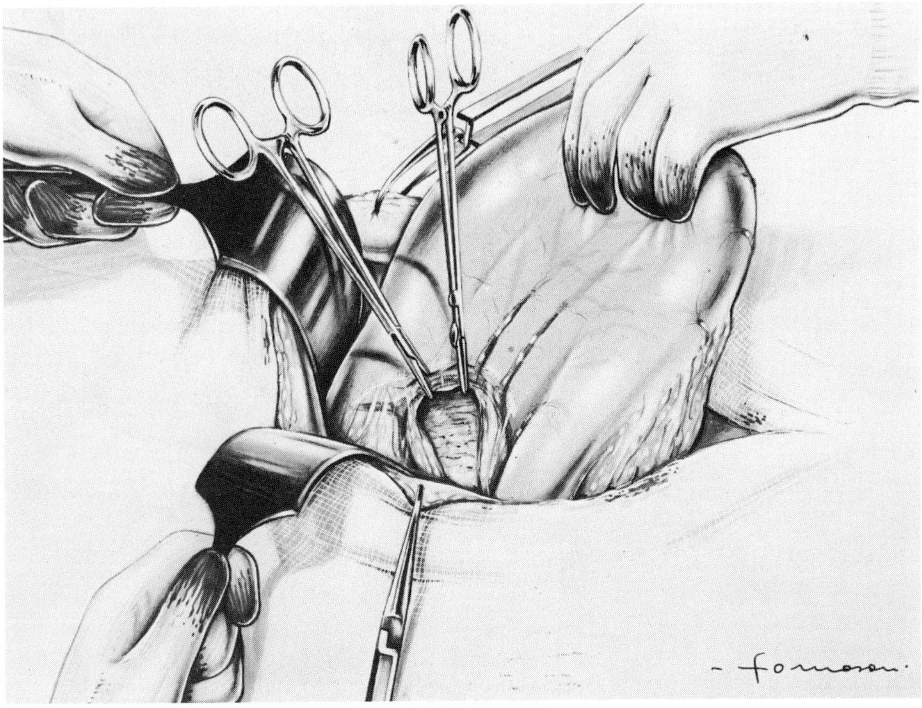

FIGURE 3. Transection of the descending ramus of the left gastric artery. At this point the lesser curvature will be transected.

for the fact that we have had no occasion to reoperate for efferent loop obstruction. This complication usually follows angulation of the efferent loop near its origin at the inferior angle of the gastric pouch. Following transection of the duodenum, traction of the stomach on the spleen ceases, because the stomach is no longer attached to the duodenum, and the spleen will shift from its usual position. Its inferior pole rotates laterally and the medial surface becomes horizontal. If the vasa brevia are not interrupted, the gastric pouch will follow the spleen in its displacement, and this will result in a change of anatomical position, with distortion at the point of anastomosis of the stomach to the efferent loop. I believe this is the reason some surgeons anastomose the efferent and afferent loops to eliminate postoperative gastric obstruction.

I think the sectioning of the vasa brevia also explains why we have not found it necessary to use prolonged gastric suction postoperatively. After the first few days, when gastric pouch atonia is frequently responsible for retention, suction is discontinued. It is important that this be done, since one is usually dealing with apprehensive patients who do not tolerate intubation well.

The Greater Omentum

In obese patients I routinely detach the omentum from the colon and then resect a segment of it with the excised portion of stomach. This maneuver prevents com-

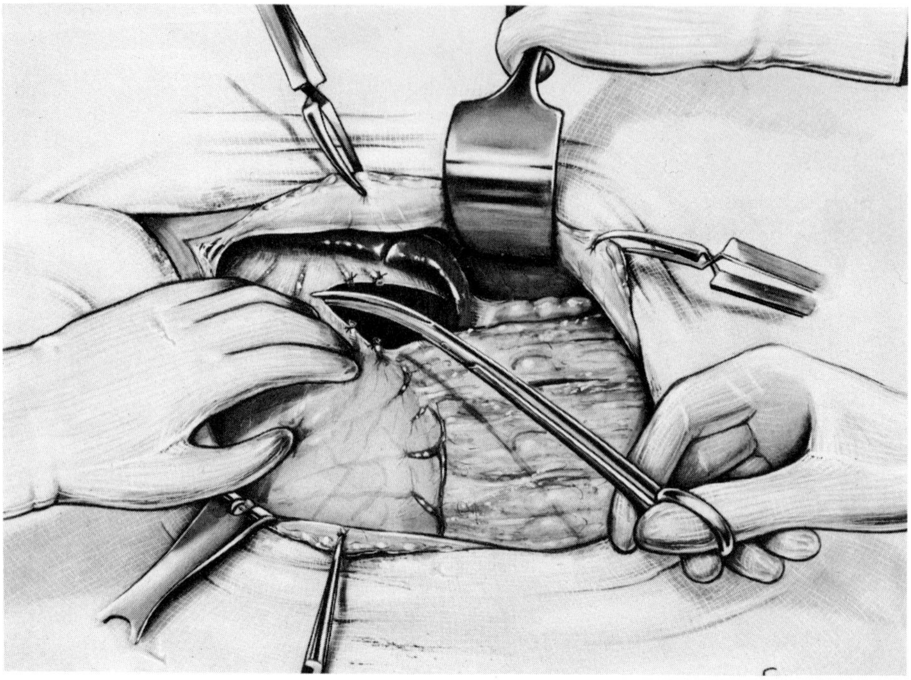

FIGURE 4. Transection of the gastrosplenic ligament to mobilize the stomach.

pression of the efferent and afferent loops (during the first few postoperative days) after an antecolic anastomosis. The omentum quickly becomes edematous in such patients, and impinges upon the two loops, especially the afferent. It is particularly important to avoid afferent loop stasis. In thin patients it is not necessary to deliver or resect any omentum.

The Type of Anastomosis

I routinely do an antecolic rather than a retrocolic anastomosis. I believe there is no difference in their effectiveness. However, an antecolic anastomosis is technically easier, can be performed more rapidly, and does not require fixation of the stomach to the mesocolon, thereby permitting the gastric pouch to move freely. This, I believe, is a most important factor in avoiding postoperative obstruction. Although it rarely occurs, one also avoids the possibility of incarcerating a loop of jejunum between the anastomosed loops and the mesocolon. The occurrence of such a complication on one occasion encouraged my abandonment of the transmesocolic anastomosis.

From the immediate as well as the long-range standpoint, it is essential that the afferent loop be long enough to be anastomosed in a fashion that does not encourage emptying of gastric contents into it. Duodenal stump leak during the immediate postoperative course is usually the consequence of an afferent loop stasis. This is an important reason for selecting an afferent loop of sufficient length to avoid compression from transverse colon or from a large residual omentum. If it is too short, it may result in fixation of the gastric pouch, or create angulation at the point of anastomosis.

The question of whether one should perform the anastomosis with the afferent loop on the lesser and the efferent loop on the greater curvature, or with the afferent on the greater and the efferent on the lesser curvature, cannot be answered categorically. It seems to me that the position of the anastomosis should be such that the stomach empties into the efferent loop at its most dependent portion and there is no restriction of the afferent loop or reflux of gastric contents into it. If the surgeon does not appreciate the need for an almost vertical obliquity of the gastric pouch (and of mobility and freedom from the spleen for the greater curvature), it is perhaps better for him to perform the anastomosis in an isoperistaltic fashion—that is, with the afferent loop on the greater curvature. With a horizontal line of gastric resection, an anastomosis with the afferent loop on the lesser curvature may not give a good functional result.

Keeping in mind the anatomical structures involved in transection of the stomach and in placing the anastomotic line, I have frequently observed radiologically the emptying of the stomach postoperatively, and have very rarely noted any passage of barium into the afferent loop. Therefore, I consider that a technical error probably has occurred in those patients in whom barium empties into the afferent rather than into the efferent loop. This finding is characteristic of the postoperative afferent loop syndrome.

A final question regarding the anastomosis is whether it should be a total or a partial stoma. I usually perform a total anastomosis; that it, I anastomose the entire end of the transected gastric pouch, even if it is very wide, to the antimesenteric portion of the jejunal loop. If we consider that the new outlet corresponds exactly to the origin of the efferent loop, it is apparent that, as in a funnel, the breadth of the receptacle portion is not as important as the caliber of the outlet.

Transection of the Duodenum

I never perform a resection when the ulcer, by penetration or its location, renders the stomach immobile. In these cases I consider it preferable to perform a gastrojejunostomy with vagotomy.

In the dissection, one must attempt a sufficiently extensive procedure to assure mobilization of the ulcer area. In difficult cases I initiate the sectioning of the duodenum by adequately mobilizing the second and third portions of the duodenum together with the head of the pancreas by the Kocher maneuver. After incision of the peritoneum over the duodenohepatic ligament, the retroduodenal portion of the common duct is identified. In doing this, one often finds that a seemingly unresectable ulcer has become resectable. The demands on the skill and experience of the surgeon are most evident in the management of the duodenal stump. I always advise our assistants to resect only those ulcers that are readily resectable.

A maneuver that may render dissection of penetrating ulcers easier consists of transecting the antrum between two gastric clamps to give mobility to the antrum and to allow one to proceed with greater facility in the dissection of the ulcer posteriorly. In difficult cases the hepatic artery is identified in the hepatoduodenal liga-

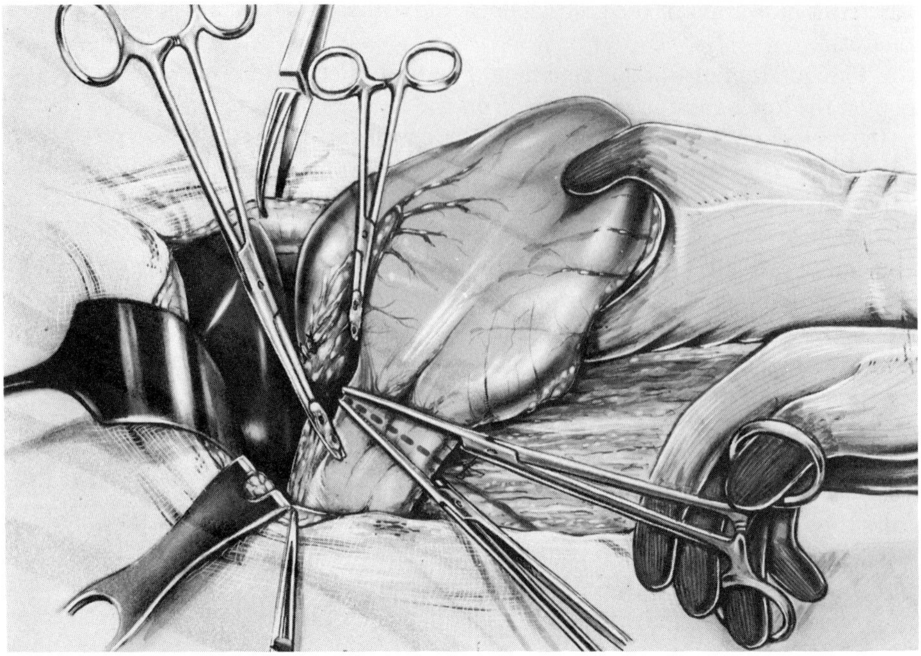

FIGURE 5. Transection of the right gastric artery directly under the line of section of the duodenum. The dashed line indicates the point of section of the duodenum.

ment prior to excision of the ulcer. I also identify the right gastric and gastroduodenal artery at their origin and individually ligate them (Fig. 5).

It is advisable to proceed along vascular lines in preparing the inferior margin of the duodenum. The gastroepiploic vein is identified first, since it is small and easily lacerated during the procedure, and is transfixed with a suture ligature. After the transection of the vein, the head of the pancreas is readily seen, together with the right gastroepiploic artery and, near its origin, the gastroduodenal artery.

One may say that every surgeon has his personal technique for closing the duodenal stump after removal of the ulcer. Almost all techniques are satisfactory, provided the anastomosis of the stomach and jejunum completely avoids stasis in the afferent loop. Such stasis is certainly the most important cause of dehiscence of the duodenal stump. If there is sufficient tissue, which is usually the case with adequate removal of the ulcer, I close the duodenal stump after transecting the duodenum along a Kocher clamp applied at the proper level (Figs. 6–8). As illustrated, a basting suture of continuous 0 catgut is applied over the clamp. Moderate traction on the suture readily closes the duodenal stump when the clamp is being removed. The stump is then further approximated with interrupted sutures. In most cases one may still further cover the stump with the peritoneum that overlies the pancreas.

Some cases, of course, present individual problems, such as the ulcer which penetrates the common bile duct, producing a choledochoduodenal fistula. If such penetration occurs in the retroduodenal segment of the common bile duct, I mobilize the duodenum inferior to the margin of the ulcer, but leave the penetration

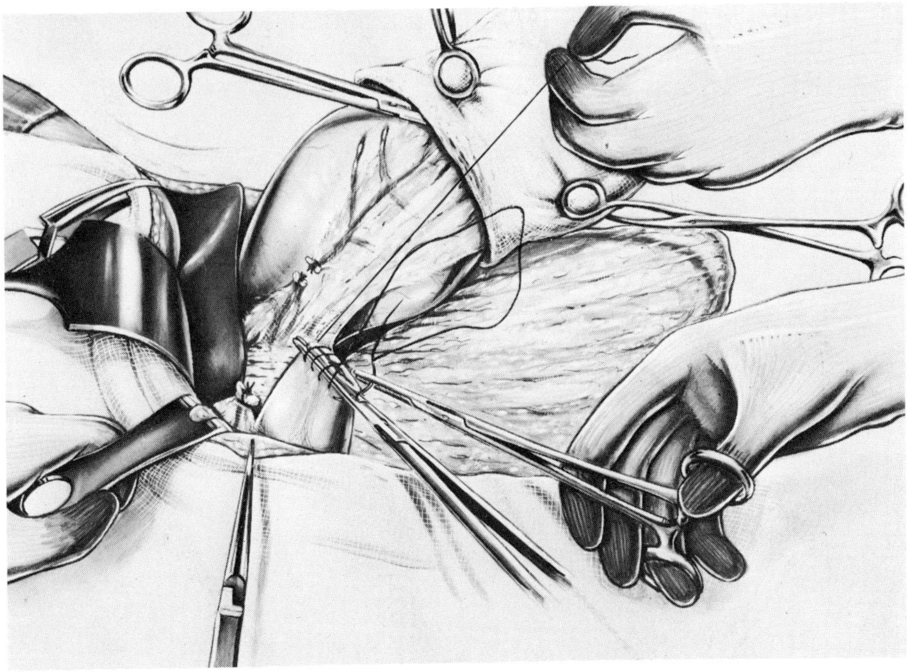

FIGURE 6. Closure of the duodenal stump with a continuous catgut suture.

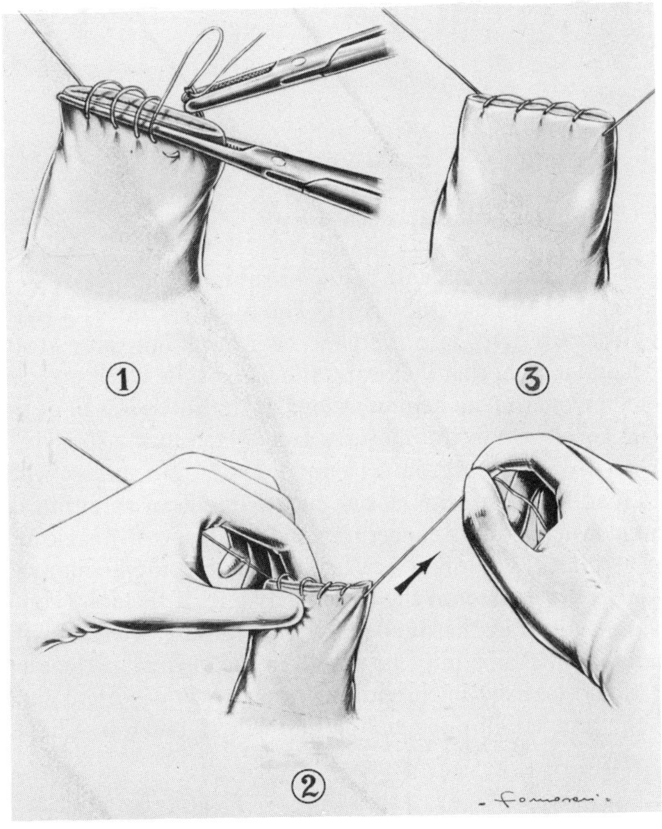

FIGURE 7. Details of the first layer of the duodenal closure.

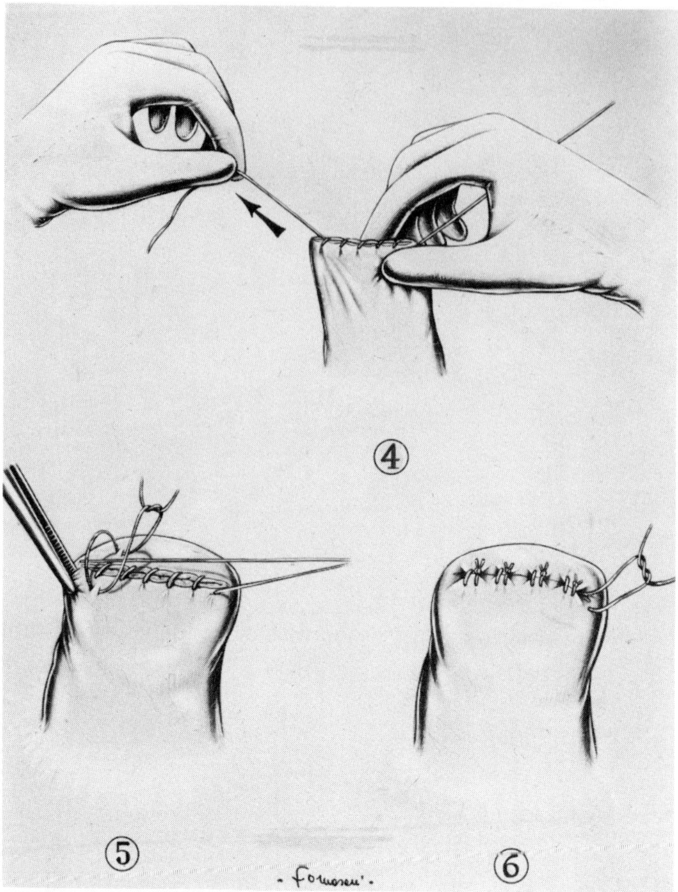

FIGURE 8. Completion of the duodenal closure.

intact, and close the duodenum with a row of sutures. A thin T tube is introduced into the common duct through the fistula. The tube is removed after two weeks.

When the ulcer penetrates into the pancreas it need not cause great concern. In freeing the mucosal margin that delineates the base of the ulcer, one can always find sufficient tissue to close the duodenum as long as the anterior wall of the duodenum offers sufficient coverage for the closure. However, broad experience and sound judgment are needed if the surgeon is to undertake radical surgery where indicated, and to effect an adequate, precise closure of the duodenal stump in difficult cases. When the surgeon has doubts concerning the adequacy of his closure, it may be wise to bring a rubber tube drain (catheter) through the abdominal wall in the subcostal region at the flank or in the midaxillary line. If the drain comes into direct contact with the sutures of the duodenal stump closure, it may contribute to dehiscence. Therefore, the tube must be placed in the vicinity of the duodenal stump but not over it, and be fixed in the desired position with a catgut suture. (Further discussion of the problem of duodenal closure will be found in Chapter 83, by Dr. Cooper.)

The Gastrojejunal Anastomosis

After the duodenum has been transected, the gastric segment is delivered through the wound and laid over the left costal arch. The two points between which the resection of the stomach is to be performed are prepared and fixed with two Allis or Chaput clamps. A loop of jejunum sufficiently long to go from the left across the midline is selected approximately 15 cm. from the ligament of Treitz, and placed in such a fashion that the afferent loop approximates the lesser curvature, passing anterior to the colon without traction (Figs. 9 and 10). I place a suture on the lesser curvature, then through the jejunal loop just posterior to the exact antimesenteric border, for one must remember that the jejunal incision must go exactly along the antimesenteric line. A similar guide suture is placed along the greater curvature and through the jejunum at the point where the efferent loop begins. Figure 11 shows clearly how the suturing is performed. This continuous suture is locked at every stitch, permitting maintenance of proper traction and thus avoiding the distraction of the approximated layers that may occur with loosely tied interrupted sutures. On completion of the seromuscular layer, the muscularis is transected with a scalpel, 0.5 cm. away from the sutures. The submucosal vessels are apparent and are individually clamped with small hemostats (Fig. 12). The gastric segment is reflected to the right, and at the level which corresponds to the line of transection

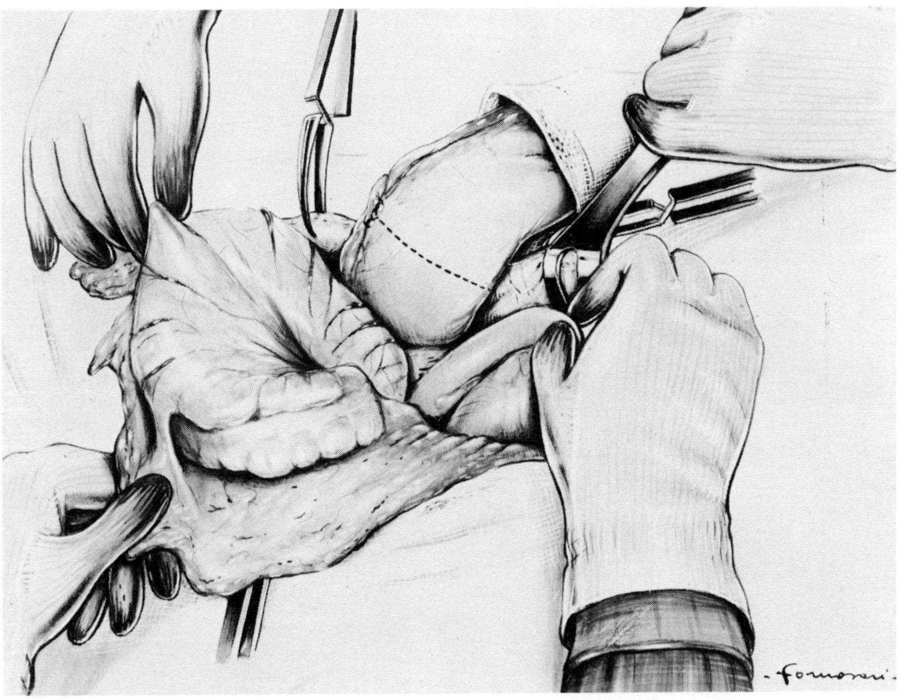

FIGURE 9. Selection of the loop of jejunum below the mesocolon. The stomach is reflected to the left of the laparotomy incision. The dashed line marks the point of gastric resection.

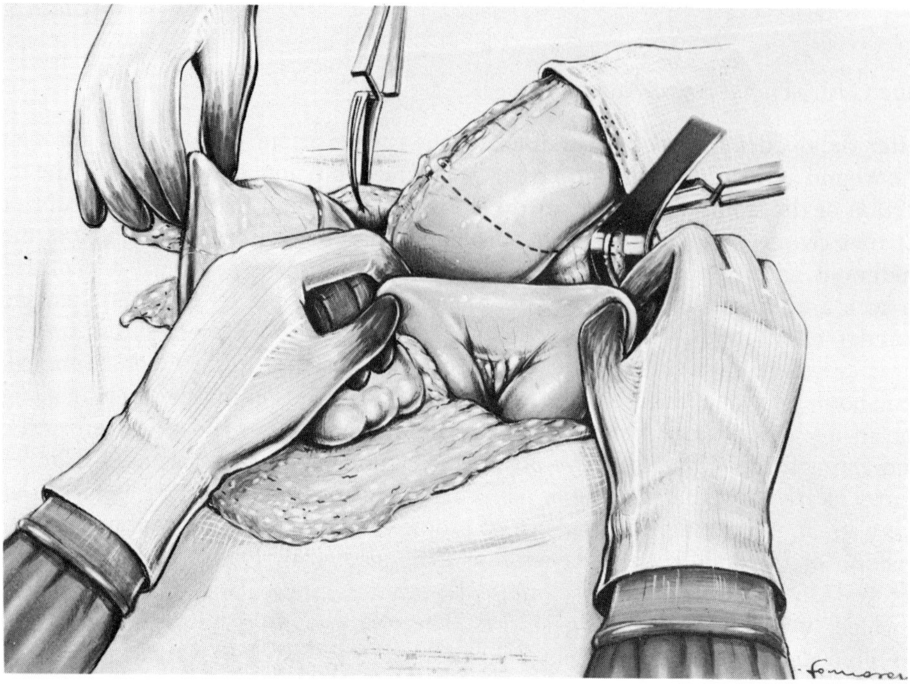

FIGURE 10. The colon has been replaced and the jejunal loop is approximated to the posterior wall of the stomach. The afferent loop is to be fixed along the lesser curvature.

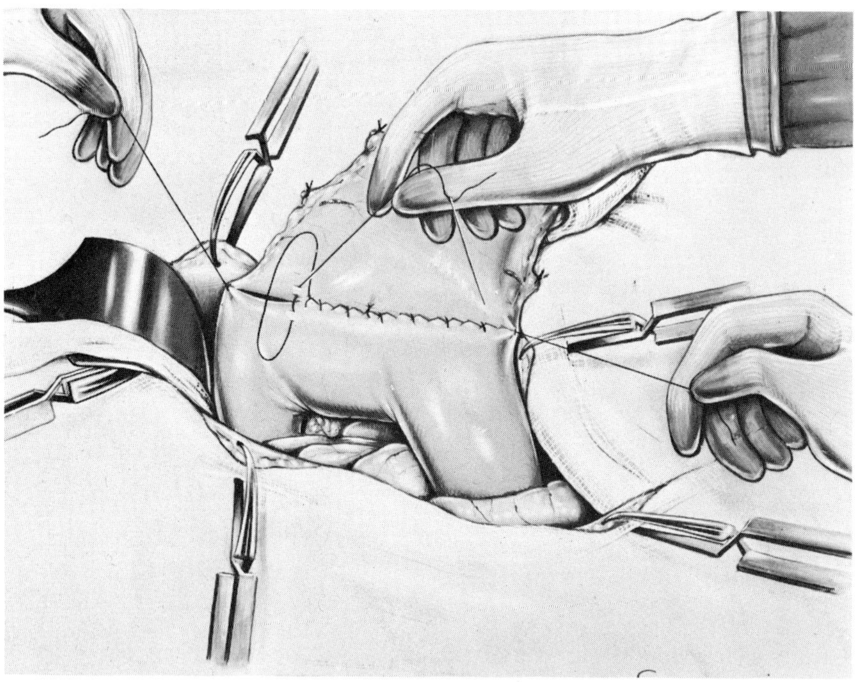

FIGURE 11. Seromuscular continuous lockstitch (first layer between stomach and jejunal loop), antecolic, with the afferent loop on the lesser curvature.

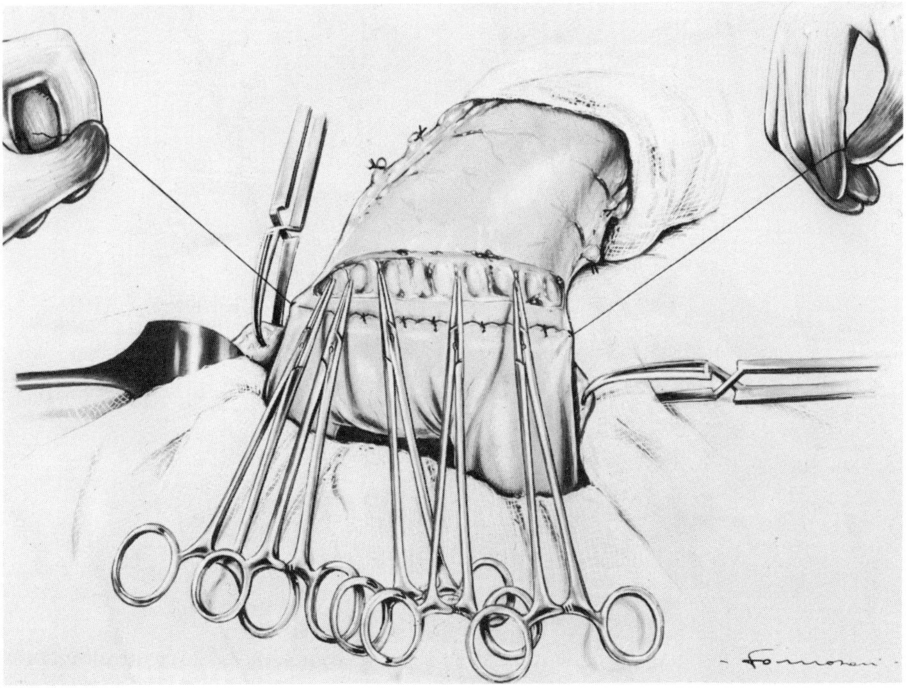

FIGURE 12. The posterior row of sutures has been completed, and the muscularis of the posterior gastric wall has been incised. Hemostasis of the submucosal vessels is being provided.

of the anterior stomach wall the muscularis of the posterior wall is transected in a similar fashion, and the vessels are clamped. The mucosa is then transected with electrocautery, first along the anterior wall and then along the posterior wall distal to the hemostats, and the operative specimen is removed (Figs. 13 and 14). The electrocautery should be used for cutting only when a nonexplosive anesthetic agent is employed. Massive coagulation is avoided, and occasionally we use catgut ligatures. The jejunum is then incised with the electrocautery. Hemostatic clamps are not necessary at this point, as hemostasis is effected satisfactorily with the electrocautery.

The length of the stoma is sutured by a continuous locking chromic catgut suture on an atraumatic needle (Figs. 15–17). This starts at the inferior angle on the greater curvature and completes the posterior row at the level of the lesser curvature, where a similar suture is continued on the anterior wall of the bowel, mucosa to serosa, and serosa to mucosa. The technique is best illustrated by the series of figures. The person inexperienced in suturing the anterior wall may have difficulty if he misjudges the length of tissue to secure with each bite, for he may find himself with excessive gastric or jejunal wall. This can be avoided by inserting three or four interrupted sutures to subdivide the gastric and jejunal walls, and approximating them in the suturing. Since one begins at the lesser curvature, misjudging the proper placing of sutures may produce a deformity near the efferent loop. Narrowing caused by serosal suturing must absolutely be avoided.

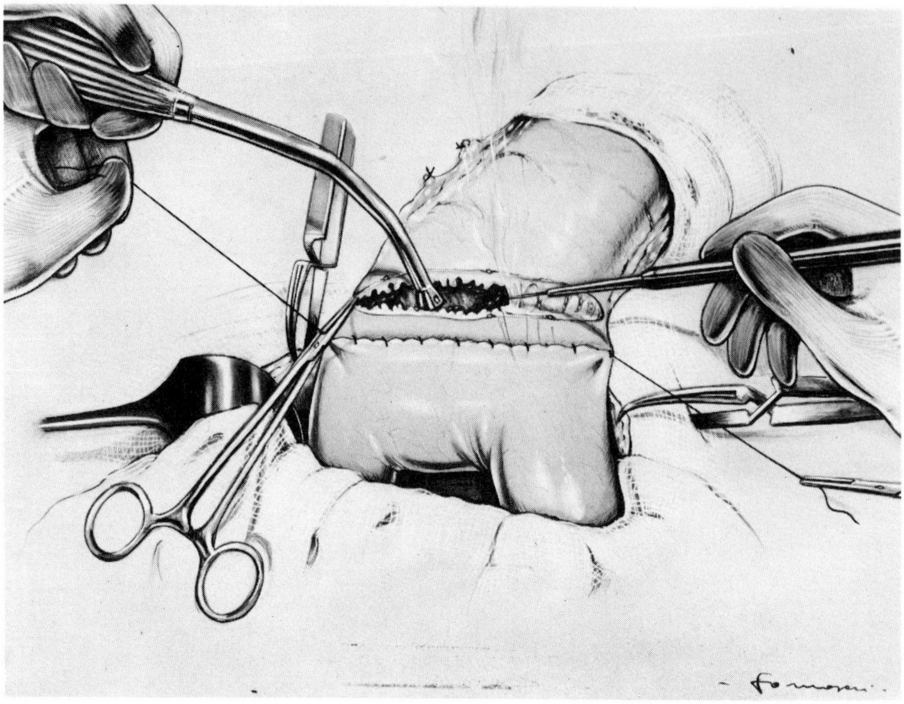

FIGURE 13. Transection of the mucosa of the posterior wall. Clamps on submucosal vessels are not shown.

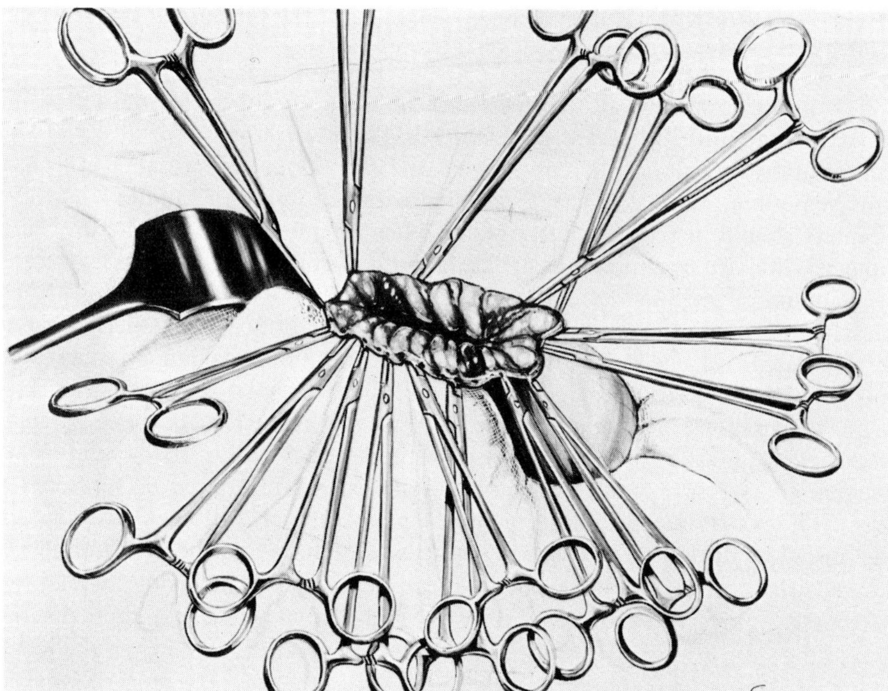

FIGURE 14. The anterior wall has been transected. The clamps provide hemostasis of the submucosal vessels.

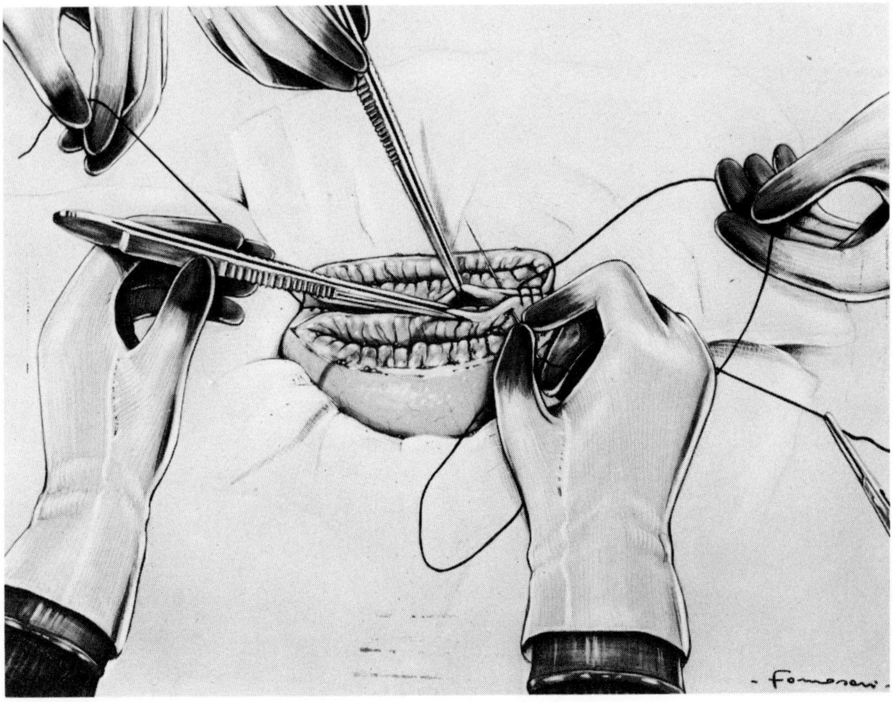

FIGURE 15. Through-and-through continuous lockstitch of chromic catgut (second posterior row of sutures).

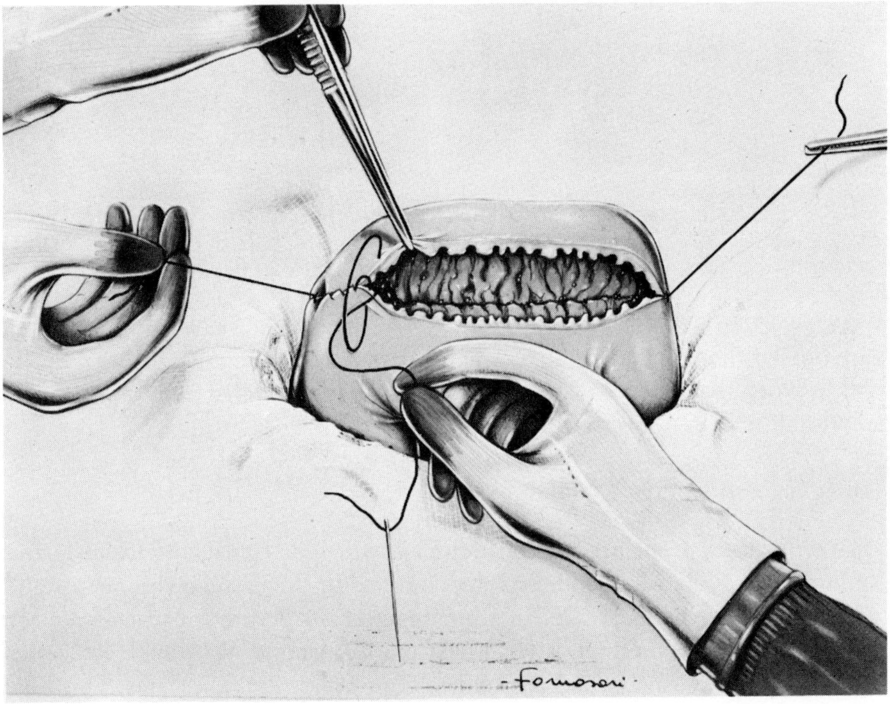

FIGURE 16. Application of the anterior row of sutures.

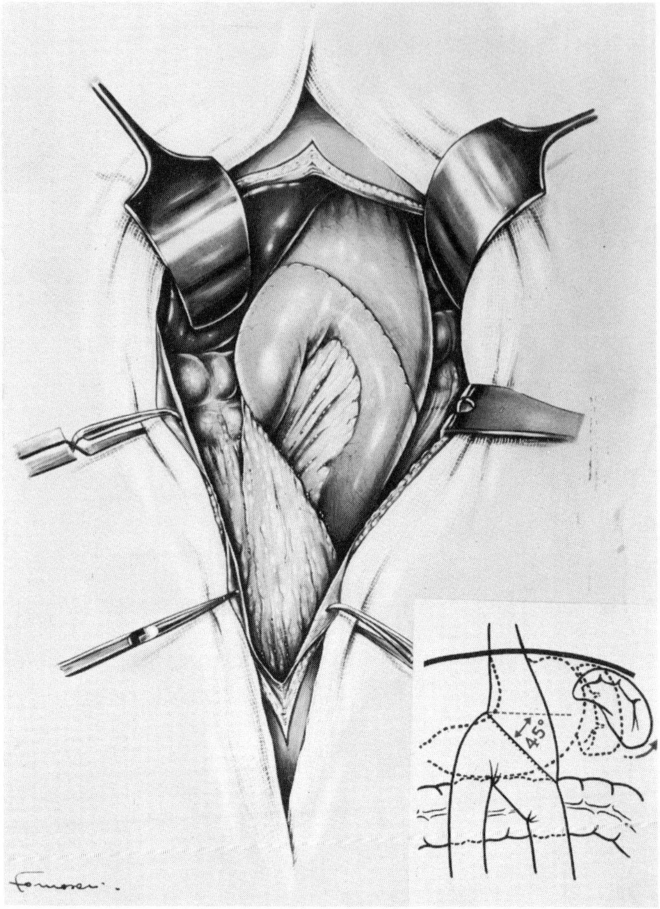

FIGURE 17. The completed anastomosis after application of the second layer of sutures. Note the position of the gastric pouch as it is mobilized from the spleen, the direction of the anastomosis, and the dependent position of the efferent loop.

Before closing the abdomen, one checks for hemostasis. It is also opportune to assure oneself that the loops are not impinged upon in the antemesocolic space. The space between the spleen and the gastric pouch becomes filled with omentum and the left half of the transverse colon.

Closure of the Abdominal Wall

In markedly obese people the peritoneum is closed with a continuous locking suture. The linea alba is closed with interrupted sutures. In thin people chromic catgut is used, and in obese patients silk. An accurate and firm closure is particularly important in these ill patients since early ambulation is desirable. We advise our patients to get out of bed on the second day, unless there are contraindications. This is generally found to be easier for men than for women.

Postoperatively the nasogastric tube is maintained for the first 48 hours. After the first several hours, in which drainage is more or less bloody, the secretion becomes bilious. After the first day the patient drinks water by the spoonful, and a balance is established between the water ingested and the liquid removed through the tube. Usually after the second day less fluid is aspirated through the tube than is taken orally. The tube is clamped before removal. It is opened after 10 to 12 hours, and if a limited or no gastric residual is present the tube is removed. I emphasize that in our entire series we have never needed to reoperate, or to maintain the nasogastric tube for longer than five days. During the first and second days, supplemental fluids are given parenterally according to general surgical principles. On the third day, liquids are taken at will and there is no need for intravenous fluids.

81. *Subtotal Gastric Resection*

EDMUND N. GOODMAN

SUBTOTAL GASTRIC RESECTION, which I recommend as the operation of choice for duodenal ulcer, incorporates the following procedures: (1) a 50 to 75 per cent resection of the stomach, (2) a subdiaphragmatic vagectomy, and (3) a Hofmeister Billroth II antecolic, isoperistaltic, short-looped gastrojejunostomy. The greater omentum is removed with the resected portion of stomach. The approach for the stomach dissection is from above downward, after division of the stomach at the planned line of resection. This facilitates dissection in the area of the duodenum and the head of the pancreas.

Subtotal gastric resection for gastric ulcer may require the same approach if the ulcer is located in the distal half of the stomach. If the ulcer is in the fundus and attached posteriorly, the dissection is facilitated by dividing the duodenum first and approaching the ulcer from below upward. Vagectomy as an adjunct is not indicated as part of the surgical treatment of the benign gastric ulcer.

Often the differential diagnosis between carcinoma and ulcer is inconclusive and therefore it is difficult to choose between subtotal gastric resection and total gastric resection for the high lesser curvature ulcer. Whether to leave the ulcer intact or remove it must often depend upon experienced clinical judgment. Even in the high gastric ulcer, one can usually remove the ulcer-bearing area by subtotal resection as described in this chapter and perform either a Billroth I or a Billroth II gastrojejunostomy as one wishes. I believe that a Billroth I type of anastomosis should not be used in the management of duodenal ulcer.

Subtotal gastric resection for carcinoma, in addition, necessitates removal of the gastrohepatic omentum and, in many cases, associated nodes, the spleen, the tail of the pancreas, and occasionally other neighboring involved structures or parts of structures that are resectable.

Technique

The patient is positioned supine with the head of the table slightly raised so as to gravitate the small intestine caudad. A nasogastric tube has already been passed into the stomach, which is suctioned clean. It is important to have had the patient's gastrointestinal tract cleaned out by catharsis before operation.

The midline incision extends from the left of the xyphoid to the right of the umbilicus. The liver is retracted to the right, using a Harrington retractor. The lesser sac is entered through an avascular area in the gastrohepatic omentum. The first assistant then places his left hand into the lesser sac, exerting caudad traction, thus exposing the branches of the left gastric artery and vein. These are dissected, clamped, cut and ligated with 3–0 silk. The area along the lesser curvature cleared by the dissection is at approximately the level of the splenic vessels.

The greater omentum is then removed from its attachment to the transverse colon (Fig. 1A) as follows. The index and middle fingers of the left hand are introduced into the lesser sac posterior to the stomach, through the cleared opening in the gastrohepatic omentum, and bluntly dissect the stomach from the transverse mesocolon, which is the posterior layer of the lesser sac and contains the midcolic artery (Fig. 2B). Following this maneuver, the operator holds the right portion of the greater omentum in his left hand, and the first assistant holds the transverse colon with his left hand and the left portion of the greater omentum with his right hand. The two-point traction exposes the relatively avascular anterior and posterior attachments of the greater omentum, which are cut from the transverse colon (Fig. 1B).

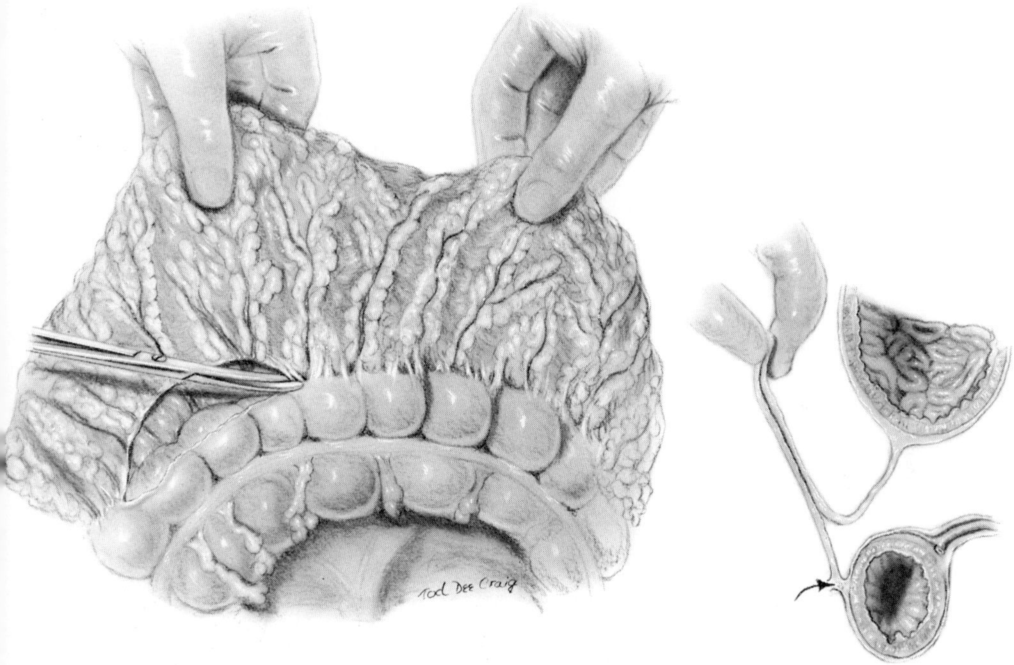

A B

FIGURE 1. (A) Dissection of the greater omentum from the colon. (*B*) Lateral view, showing the plane of dissection. The arrow shows the anterior attachment open. The posterior attachment to the colon will also be incised and the omentum reflected off the mesocolon.

The left gastroepiploic vessels are then dissected, clamped, cut, and tied on the greater curvature of the stomach, at approximately the upper one-quarter.

The level of transection of the stomach is then decided. In the majority of my cases, 60 to 75 per cent of the distal stomach is removed (Fig. 2A). A Payr clamp is placed across the stomach at the desired level and clamped approximately at a 45-degree angle from the greater curvature (Fig. 3). Though at present a 50 per cent resection or antrectomy with vagectomy is popular, I still remove 60 to 75 per cent of the stomach since, in my own series of cases, there has not been significant dumping or weight loss and I believe the greater resection affords better insurance against recurrence. Furthermore, it also has been noted radiologically that after a few months the gastric pouch dilates some 25 to 50 per cent. Angulating the gastrojejunostomy also decreases the stomach emptying time.

Subdiaphragmatic Vagectomy

Vagectomy is the next procedure in the operation for duodenal ulcer. Caudad traction on the Payr clamp flattens the fundus of the stomach and thus exposes the esophagus and the diaphragmatic crura. A Harrington retractor is placed in the region of the left crus of the diaphragm. The left triangular ligament of the liver is cut, and also the posterior parietal peritoneum over the esophagus. Palpation of the inlying nasogastric tube assists in identifying the position of the esophagus before the peritoneum is incised. The right hand, utilizing the first and second fingers, bluntly dissects the lower esophagus. When a finger is initially passed behind the esophagus, care is taken to dissect posterior to the right vagus, which should be identified as one frees the lower esophagus. Downward traction applied to the Payr

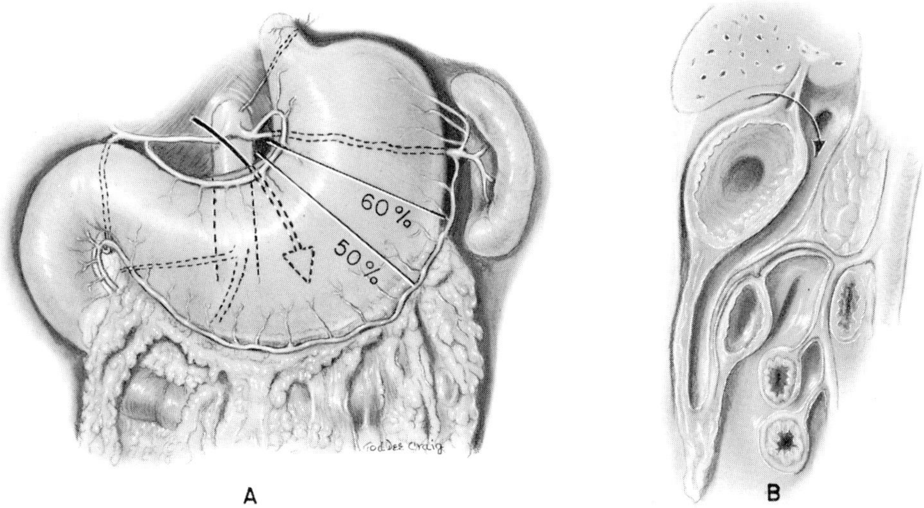

FIGURE 2. (*A*) The approximate levels for stomach resection. (*B*) Sagittal view showing entrance into the lesser sac, which is accomplished prior to dissection of the greater omentum off the colon.

clamp accentuates the tougher consistency of the vagi, which are partly separated from the esophagus by blunt finger dissection. The nerves are then held in the second and third fingers of the right hand. A Wylie clamp is applied to the nerve, and further dissection is done to free the distal 6 to 8 cm. This allows the resection of approximately a 4 cm. length of nerve between ligatures of fine silk. The distal ligatures are tied close to the stomach wall.

Transection of the Stomach

The stomach is next transected between the Payr clamp and a noncrushing horizontally grooved intestinal clamp placed above the Payr for a distance of 4 cm. on the greater curvature portion of the stomach (Fig.3). The lesser curvature portion of the stomach not included in the intestinal clamp is closed with a running 3-0 catgut suture. The first assistant cuts over the Payr clamp, while holding tension on the suture with his other hand. The second assistant manipulates the Payr clamp so as to expose the posterior portion of the stomach and thus facilitate the use of a straight needle for rapid and accurate closure. A second layer of interrupted silk sutures approximates the serosa.

Dissection of the Distal Stomach and the Duodenum

The dissection of the distal stomach and the duodenum is done by manipulating the distal stomach to expose in turn the branches of the right gastric artery and

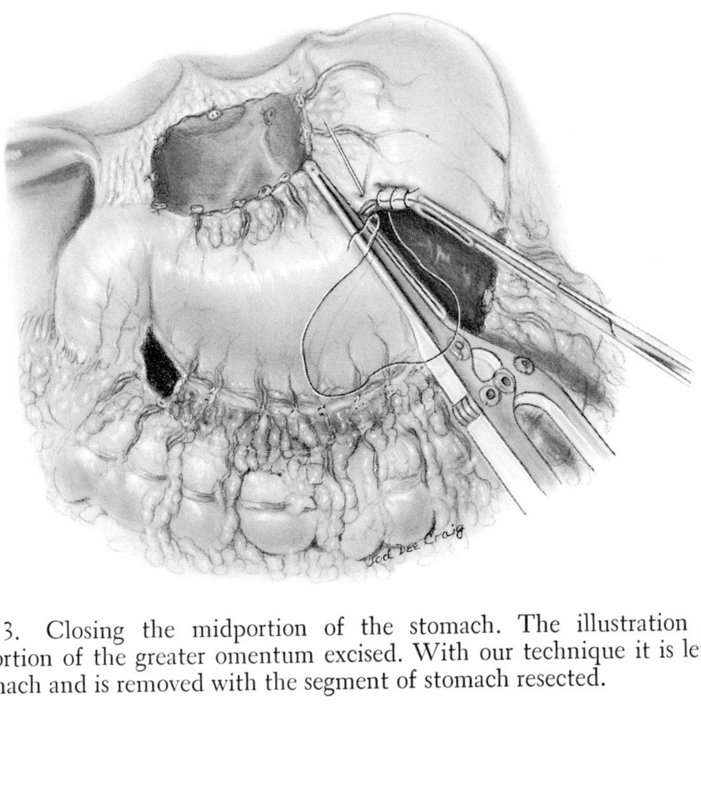

FIGURE 3. Closing the midportion of the stomach. The illustration shows the anterior portion of the greater omentum excised. With our technique it is left attached to the stomach and is removed with the segment of stomach resected.

veins, the right gastroepiploic vessels, and the posterior part of the pylorus and duodenum and the attachments to the pancreas (Fig. 4). In freeing the capsule of the pancreas from the posterior duodenum, straight Halsted clamps should be applied on the small vessels going to the duodenum. One should cut over the clamps and never attempt to underclamp a vessel, since bleeding will surely occur, due to tearing of deeper vessels abundant when this area is inflamed and indurated. The duodenum is cleared for the desired length, which usually includes the ulcer. A straight clamp is then placed across the duodenum and the duodenum is transected distal to the clamp. The distal transected duodenal stump is not clamped.

Ideally, closure of the duodenal stump includes (1) approximation of mucosa to mucosa, without tension, using silk suture material; (2) reinforcement of the mucosal approximation with a layer of interrupted silk sutures approximating seromuscular to seromuscular tissue, or seromuscular to pancreatic capsular tissue; and (3) subsequent construction of a short-looped duodenal-jejunal afferent limb which readily empties the pancreatic and biliary flow into the efferent limb, thereby preventing stasis and back pressure on the duodenal stump closure. (This is facilitated by the removal of the entire greater omentum.)

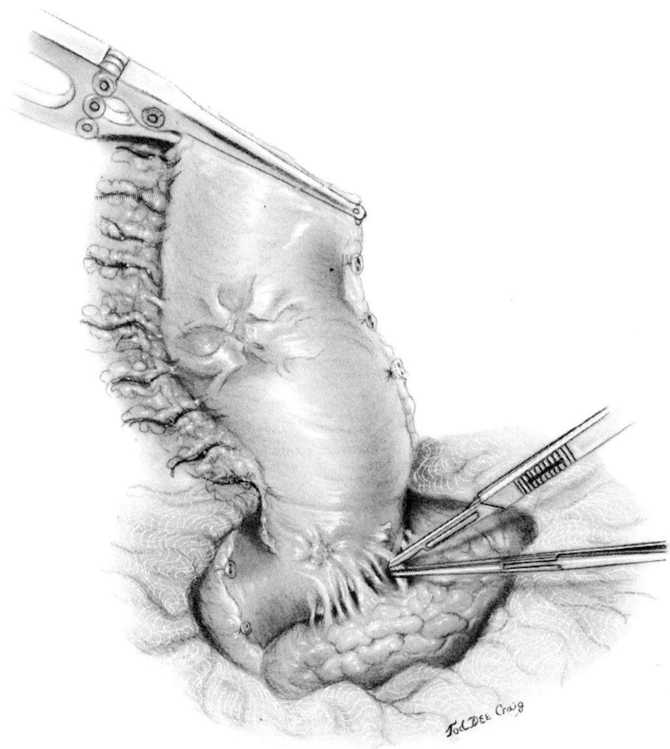

FIGURE 4. The manipulation of the stomach facilitating the posterior dissection of the duodenum from the pancreas and from other attachments in the lesser sac.

However, when the duodenum is edematous and scarred, so that dissection might easily injure the common bile duct, it is better to avoid extensive dissection and perform a duodenostomy about a mushroom catheter (Fig. 5A, B). The technique may involve leaving a portion of the pylorus, reaming out the mucosa, or dissecting the duodenum as shown. H. Harvey described this technique in 1961. This method affords a relatively safe duodenal closure and does not lengthen the morbidity. In fact, it may be a life-saving measure.

If a posterior ulcer has penetrated into the pancreas, the ulcer may be excluded by this technique if satisfactory duodenal wall can be freed distal to the ulcer without dissecting into pancreatic tissue (Fig. 5C). The closure may be safeguarded by a sump drain adjacent to the closure.

If hemorrhage has been one of the major indications for operation for duo-

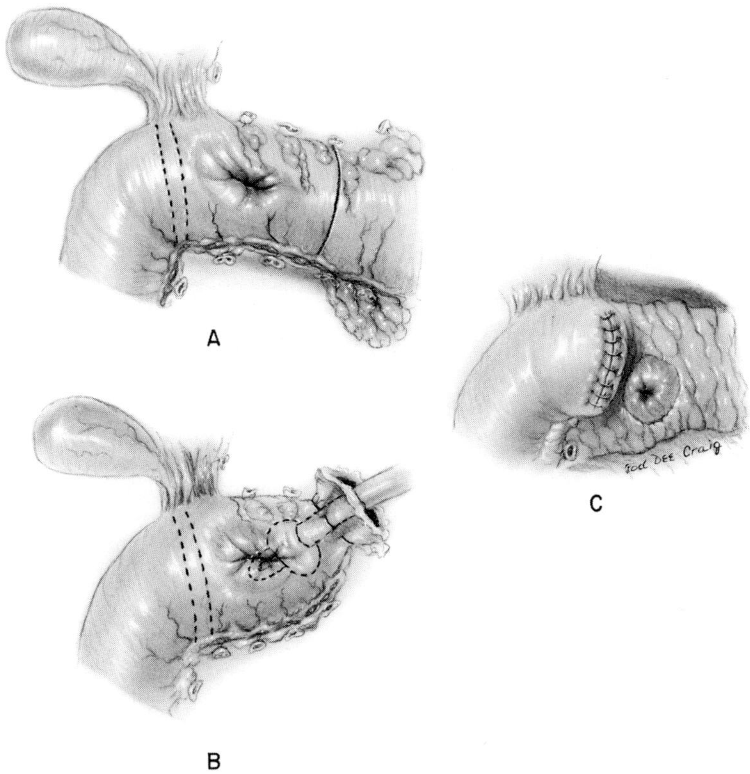

FIGURE 5. (A) Ulcer area, showing shortening of the duodenum in the region of the common duct. The dashed line represents the direction of the common duct. The figure reveals how the duct may be pulled near the ulcer area and could be injured if an attempt were made to remove the ulcer. (In the illustration the first portion of the duodenum has been elongated.) Care should be taken not to devascularize the portion of the pylorus being left in situ. (*B*) Method of leaving the ulcer and draining the duodenal stump with duodenostomy by means of a catheter. We usually employ a mushroom catheter as shown. It is usually removed on the eleventh or twelfth day. (*C*) Exclusion of the ulcer.

denal ulcer, exposure of the ulcer and ligation by figure-of-eight silk suture of the bleeding area is important, especially in patients over 50, if the ulcer cannot be removed.

Gastrojejunostomy

An antecolic, isoperistaltic, short-looped gastrojejunostomy is performed. Having removed the entire greater omentum, and having cleaned out the colon prior to operation, one can easily estimate the length of the short loop. The anastomosis is planned with a stoma 3 to 4 cm. in length (Figs. 6 and 7). The posterior layer of interrupted silk sutures approximating the serosa of the jejunum to the serosa of the stomach must have the jejunal sutures well toward the mesentery on the posterior side as this will place the stoma properly when the anterior layer is approximated.

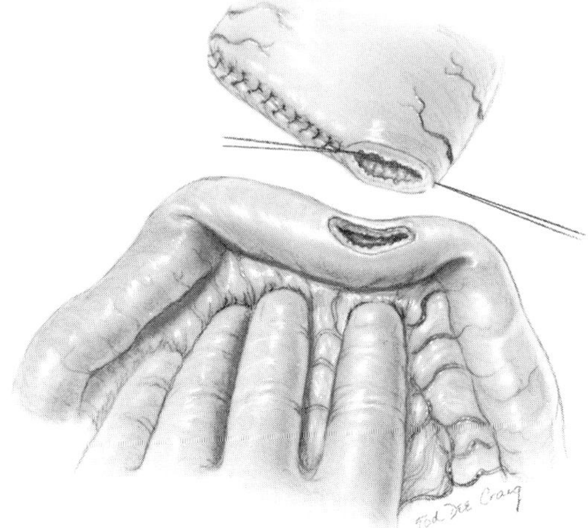

FIGURE 6. The placing of the stoma of the gastrojejunostomy so as to prevent twist of the jejunum. Usually the posterior layer of serosal sutures is placed before the jejunum is incised.

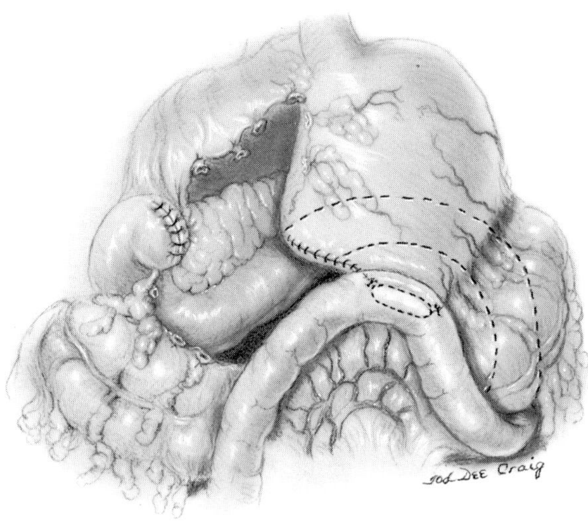

FIGURE 7. Completed anastomosis – short-looped antecolic gastrojejunostomy.

The inner layer of the anastomosis is accomplished with 3–0 catgut. A Penrose drain is placed along the esophagus and lesser curvature and over the duodenal stump.

The abdomen is closed using a continuous 0 chromic catgut suture for the peritoneum, and interrupted 0 chromic catgut sutures for the linea alba. In obese patients or in those with carcinoma, 3–0 Surgilon twisted steel wire, interrupted sutures are used. The skin is closed with a continuous No. 35 stainless steel wire.

Reference

HARVEY, H. Safety in performing partial gastrectomy for gastric ulcer. *Ann. Surg.* 153:256, February 1961.

82. *Benign and Malignant Lesions of the Stomach*

KOMEI NAKAYAMA

Specially Designed Instruments

My aim as a surgeon has been to develop procedures that are simple, practical, and efficient as well as anatomically and physiologically sound. The specially designed instruments we employ in performing gastric, hepatic, or pancreatic surgery are aids to that end. The gastric clamp is a large but relatively simple instrument (Fig. 1A). It serves four purposes: (1) by crushing the stomach it makes the line of resection relatively avascular; (2) it inserts two rows of clips along the line of resection; (3) by sealing both margins of the divided stomach, it reduces the degree of contamination; and (4) it allows a blade, for division of the stomach, to be passed through a slit provided in the clamp. The action of the clamp is similar to that of the common office stapler. Intermittent pressure on each bar sets the double row of clips in place.

The duodenal clamp we use (Fig. 1B) is similar to others such as the Carmalt or Allen. The jaws of our instrument are narrower.

Our two types of crushing clamps vary only in size. One is used on the pancreas and the other on the liver (Fig. 1C) in partial resection of the organ. They have two oval bars which act as jaws. When the clamp is closed tightly the bars approximate each other. Absence of sharp edges makes these clamps especially suitable for the friable tissues of liver and pancreas.

For suture material we at present use silk exclusively: fine silk for anastomoses, medium silk for mass ligations of the omental vessels, and heavy silk for fascia and for mass ligatures in pancreatic and liver resections.

Technique

A midline abdominal incision, extending from the xyphoid to a point approximately 3 cm. to the left of and inferior to the umbilicus, is employed in all our upper gastrointestinal procedures.

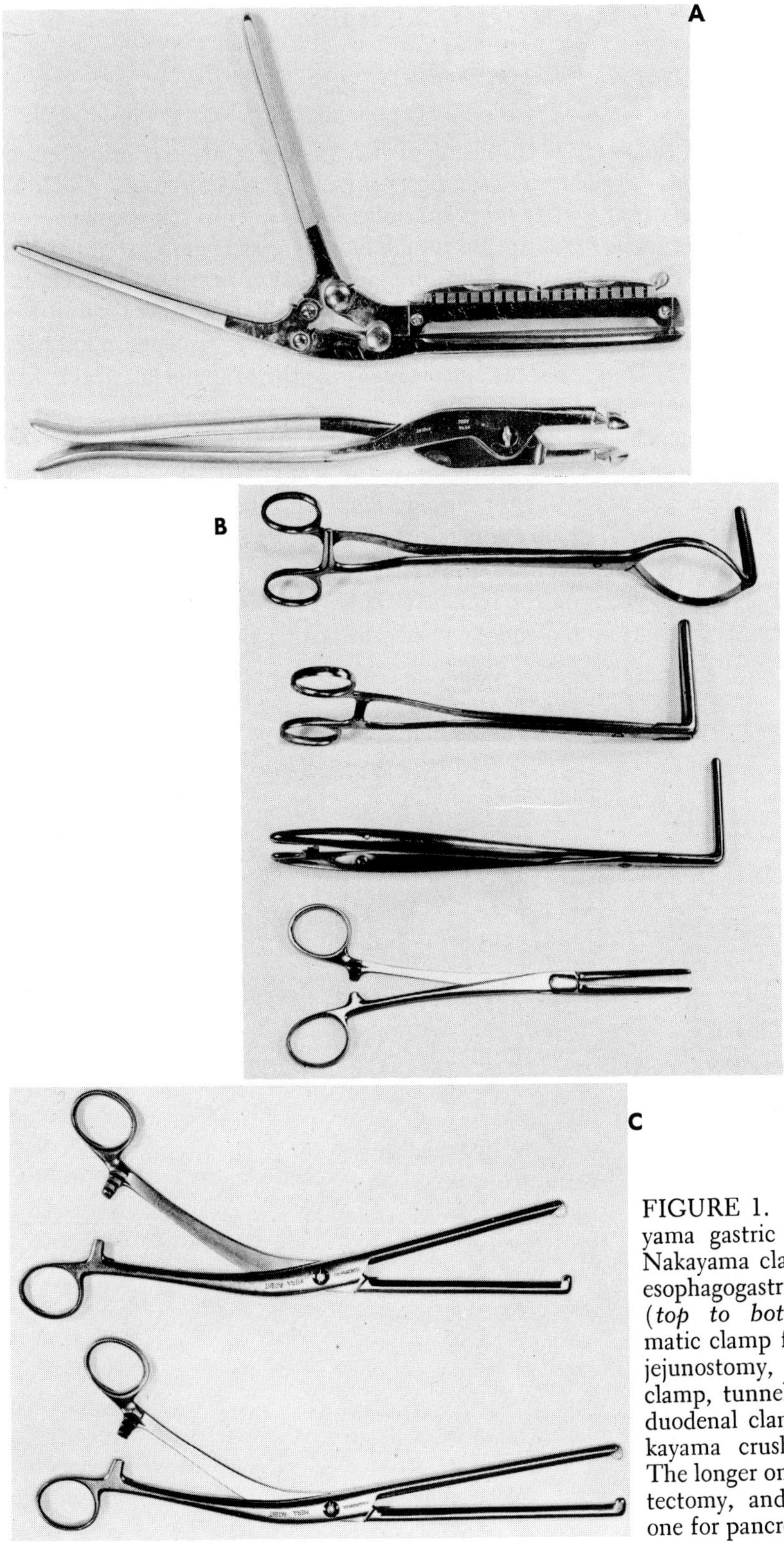

FIGURE 1. (*A*) Nakayama gastric clamp. (*B*) Nakayama clamps used in esophagogastric surgery: (*top to bottom*) atraumatic clamp for esophagojejunostomy, right-angle clamp, tunnel clamp, and duodenal clamp. (*C*) Nakayama crushing clamps. The longer one is for hepatectomy, and the shorter one for pancreatectomy.

Benign Lesions

Vagotomy as part of the surgical treatment of benign peptic ulcer is discussed in other chapters. I will review the technical aspects of gastric resection alone.

SUBTOTAL GASTRECTOMY. *Modified Billroth I Gastrectomy.* It has been our experience with peptic ulcer that the Billroth I type of gastrectomy is widely applicable and gives satisfactory results. Since our modification nearly completely relieves the shortcomings of the conventional Billroth I methods, the location of the lesions and the extent of resection do not present problems, except on rare occasions when there is a large duodenal ulcer involving the ampulla of Vater or a gastric ulcer encroaching upon the esophagus.

The normal stomach is fixed at two points, one at the esophagus and the other at the duodenum. In partial gastrectomy, the fixation at the pyloric end is destroyed. Therefore I compensate for this by employing fixation sutures. These pass from the posterior wall of the stomach through the pancreatic capsule adjacent to the duodenum. They should be inserted very carefully. Shallow but wide bites of tissue should be taken on the pancreatic side. The bites should include the tissues overlying the pancreas, and should avoid penetrating the pancreatic tissue to

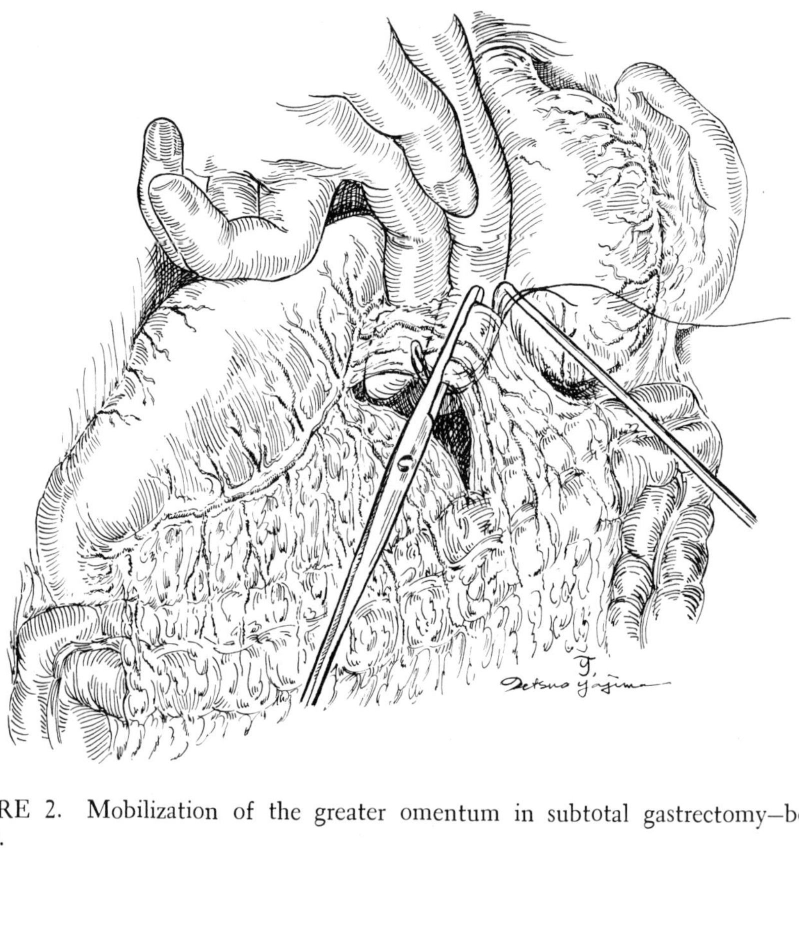

FIGURE 2. Mobilization of the greater omentum in subtotal gastrectomy—benign lesions.

a depth that could result in leakage of pancreatic juice. These fixation sutures serve several purposes: they seal the anastomosis posteriorly, they support the stomach, they relieve tension on the anastomosis, and they fix the distal end of the stomach so that the postoperative function will approximate the normal. The usual posterior serosal row of inverting sutures is eliminated, and the likelihood of postoperative stenosis at the anastomosis is greatly reduced. This principle of fixation is employed in all our upper gastrointestinal techniques, which in other respects involve only minor variations from traditional methods.

An opening is made in the midportion of the greater omentum, and the posterior surface of the stomach is explored. The greater omentum is divided. Ligatures on the omentum are placed distal to the gastroepiploic arch (Fig. 2). Silk ligatures are used on the colic side, but hemostats are left in place on the gastric side to save time. Care is taken to avoid injuring the middle colic artery. The mesocolon is separated from the posterior leaf of the greater omentum by blunt dissection. Adhesions, which are rather common over the posterior aspect of the stomach, are also freed. As the dissection proceeds toward the pylorus, the first portion of the duodenocolic ligament is freed and divided. Traction on the duodenal side of the cut ligament exposes the right gastroepiploic artery. This is ligated adjacent to the duodenum and as close to its origin as possible (Fig. 3). Small vessels at the inferior margin of the duodenum may require ligation for adequate mobilization. The stomach is elevated and the surgeon's left hand is passed behind the antrum. The lesser omentum is opened by the fingers of the left hand, and the right gastric artery

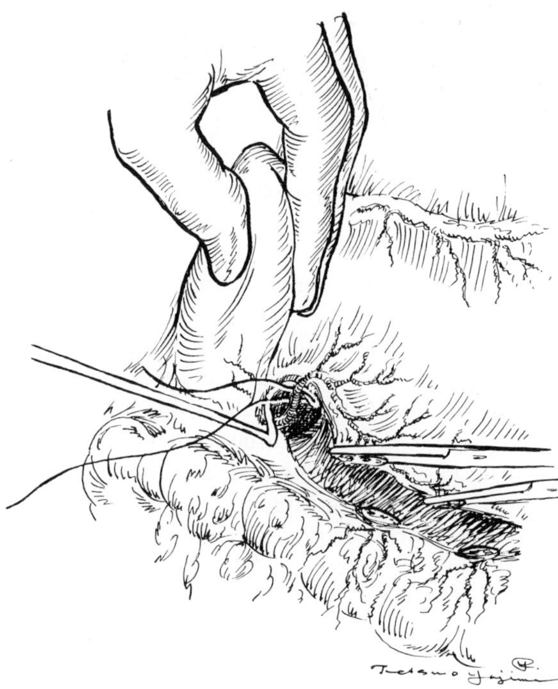

FIGURE 3. Ligation of the right gastroepiploic artery–benign lesions.

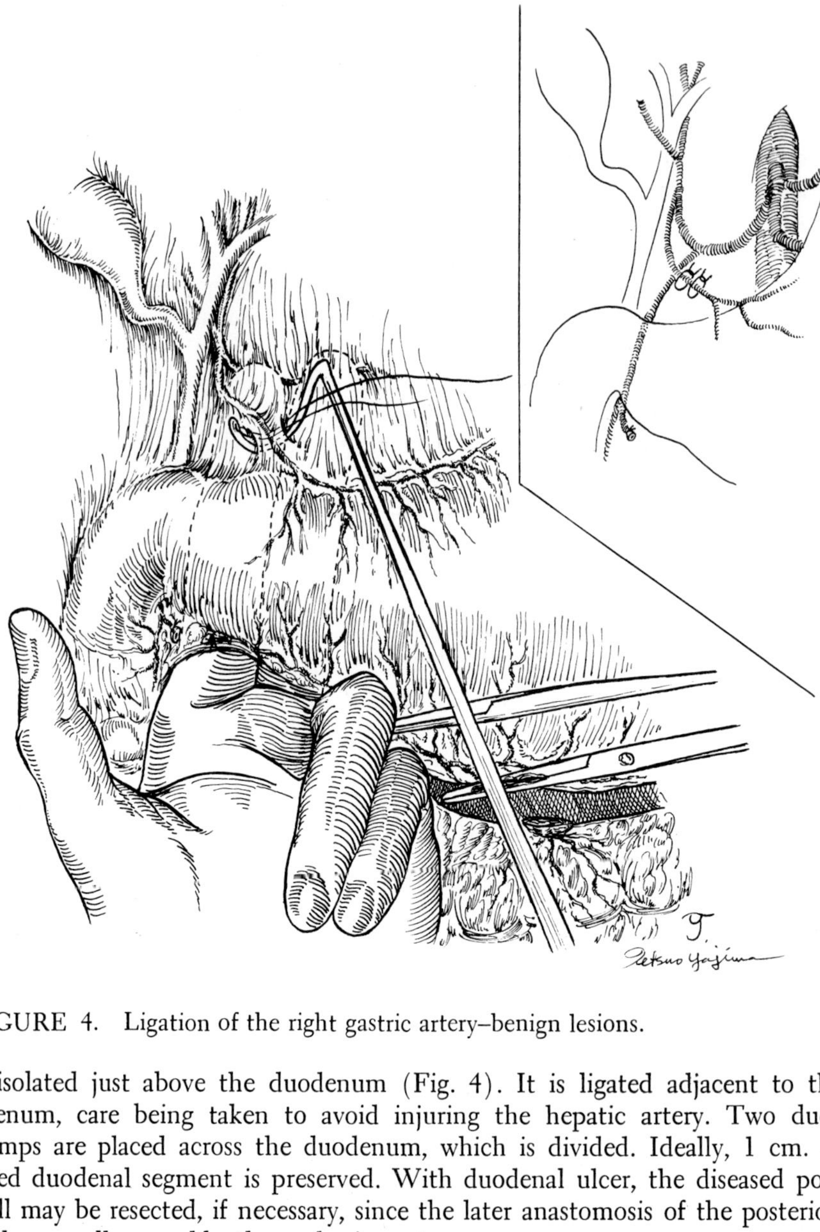

FIGURE 4. Ligation of the right gastric artery–benign lesions.

is isolated just above the duodenum (Fig. 4). It is ligated adjacent to the duodenum, care being taken to avoid injuring the hepatic artery. Two duodenal clamps are placed across the duodenum, which is divided. Ideally, 1 cm. of the freed duodenal segment is preserved. With duodenal ulcer, the diseased posterior wall may be resected, if necessary, since the later anastomosis of the posterior wall is always well secured by the anchoring sutures.

The pyloric end of the stomach is retracted upward and the inferior branches of the left gastric artery with its accompanying veins are doubly ligated on the lesser curvature just distal to their bifurcation (Fig. 5). A third ligature is placed distal to the planned line of resection, since a hemostat at that point would interfere with the proper placement of the gastric clamp. The vessels are then divided. The line of resection is prepared by stripping the fat and dividing other vessels crossing that area. We usually remove approximately 70 per cent of the stomach.

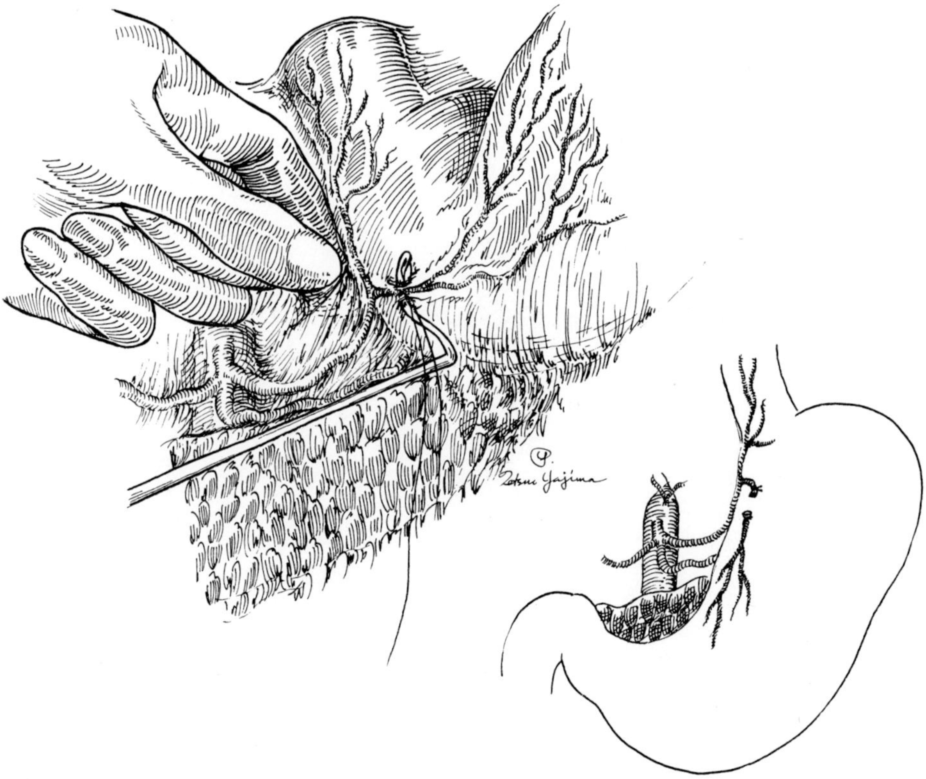

FIGURE 5. Ligation of the left gastric artery–benign lesions.

The greater curvature is mobilized to the planned point of resection by ligation and division of the greater omentum. The short gastric arteries in the gastrosplenic ligament are preserved. Adhesions over the posterior aspect of the fundus are freed by blunt dissection. The stomach is held up and a duodenal clamp is placed perpendicular to the greater curvature at the site of the intended gastroduodenostomy. The gastric clamp is applied just distal to the duodenal clamp (Fig. 6). The staples are inserted and the stomach divided. The cut margin of the gastric remnant is treated with tincture of iodine. Traction is placed on the stomach by means of the duodenal clamp, and the row of staples above the duodenal clamp (the lesser curvature side) is reinforced with a continuous running seroserosal suture, which inverts the row of clips. The suture is tied when it reaches the tip of the duodenal clamp. The remainder of the procedure is facilitated by performing a rather extensive Kocher maneuver freeing the lateral attachments of the second portion of the duodenum.

Four sutures attaching the gastric remnant to the head of the pancreas are now placed (Fig. 7). The primary purpose is to eliminate any undue tension at the gastroduodenostomy. Accurate positioning of these fixation sutures is of the utmost importance. The first stitch picks up the sealed margin of the gastric remnant, about 1.5 cm. from the anastomosis, and the pancreatic capsule, about 0.5 to

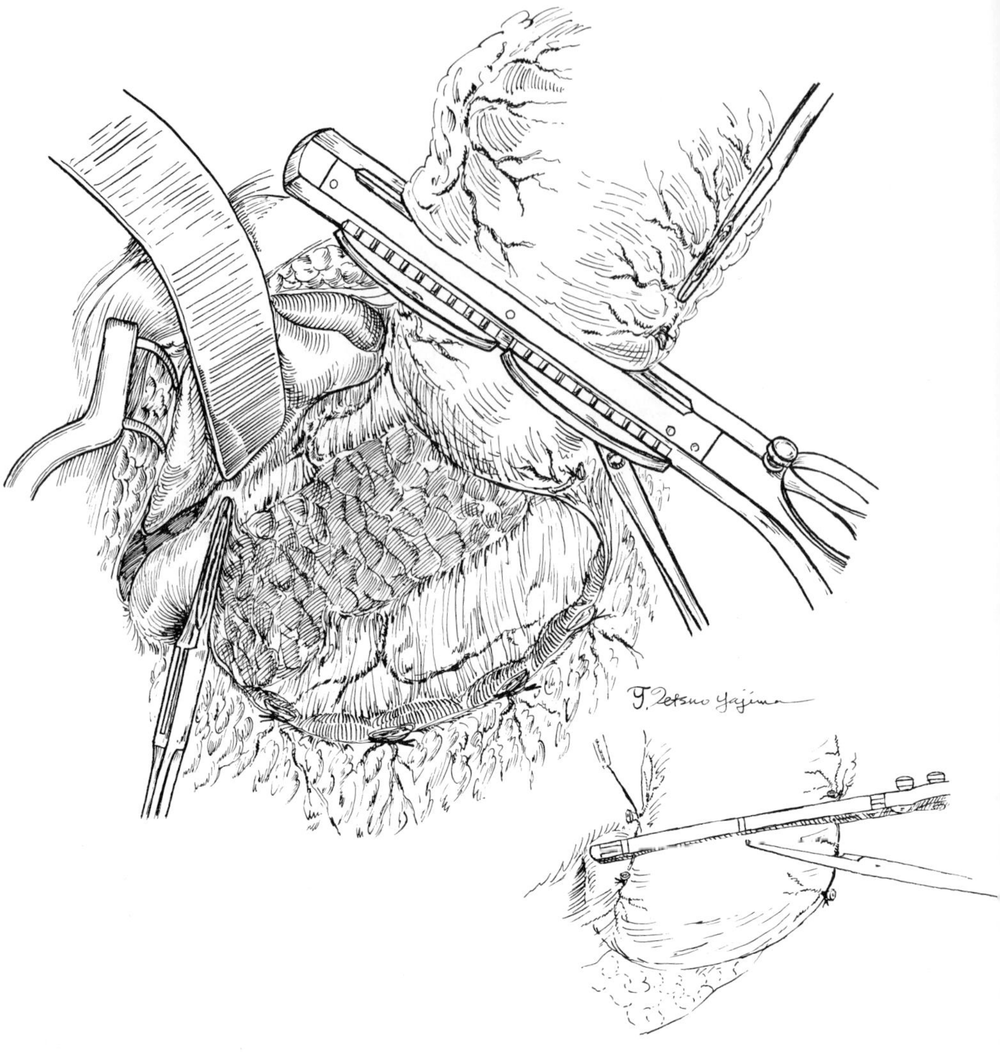

FIGURE 6. Application of the gastric clamp for resection of the stomach.

1 cm. from the superior border of the duodenum. The next two sutures are placed parallel to the duodenal clamp through the posterior serosa of the stomach, about 1.5 cm. from the duodenal clamp. The fourth suture should be placed about 0.5 cm. posterior to the lower margin of the gastric remnant. These sutures are passed through the pancreas 1 cm. from the duodenal stump in the same plane as the long axis of the duodenum. The third suture should be placed just to the right of the ligated right gastroepiploic artery, if possible, to keep the arterial stump away from the posterior anastomosis line. The fourth suture is passed through the pancreas inferior to and beyond the duodenal stump. It should be approximately 1.5 cm. to the right of the ligated right gastroepiploic artery. These sutures should be shallow but the bite should be wide (about 1 cm.). All sutures are placed before they are

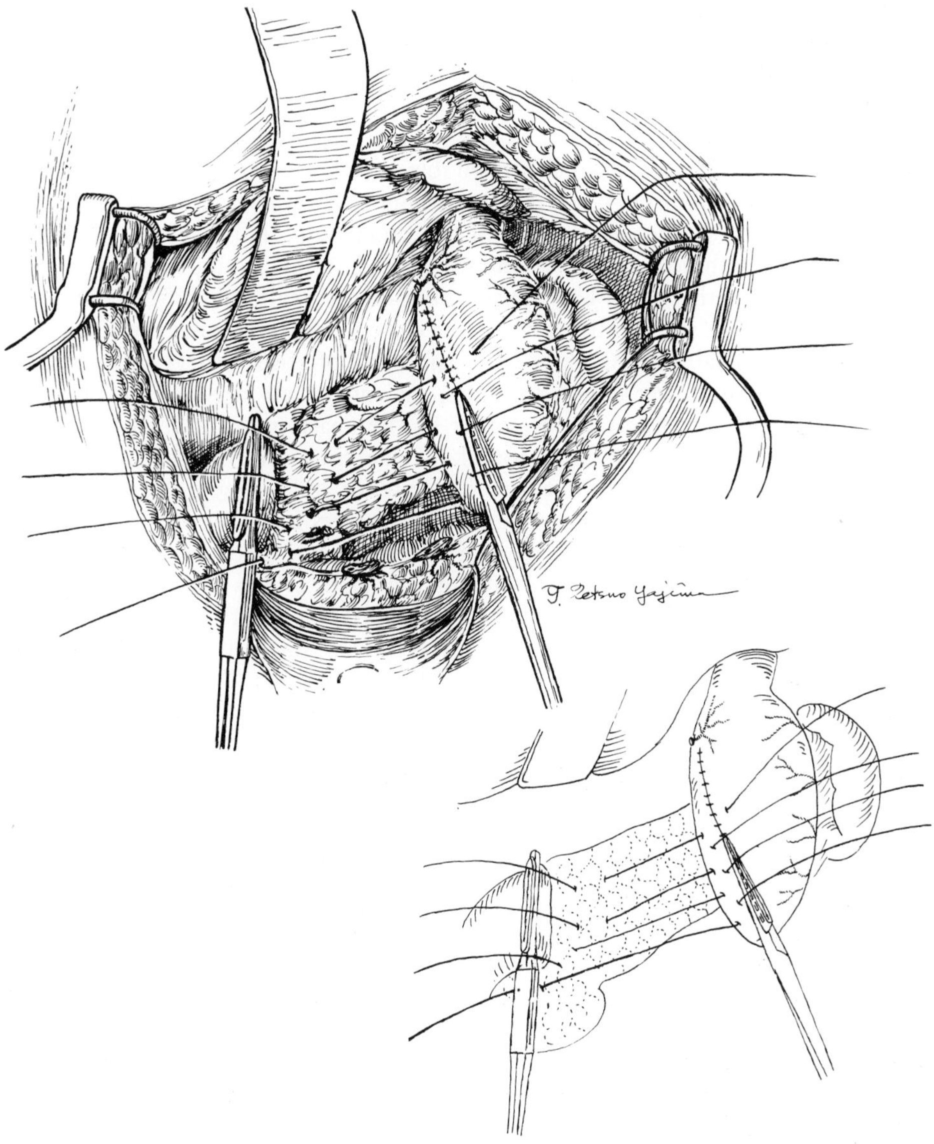

FIGURE 7. Placing of four fixation sutures in the simplified Billroth I type of gastrectomy.

tied. If bleeding is encountered while one is passing a suture through the pancreas, that suture should be tied at once.

The contents of the gastric remnant is aspirated by a nasogastric tube, which has been in place. An atraumatic intestinal clamp is placed across the stomach to prevent spillage and to reduce bleeding. The tissue distal to the duodenal clamp, on the stomach, is trimmed away. Both duodenal clamps are then released. Usually, the inferior corner of the duodenum is grasped and the midanterior edge of the gastric stoma is picked up to facilitate placement of the posterior through-and-through row of suture. A long strand of fine silk which will be the anterior serosal suture is placed through the closed gastric edge (approximately 0.5 cm. from the anastomosis) and then through the head of the pancreas above the first fixation suture. It is left untied. It is placed at this time because it would be difficult to do so after placement of the through-and-through row of sutures (Fig. 8A).

The through-and-through row of silk is begun at the upper corner of the gastric stoma and carried through the corner of the duodenum. This stitch is placed so that the knot is within the lumen of the stomach. The silk should be a long strand with a needle on either end. The upper corner of the anastomosis is a potentially weak point. The first stitch must therefore be close to the seroserosal row of sutures that covers the metal staples, and a fairly large bite of tissue is taken. The silk is then run in a simple over-and-over fashion, picking up all layers of the stomach and the duodenum, to the inferior corner of the anastomosis. The last stitch is locked and tagged by a clamp, but not tied. The anterior wall is closed similarly, no attempt being made to invert the edges. The anterior and posterior strands are tied together and tagged. The through-and-through sutures are placed so that a relatively larger portion of the serosa than of the mucosa is taken (Fig. 8B). These sutures are placed close together (0.5 cm.) and a larger bite is taken on the gastric side than on the duodenal side. Sufficient tension is applied to the sutures to accomplish proper hemostasis. When the duodenum is small, it is usually divided obliquely, and its inferior corner is pulled down while the through-and-through sutures are being placed. If this does not give the required dimension, a small incision is made perpendicular to the stump near its inferior margin. It will be noted that often some of the gastric mucosa everts through the suture line. This should be trimmed away. The anterior serosal suture, which has already been started, is now completed. Traction on the tagged ends of the through-and-through sutures will rotate the anastomosis and expose the superior surface of the duodenum. The suture that was passed through the stomach and the head of the pancreas is now carried through the serosa of the superior surface of the duodenum and tied (Fig. 8C). The serosal row is a Lembert suture. The bites on the gastric side are larger than those on the duodenal side so that the anastomotic line will be covered with gastric serosa (unless the gastric serosa is fragile). The last stitch picks up the inferior border of the stomach (slightly posterior to the attachment of the greater omentum on the greater curvature), the head of the pancreas (slightly to the right of and inferior to the fourth fixation suture), and the inferior border of the duodenum, sealing the anastomosis completely (Fig. 8D).

We have found that if the anastomosis lies to the left of the vertebral column and at approximately a 45-degree angle, there will rarely be postprandial symptoms (Fig. 9). The Kocher maneuver may require an extension to permit this placement.

Billroth II Gastrectomy. In very rare circumstances, we have occasion to perform a Billroth II gastrectomy for benign lesions. When this type is indicated, a retrocolic anastomosis is usually performed without enteroenterostomy. The stomach is transected with our gastric clamp, and the lesser curvature side of the gastric remnant is closed as in the Billroth I procedure. A proximal jejunal loop is brought

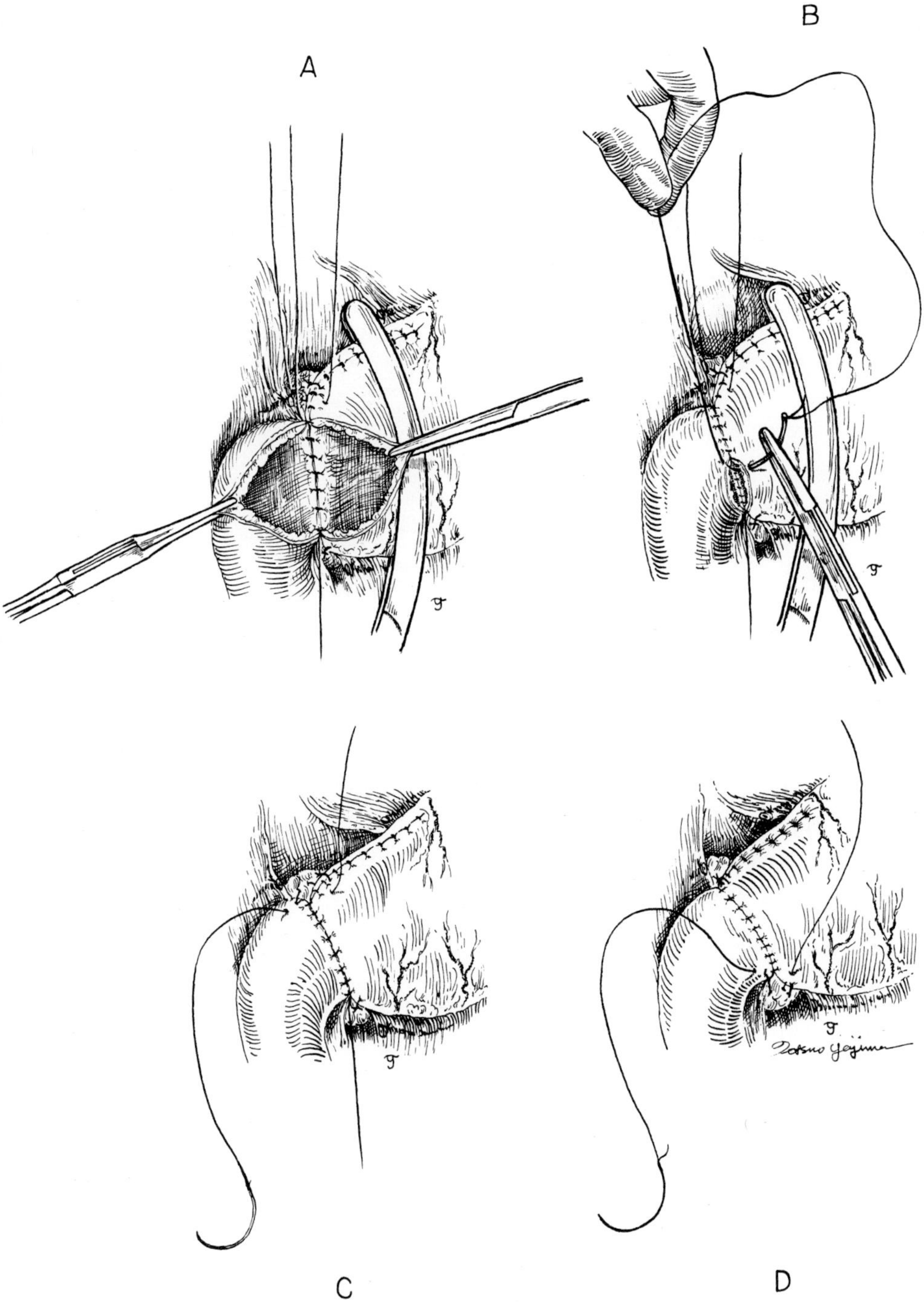

FIGURE 8. Technique of gastroduodenostomy in the simplified Billroth I type of gastrectomy. (*A*) Placement of silk strand to be used for the anterior serosal suture. (*B*) Placement of through-and-through suture. (*C*) Completion of the anterior serosal suture. (*D*) Final stitch sealing the anastomosis.

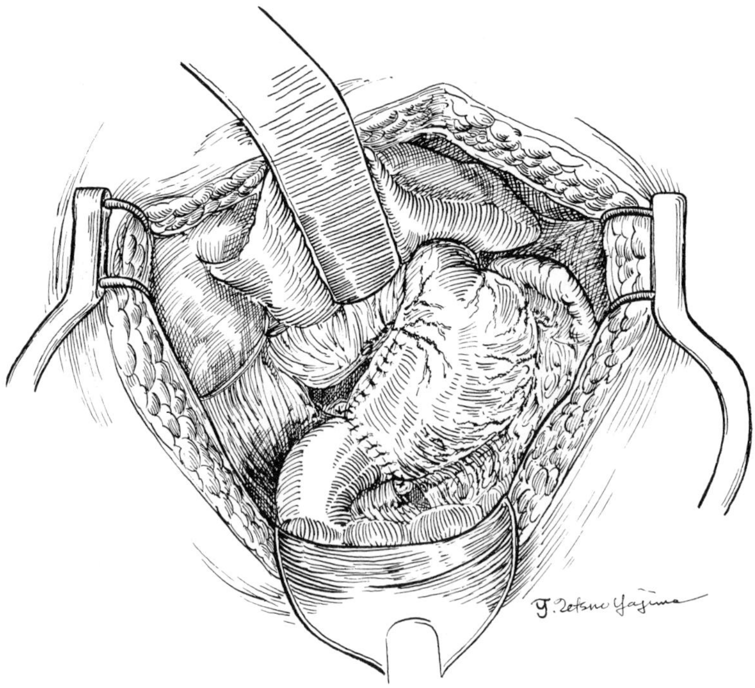

FIGURE 9. Completed anastomosis.

through a rent in the transverse mesocolon. The afferent limb is fixed to the sealed gastric margin for a few centimeters (for a better evacuation of gastric contents), while the efferent limb is anastomosed to the greater curvature side. A two-layer anastomosis is performed. The stomach is fixed to the opening in the mesocolon. Treatment of the duodenal stump is covered under Total Gastrectomy.

Malignant Lesions

Subtotal Gastrectomy. It has been our experience, in treating carcinoma of the pylorus and some carcinomas of the body of the stomach, that subtotal resection, extirpation of the regional lymphatics, and excision of the greater omentum will yield survival rates equal to those of total gastrectomy, provided a wide margin of normal tissues is taken. The postoperative status of patients having subtotal resections is far superior to that following total gastrectomy.

When a malignant neoplasm is found and subtotal resection is decided upon, the greater omentum is freed from the transverse colon (Fig. 10). The marginal arteries are preserved and little bleeding will be encountered. Freeing the omentum from the gastrosplenic ligament to the first portion of the duodenum is usually adequate. The procedure continues as for benign lesions except for the removal of lymph node metastases. Subpyloric lymphatics are often involved; these should be removed en bloc (Fig. 11). Along the celiac axis, metastatic nodes are rather frequent. They are freed from their medial attachments and dissected toward the

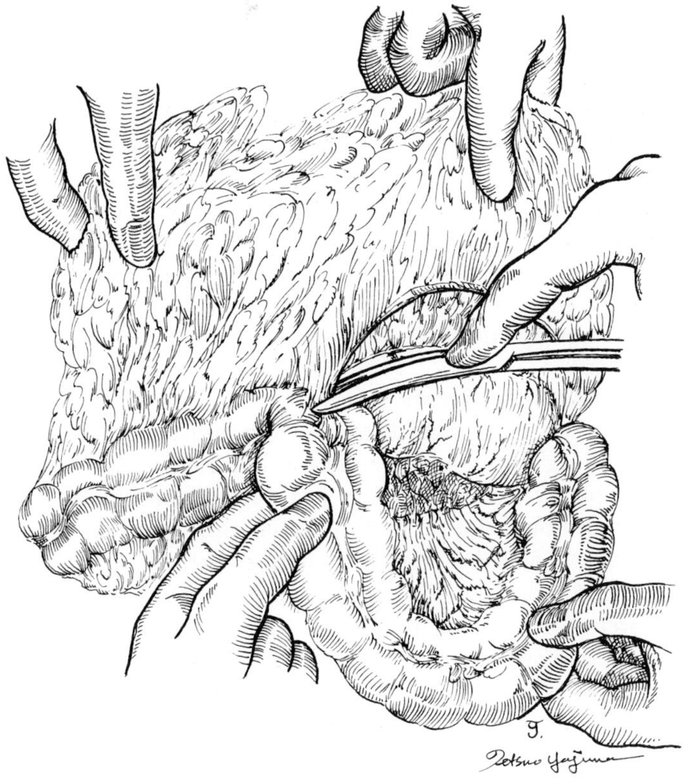

FIGURE 10. Mobilization of the greater omentum in subtotal gastrectomy for malignant lesions.

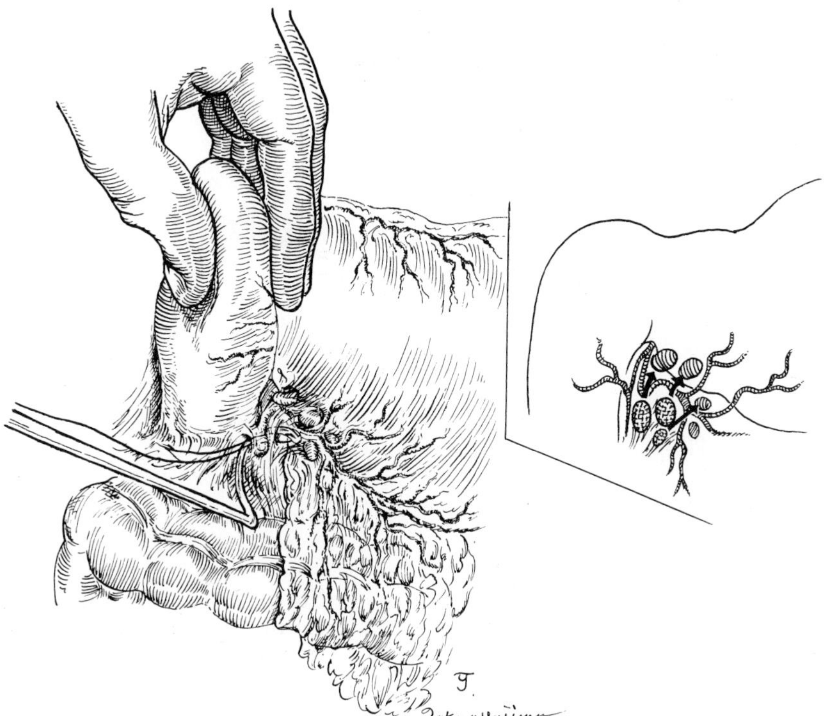

FIGURE 11. Ligation of the right gastroepiploic artery and dissection of subpyloric nodes—malignant lesions.

lesser curvature so that they may be removed en bloc with the stomach and greater omentum (Fig. 12). The left gastric artery is ligated and divided as close to its origin as possible (Fig. 13). Occasionally, metastatic lymph nodes will be found in the porta hepatis, the paracardiac lymphatics, and the gastrosplenic ligament. Division of the vagus nerve at the cardiac end allows delivery of the cardiac portion to a considerable degree, and mobilization of the paracardiac lymphatics is greatly facilitated (Fig. 14). To achieve a possible cure, these metastatic sites must be removed en bloc, if feasible. Continuity of the gastrointestinal tract is re-established by gastroduodenostomy or gastrojejunostomy as in subtotal gastrectomy for benign lesions.

Resection of the Cardia of the Stomach. This operation will rarely be indicated for benign lesions. Malignant diseases of the cardia and of the distal end of the esophagus (the lower 3 cm.) may be effectively treated in this manner. Preservation of a portion of the stomach, in this instance the antrum, greatly improves the postoperative nutritional state. For this reason this operation is preferable to total gastrectomy and should be performed whenever there is a choice between them. When this operation is applied to benign lesions the only variation is the omission of the steps for handling metastatic lymphatics or invaded adjacent organs. The operation for malignant disease will be described.

With malignant lesions the usual abdominal incision is made and resectability is determined. An opening in the anterior leaf of the greater omentum will be helpful in deciding operability and the extent of the procedure. Once a radical

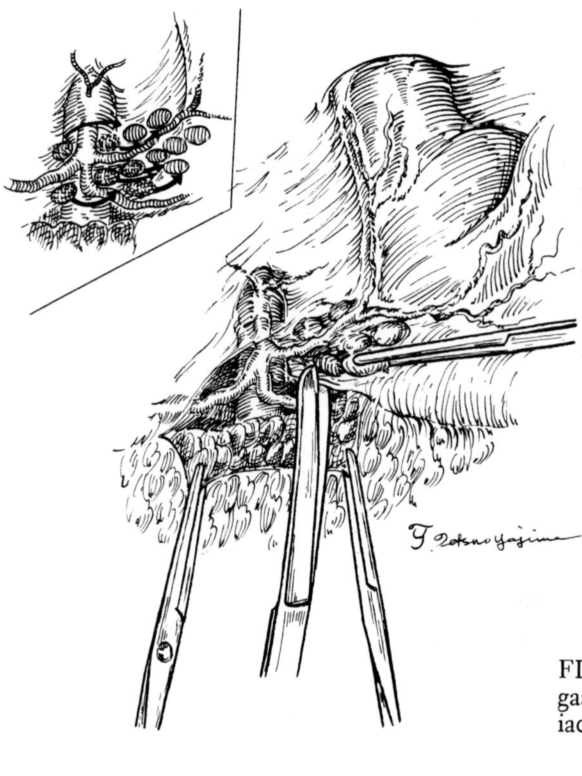

FIGURE 12. Ligation of the left gastric artery and dissection of celiac nodes—malignant lesions.

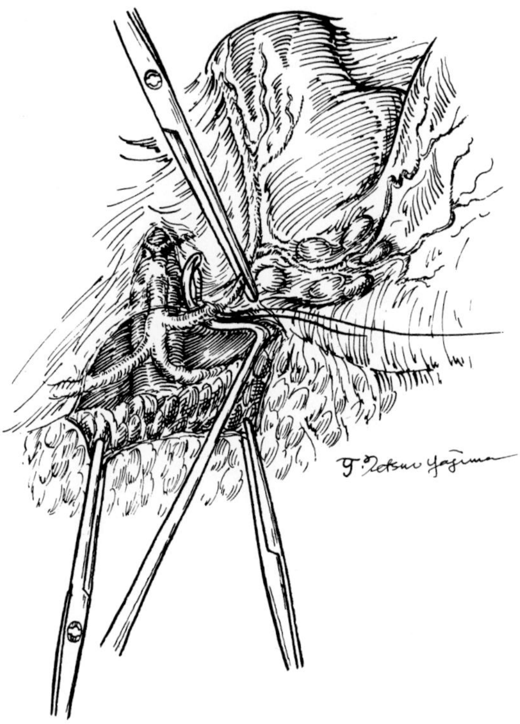

FIGURE 13. Division of the left gastric artery—malignant lesions.

operation is decided upon, the greater omentum is freed from its attachments to the transverse colon. The detachment is carried out from the midtransverse colon to the splenic flexure. When there is rather marked infiltration of the omentum more of the structure may be removed. The line of transection of the stomach is determined and the vessels of the greater and lesser curvatures at that line are

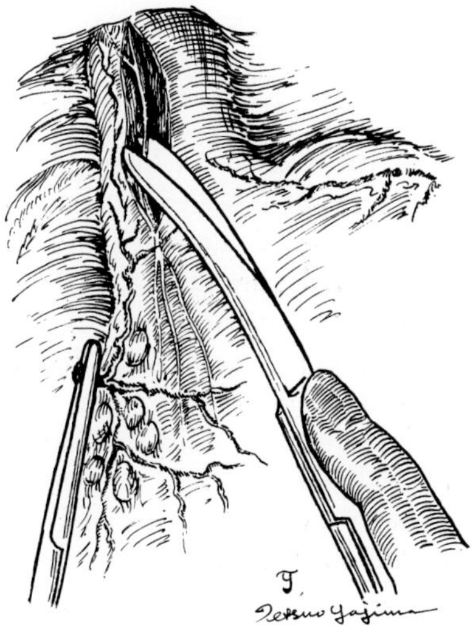

FIGURE 14. Division of the vagus nerve to deliver the cardiac end for easier manipulation in cases of malignant lesions.

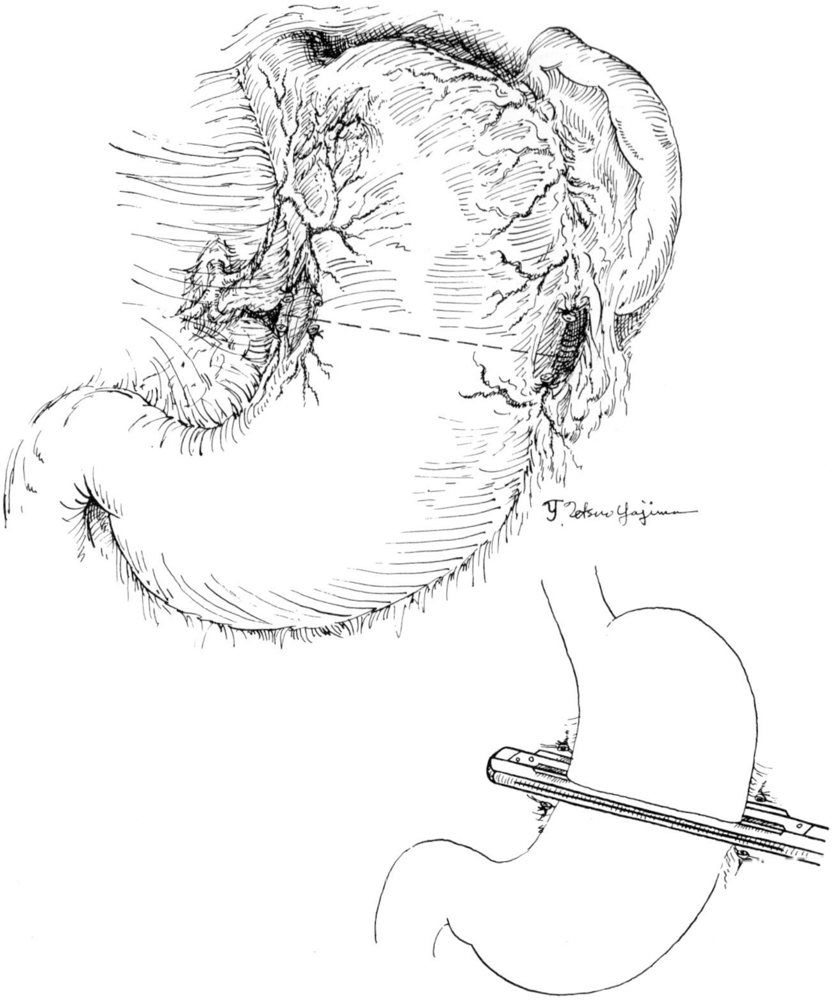

FIGURE 15. Application of the gastric clamp for resection of the cardiac portion of the stomach.

ligated (Fig. 15). The gastric clamp is applied across the transection line and the stomach is divided. The stapled margin of the distal segment is sealed with an inverting, continuous, seroserosal row of suture. The celiac axis is identified and the left gastric artery is doubly ligated at its origin. Involved nodes are dissected toward the stomach and removed with as much lesser omentum as is necessary. As the dissection continues along the lesser curvature toward the esophageal hiatus, the inferior phrenic artery is encountered. This is ligated and divided. The right vagus nerve is divided as high as possible at this point, and downward traction on the stomach delivers the lower esophagus into the abdominal cavity. This allows better exposure of the paracardiac lymph nodes, which are usually involved and should be removed. The peritoneal reflection from the diaphragm over the esophagocardiac junction is divided, preserving as much tissue as possible, so that it may be used for the anterior serosal covering of the anastomosis. The gastrosplenic ligament is divided close to the spleen. Very little mobilization of the esophagus passing through the hiatus is necessary for the intraabdominal procedure. The esophagus is held in the abdomen by traction and a right-angle clamp with longitudinal striations is placed across it proximal to the cardiac junction. A second clamp is placed just distal to the first clamp, and the esophagus is then divided between these instruments. It should be remembered that no more than the distal 3 cm. of the esophagus may be removed by the abdominal route. The divided margins of the esophagus are treated with iodine solution, and the resected specimen is delivered.

We employ several types of anastomosis in restoring the continuity of the gastrointestinal tract following this procedure and following total gastrectomy: esophagogastrostomy, Billroth II, jejunal transplant, Roux en Y, esophagojejunostomy and most recently our new beta anastomosis. We will describe first our technique of esophagogastrostomy and then our use of esophagojejunostomy. Esophagogastrostomy is the simplest repair, but in our experience shows a slightly higher incidence of postoperative stenosis than esophagojejunostomy.

Esophagogastrostomy. The distal segment of the stomach has already been sealed with a row of inverting sutures. When esophagogastrostomy is anticipated, a duodenal clamp is placed on the greater curvature side of the stomach prior to the transection of that organ. The clamp marks the stoma of the gastric side of the anastomosis, and the inverting suture row that seals the distal segment is not carried beyond the tip of this clamp. The duodenal clamp is replaced with a right-angle clamp, and the redundant tissues and clips which are at the side of the intended anastomosis are trimmed away before one begins the anastomosis. The stump of the gastric remnant is then approximated to the stump of the esophagus. Three fixation sutures are placed (Fig. 16). They relieve tension on the anastomosis. The sutures pass through the stomach about 1 cm. distal to the blade of the right-angle clamp and parallel to the line of the anastomosis. On the esophageal side the first and third should pick up tissue of the crura of the diaphragm and the peritoneal reflection of the diaphragm posteriorly. The second (central) suture should pick up the peritoneum of the diaphragm and the posterior wall of the esophagus, about 2 cm. proximal to the anastomosis. We have found it easier to place the posterolateral suture first, then the second directly behind the anastomosis, and the third posteromedially. All the sutures are placed before they are tied. The bites should be wide and shallow. If a suture is passed too deeply through the diaphragm, one may pick up the pericardium. This should be avoided.

Positioning the stomach for this anastomosis is of major importance. The posterior wall of the anastomosis will be the most vulnerable area, because of the small number of sutures placed in the serosal layer—only the three fixation sutures. For this reason, the greater curvature edge of the anastomosis on the gastric side should be brought posterior. This area will have the best blood supply, and therefore healing should be most rapid in it. The middle fixation suture is cut after being tied. The other two are tagged for orientation purposes. The right-angle clamps are removed. Although most surgeons use interrupted sutures,

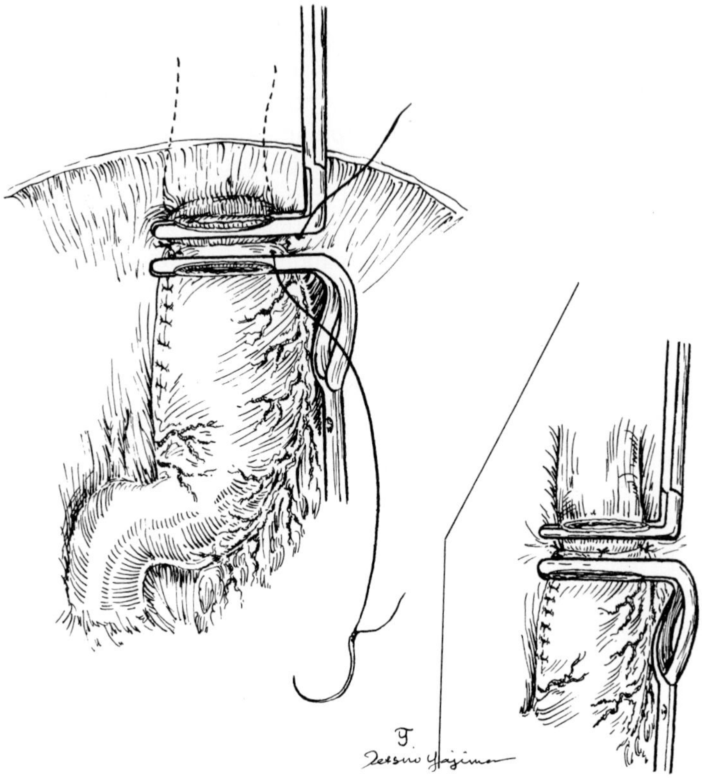

FIGURE 16. Placing of the three fixation sutures in esophagogastrostomy.

we prefer a continuous through-and-through suture of fine silk for the inner layer of the anastomosis (Fig. 17A). We usually begin the anastomosis near the mid-point of the posterior wall. After the first stitch is taken the tie is made in the middle of the silk strand. A rather large bite is required on the esophageal side to prevent the sutures from tearing out. When the posterior wall has been completed, the suture is locked at either end. At this time, the anesthetist passes a rubber tube of large caliber (about No. 30 French) via the mouth through the anastomosis and into the stomach (Fig, 17B). The anterior through-and-through suture is then completed, and the two ends of the silk strand tied together at the medial end of the anastomosis. The rubber tube acts as a splint, insuring adequate patency of the anastomosis. We have found this splinting to be very valuable in avoiding post-operative stenosis, which has, in the past, been a problem with esophagogastrostomy. A polyvinyl tube is passed through the rubber tube and left in place in the stomach when the rubber tube is removed at the completion of the anastomosis.

The anterior serosal layer is now placed. Traction on the tagged end of the through-and-through suture exposes the medial angle of the anastomosis. The serosal layer is started just anterior to the medial fixation suture. It then picks up the gastric serosa and the peritoneal reflections of the diaphragm (Fig. 17C). We have found it unnecessary to pick up the esophagus with this row of suture as the fixation suture and the through-and-through sutures are adequate to prevent the esophagus from retracting. The row is completed adjacent to the lateral fixation suture, thus sealing the anastomosis anteriorly. On occasion, when the anterior

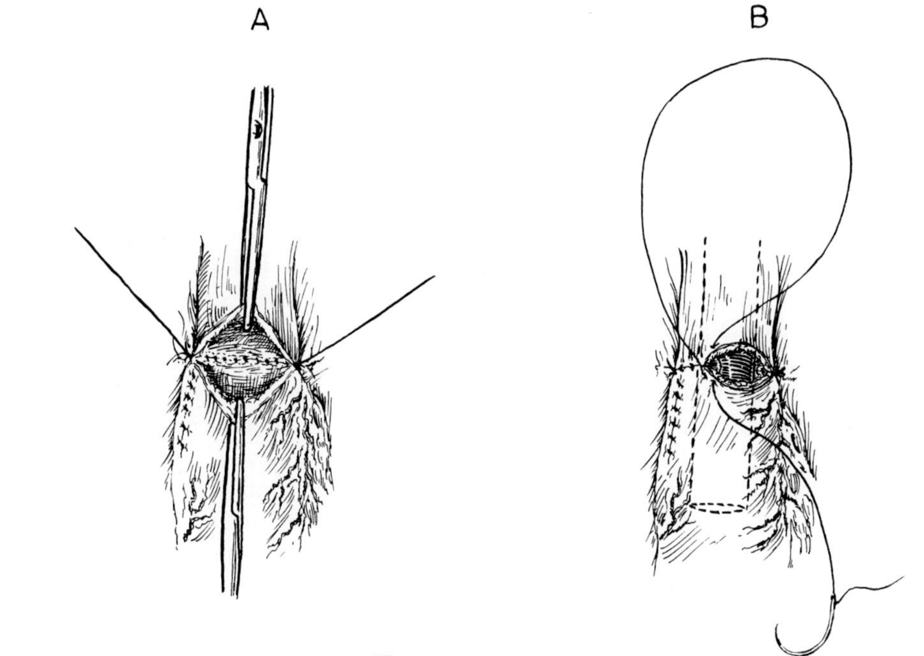

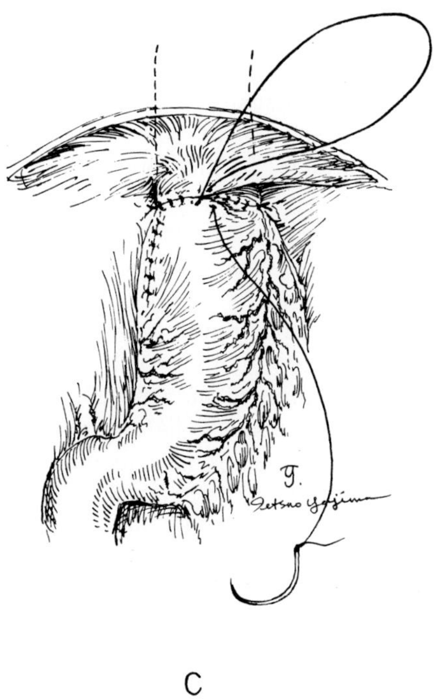

FIGURE 17. A large rubber tube is placed beyond the anastomotic site as a splint to secure adequate patency in esophagogastrostomy. (*A*) Suture of the posterior wall. (*B*) Insertion of the tube. (*C*) Suture of the serosal layer.

serosal row appears to be somewhat weak, we place one or two interrupted sutures through the gastric serosa and gastrohepatic ligament at the medial angle of the anastomosis.

Esophagojejunostomy. We have recently employed gastrostomy as an adjunct procedure to esophagojejunostomy in the poor risk patients with malignant lesions of the cardia (Fig. 18). In such cases, the greater curvature side of the gastric remnant is brought through a stab wound in the upper abdomen to the right of the umbilicus. The gastrostomy is fixed to the abdominal wall and opened on the first postoperative day. A feeding tube is inserted, and feeding may start on the second postoperative day. Once the patient passes flatus, rather large feedings through the gastrostomy may be given without hesitation. The nasointestinal tube may be removed early in the postoperative period. There is evidence that the preservation of the antrum by gastrostomy is beneficial not only to aid in intestinal absorption but also to avoid the anemic state that may follow total gastrectomy.

The esophagojejunostomy may be established in many different ways. Here, we will describe our technique for the Roux en Y.

The jejunum is divided approximately 40 cm. distal to the ligament of Treitz. The exact site is determined after examining the arterial arcades. The proximal end of the jejunum is anastomosed to the distal jejunal segment between 30 and 50 cm. from the proposed esophagojejunostomy.

Esophagojejunostomy is performed in a manner similar to the accomplishment of esophagogastrostomy. Three fixation sutures are placed posteriorly, through-and-through sutures are placed across the anastomosis line, using a rubber tube splint, and the anterior serosal row is placed as described in the preceding section. A key point in the success of this anastomosis is the rotation of the jejunum so that the mesenteric border, which has the best blood supply, is posterior at the anastomosis. The Roux limb must be anastomosed sufficiently distal to the anastomosis (at least 30 cm.) to prevent regurgitation to that vulnerable area. The defect which has been made in the mesentery should be closed with a few interrupted sutures, caution being taken not to compromise the blood supply. The indwelling tube should reach through the anastomosis and lie just proximal to the enteroenterostomy.

The postoperative nutritional state of patients who have undergone this procedure has been very encouraging. This technique of reconstruction may be applied to total gastrectomy as well.

Total Gastrectomy. Almost invariably, total gastrectomy is performed for large and unusually invasive malignant lesions. These tumors usually arise in the body or fundus of the stomach. It is only in unusual circumstances that growths arising from the pyloric regions, if resectable, cannot be appropriately removed by partial resection. On rare occasions benign lesions may require total resection. When the tumor is benign it is not necessary to remove the regional lymphatics and the entire omentum. Here we will describe the operation for malignant growths.

The abdomen is opened in routine fashion, and resectability is determined. If the tumor has not invaded beyond a point which will interfere with an adequate resection of uninvolved esophagus transabdominally, the procedure may be continued by this route. Peritoneal seeding of the pelvis or the mesentery indicates incurability. However, direct invasion of the liver or pancreas does not necessarily carry the same prognosis.

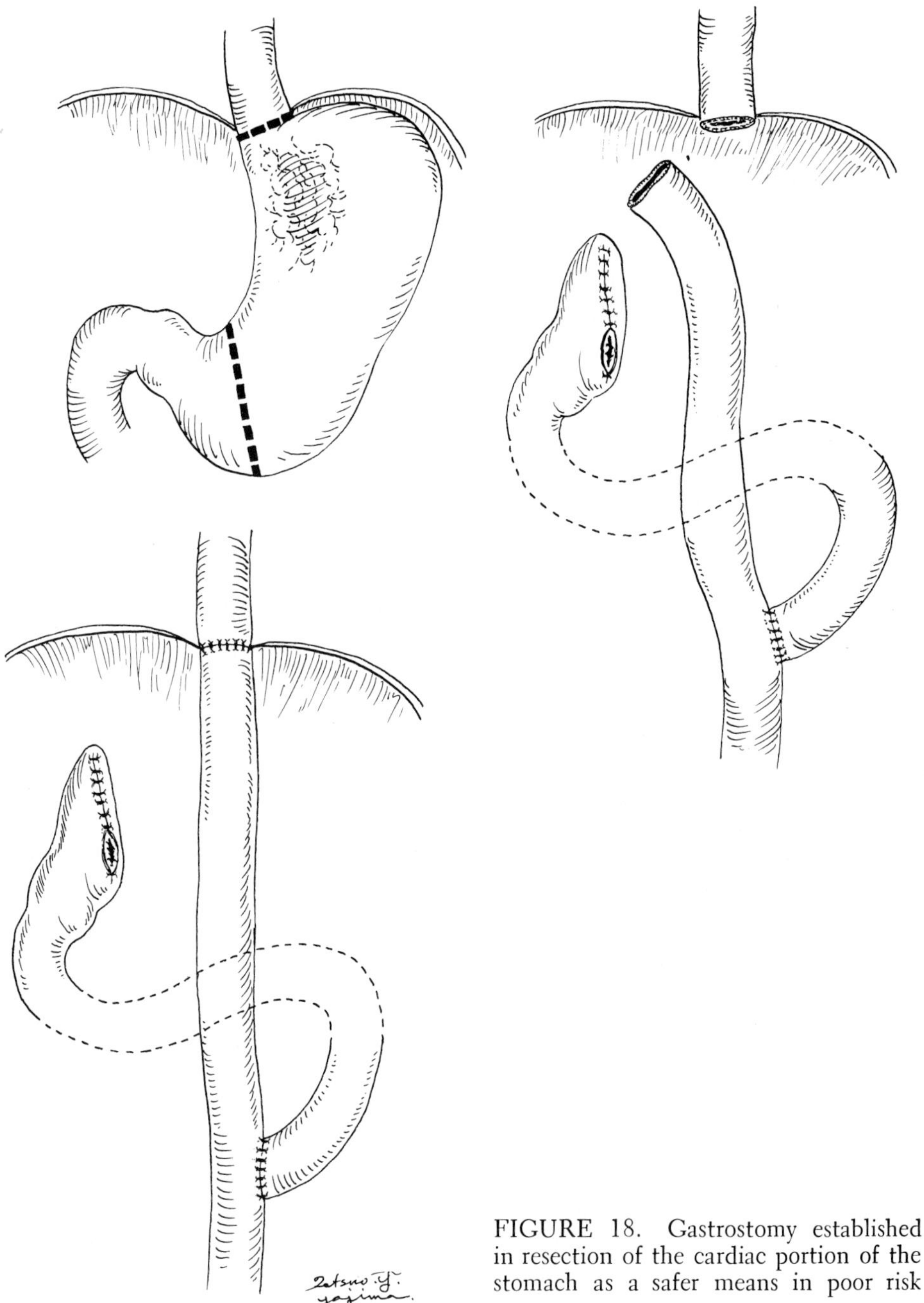

FIGURE 18. Gastrostomy established in resection of the cardiac portion of the stomach as a safer means in poor risk cases.

The resection is started by detaching the entire greater omentum from its colic attachments. The operator's hand is passed posterior to the stomach and the lesser omentum is opened near the pylorus. The right gastroepiploic and gastric arteries are ligated as in subtotal gastrectomy, but with sufficient margin to allow complete removal of any tumor in this region. If esophagoduodenostomy or interposition of a jejunal loop (or segment) is to be performed, the duodenum is divided between our duodenal clamps. When another form of reconstruction is to be done, we usually employ a small version of our gastric clamp. This places a row of metal staples through the duodenal stump, and our first layer of the closure is complete. The closure is then completed with one or two rows of serosal sutures. The duodenal stump is buried in the head of the pancreas by the last row of sutures. Mobilization of the stomach is carried out as in all resections for malignant growths. A right-angle clamp is placed above the esophagogastric junction and a second clamp just distal to it. The resection is completed by sectioning the esophagus between these clamps. When involved, segments of the liver and/or pancreas are resected en bloc, as usual.

For reconstruction, we have made it a practice to use one of the following procedures: esophagojejunostomy (Billroth II type), esophagoduodenostomy, esophagojejunostomy with a jejunal transplant, or Roux en Y esophagojejunostomy (straight, looped, or beta). Choosing the method for reconstruction involves comparison of the alternatives. Each procedure has advantages.

Esophagojejunostomy (Billroth II Type). With this method, postoperative esophagitis due to reflux of duodenal juices may occur, and intestinal absorption is slightly poorer than in reconstructions in which food passes through the duodenum.

A segment of jejunum approximately 50 cm. distal to the ligament of Treitz is selected for the anastomosis (Figs. 19 and 23A). A loop at least 30 cm. in length is necessary to prevent the reflux of duodenal juices. The loop is usually brought up in a retrocolic manner, and at the anastomotic site the efferent limb is arranged to lie anteriorly. An enteroenterostomy is established. The anastomosis is done with two continuous rows of silk suture, one serosal inverting layer and one layer of through-and-through sutures. The stoma at the enteroenterostomy should measure about 5 cm. An atraumatic clamp is placed across the jejunum just distal to the site of the anticipated esophagojejunostomy. The jejunum is then approximated to the esophagus, and three fixation sutures are placed. These sutures must not encroach upon the mesentery of the jejunum and impair blood supply. They pass from the posterior serosa of the jejunum to the peritoneal reflections of the diaphragm and through the muscular wall of the esophagus. The posterior layer of through-and-through sutures is placed, after an opening in the jejunum has been made at right angles to the long axis of the jejunum (a small incision is adequate, because it is easily dilated). A large rubber tube splint is passed into the efferent limb of the jejunum, and the anterior row of through-and-through sutures is placed. The anterior serosal layer picks up the anterior and lateral serosa of the jejunum and the peritoneum of the diaphragm. The esophagus is avoided in this final row of suturing. The polyvinyl tube is allowed to remain through the anastomosis and beyond the enteroenterostomy.

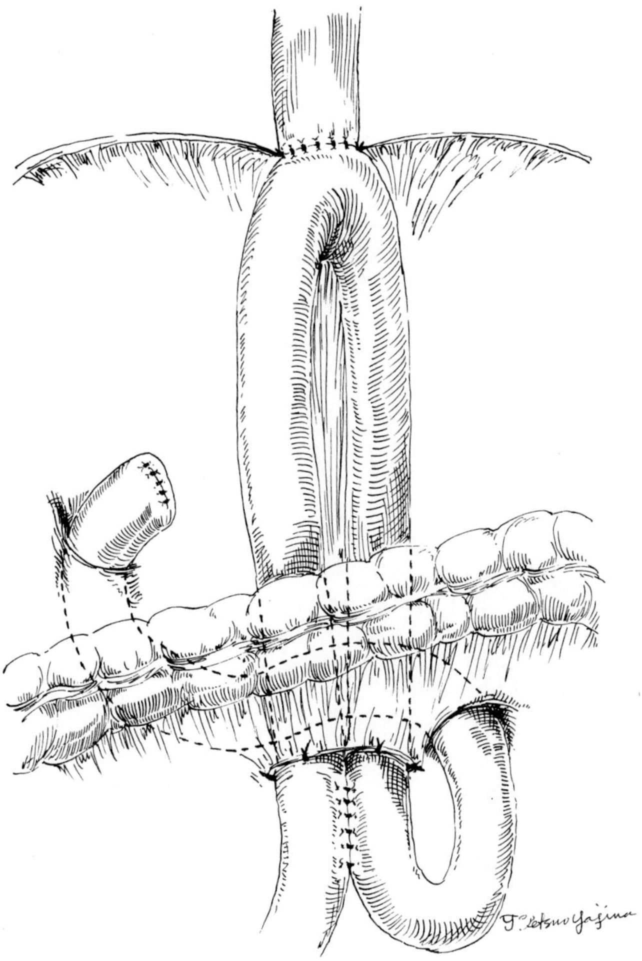

FIGURE 19. Billroth II type of reconstruction in total gastrectomy.

Esophagoduodenostomy. This is the simplest technique for repair, but requires that the pancreas be relatively normal and mobile. It should not be performed when the operation has included a resection of a portion of the pancreas. Intestinal absorption is adequate, but postoperative esophagitis may occur.

Three fixation sutures are placed between the capsule of the head of the pancreas and the diaphragm just below the esophageal hiatus (Fig. 20). Supplementary fixation sutures are placed to the left of these initial anchoring sutures. These serve to fix the body of the pancreas to the diaphragm. The anterior and posterior through-and-through layers are placed in the usual manner. A large rubber tube is used as a splint. The anterior serosal layer is begun at the right corner of the anastomosis and placed in continuous fashion toward the left. Approximately two-thirds of this layer can be placed in the usual manner, but as the terminal portion is approached, it becomes difficult to approximate the serosa

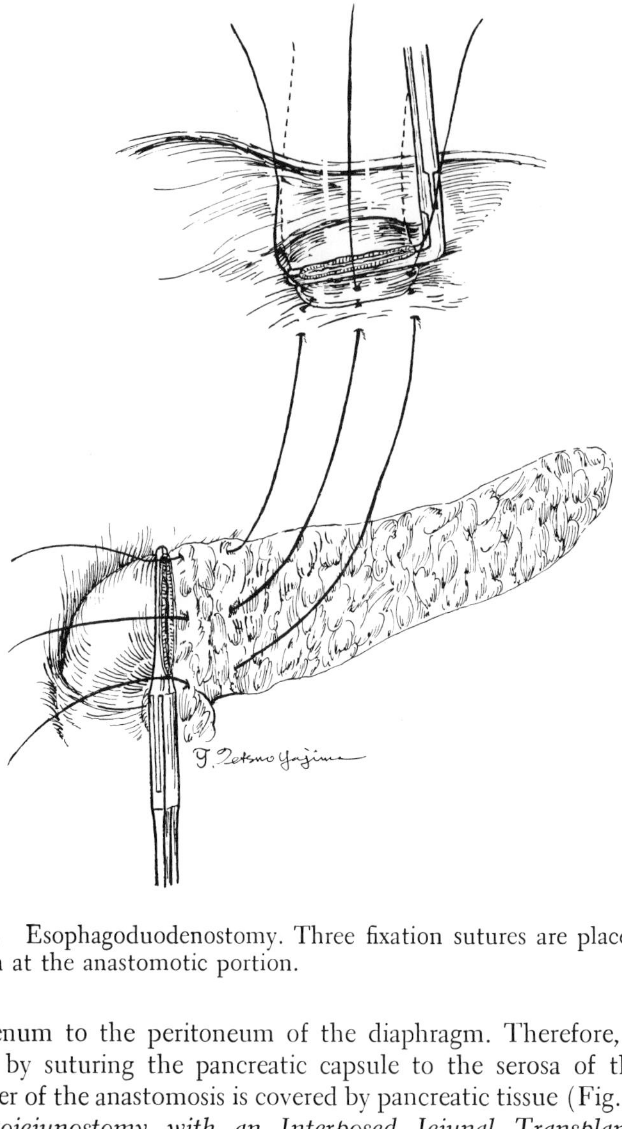

FIGURE 20. Esophagoduodenostomy. Three fixation sutures are placed to eliminate undue tension at the anastomotic portion.

of the duodenum to the peritoneum of the diaphragm. Therefore, we close this final portion by suturing the pancreatic capsule to the serosa of the diaphragm. The left corner of the anastomosis is covered by pancreatic tissue (Fig. 21).

Esophagojejunostomy with an Interposed Jejunal Transplant. This procedure is accompanied by slightly greater operative stress than the others. It is our opinion, however, that it is the most physiological reconstruction; it produces the least postoperative esophagitis and the best intestinal absorption. We have reserved this procedure for use in good risk patients when we feel the malignant growth has been removed.

A segment of about 30 to 40 cm. is isolated from the proximal jejunum; its vascular pedicle is preserved (Fig. 22). An appropriate segment can usually be obtained approximately 60 cm. below the ligament of Treitz. The segment is brought up through an opening in the transverse mesocolon. A jejunal loop is fashioned, using the proximal end of the transplant. This yields a food reservoir post-

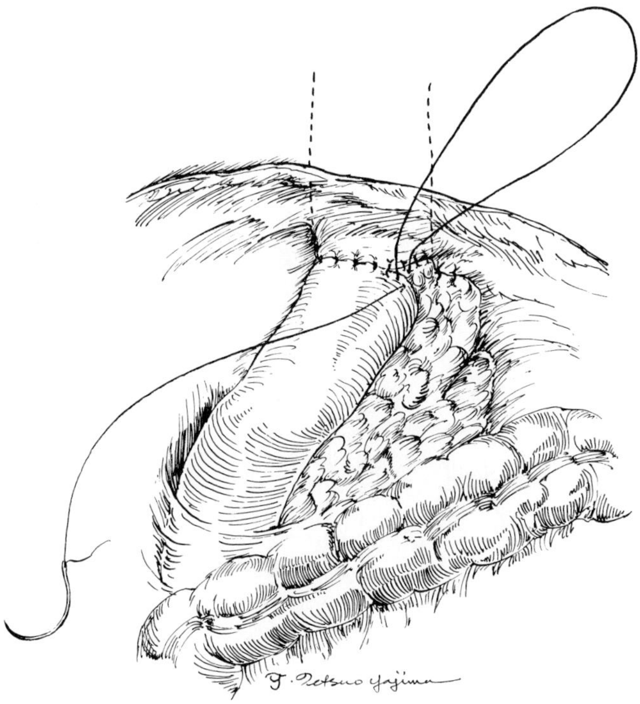

FIGURE 21. Completion of esophagoduodenostomy.

operatively. An end-to-side esophagojejunostomy is carried out. The distal end of the isolated segment is anastomosed to the duodenum, employing a routine two-layer anastomosis. End-to-end anastomosis of the jejunal stumps below restores the continuity of the intestinal tract.

Roux en Y Esophagojejunostomy. The main advantage of this mode of reconstruction is less regurgitation of duodenal juices than in the Billroth II type (Fig. 23B, C). If leakage occurs at the esophagojejunostomy, smaller amounts of duodenal juices are present at the anastomotic portion. This technique has been described in connection with resection of the cardiac end of the stomach. The only difference is that the duodenal stump is closed in total gastrectomy, and there is a gastrostomy with resection of the cardia (Fig. 23B).

Recently we have constructed a jejunal loop proximally and performed end-to-side esophagojejunostomy, since it has been shown that the end-to-side anastomosis does not compromise the blood supply at the primary anastomotic site (in contrast to the end-to-end anastomosis). The loop is formed from the proximal end of the segment of jejunum and is anastomosed to the esophageal stump exactly as in the Billroth II type end-to-side esophagojejunostomy (Fig. 23C).

The Roux en Y mode with jejunal loop has been very satisfactory. This method, however, requires three anastomoses. Aiming at its simplification, I have developed a new method, our beta anastomosis (Figs. 23D and 24). In this procedure, an anastomosis is done only twice. In order not to compromise the blood

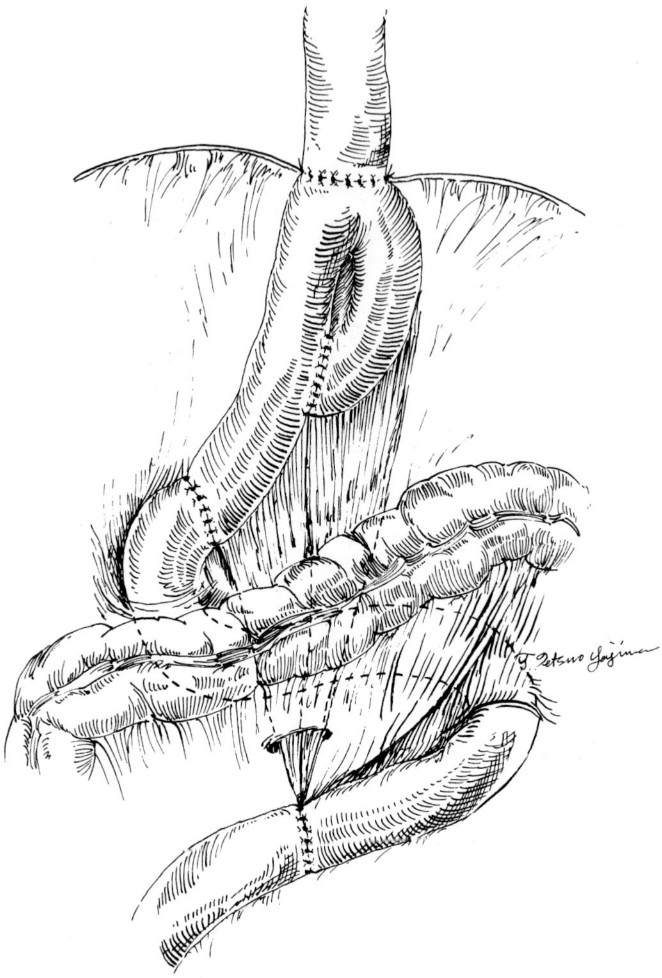

FIGURE 22. Esophagojejunostomy with an interposed jejunal transplant.

supply to the enteroenterostomy, the jejunum is not completely divided. All the steps except for the enteroenterostomy resemble those in Roux en Y with jejunal loop. The results thus far obtained have been satisfactory.

RESECTION OF THE PANCREAS, LIVER, OR COLON. *Pancreas.* When the tail of the pancreas is involved by tumor growth, resection of the tail of the pancreas and the spleen is indicated. Once the stomach has been divided, the pancreas is readily exposed. The upper and lower peritoneal attachments of the body of the pancreas are freed. The pancreas is freed from its posterior attachments by blunt dissection. The pancreatic crushing clamp is then placed just proximal to the proposed resection of the pancreas. The clamp is closed and the parenchyma of the pancreas is crushed, but the capsule remains intact. A second crushing clamp is placed across the pancreas, just distal to the first clamp. The pancreas is divided by scalpel. The usual transection line is within a few centimeters of the

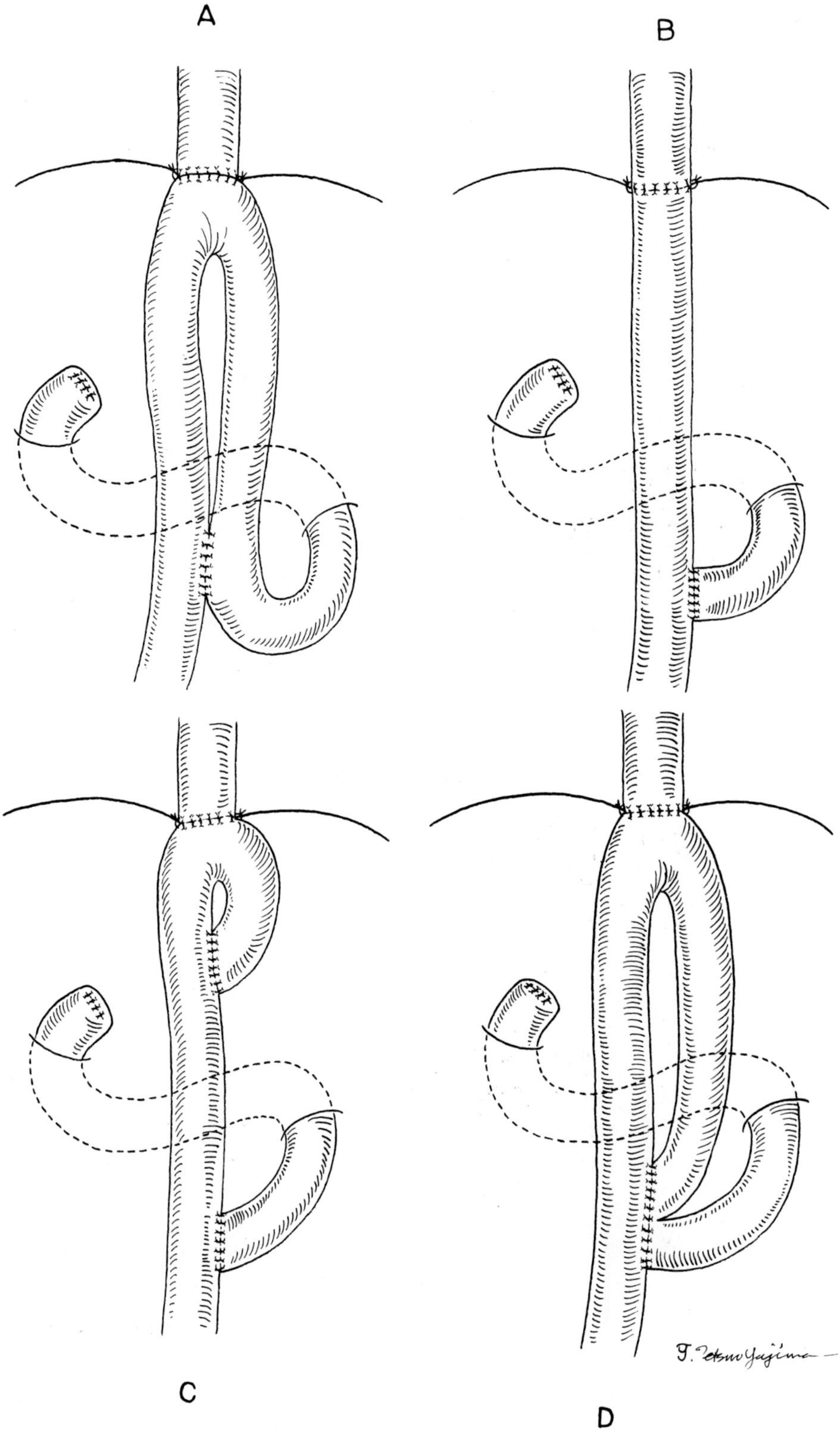

FIGURE 23. (*A*) Billroth II type of esophagojejunostomy. (*B*) Roux en Y esophagojejunostomy with a straight jejunal segment. (*C*) Roux en Y esophagojejunostomy with a looped jejunal segment. (*D*) Beta esophagojejunostomy.

celiac axis (Fig. 25). After the pancreas has been divided, the cut ends of the splenic artery and vein can be identified in the pancreatic stump. A ligature is placed about each of these structures. When the resection must be done to the

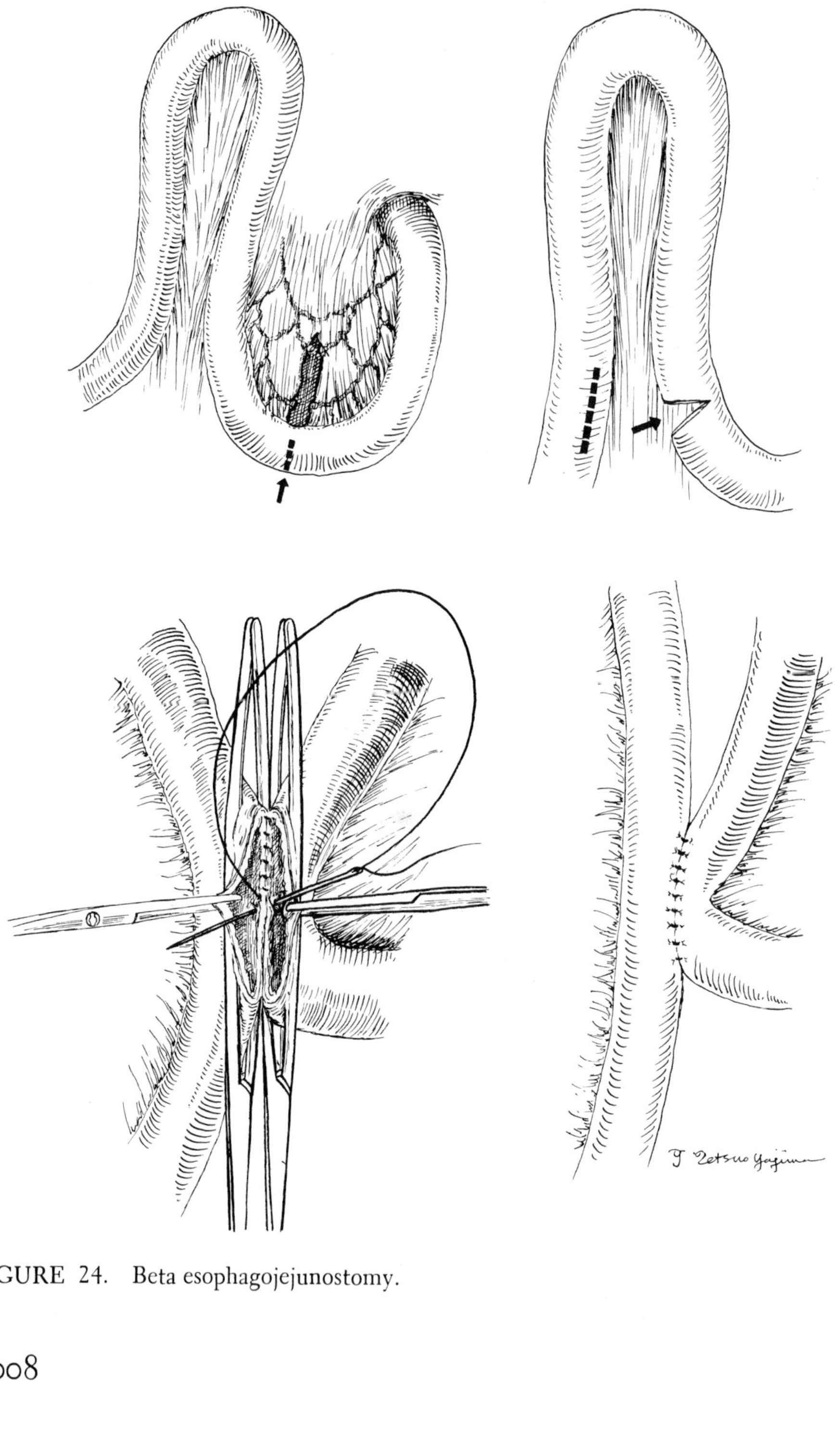

FIGURE 24. Beta esophagojejunostomy.

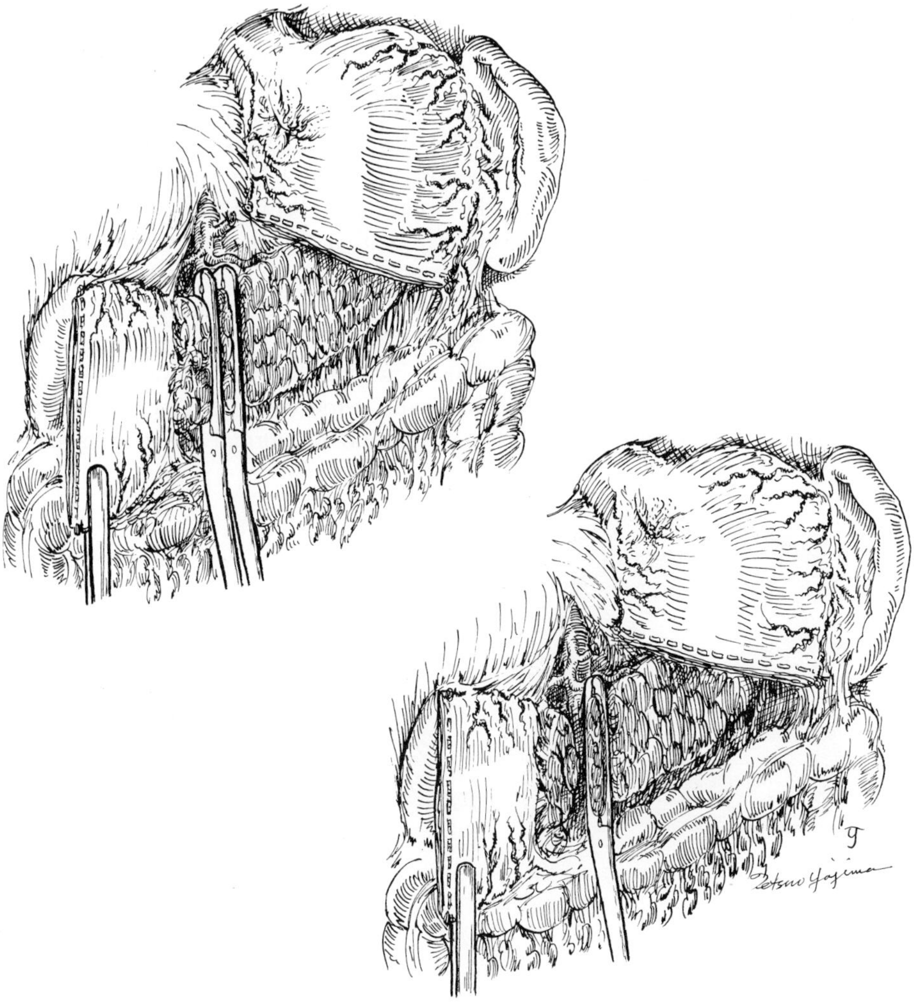

FIGURE 25. Two steps in simplified pancreatic resection with Nakayama crushing clamps.

left of the celiac axis, it is better to ligate the splenic artery prior to transection of the pancreas. (The splenic artery runs along the upper margin of the pancreas in this portion.) A very heavy silk ligature is now passed around the entire pancreas just proximal to the first crushing clamp. As the ligature is slowly tied, the crushing clamp is gradually released. This tie must be applied very tightly. The pancreatic tail is freed en bloc with the spleen and the stomach. Sufficient time will now have elapsed for the vessels to retract, and the pancreatic tissue is trimmed away. A margin of about 0.5 cm. remains distal to the ligature. If one is concerned about the security of this ligature, interrupted silk sutures through the cut end of the pancreas should be employed. The abdomen is drained.

Liver. When direct invasion of the liver occurs, it usually involves a portion of the left lobe. One or two crushing clamps are placed across the liver medial to the malignant growth. The number of clamps depends upon the size of the segment to be resected. The resection is carried out using sharp dissection on the gastric side of these clamps. Large vessels or bile ducts which can be identified in the transected remnant are ligated with horizontal mattress sutures of fine silk. Two or three are usually sufficient. Two or three very heavy silk sutures are then passed through the midportion of the stump just behind the crushing clamp. These are carried anteriorly and posteriorly so that together they encompass the entire liver mass (Fig. 26). The clamps are released gradually as the heavy ligatures are slowly tied very tightly. No further treatment is necessary. With a resection the abdomen is drained.

Colon. When the transverse colon is involved by tumor growth that is an extension of a primary gastric malignant lesion, it too must be removed. Sufficient colon should be removed so that a wide margin of normal tissue is taken. In

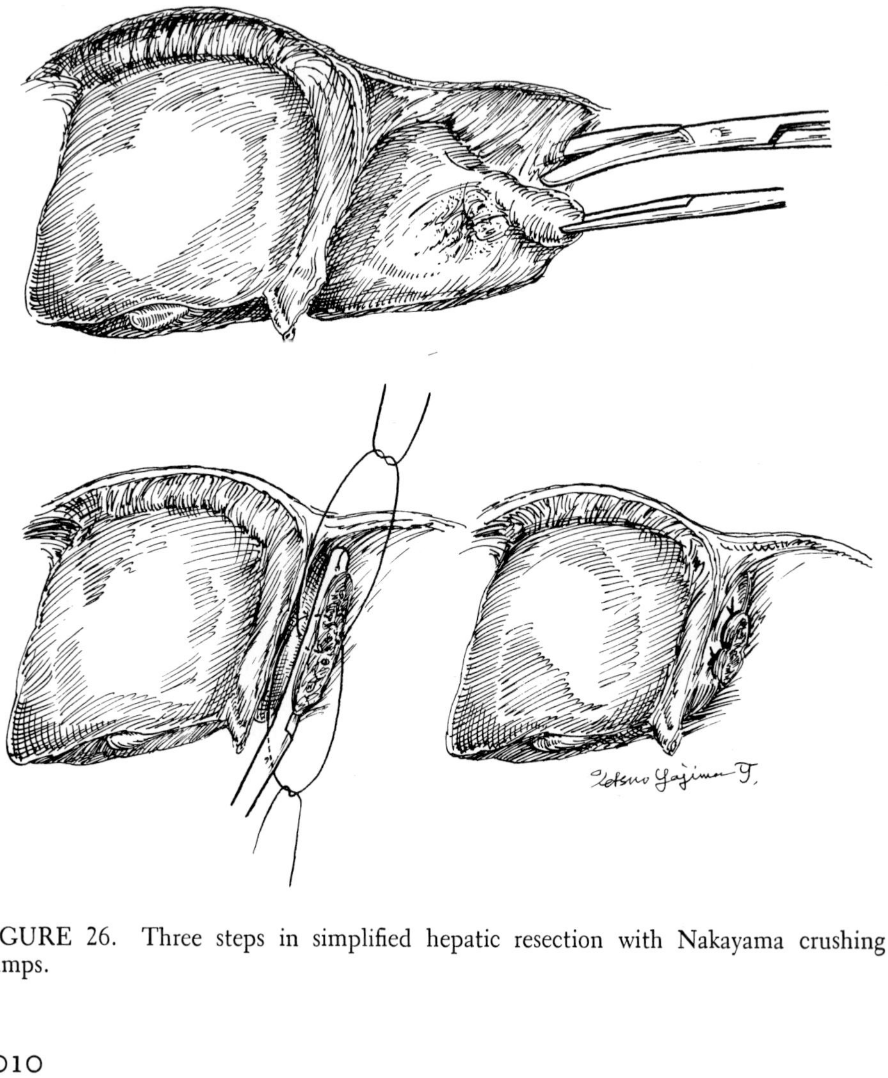

FIGURE 26. Three steps in simplified hepatic resection with Nakayama crushing clamps.

poor risk patients, we usually perform a right-sided colostomy. The distal stump of the descending colon is closed and allowed to remain in the abdomen. When the continuity of the colon is to be re-established, we have found that end-to-side anastomosis is preferable to end-to-end in the majority of these cases. Such an anastomosis must be kept well away from any other anastomosis in the upper abdomen. Usually we prefer closure of the distal stump of the descending colon and anastomosis of the stump of the ascending colon to the side of the sigmoid. We consider it important to have a colon tube passed through this anastomosis in order to decompress this area. Such a tube is left in place until good peristaltic action is observed.

Postoperative Period

In the postoperative period we employ an indwelling polyvinyl tube. In subtotal resections, this tube is placed in the gastric remnant, proximal to the anastomosis. It serves to decompress the stomach and to prevent leakage. The tube is removed when the patient passes flatus, usually on the third or fourth postoperative day. If the volume of drainage from the tube is excessive, it is kept in place until the amount is adequately reduced.

During a total gastrectomy, a cardiectomy, etc., the tube is passed through the anastomosis so that it may be used for feeding after peristalsis has been re-established. Tube feeding usually starts on the third postoperative day. The tube can usually be removed safely around the tenth postoperative day. It seems wise to delay slightly the progress of feedings in esophagogastrostomy as compared with esophagojejunostomy. The position of the tube should be changed by a few centimeters every second or third day to eliminate the possibility of traumatic perforation of bowel.

If leakage from the anastomotic site is suspected, it must be investigated immediately. Methylene blue and aqueous radiopaque substances are the agents we use. If significant leakage is demonstrated, a jejunostomy is performed immediately and the abscess drained. Ideally, the jejunostomy should be 70 to 100 cm. distal to the ligament of Treitz. When extensive adhesions have been found, due to previous surgery, it is preferable to introduce an oral jejunal feeding tube sufficiently distal to the anastomosis. Ten days to two weeks are allowed to pass before the anastomosis is re-evaluated by x-ray. If the leak has sealed, oral feedings are begun gradually.

ACKNOWLEDGMENTS

I wish to thank my assistants, Dr. Hiroyasu D. Makino and Dr. Tatsuo Tamiya, for their aid; Dr. Paul Williams of Bay Village, Ohio, for his help in preparing the chapter; and Tetsuo Yajima for making the illustrations.

83. Duodenal Closure After Gastrectomy

PHILIP COOPER

IN DEALING with the stump of a normal duodenum or one with limited pathology, an adequate length of duodenum can be readily mobilized and transected, and the end closed without difficulty. This would be the situation when a gastrectomy is being performed for a benign or malignant lesion of the stomach, or for a small or uncomplicated duodenal ulcer. However, in the presence of a large, a complicated, or a penetrating duodenal ulcer, the technique of dissection and the closure of the stump would of necessity be more involved and be influenced by the operative findings.

The pathological findings in chronic duodenal ulcer vary because of the type, extent, and location of the ulcer, and also because of the associated pathology. There may be considerable scarring and shortening of the first part of the duodenum. Periduodenal inflammation and induration may be associated with the ulcer. Ulcers which cause stenosis of the duodenal lumen may or may not produce a pseudodiverticulum or pseudodiverticula proximal to the stenotic area. Large posterior wall ulcers frequently penetrate through the entire thickness of the viscus, and form a base composed of thickened pancreatic capsule, pancreatic substance, or other tissue or structure, depending on the direction of the penetration. Multiple duodenal ulcers may involve both the anterior and posterior walls.

Given the present acceptance of vagotomy with pyloroplasty or gastroenterostomy as reasonable operative procedures for duodenal ulcer, one should carefully evaluate the pathology and the technical problems involved in mobilization of the duodenum, prior to or while proceeding with the dissection, and determine operability before one is committed to sectioning of the duodenum. It is necessary to appraise the situation meticulously, for often the pathological changes may appear more complex than they actually are. In general, a duodenal stump can be safely dissected and closed if the anterior wall and the superior and inferior borders of the duodenum are relatively free of disease and are pliable. Conditions are also favorable for closure, when the superior or inferior border has been replaced by an ulcer, as long as the anterior and posterior duodenal walls are in reasonable condition. Some thickening and induration of the anterior wall in the presence of a large posterior ulcer does not preclude a secure closure, provided that the anterior wall can be properly inverted as the interrupted sutures are tied. If the anterior wall is markedly indurated, a satisfactory inversion of the wall is not possible.

Closure of the duodenal stump is hazardous if an ulcer has replaced both the posterior wall and the superior or inferior border. In that situation, gastric resection should not be contemplated. A vagotomy and gastroenterostomy would be indicated. These problems will be discussed in more detail in the following section.

Technique

The approach to the duodenum in doing a gastrectomy for a nonmalignant lesion may be considered as starting with the grasping of the greater curvature part of the stomach with the fingers of the right hand, while the index finger of the left hand is inserted through the avascular area in the gastrohepatic ligament. The finger is passed behind the stomach through a free area, or through a finely adherent area which responds to gentle blunt dissection. The finger is kept close to the stomach wall until it appears under the gastrocolic ligament. It is then withdrawn, to be joined by the middle finger (Fig. 1). Both fingers are then advanced to the gastro-

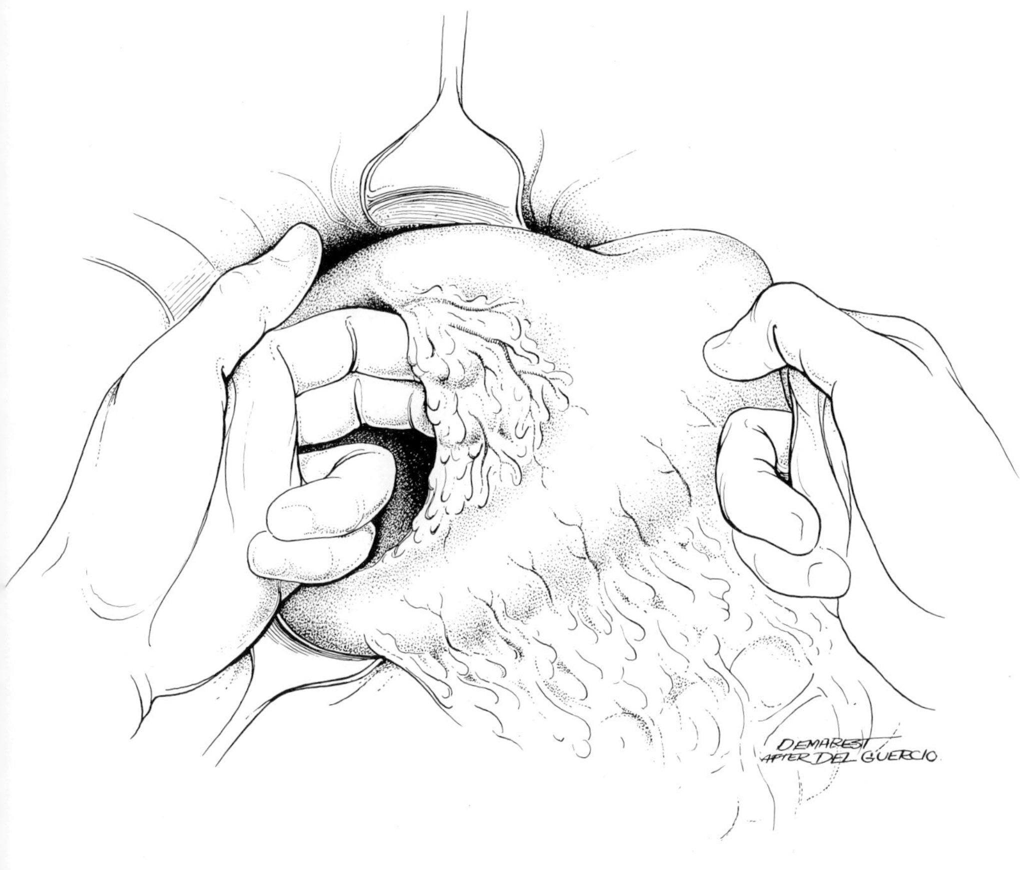

FIGURE 1. The stomach is mobilized by carefully passing two fingers of the left hand posteriorly while the stomach is grasped and supported on the greater curvature by the fingers of the right hand.

colic ligament, and spread; and the ligament is opened by the insertion of a clamp between the two fingers. The opening is made through an avascular area, usually beyond the gastroepiploic vessel arcade. The incision is made *within* the arcade in the obese patient, because there is less fat to contend with in this area, and the blood supply to a thick, fatty greater omentum is better preserved. A Penrose or narrow gauze drain is then grasped between the two fingers, pulled behind the stomach, drawn through the opening in the gastrohepatic ligament, and then clamped with a Kelly hemostat. The drain is used for traction purposes until the duodenum is transected. Grasping the anterior stomach wall with a large Babcock clamp also assists in the establishment of proper tension for the dissection.

The approach to the duodenum in doing a gastrectomy for a malignant lesion of the stomach would be the same as that just described, except that the gastrocolic ligament would not be opened. The fingers passed behind the stomach would by careful blunt dissection free the gastrocolic ligament from the transverse mesocolon. It is important to limit this blunt dissection to the freeing of fine adhesions. If a firm adhesion is encountered, it is bypassed to be freed later when the area is exposed. The greater omentum is then elevated and dissected off the transverse colon by scissors. A few small vessels requiring ligation are encountered. The Penrose or gauze drain is then passed behind the stomach and the omentum and clamped with a Kelly hemostat.

In doing a gastrectomy for a duodenal ulcer, I prefer not to excise the greater omentum, unless I am concerned about its vascular status after the gastrocolic ligament has been incised, or unless the bulk of the omentum would interfere with the establishment of a satisfactory antecolic gastrojejunostomy. In the latter situation only a segment of the omentum is removed, enough to allow the jejunal loop to rest on the transverse colon without excessive tension being applied to the line of anastomosis.

Since the major problems in duodenal closure occur when a duodenal ulcer is present, the discussion that follows will concern the dissection, transection, and closure of the duodenal stump in the surgical management of that disease.

As already noted, incision beyond rather than within the gastroepiploic vascular arcade is usually accomplished. Following the application of tension to the Penrose or gauze drain, further dissection and incision of the gastrocolic ligament is facilitated by placing the index and middle fingers of the left hand under the ligament and inserting a clamp between them. The defect is enlarged by opening the clamp. Two clamps are then applied, and the tissue is cut and ligated (Fig. 2). The same maneuver is repeated until the proper length of ligament has been incised.

As the dissection brings one near the duodenum, the peritoneum on the anterior aspect of the gastrocolic ligament is incised, and the colon is bluntly displaced downward. This exposes a relatively avascular fatty layer between the vascular arcade above and the transverse colon below. Another advantage of this maneuver is that the subpyloric lymph nodes are left attached to the stomach and duodenum. The greater curvature of the stomach is now elevated, and the peritoneum covering the posterior aspect of the gastrocolic ligament is incised. Not

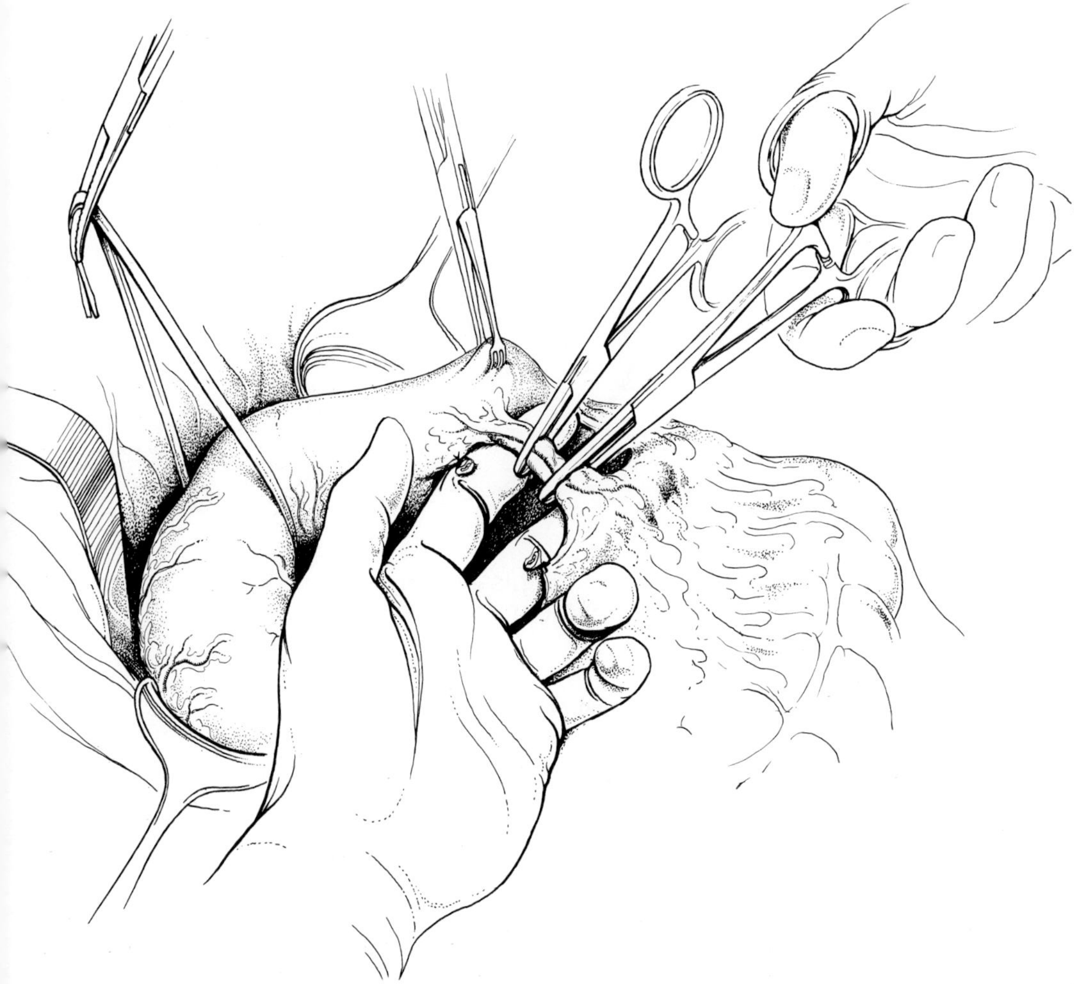

FIGURE 2. Application of clamps and cutting of the gastrocolic ligament vessels as they are delivered and supported by the index and middle fingers of the left hand.

infrequently there are adhesions extending from the pancreas and mesocolon to the stomach and duodenum. They should be carefully freed. This will further mobilize the mesocolon and protect it and its enclosed vessels from possible injury. The fatty tissue, the remnant of the gastrocolic ligament, now is a tenuous structure which is relatively avascular. This fatty layer is incised.

The right gastroepiploic vessels are now exposed, and are ligated at their origin from the gastroduodenal vessels (Fig. 3) unless the landmarks are somewhat obscured by extensive induration or scarring in that area. In that situation, one proceeds slowly along the lower border of the duodenum, dissecting, cutting, and ligating the branches rather than the main trunk of the gastroepiploic vessels. With care, the inferior border and the lower posterior wall of the duodenum can be dissected free, unless they are actually replaced by the ulcer crater.

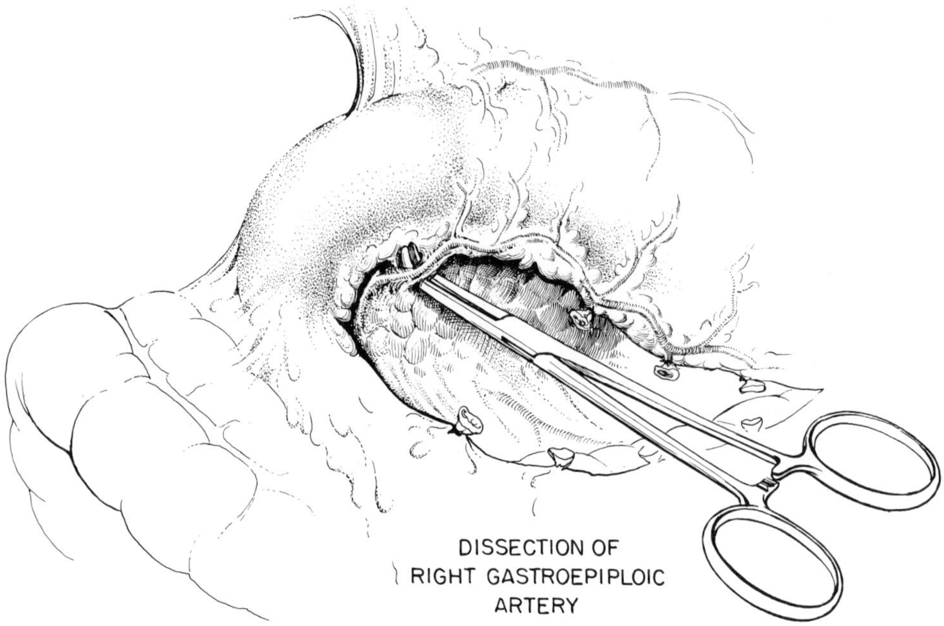

FIGURE 3. Dissection and ligation of the right gastroepiploic artery.

Following the dissection of the inferior border and the lower posterior wall, one exposes the superior border of the duodenum. The right gastric vessels are freed by cautiously inserting a right-angle clamp near the wall of the duodenum just beyond the pyloric ring. This can be accomplished with greater safety, particularly when the neighboring tissues are indurated, by applying the index finger against the end of the clamp as it is being gently advanced through the tissue. The right gastric vessels are then doubly ligated with 00 silk and cut. Ligating these vessels early in the duodenal dissection allows one to judge better the extent of mobilization of the posterior duodenal wall necessary for an adequate duodenal closure. This sequence can be readily followed in dissecting the duodenum with an uncomplicated ulcer, but may require alteration if the location, the extent of the ulcer, or the associated inflammatory reaction makes it advisable.

If there is only a short segment of relatively normal posterior wall of duodenum distal to an ulcer, the posterior wall can be further mobilized by ligation of lateral branches of the gastroduodenal vessels (Fig. 4). A satisfactory method is to free the branches partially, apply mosquito clamps, cut the vessels, and finally ligate them with fine silk. Dissection into the substance of the pancreas is neither necessary nor advisable. It may result in acute pancreatitis, a pancreatic fistula, or a "blown" duodenal stump.

If the duodenal dissection appears difficult or hazardous, or if the exposure is limited, it may be advisable to apply appropriate clamps and to transect the stomach early in the procedure. This will improve the exposure of the posterior

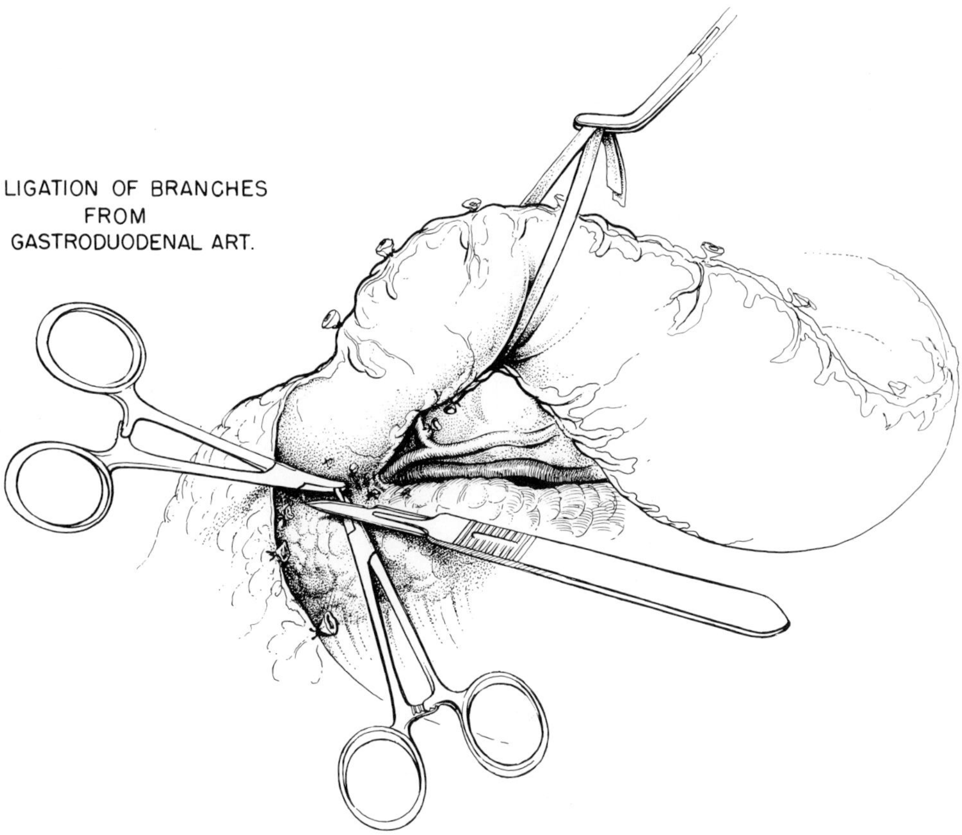

FIGURE 4. Exposure, partial freeing, clamping, and cutting of branches of the gastroduodenal vessels to further mobilize the posterior wall of the duodenum.

wall of the duodenum and allow one to proceed with the dissection with greater safety and confidence .

It is most important to avoid any excessive freeing of the duodenum, since excessive dissection may jeopardize the blood supply of that structure. In order to limit the extent of the final mobilization, it is well to preserve as much of the duodenum as possible until a decision as to the method of closure has been reached. The maximum length of duodenum can be best obtained after the structure has been partially mobilized, by applying a small Payr clamp immediately proximal to or on the pylorus. This forces the pylorus forward, and it then can be palpated readily through the anterior duodenal wall. The anterior wall of the duodenum is incised transversely close to the pylorus. The posterior wall can then be cut with scissors, next to the pylorus, under direct vision (Fig. 5). This technique is not feasible or necessary if the posterior wall has been disrupted in freeing a posterior wall ulcer.

The end of the closed duodenal stump should rest at a level slightly above the anterior surface of the pancreas. Mattress sutures, if used, should be ade-

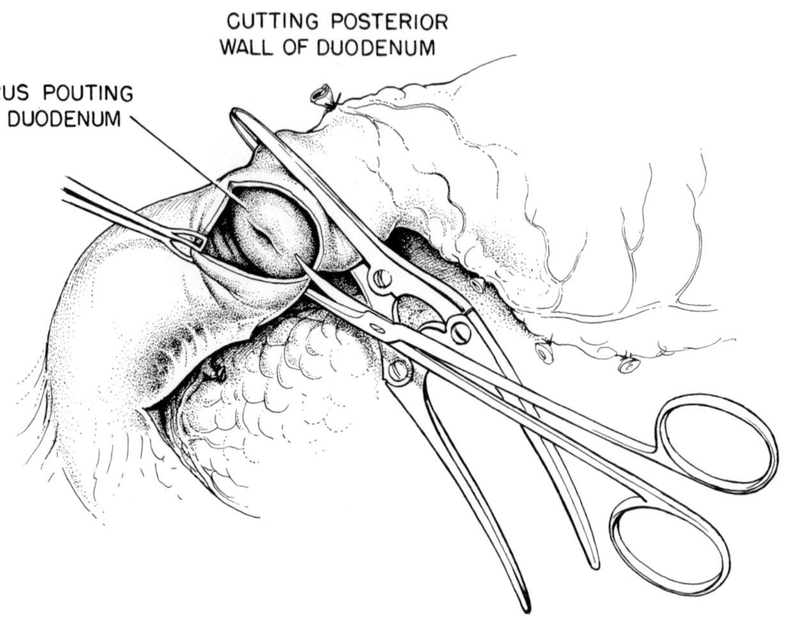

FIGURE 5. A Payr clamp has been applied to the region of the pylorus, and the anterior duodenum incised transversely at its most proximal point. The posterior wall is being sectioned next to the pylorus.

quately spaced, and too numerous sutures avoided so as not to jeopardize the blood supply of the duodenal stump.

The Normal Duodenum or the Duodenum with Limited Ulcer Pathology

Care should be taken to free the duodenum only to the extent required for a secure closure. In the absence of pathology, or in the presence of limited pathology, one may be unwittingly drawn into freeing the duodenum extensively. This could result in serious devascularization of the stump. The insertion of too many sutures in the stump closure tends to aggravate this problem.

If an adequate length of satisfactory anterior and posterior wall is mobilized, the two walls may be approximated by either an open or a closed technique. An open technique is preferred, because it more efficiently prevents later bleeding from the inverted end of the bowel. This rarely occurs with either method, but is a greater hazard following a closed method.

In the usual closed method, two clamps are applied, and the duodenum is cut between the clamps. A continuous Cushing suture is placed distal to the clamp, and the duodenum is inverted as the clamp is removed. A second layer of interrupted Lembert sutures is then placed. A third layer may be applied by suturing the seromuscular layer of the anterior duodenal wall to the peritoneum and areolar tissue covering the pancreas. Silk is used in all layers.

In the open method, if the anterior and posterior duodenal wall are pliable

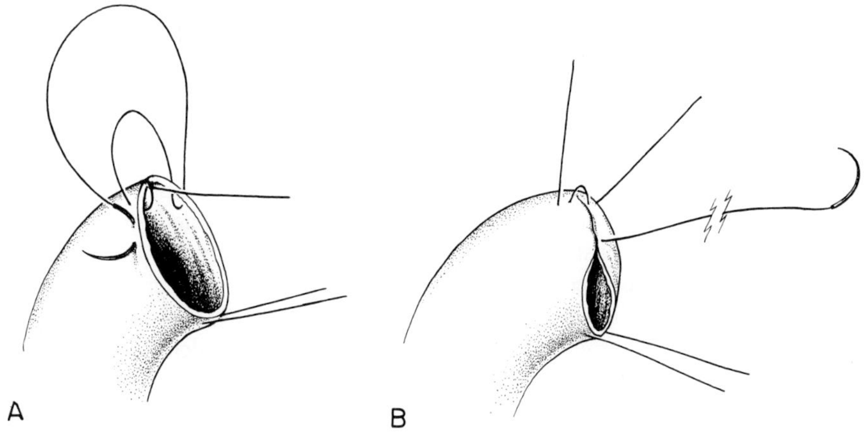

FIGURE 6. (*A*) Method of starting the inversion suture, by applying tension to one strand and taking a few bites in the duodenal wall with the other strand of the continuous suture. (*B*) Continuation of the Connell suture, and early insertion of the first suture of the second layer.

and of adequate length, the stump is closed with a continuous Connell suture. It is helpful to insert the first bite through the duodenal wall at the upper border, to tie the suture, and then to gently pull the short strand of the suture toward the lumen while the other strand is being used to take appropriate bites in the bowel wall (Fig. 6A). The short strand of the suture, while under tension, is cut after two to three bites have been taken. This method of starting the suture helps to invert the upper end of the duodenum. At this time the first interrupted Lembert suture of the second row of sutures is placed (Fig. 6B). The last two to three bites of the Connell suture are not drawn tight until the last bite has been taken. This allows the lower end of the stump to be inverted easily. The closure is reinforced by completing the layer of interrupted Lembert sutures. As in the closed method, a third layer may be placed, and all sutures are of silk. If there is any doubt as to the advisability of using continuous suture because of the limited length or the friable condition of the posterior wall, it should not be employed, and interrupted silk sutures should be used in all layers.

The Duodenum with an Involved, Complicated, or Penetrating Ulcer

Additional problems do arise when the ulcer is acute or extensive, or involves neighboring structures. The severity of an associated acute inflammatory process may frequently be reduced if definitive surgery is delayed for three to four weeks, or longer, following an acute exacerbation of the disease. If a marked inflammatory response is still present at the time of surgery, one may choose to do a pyloroplasty or a gastroenterostomy, and a vagotomy, or proceed with the duodenal dissection if it can be accomplished safely. In the latter situation one follows proper tissue planes and dissects close to the duodenum to simplify and to avoid complicating the procedure. This comment has particular reference to the freeing of the superior and inferior borders of the duodenum from their blood supply. Small bites of tissue should be taken, and promptly ligated.

Indurated tissue extending from the duodenum can usually be handled without excessive difficulty if it is dissected slowly and cautiously, employing both sharp and blunt methods, including the thinning of tissues by finger pressure or by blunt use of instruments. It should rarely be necessary to open the common duct and insert a T tube prior to the final dissection of the duodenum.

If there is a large posterior ulcer involving the pancreatic head, and the duodenum *distal* to the ulcer *cannot* be mobilized without incising pancreatic tissue, the following technique is recommended. It requires a reasonably pliable anterior wall. With this method the distal margin of the ulcer is not utilized, and in most cases it has been found unnecessary to use the proximal margin of the ulcer for the closure. As the dissection is carried posteriorly on to the duodenum, the ulcer crater is intentionally entered and the contiguous duodenal wall trimmed and excised as indicated in Figure 7A. Thick, indurated, edematous duodenal wall adjacent to the ulcer may be removed, provided the wall along the superior and inferior borders of the duodenum remains intact. Only enough anterior wall should be left to permit closure without undue tension.

The closure is accomplished with two layers of interrupted 4–0 or 3–0 silk. The sutures on the pancreatic side are placed superficially, the first layer through the thickened scar tissue which usually borders the ulcer crater, and the second layer through peritoneum and areolar tissue overlying the pancreas (Fig. 7B, C). An adequate bulk of tissue for proper support for the second layer can usually be obtained on the pancreatic side by taking multiple diagonal bites. Above and below the ulcer crater the seromuscular layers of the duodenal wall may be incorporated in the first row of sutures, and as one approaches the superior or inferior border, the sutures can often be placed in the duodenal wall alone. By placing the sutures very superficially in the pancreas, the hazards of deep penetration into that organ are avoided. In the anterior duodenal wall, Lembert or Cushing mattress sutures may be used, depending on the width of the wall which has to be turned in. If it is edematous or thickened, one may be able to invert it by inserting the Lembert sutures partially through the thickness of the wall. If they are inserted through the entire thickness of an indurated wall, inversion may prove difficult or impossible.

This approach to the closure of the duodenum with a large posterior wall ulcer allows a safe, rapid, and limited dissection of the duodenum and avoids trauma to the pancreas. The dissection must be carried out meticulously and an adequate blood supply to the duodenal wall retained. If one is at all concerned about the security of the closure, two Penrose drains may be inserted near the duodenum.

In rare instances the major part of the posterior wall is replaced by the ulcer, and the anterior wall is considerably thickened and indurated. Here it is advisable to close the duodenum around a Foley catheter. The closure is accomplished as thoroughly as possible with interrupted silk sutures, and the greater omentum is placed around the catheter, which is brought through a stab wound in the abdominal wall. Penrose drains are inserted near the duodenal closure and brought out through a separate stab wound. Some prefer to bring the Foley catheter through the lateral duodenal wall rather than through the end of the stump. This may be feasible if the duodenal stump closure is fairly secure. It is

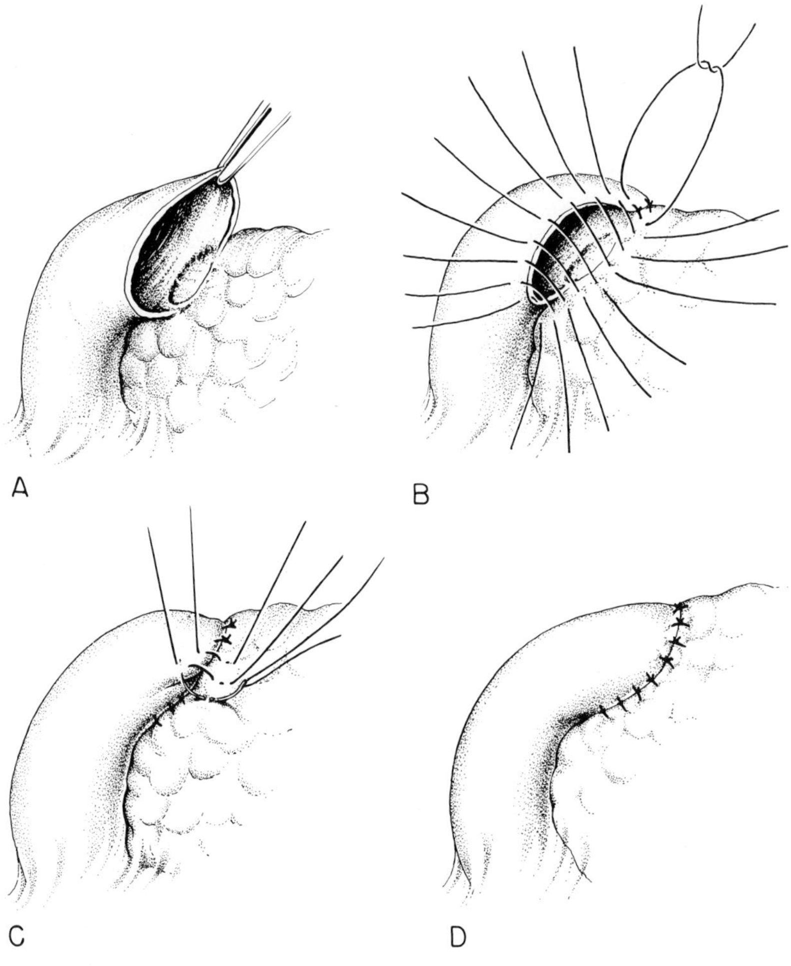

A B C D

FIGURE 7. The large posterior wall ulcer. (*A*) The posterior wall of the duodenum has been separated from the proximal border of the ulcer by blunt dissection. The remainder of the posterior wall is then sectioned as indicated. (*B*) Placing of the first layer of sutures, first in the scar tissue *near* the ulcer crater, and then in the anterior wall of the duodenum. The first layer of the closure can usually be completed with fewer sutures than are shown in this figure. Above and below the ulcer, the posterior duodenal wall may be incorporated in the sutures if it appears suitable. (*C*) Placing of the second layer of sutures, first in peritoneum and areolar tissue over the pancreas and then in the anterior duodenal wall. Note the method of taking multiple bites with each suture through the tissues over the pancreas, while avoiding penetration of pancreatic glandular tissue. (*D*) Completed closure.

doubtful whether that method would be advisable if the stump closure is unsatisfactory. We have rarely found it necessary to do a catheter duodenostomy.

If the operation is for a bleeding duodenal ulcer, and the ulcer cannot be removed without incising pancreas, it is left in situ and the vessel or the area of the vessel in the ulcer crater is sutured with one or two mattress or figure-of-eight sutures of 00 silk. The remainder of the stump closure is the same as that previously described.

The ulcer which has produced a pseudodiverticulum or pseudodiverticula in the proximal duodenum (Fig. 8A) occasionally is troublesome. If an attempt is made to close the duodenum through or proximal to the pseudodiverticulum, one may have difficulty with the inversion of the bowel wall because the ulcer has produced stenosis of the duodenum distal to the pseudodiverticulum. Usually, it is best to dissect the pseudodiverticulum free unless dissection would result in injury to the common duct or probably create other hazards. The dissection can usually be accomplished by staying close to the pseudodiverticulum, clamping, cutting, and tying the small blood vessels running to that structure. The pseudodiverticulum is then excised. At times, it may be advisable to leave a small border of the diverticulum next to the stenotic area for more secure placement of the sutures (Fig. 8B).

It is frequently unnecessary and it may be unwise to remove an obstructing stenotic ulcer completely. By cutting *through* but not beyond the distal end of the stenotic area and freeing the duodenum for a short distance beyond, one is usually able to close the duodenum by two layers of a few interrupted Lembert or mattress sutures of silk (Fig. 9A, B, C, D), because of the small opening in the duodenum.

An ulcer may involve predominantly the superior border, and the pathology

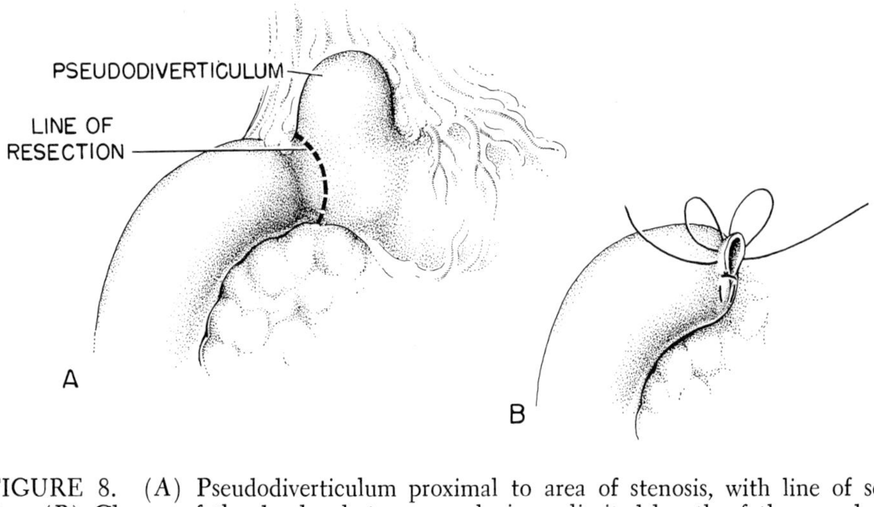

FIGURE 8. (A) Pseudodiverticulum proximal to area of stenosis, with line of section. (*B*) Closure of the duodenal stump employing a limited length of the pseudodiverticulum. Interrupted Lembert or mattress sutures may be used instead of the purse-string sutures shown in this illustration. A second layer of interrupted Lembert sutures is used to reinforce the closure.

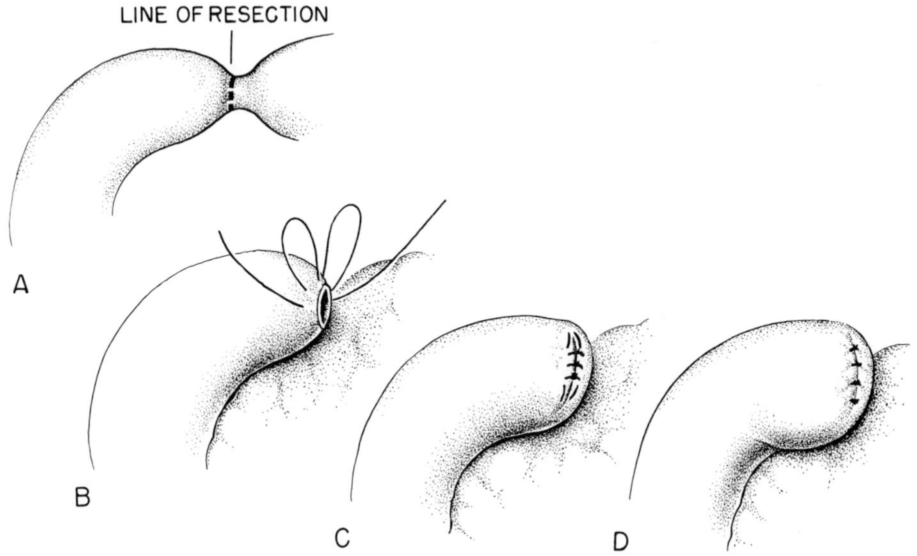

FIGURE 9. (*A*) Stenotic ulcer, with line of section. (*B*) Start of the first layer of the closure. (*C*) Completed first layer of the closure. Interrupted Lembert or mattress sutures may be used instead of the purse-string sutures shown in the illustration. (*D*) Completed closure of the duodenum.

may extend close to the common duct. In this situation the duodenum is transected through the distal border of the ulcer, and the distal duodenum is not freed or is freed to a very limited extent beyond the edge of the ulcer. The closure is started by placing a suture first in the posterior wall, then in the scar tissue which represents the distal border of the ulcer, and finally in the anterior wall of the duodenum (Fig. 10). After this suture has been tied, another suture is used to ap-

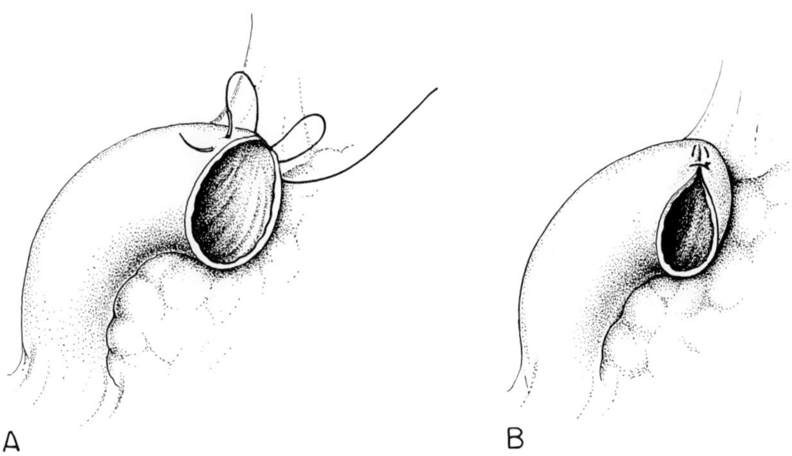

FIGURE 10. (*A*) Superior border ulcer. Insertion of the first suture, incorporating the distal edge of the ulcer. (*B*) First suture tied.

proximate the anterior and posterior walls above the previous suture. This maneuver usually closes the upper end of the duodenum satisfactorily. The remainder of the duodenum is closed by Lembert sutures. Another layer is inserted by suturing the anterior to the posterior wall of the duodenum by a second row of Lembert sutures, or by suturing the anterior wall of the duodenum to the peritoneum and areolar tissue on the pancreas. A similar approach is used to handle an ulcer along the inferior border of the duodenum or the small posterior wall ulcer which creates a narrow scarred defect in the posterior duodenal wall (Fig. 11), when dissection beyond the ulcer is not feasible.

The very large posterior ulcer which involves either the superior or the inferior border of the duodenum, or both, presents a serious problem. The duodenum when freed not only lacks the posterior wall but also has a disrupted superior or inferior border. If the potential problem is recognized early, it can be handled by doing a vagotomy and gastroenterostomy, instead of a gastrectomy. If dissection has been accomplished to a point where sectioning of the duodenum is necessary, a large catheter is inserted into the stump of the duodenum and closure is accomplished by interrupted silk sutures around the catheter. Penrose drains should be placed near the duodenum. The catheter and the Penrose drains are brought out through separate stab wounds in the abdominal wall. Consideration should be given to T tube drainage of the common duct, to divert the bile temporarily from the duodenum; and to the possible placement of a soft sump drain near the duodenal stump.

If one has committed himself technically to a partial gastrectomy and if further dissection of the duodenum appears hazardous, one may, on occasion, choose to leave in a distal segment of the stomach, according to methods advocated by Devine, Bancroft, Harvey, and others. For maximum safety, the decision to utilize this type of closure should be made prior to dissection of the duodenum,

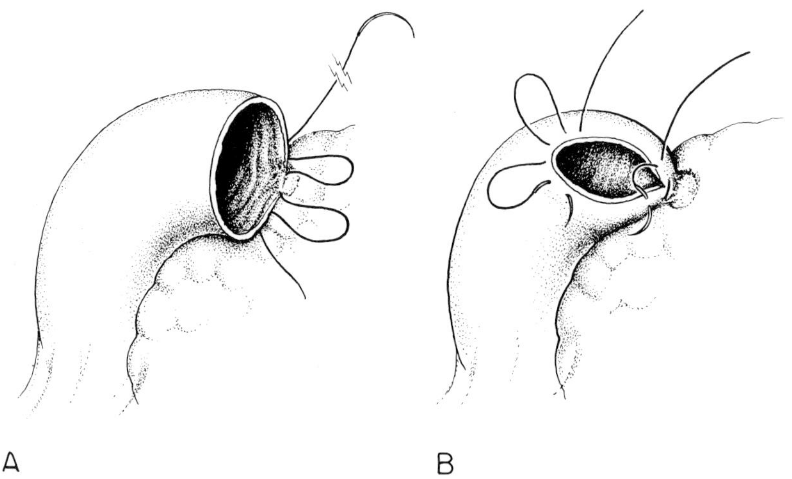

FIGURE 11. (*A*) Small posterior wall ulcer. Insertion of the first suture, incorporating the distal edge of the ulcer. (*B*) Method of inserting additional sutures of the first row of sutures.

for the blood supply to the prepyloric region of the antrum should be preserved. In the currently recommended method the antrum is divided 3 to 4 cm. from the pylorus, and the gastric mucosa down to the level of the pyloric ring is excised, after being freed by dissection along the plane of the submucosa. The mucosa at that point is closed by interrupted silk sutures, and the muscular walls of the stomach are approximated with one or two rows of horizontal mattress sutures placed in the manner of a quilting stitch. Harvey suggested oversewing but not inverting the antral stump with interrupted sutures. If one prefers to invert the end of the stump, a larger segment of stomach must be preserved. If there has been some questionable interference with the blood supply of the gastric stump, a No. 12 or No. 14 catheter is inserted through the end of the stump, into the duodenum, and the other end of the catheter is brought out through a stab wound in the abdominal wall. A Penrose drain is placed near the gastric stump and brought out alongside the catheter. This will establish a temporary fistula which should heal without too much difficulty. We have found it necessary to retain a segment of distal stomach after gastrectomy in less than 1 per cent of our patients and we believe that this approach should be rarely utilized.

In the literature many techniques have been recommended for handling specific problems of duodenal closure. The methods described in this chapter can be applied in most situations the surgeon is likely to encounter, although minor variations may be necessary.

Drainage After Duodenal Stump Closure

Although I rarely insert drains to the periduodenal area after gastrectomy, I wish to emphasize that these drains usually do not cause complications, and if one has any concern as to the security of the closure, he should not hesitate to place two Penrose drains near the duodenum and bring them out through a separate stab wound. Two drains rather than one are preferred, because they establish a larger drainage tract.

One should also take proper precautions, in performing the gastrojejunostomy, to avoid producing partial obstruction to the proximal jejunal loop. If one employs an antecolic anastomosis in the obese patient, it is frequently advisable to resect the omentum in the area where the jejunal loop eventually rests.

If a catheter is inserted into the end of the duodenum or through the end of a gastric stump, it is usually left in situ for 10 to 12 days. Dependent tube drainage or suction is attached, depending on the volume of drainage.

If limited leakage occurs postoperatively from a duodenal stump, it may be adequately handled by the Penrose drains if such drains were inserted at the time of surgery. If drains were not inserted, or if the drainage is excessive, or if the general or local clinical findings imply inadequate drainage, the area of the duodenal stump should be promptly explored and proper drainage established. This may require the insertion of a sump drain. If one suspects an accumulation of fluid along the right colon or in the pelvis, a McBurney incision should also be accomplished for exploration, aspiration, and drainage. Proper attention should be given to the fluid and electrolyte problem, and to the use of antibiotics. If adequate drainage is maintained, and additional complications such as a pancreatic fistula or erosions of blood vessels do not occur, the fistula usually closes spontaneously.

References

BANCROFT, F. W. A modification of the Devine operation of pyloric exclusion for duodenal ulcer. *Am. J. Surg.* 16:223, August 1932.

COOPER, P. Duodenal closure after gastrectomy for duodenal ulcer. *Surgery* 50:425, August 1961.

GINZBURG, L. Management of the difficult duodenal stump. Technical considerations. *S. Clin. North America* 34:473, April 1954.

HARVEY, H. D. Safety in performing partial gastrectomy for peptic ulcer. *Ann. Surg.* 153:256, February 1961.

NISSEN, R. *Duodenal and Jejunal Peptic Ulcer, Technique of Resection.* New York: Grune & Stratton, 1945.

84. A Method of Handling the Jejunal Loop in Subtotal Gastrectomy with a Posterior Anastomosis

J. ENGLEBERT DUNPHY

SUBTOTAL GASTRECTOMY with removal of two-thirds of the stomach and reconstruction by a gastrojejunal anastomosis is a well-established operation. It has acquired over the years an excellent reputation in the treatment of both gastric cancer and duodenal or gastric ulcer. Although lesser procedures such as 50 per cent gastrectomy and vagotomy, or pyloroplasty and vagotomy, have a somewhat lower mortality and for this reason are currently popular, it remains to be seen whether they will provide as effective long-range control of the ulcer diathesis as a 60 per cent subtotal gastric resection.

There are many advantages to carrying out a posterior anastomosis of jejunum to stomach, but because of certain disadvantages there has been a tendency to abandon the posterior anastomosis for the somewhat simpler anterior anastomosis. The chief disadvantages ascribed to the posterior anastomosis are: (1) The stomach, which has been pulled through the rent in the mesocolon, tends to slip upward, thus producing postoperative obstruction. (2) In some patients, the transverse colon must be dislocated well up into the upper abdomen in order to permit the stomach to be brought through the rent in the mesocolon. This places the stomach and colon in close proximity and favors the development of a gastrojejunocolic fistula if a marginal ulcer should develop. (3) A loop of jejunum enters and leaves the stomach in the free peritoneal cavity, behind which herniation or volvulus may occur. (4) If there is a need, either early or late, for reoperation, the anastomosis is in an inaccessible position. Because of these disadvantages, anterior anastomosis is more commonly used.

One difficulty with anterior anastomosis is that the proximal limb of the loop is apt to be longer than is necessary with posterior anastomosis. There is also no bar to herniation behind the loop. Moreover, if the mesocolon is heavy it tends to drag against the proximal limb unless this is made quite long.

The method described in this chapter avoids all the difficulties encountered in the conventional performance of either a posterior or an anterior anastomosis.

In this procedure the afferent limb can be made quite short without the slightest tension. There can be no slipping of the attachment of the mesocolon to the stomach, because the colon is left in its normal position and the stomach is allowed to retract comfortably well up into the left upper quadrant of the abdomen. Herniation behind the anastomosis is impossible. Finally, the anastomosis itself presents readily for inspection or exposure in the event of an immediate or late postoperative complication.

Technique

The steps of this procedure are illustrated in Figures 1 through 8. After completion of the resection of the stomach, the first step in proceeding to the anastomosis is to mobilize the proximal jejunum at the ligament of Treitz. This is illustrated in Figure 1. Gentle dissection to the right mobilizes the fourth portion of the duodenum in an avascular area. Care should be taken not to injure the inferior mesenteric vein, which is to the left, or the superior mesenteric artery and vein, which are to the right. Ordinarily these three structures are well out of the field of the dissection, and very adequate mobilization of the bowel can be obtained so that the fourth portion of the duodenum and the proximal jejunum are displaced into the lesser peritoneal sac directly across the body of the pancreas.

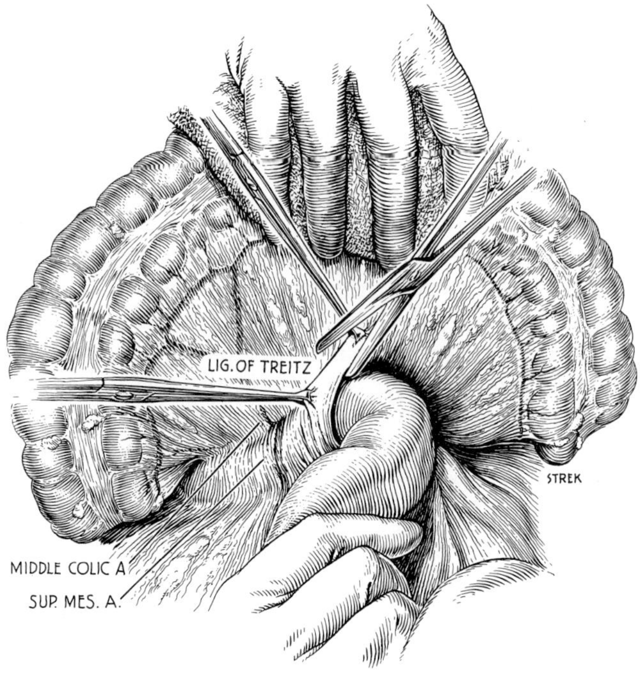

FIGURE 1. Exposure and incision of the ligament of Treitz. (All figures in this chapter are reproduced by permission of *Surgery, Gynecology and Obstetrics* from Dunphy, J. E., *Surg., Gynec. and Obst.*, 110:108, January 1960.)

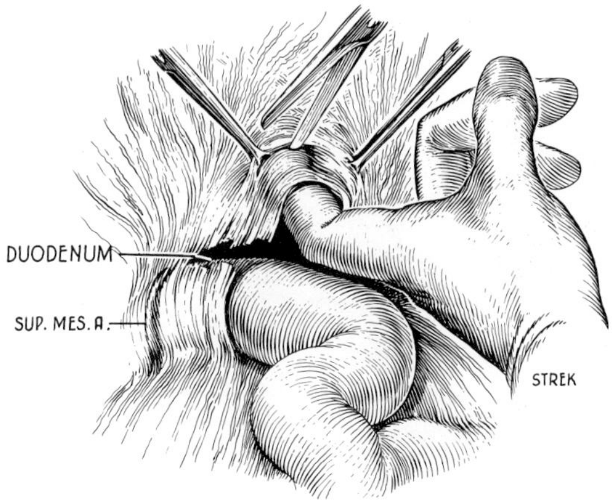

FIGURE 2. Mobilization of the root of the mesocolon.

The extent of the mobilization is shown in Figure 2. In the thin patient, practically no dissection is required, and in many instances the proximal jejunum and fourth portion of the duodenum lift up readily into the lesser sac with minimal dissection. In the obese person, a fair amount of cautious mobilization is necessary.

Figure 3 depicts the dissection just prior to bringing the bowel through the opening at the root of the mesocolon. The dissection as shown lies directly on the pancreas, and the opening is well away from the transverse colon.

A loop of the fourth portion of the duodenum and proximal jejunum is now drawn through the rent in the mesocolon as shown in Figure 4. Because of the mobilization, the fourth portion of the duodenum is not angulated and passes directly to the anastomosis, which can now be performed in any of the conventional fashions (Fig. 5).

Most of the time the afferent limb will be found to pass conveniently to the

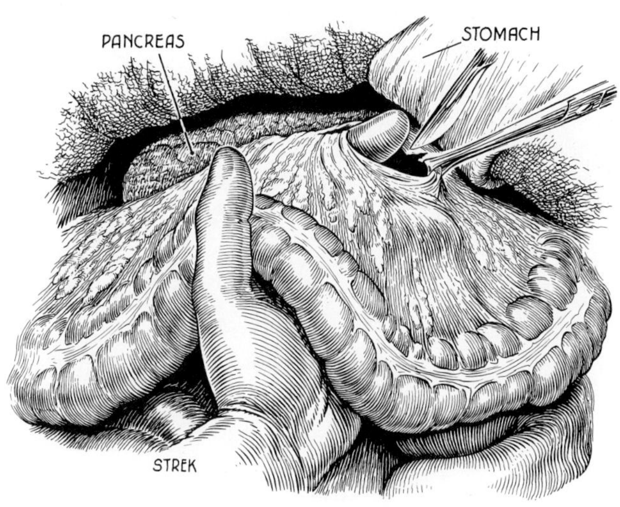

FIGURE 3. Further dissection at the root of the mesocolon.

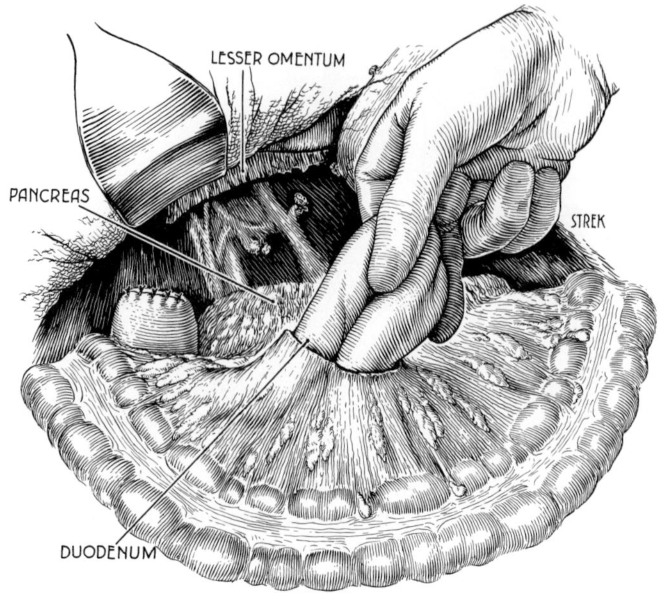

FIGURE 4. Distal duodenum and proximal jejunum drawn through the opening in the mesocolon.

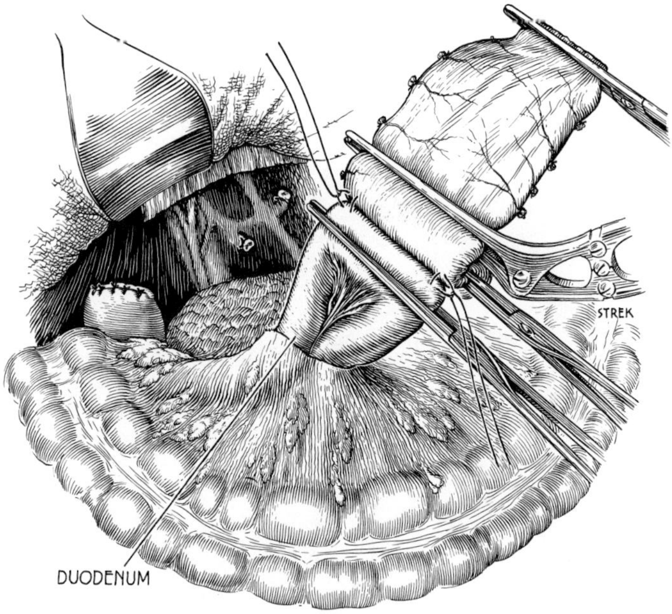

FIGURE 5. Anastomosis of duodenojejunum to stomach.

lesser curvature, but at other times it will fit more appropriately to the greater curvature. The essential point is to avoid any tension or angulation of the bowel. It makes no functional difference whether the anastomosis is completed in an anti-peristaltic or isoperistaltic fashion.

The completed anastomosis is depicted in Figure 6. It can be seen that the afferent limb lies completely in the lesser peritoneal cavity while the efferent limb and its mesentery pass through the opening in the mescolon to the stomach. It is now necessary to reconstruct the loose areolar and fatty tissue of the ligament of Treitz against the efferent limb and its mesentery to prevent the passage of any adjacent loop of bowel through the rent in the mesocolon and also to fix the efferent limb at the point where it passes through the opening. This is done with three or four carefully placed silk sutures. At the completion of this procedure, when the surgeon lifts up the mesocolon, only one limb is seen to pass through it into the peritoneal cavity. Indeed, it is difficult to tell that a gastric resection has been performed if one looks at the ligament of Treitz.

On the upper side of the mesocolon one finds the loop of bowel passing from the fourth portion of duodenum to the stomach and then back to the opening in the mesocolon. The loop is left sufficiently long to lie without tension in the lesser peritoneal cavity. The view is shown from both sides in Figure 6, (*A*) from above and (*B*) from below the mesocolon.

As aids to understanding, the relationships are shown diagrammatically in Figures 7 and 8. The preoperative situation is shown in Figure 7. The duodenum lies entirely posteriorly. The postoperative situation is depicted in Figure 8. As can be seen, the fourth portion of duodenum and the jejunal limb now occupy the same posterior position in the lesser sac. In practice the mesocolon can be laid across the loop at any convenient point, so that there is no tension whatsoever on the anastomosis.

At the completion of the operation, the stomach is allowed to retract into

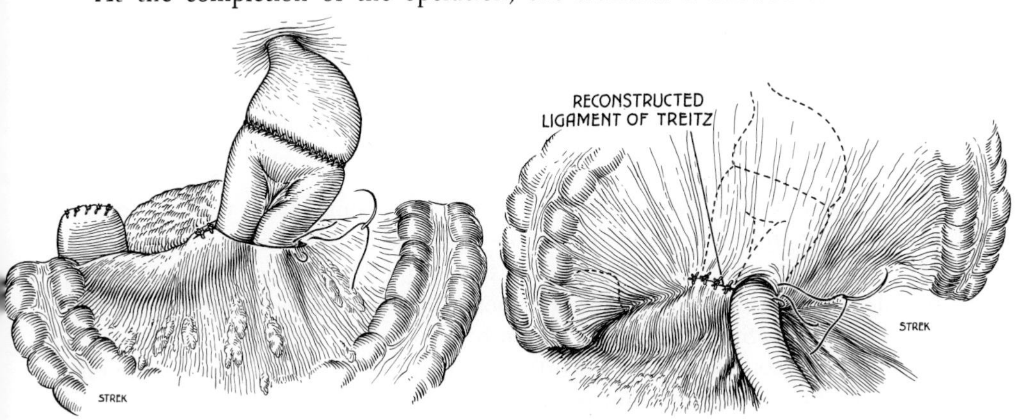

A **B**

FIGURE 6. (*A*) Completed anastomosis. (*B*) Reconstruction of the ligament of Treitz.

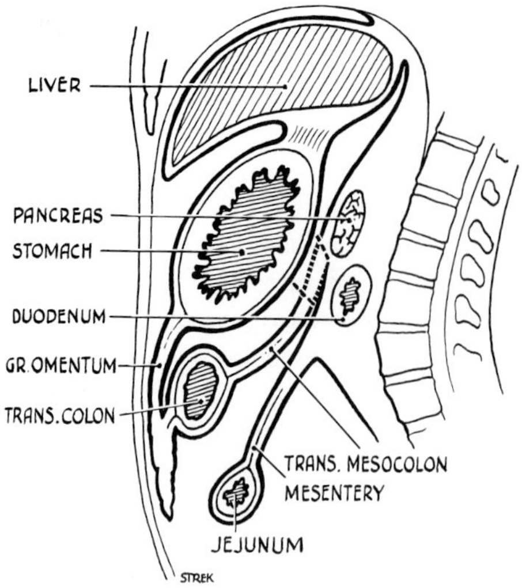

FIGURE 7. Preoperative relationship of the duodenum and the jejunum.

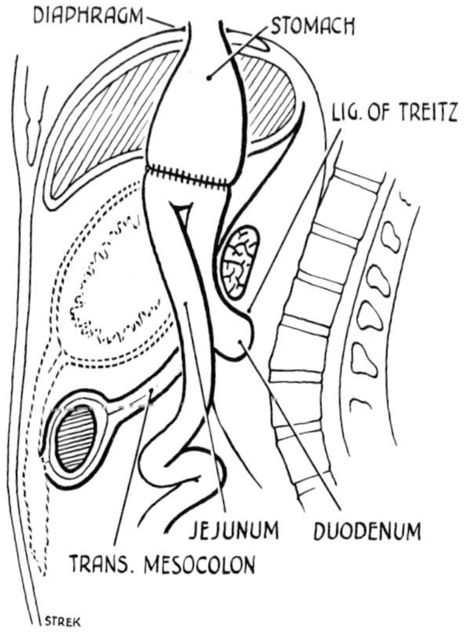

FIGURE 8. Postoperative relationship of the duodenum and the jejunum.

the left upper quadrant, where the anastomosis rests comfortably without tension. It is well away from the transverse colon and readily accessible to the operator in the event that reoperation for any reason might be required. Only one limb of bowel passes through the mesocolon; hence, there is no possibility of a gastrojejunal herniation. Since the proximal limb lies entirely above the mesocolon, it is not subject to compression or distortion by the drag of the colon, and the efferent limb lies in a similar position passing through the mesocolon so far posteriorly that it also is free of tension or rotation.

An extensive experience with this procedure has been without complications related to postoperative obstruction or the so-called afferent loop syndrome. The incidence of postoperative dumping and other undesirable sequelae of gastrectomy has been very low.

85. *Gastrostomy, Pyloroplasty, and Operative Treatment of Perforated Peptic Ulcer*

PETER A. ROSI

Gastrostomy

GASTROSTOMY FEEDING, through either a temporary tube gastrostomy or a permanent tubulovalvular fistula, has long been an accepted treatment for patients who cannot swallow because of neurogenic disturbances or organic obstruction of the upper stomach and esophagus. Temporary gastrostomy is of value for short-term feeding of patients undergoing resections of the esophagus and stomach. Also, in recent years, temporary tube gastrostomy, which is associated with little discomfort to the patient, has been replacing nasogastric suction for postoperative decompression of the stomach.

Temporary gastrostomies, which are usually performed by means of a catheter placed into the stomach and brought out of the peritoneal cavity through a stab wound in the abdominal wall, are lined by a serosal membrane that forms around the catheter. After removal of the catheter, the sinus tract immediately closes.

In patients who require long-term feeding, a permanent gastrostomy is often necessary. Permanent gastrostomies are usually formed by constructing from the wall of the stomach a mucosa-lined tube which is brought out to the skin through a stab wound in the abdominal wall. The advantage of this type of gastrostomy is that it eliminates the indwelling catheter of the temporary gastrostomy. A catheter is inserted into the stomach through the gastrostomy tube only at the time of feeding and is then withdrawn. The disadvantages of a permanent gastrostomy are that it is more difficult to perform than a temporary gastrostomy and the operation usually requires a general anesthetic, whereas temporary gastrostomies can be simply performed under local anesthesia. Also, if the need for a permanent gastrostomy is eliminated, a second laparotomy is necessary in order to remove the mucosal tract.

Technique

Temporary Gastrostomy. There are many methods of establishing a temporary tube gastrostomy. The one originally described by Stamm is the simplest and most frequently performed for temporary feeding or decompression of the stomach. The stomach is exposed through a left paramedian or transverse left upper abdominal incision, as shown in Figure 1, and a tube is inserted.

Of the many types of gastrostomy tubes, such as urethral, mushroom, or balloon catheters, the Foley balloon catheter is the most effective since the inflated balloon prevents the catheter from being accidentally pulled out of the stomach. If the catheter for some reason needs to be changed, the balloon is deflated, the catheter is removed, and a new catheter is immediately inserted into the stomach and the bag inflated.

The technique for performing a gastrostomy is as follows. A purse-string suture of a nonabsorbable material, such as 3–0 silk or dacron, is placed at the site of the proposed gastrostomy, which is preferably near the greater curvature of the stomach. A No. 20 to 24 Foley catheter is inserted into the stomach through a

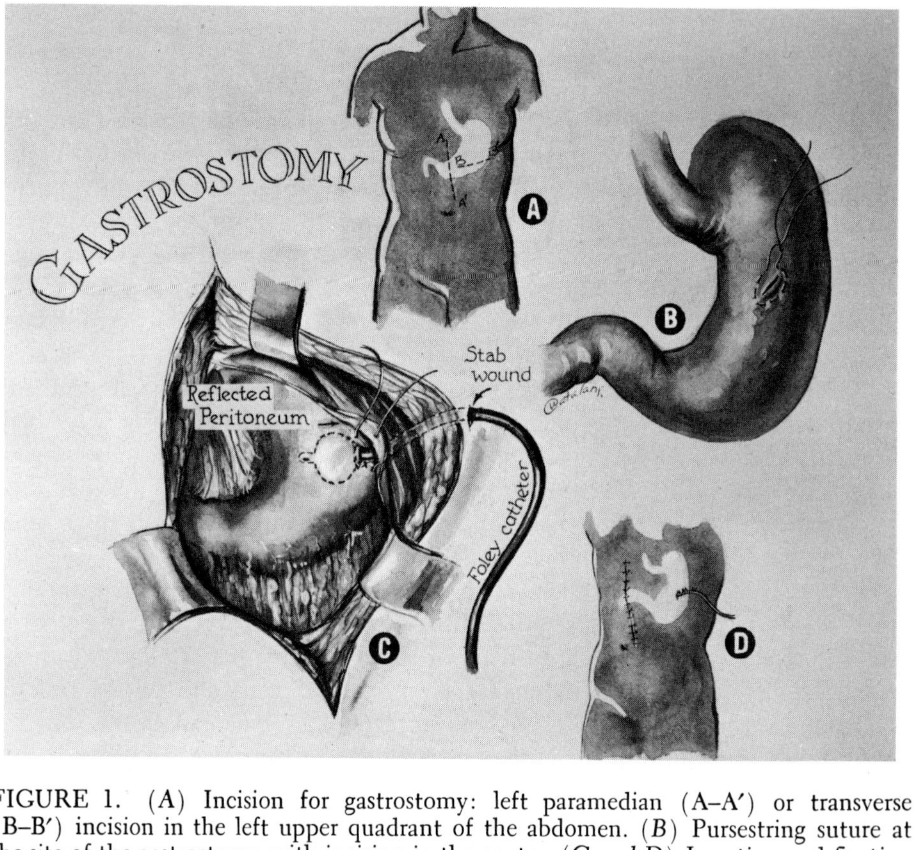

FIGURE 1. (*A*) Incision for gastrostomy: left paramedian (A–A′) or transverse (B–B′) incision in the left upper quadrant of the abdomen. (*B*) Pursestring suture at the site of the gastrostomy, with incision in the center. (*C and D*) Insertion and fixation of the Foley catheter.

stab wound in the center of the purse-string suture, which is drawn taut against the catheter and tied. The balloon of the Foley catheter is inflated with about 10 to 20 ml. of sterile saline. A second purse-string or several interrupted sutures are placed into the stomach adjacent to the catheter to provide additional security of the stab wound in the stomach against leakage. The stomach is then replaced into its normal position in the left upper quadrant of the abdomen, and the catheter is brought out of the peritoneal cavity through a stab wound in the abdominal wall, as closely as possible to the gastrostomy opening in the stomach.

The stomach is drawn up to the abdominal wall by traction on the Foley catheter. The stomach adjacent to the gastrostomy is fixed to the peritoneum at the site of the stab wound with interrupted 4–0 silk or dacron sutures. This maneuver further seals off the gastrostomy fistula from the peritoneal cavity and reduces the incidence of peritonitis from leakage around the gastrostomy stoma, which has been reported as an infrequent complication following tube gastrostomy.

If the stomach is not sufficiently mobile to be brought up to the abdominal wall, the catheter passes through the unprotected peritoneal cavity to the stab wound in the abdominal wall. Some protection of the peritoneal cavity from leakage may be obtained by surrounding the catheter with omentum or by drawing the catheter through a channel made between the peritoneum and the abdominal wall.

To prevent accidental withdrawal of the gastrostomy tube, the Foley catheter is fixed to the skin with two steel wire sutures that are tied around the catheter in the form of a "Chinese basket stitch." Stainless steel wire sutures are preferred for this purpose because of their greater strength and because of the minimal skin reaction around the wire suture, which may have to remain in place for two or more weeks.

Postoperatively, constant low vacuum suction is immediately applied to the gastrostomy tube. If the gastrostomy tube is for postoperative decompression, the tube is clamped after peristalsis has been established. If the tube is to be used for feeding, suction is likewise continued until all signs of the immediate postoperative ileus have disappeared and sufficient time has elapsed for fibrinous exudate to form around the gastrostomy tube and between the stomach and abdominal wall. This period may vary from three to seven days.

Tube feeding should be delayed until the gastrointestinal motility returns to normal. If tube feeding is begun before this occurs, the feeding may increase the pressure in the stomach and may predispose to leakage around the gastrostomy tube, with resultant peritonitis. In young patients, feeding may be started from five to seven days postoperatively, but in older and often debilitated individuals with poor healing capabilities, feeding is better delayed for seven to ten days after surgery.

Once the tube gastrostomy is no longer necessary, the tube is removed. The serosa-lined sinus tract immediately closes. When tube gastrostomies have been used for decompression in lieu of nasogastric suction, the tubes have sometimes been removed after four to five days. However, instances have been reported of development of peritonitis after early removal of the tube. To prevent this complication, decompression tubes are clamped and left in place for about seven to ten days. If the patient has had a vagotomy, the tube is left in place until pyloric balance studies show that gastric stasis has disappeared.

In patients in whom the stomach was not sufficiently mobile to be brought up to the abdominal wall, a long, poorly protected fistulous tract which crosses the peritoneal cavity develops around the tube. In such instances it is wise to leave the tube in place until a well-established fibrous fistulous tract forms. Depending on the age of the patient, this may require as long as 21 to 30 days and often as long as six to eight weeks. A good axiom for removal of gastrostomy tubes is: A clamped gastrostomy tube that is left in place does no harm, but removal of a tube before a fistulous tract has been established may lead to disastrous peritonitis.

PERMANENT GASTROSTOMY. Permanent gastrostomy for long-term feeding of patients with obstruction in the upper stomach or esophagus is infrequently performed since many of the neoplasms are either removed surgically or palliated by radiotherapy. In selected patients in whom prolonged gastrostomy feeding is required, a permanent type of gastrostomy with a mucosa-lined tract is indicated since, unlike the serosa-lined tract of the temporary gastrostomy, the mucosa-lined tract does not close spontaneously and does not require continued intubation.

The basic operation for a permanent gastrostomy is the construction, from the stomach wall, of a tube that can be brought out to the abdominal wall. The tubes developed by the early gastrostomy technique had the disadvantage that gastric contents often leaked backward through the tube and onto the abdominal wall, where it often produced a severe inflammation of the adjacent skin. The fashioning of a valve-like fold at the origin of the tube from the stomach wall, as popularized by Spivak, prevents this complication.

The basic feature of a tubulovalvular gastrostomy (shown in Figure 2) is the construction of a valve parallel with and about 2 cm. from the lesser curvature of the pars media of the stomach. The valve is made by folding the stomach wall with interrupted 4–0 silk sutures over a No. 14 French urethral catheter. A flap of stomach wall for the proposed tube is fashioned from the base of the valve toward the greater curvature. It should be long enough to go through the abdominal wall. The flap is then displaced upward toward the lesser curvature, thus exposing the mucosal aspect of folded stomach wall that will form the doughnut-like valve at the base of the tube when opposite ends of this infolding are approximated by a 4–0 silk seromuscular suture. The defect in the stomach wall is repaired with a layer of continuous catgut sutures reinforced with interrupted 4–0 silk sutures.

A tube is then constructed from the isolated flap of the anterior stomach wall by approximating the mucosal and seromuscular layers with a continuous non-inverting stitch of 4–0 catgut reinforced with interrupted 4–0 silk seromuscular sutures, the last of which is placed near the stoma and left long so that it may act as a guide and tractor in bringing the tube onto the abdominal wall through a stab wound in the left upper quadrant.

The stab wound in the abdominal wall is placed where there is the least distance between the abdominal wall and the site of the origin of the tubulovalvular gastrostomy from the stomach. A circular piece of skin of about the diameter of

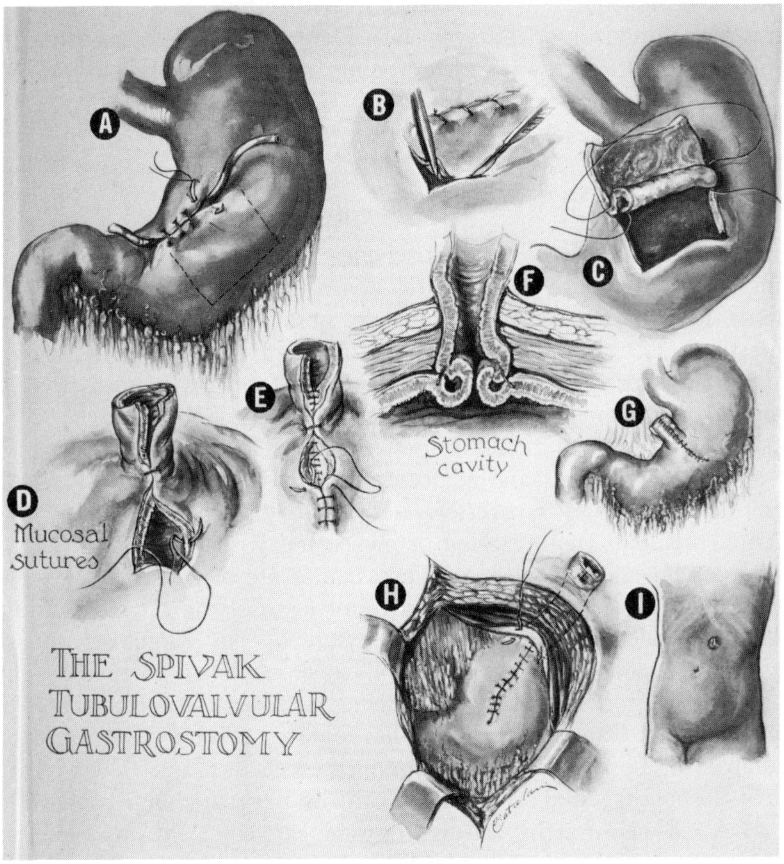

FIGURE 2. (A) Inversion of a fold of stomach wall over the catheter. (*B*) Cutting the flap of stomach wall for the tube. (*C*) Upward displacement of the flap, exposing the gastric fold at its base. (*D and F*) Formation of the doughnut-like valve. (*E and G*) Repair of the defect in the stomach wall. (*H*) Suture of the stomach wall and fixation of the tube to the skin. (*I*) The completed tube.

the gastrostomy tube is excised at the site of the stab wound in order to prevent postoperative stricture of the stoma. A similar circle is excised from the anterior and posterior rectus fascias and the peritoneum.

After the tube has been drawn through the abdominal wall, the stomach at the base of the tube is attached to the peritoneum surrounding the stab wound with interrupted 5–0 silk sutures. The stoma is also attached to the subcutaneous tissues and derma of the skin with interrupted 5–0 silk sutures.

When the operation is completed the tube should accommodate a No. 14 to No. 16 French catheter.

The postoperative care of these patients consists of gastric decompression by continuous nasogastric suction or by intermittent suction through a No. 14 French catheter that is passed into the stomach through a tubulovalvular gastrostomy about every 6 to 12 hours.

When the stomach has recovered its normal tone and peristalsis, decompression is discontinued and feeding is started. A catheter is inserted into the stomach through the gastrostomy only for feeding, after which it is removed.

Pyloroplasty

Plastic reconstruction of the pylorus whenever possible is the best method of correcting gastric stasis that occurs after neurogenic or scar tissue obstruction of the pylorus. Pyloroplasty, by maintaining the normal passage of food through the gastrointestinal tract, is followed by little if any disturbance in gastrointestinal physiology and is particularly suited for the relief of gastric stasis that follows vagotomy in the treatment of peptic ulcer.

The pyloroplasty operation first described by Heineke-Mikulicz, which consists of incising the pylorus and adjacent stomach and duodenum longitudinally and repairing the incision transversely, is the simplest procedure and, with minor modifications, remains the operation of choice today. The operation entails little risk to the patient and, except for the occasional case of postoperative stenosis at the site of anastomosis that occurs as a result of infolding a large diaphragm of stomach and duodenal wall during the closure of the pyloroplasty incision, is followed by few complications. To avoid such infolding, Weinberg suggested closure of the incision in one layer, utilizing interrupted nonabsorbable sutures and a noninverting Gambee stitch. He has reported the largest series of patients operated upon in this manner, and has obtained excellent results. The advantages of the type of closure suggested by Weinberg can also be secured by a two-layer closure with interrupted noninverting sutures of fine catgut in the mucosa and nonabsorbable sutures in the seromuscular layer.

Pyloroplasty with vagotomy and transfixion of bleeding vessels is receiving increasing acceptance for the treatment of bleeding duodenal ulcer. In these cases the pyloroplasty incision which exposes the lower portion of the stomach and duodenum permits careful inspection of this area for bleeding, allows access to the majority of bleeding peptic ulcers, and permits transfixion of the eroded vessel. Since the operation has a low operative risk and morbidity, many patients with actively bleeding peptic ulcer who might not be able to withstand a gastric resection can be operated upon early during the bleeding episode with immediate control of the hemorrhage.

Technique

The type of abdominal incision that is most suitable for performing a pyloroplasty depends upon the habitus of the patient and the angle of the costal arch. Thin persons, who usually have an acute angulation of the costal arch, are more easily operated upon through a right paramedian incision, whereas stout, obese individuals with a broad costal arch are better operated upon through a transverse incision at about the level of the midepigastrium (Fig. 3).

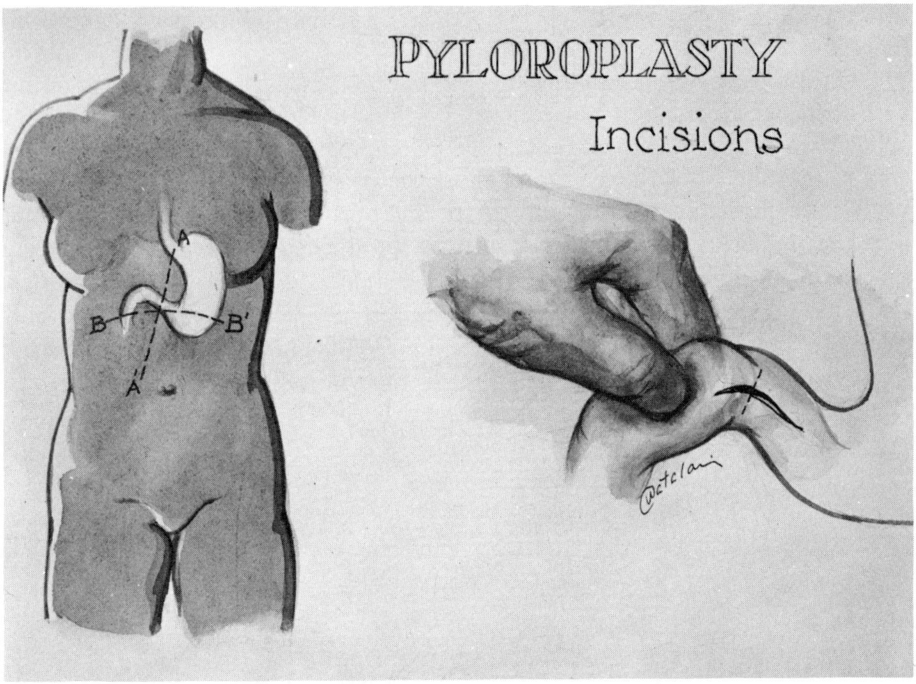

FIGURE 3. A–A′: Right paramedian incision. B–B′: Transverse abdominal incision that may be arched upward. The incision extends through the pylorus and into the lower 3 cm. of the stomach and upper 2 cm. of the duodenum.

If the pyloroplasty is performed in conjunction with vagotomy for the treatment of duodenal ulcer, the vagotomy is done first in order to prevent contamination of the esophageal hiatus and mediastinum.

If the pyloroplasty is performed for the control of a hemorrhage, the pyloroplasty is done first in order to establish the diagnosis of a duodenal ulcer, if one is present, before the vagus nerves are divided. This procedure avoids a needless vagotomy if the exploration of the area of the pylorus fails to reveal an ulcer.

The technique of pyloroplasty consists first of the identification of the duodenum and the pyloric ring. In most instances this area is free of adhesions and there is good visualization and sufficient mobility of the stomach and duodenum for performing the pyloroplasty without tension on the suture line. In some instances, as a result either of the habitus of the patient or of adhesions around the duodenum, there is not enough mobility of the stomach or duodenum for a pyloroplasty. In these patients the duodenum is mobilized by the Kocher maneuver; that is, by cutting the lateral peritoneal reflection and freeing the duodenum from the posterior abdominal wall. In patients with a long history of duodenal ulcer, and particularly if scar tissue deformity and contracture of the first portion of the duodenum are present, mobilization of the duodenum will fail to give sufficient freedom of the pyloric region to permit a Heineke-Mikulicz pyloroplasty to be performed with any degree of safety from postoperative stenosis of the stoma. When this condition exists, pyloroplasty should be abandoned in favor of some other procedure.

Once the indication for a pyloroplasty has been established, the operation can be carried out according to the following technique (Fig. 4). Two guide sutures, about 1 cm. apart, are placed through the pyloric sphincter in a relatively avascular area in the middle of the anterior wall of the pylorus. A longitudinal incision is made through the pyloric ring into the pyloric canal. The incision is extended up into the stomach for about 3 cm. and into the duodenum for about 2 cm. The mucosa of the duodenum is inspected for ulceration, and the second portion of the duodenum is examined for the possibility of a stenosis which might lead to postoperative complications. The gastric mucosa is carefully inspected. Traction is made upon the two original guide sutures through the pyloric sphincter in order to con-

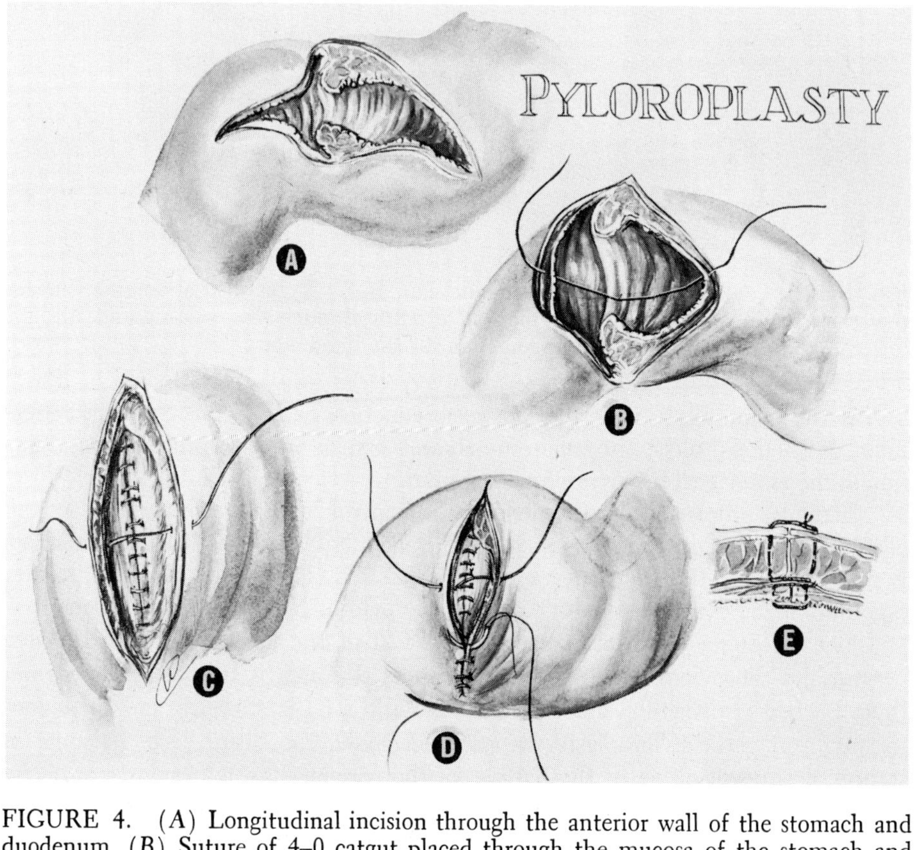

FIGURE 4. (*A*) Longitudinal incision through the anterior wall of the stomach and duodenum. (*B*) Suture of 4–0 catgut placed through the mucosa of the stomach and duodenum at the ends of the longitudinal incision. The suture, when tied, equally divides the now transverse incision. (*C*) Approximation of the remaining mucosa of the stomach and duodenum with interrupted 4–0 catgut sutures. (*D and E*) Approximation of the cut edges of the seromuscular layer of the stomach and duodenum, without inversion, with interrupted 4–0 silk sutures placed about 2 mm. from the cut edge and about 3 mm. apart. The completed anastomosis widens the pyloric canal to about 2 to 3 cm.

vert the longitudinal incision into a transverse opening. The now transversely placed incision may be closed either in two layers by suturing the mucosa and seromuscular layers separately, or in one layer with a noninverting Gambee stitch. If there is edema in the region of the pylorus because of an active duodenal ulcer, a two-layer closure with interrupted stitches of 4–0 catgut in the mucosa and 4–0 silk in the seromuscular layer may be technically more desirable.

In performing a two-layer closure, the first suture is placed through the opposite ends of the original longitudinal incision so as to divide the now transversely placed incision into equal parts. The remaining mucosa is repaired with 4–0 catgut sutures placed about 3 mm. apart, from the greater to the lesser curvature. Upon completion of the mucosal anastomosis the defect in the seromuscular layer of the adjoining stomach and duodenum is repaired in a similar manner with 4–0 silk sutures. When these sutures are tied, they simply approximate the cut edges of the mucosal and seromuscular layers of the stomach and duodenum; there is no inversion of the suture line and no reduction in the size of the stoma.

If the alternative method of one-layer closure of the pyloroplasty incision is chosen, the cut edges of the wall of the stomach and duodenum are approximated by interrupted Gambee stitches (Fig. 5) with a 4–0 silk suture. The first suture is

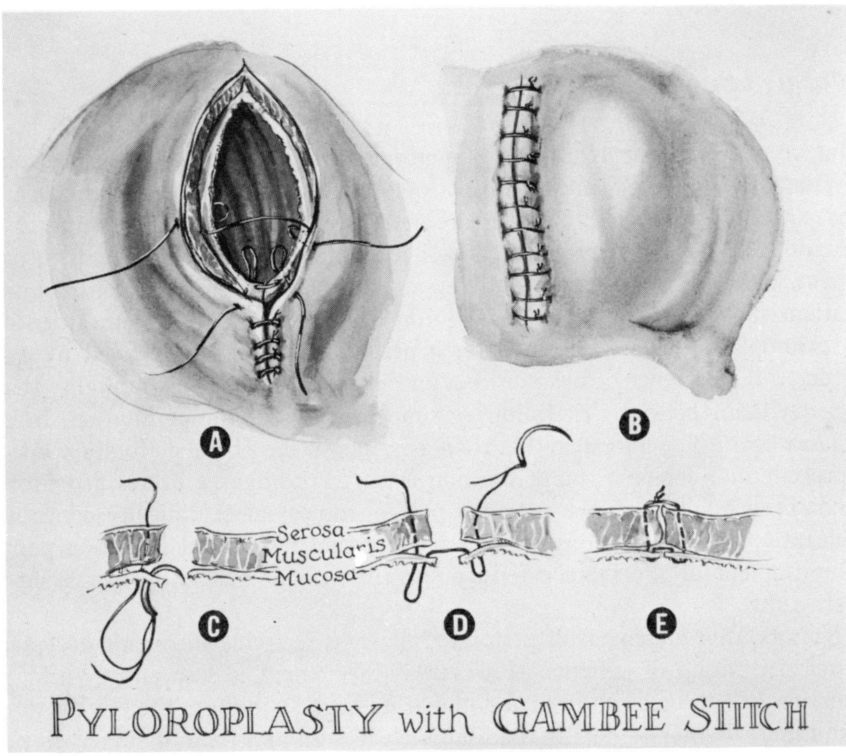

FIGURE 5. Pyloroplasty closure with Gambee suture. (*A, C, and D*) Steps in placing a Gambee stitch. (*B*) When tied, the sutures approximate the cut edges of the stomach and duodenum without inversion. (*E*) Cross-section of the Gambee stitch.

placed through the ends of the original longitudinal incision to divide equally the now transversely placed incision. The remaining sutures are placed from the greater to the lesser curvature. The sutures are placed about 3 to 4 mm. from the cut edge of the stomach and duodenum and about 3 mm. apart. The course of the sutures is from the serosa of the stomach through the entire wall of the stomach and back through only the mucosa of the stomach, then over to the duodenum through the mucosa of the duodenum into the lumen of the duodenum and then back out through the seromuscular layers (Fig. 5A, C, D). When these sutures are tied the cut edges of the mucosa and seromuscular layers of the stomach and duodenum come together without any tendency toward inversion of the wall of the stomach and duodenum at the site of anastomosis (Fig. 5B). This avoids the development of a diaphragm which, by decreasing the size of the stoma, may lead to a post-operative stenosis. Upon completion of the anastomosis the pyloric segment is covered by the adjacent gastrocolic or greater omentum.

The postoperative care of patients with pyloroplasty consists of decompression of the stomach either by means of a nasogastric tube or, as is currently popular in many clinics, by means of a Foley catheter gastrostomy. After normal peristalsis and gastric motility has returned, the patients are given feedings which are gradually increased up to a general diet.

Perforated Peptic Ulcer

During recent years the treatment of perforated peptic ulcer has shifted from a predominantly simple closure of the perforation to ulcer-curative operations in selected patients. Although the immediate mortality following simple closure of the perforation has been low, the incidence of recurrent ulcer disease, such as intractable pain, bleeding, obstruction, and reperforation, has been high. Ulcer-curative operations such as gastric resection, vagotomy and antral resection, and vagotomy with pyloroplasty, when performed for a perforated ulcer, are followed by a low postoperative recurrence of ulcer disease, and in selected cases by a mortality that is no greater than the mortality following simple closure of the perforation. In general, ulcer-curative operations rather than a simple suture of the perforation may be the procedure of choice if the perforation is of recent origin, a bacterial peritonitis has not been established, the patient's past history of ulcer difficulty contributes significantly to the indications for such surgery, and his general condition permits accomplishment of the more extensive surgery without materially increasing the operative risk.

Nonoperative treatment of perforated ulcers is receiving increasing acceptance in a selected group of patients. However, if the patient is seen shortly after the perforation has occurred and the abdominal findings are diffuse, there is no way of determining whether or not the perforation will seal, and prompt surgery is probably indicated. If the abdominal findings when the patient is admitted to the hospital are limited to the right side or to the right upper quadrant of the abdomen, it is reasonable to observe the patient for several hours and then make the final decision on the type of therapy. If the patient's history when he is first seen is consistent with a perforation from 8 to 12 hours old and the abdominal findings are limited, it may be assumed that the perforation has sealed. Nonoperative treatment may be initiated and the patient carefully observed.

Clinical observation has shown that the conservative treatment of perforated ulcer with nasogastric suction and intravenous fluids and antibiotic drugs has, in general, been effective for patients who have had no previous history of ulcer disease and in whom the perforation has been sealed off from the peritoneal cavity by fibrinous exudate. Although the incidence of recurrent ulcer disease is low after surgical treatment of acute ulcers, conservative treatment, if it appears feasible and safe, is now considered more desirable than surgical closure of the perforation, which some surgeons believe may convert into a chronic ulcer.

Simple closure of the perforation, rather than an ulcer-curative operation, is the procedure of choice in the treatment of perforated acute and chronic ulcers with associated bacterial peritonitis. Simple closure is indicated also for perforated acute and chronic ulcers in the poor risk and elderly patient who would not withstand an ulcer-curative operation, and for perforated drug-induced or stress ulcers.

Perforated benign gastric ulcers may be treated by simple closure. However, since gastric ulcers are often malignant, the better procedure is to excise the ulcer for biopsy purposes and close the resultant defect in the stomach with a through-and-through nonabsorbable suture. In selected patients who are in good condition and have no bacterial peritonitis, a gastric resection may be done at this time without increasing the operative risk.

Perforated gastrojejunal ulcers in the absence of obstruction are best treated by simple closure of the perforation and vagotomy.

Technique of Repair

The majority of perforated ulcers occur in the anterior wall of the first portion of the duodenum and lower portion of the stomach within a radius of about 4 cm. from the pylorus. Since perforations usually occur in this restricted area, the abdominal incisions for the repair of perforated ulcers should be planned with this fact in mind (Fig. 6). The choice of the incision is also influenced by the general condition of the patient and the type of anesthesia. If there are no contraindications for general or spinal anesthesia, a right paramedian or transverse upper abdominal incision that is curved upward toward the costal arch will give adequate exposure of the upper abdomen. Perforated ulcers in poor risk patients who might not withstand a general or spinal anesthetic can be closed under local anesthesia through a long right paramedian muscle- and fascia-splitting incision. It begins at the xyphoid and extends to the right of the umbilicus. The anterior rectus sheath is divided about a centimeter from the midline. The right rectus muscle is retracted laterally; the posterior rectus sheath and the transversalis muscle are divided transversely at a point midway between the xyphoid and the umbilicus. Retraction of the upper edge of the incision and the right lobe of the liver, which may cover the pylorus and duodenum, easily exposes the site of the perforation.

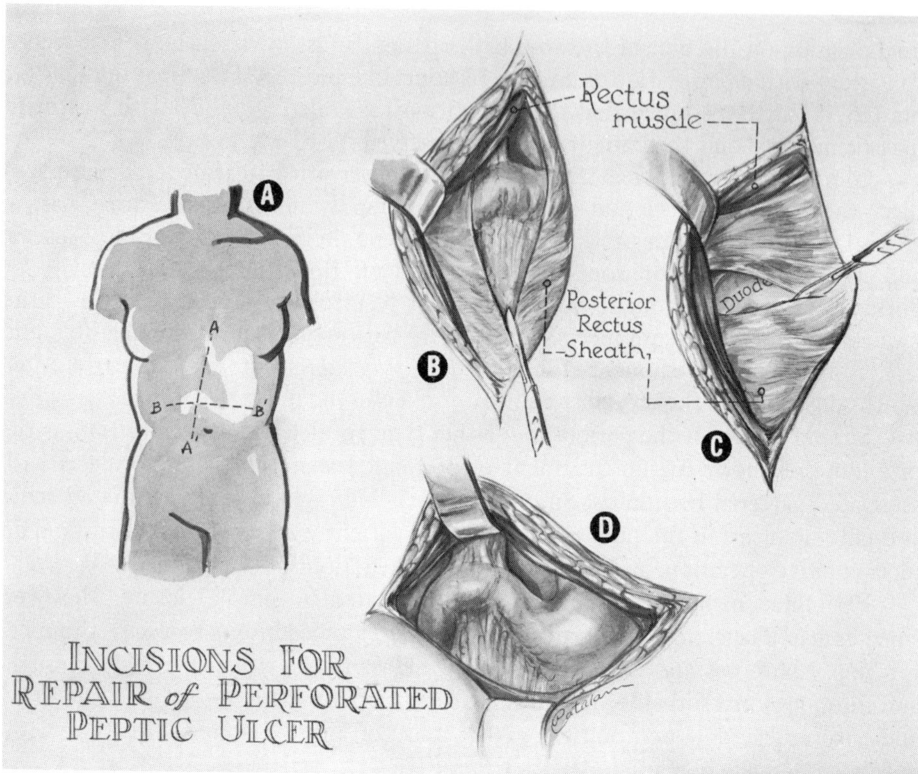

FIGURE 6. (*A*) Right paramedian, A–A′, and transverse incision, B–B′, for repair of perforated peptic ulcer. (*B*) Right paramedian incision. The anterior rectus fascia is incised longitudinally, the rectus muscle is retracted laterally, and the posterior rectus sheath is incised longitudinally. (*C*) Muscle and fascia-splitting incision. Through a long right paramedian skin incision the anterior rectus fascia is incised longitudinally, the rectus muscle is retracted laterally, and the posterior rectus sheath is incised transversely at a point midway between the xiphoid and umbilicus. (*D*) Transverse abdominal incision in the right upper quadrant. All the layers of the abdominal wall are cut transversely.

When the peritoneal cavity of a patient with a perforated duodenal ulcer is entered, the peritoneal exudate is thoroughly aspirated. The duodenum and pylorus and lesser curvature of the stomach are then explored for perforations. These are usually single, but multiple simultaneous perforations can occur. The techniques for closure of perforations are shown in Figure 7. If the perforation is small, about 2 to 3 mm. in diameter, and in the anterior wall of the duodenum, it is closed with a through-and-through stitch of three or more 4–0 silk sutures, or with cotton and dacron sutures, which are equally suitable for this purpose. Large perforations, which often occur in long-standing ulcerations, may have indurated and friable edges. If this condition exists, the sutures are placed wide of the perforation into relatively normal tissue, often 4 to 8 mm. from the cut edge of the perforation. When these sutures are tied, care is taken not to tear the edematous and friable bowel at the edge of the perforation. The closed perforation is then

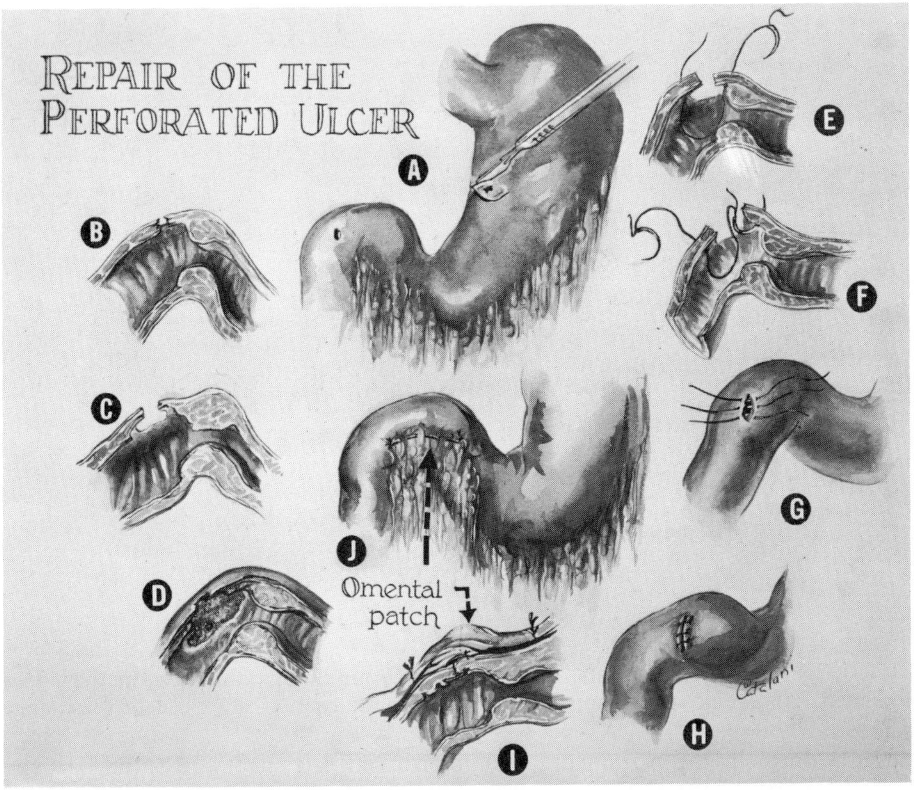

FIGURE 7. (*A*) Excision of perforated gastric ulcer for biopsy. Perforated ulcer in first portion of the duodenum. (*B*) Acute ulcer with minimal induration in the anterior wall of the duodenum. (*C*) Perforation in a large chronic ulcer in the anterior portion of the duodenum. The edge of the perforation is friable and indurated. (*D*) Perforation in a large chronic ulcer in the posterior wall of the duodenum, extending up and around to the anterior wall of the duodenum. (*E*) Closure of an acute ulcer with through-and-through silk sutures. (*F*) Closure of a large perforation with friable indurated edges by means of interrupted silk sutures placed into normal tissues. Often this is done by placing needles at both ends of the suture, which can then be brought wide of the perforation by utilizing the opening of the perforation for inserting the sutures. (*G and H*) Closure of the perforation with interrupted silk sutures. (*I and J*) Use of adjacent gastrocolic or greater omentum to cover the site of the perforation. The covering is kept in place by interrupted silk sutures.

covered with adjacent greater omentum, which is held in place by interrupted silk sutures.

The upper abdomen is irrigated with normal saline solution. The remaining areas of the peritoneal cavity, such as the subphrenic spaces and pelvis, are aspirated in order to remove as much as possible of the inflammatory exudate that has spread throughout the peritoneal cavity. Following this procedure, noncollapsible thick plastic tubes with multiple perforations are placed in the subphrenic areas and in the pelvis (Fig. 8). The abdominal wall is then closed with interrupted

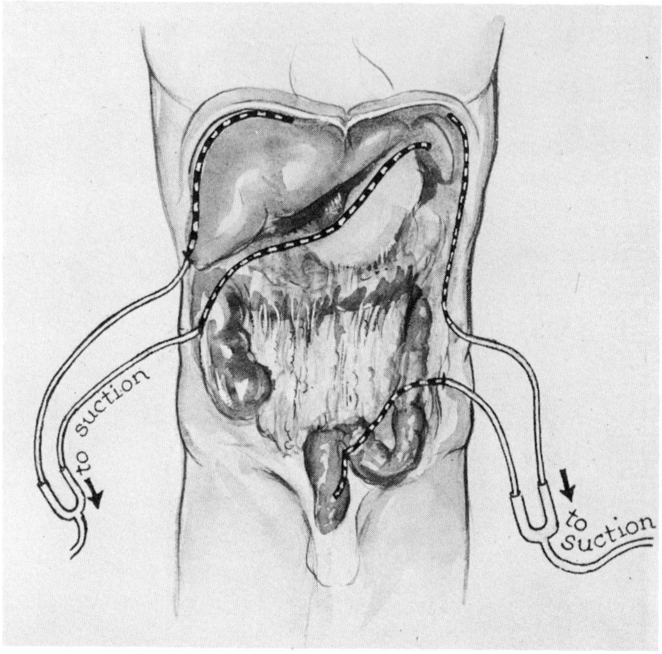

FIGURE 8. Position of plastic tube drains, with multiple perforations, in the upper abdomen, subphrenic spaces, and pelvis. High vacuum suction is applied to the drains.

catgut sutures in the peritoneum and interrupted 4–0 steel wire sutures in the anterior sheath of the rectus fascia.

Postoperative Management

Postoperative care consists of supportive treatment with intravenous dextrose and electrolytes. Continuous nasogastric suction is used for gastric decompression. High suction is applied to plastic tubes that were placed throughout the peritoneal cavity. Intravenous fluids and nasogastric suction should be continued until the patient has become afebrile for three consecutive days.

The patient is then placed on a liquid diet. Antibiotics are administered orally, and continued until the patient has been afebrile for one week. The diet is gradually increased as the patient tolerates additional food. The drainage tubes in the peritoneal cavity are left in place for about 10 to 14 days, or just as long as exudate is being obtained from the peritoneal cavity.

XV. THE SMALL BOWEL, COLON, AND RECTUM

86. *Regional Enteritis*

JOHN H. GARLOCK

BY AND LARGE, the most difficult part of the surgical treatment of regional enteritis is the proper selection of the patient and the timing of the intervention. The well-known increasing incidence of recurrence (usually at or near the new suture line) found as the period of follow-up is extended has necessitated an intense reappraisal of the many factors which could contribute to the recurrence. Although nothing is known concerning the cause of this unusual disease, enough clinical and morbid anatomical experience has been accumulated to offer a fairly clear-cut picture of its life history. At Mount Sinai Hospital, we have recently completed a six-year intensive study of the possible viral cause of ileitis and have reached the conclusion that this source can finally be unequivocally excluded. This is an important negative finding because, for many years, the virus group has been repeatedly singled out as the probable cause of the disease.

The proper selection of the patient and the timing of the operation must be considered in the light of the pathological life history of the disease. Although it is difficult to prove, I have for some years believed that enteritis starts as a fairly diffuse disease involving, in varying degrees, most of the small bowel. The major localization takes place usually in the terminal part of the ileum and occurs at an early stage. It is very difficult, if not impossible, to say how much time elapses before the minimal changes in the remainder of the bowel disappear and heal. But we do know, from our large experience at Mount Sinai Hospital, that if operation is undertaken for the more obvious distal disease before complete healing of the minimal proximal involvement, the recurrence rate eventually is very high. From an appraisal of hundreds of patients with regional enteritis, we have come to believe that the longer operation is deferred, the lower will be the recurrence rate. We attempt to wait for the disease to become "burnt out"—that is, until the x-ray films disclose sharp localization to the distal ileum with obvious cicatrization and stricturing. Prior to this late stage of the disease, it is impossible for the surgeon to detect minimal mucosal involvement proximal to the obviously diseased segment. This is what makes for the so-called recurrence, because the surgeon inadvertently leaves behind what he cannot recognize in the gross as minimal disease.

Not infrequently, the surgeon's hand is forced by circumstances beyond his control, before the cicatricial stage of the disease is reached. Persistent fever with manifestations of toxemia, rapid loss of weight and anemia, severe enteritic symptoms, a rapidly enlarging mass, profuse intestinal bleeding, singly or combined, may necessitate earlier intervention. In such circumstances, a higher recurrence rate must be expected. The immediate result is often brilliant: subsidence of fever, gain in weight, and restoration of well-being. However, it is impossible to predict what the immediate and late response will be. On the other hand, in the "burnt out" stage, the surgeon can usually be more positive in his prognosis for a salutary response.

Ileotransverse Colostomy with Exclusion versus Ileocolic Resection

The "Mount Sinai operation," as it is frequently labeled, or ileotransverse colostomy with exclusion (Fig. 1), came into being rather fortuitously. A quarter century ago, soon after Crohn and his co-workers made their famous contribution, the usual operation for ileitis was ileocolic resection, with removal of the diseased ileum and a liberal segment of normal ileum and the ascending colon. In those years, we encountered more of the severe complications of ileitis than are noted today. Extensive retroperitoneal inflammation, multiple abdominal wall fistulas, multiple intraabdominal abscesses, and internal fistulas with other organs were not exceptional. Following ileocolic resection under such circumstances, it is small wonder that the morbidity was considerable and the operative mortality was close to 15 per cent.

To obviate or, at least, to decrease this incidence, a two-stage ileocolic resection was developed. At the first-stage operation, the ileum, well proximal to the

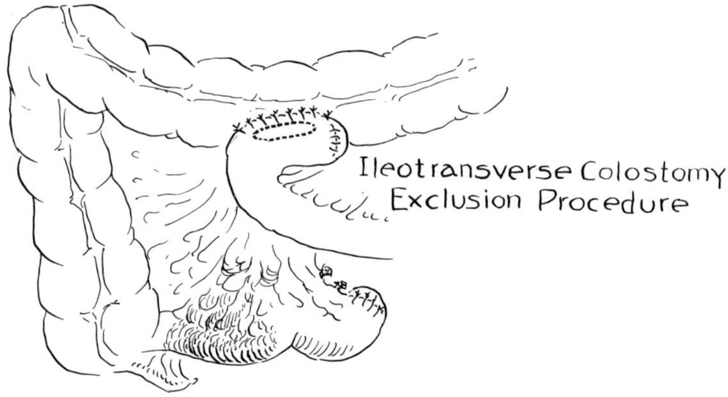

FIGURE 1. Operation of ileotransverse colostomy with exclusion. Complete division of the ileum well proximal to the diseased segment is an essential step. It is probably better to place the anastomosis in the transverse colon in an isoperistaltic direction. On rare occasions in the presence of acute obstruction, it may be desirable in the interests of safety to make the anastomosis in continuity.

diseased segment, was divided and both ends were closed by inverting sutures. A side-to-side anastomosis was then made between the proximal end of ileum near its inverted portion and the transverse colon. When the second stage was undertaken three to six months later, it was noted in approximately 9 of 10 patients that the previously diseased segment was now represented by an attenuated fibrotic cord, the markedly enlarged mesenteric nodes had disappeared, and the abdominal wall fecal fistulas had healed spontaneously. I remember one patient with 27 abdominal wall fistulas, all of which closed spontaneously after this first-stage operation.

Quite naturally, these repeated observations led to the conclusion that the second stage was not necessary and that the operation of ileotransverse colostomy with exclusion should be adopted as the procedure of choice for regional or terminal ileitis. The operation has much to commend it. Firstly, as far as I am able to determine, there has been no death following it in our hospital since its adoption as a primary procedure. Secondly, the late recurrence rate has been appreciably lower than that following the one-stage ileocolic resection as practiced at that time. And thirdly, when resection became necessary (in about 8 per cent of the patients) the technical difficulties were far less formidable than those encountered in the one-stage procedure.

In recent years, I have returned to the one-stage resection operation, but with important reservations as to the circumstances in which it is applicable, and with changes in technique based on physiological reasons. I have returned to the camp of the "resectionists" not because I expect any reduction in the recurrence rate (in fact, there has been none), but because of the great desirability of restoring to the ascending colon and proximal transverse colon the physiological process of water absorption in the hope of eliminating the diarrhea which frequently persists after the ileocolostomy operation. This objective has been achieved in great part.

I therefore recommend primary resections for the relatively uncomplicated cases of terminal ileitis without extensive retroperitoneal involvement and in the absence of internal and external fistulas. The majority of our patients fall into this category. I stress repeatedly, however, that if the surgeon has any doubts as to the extent of involvement beyond the confines of the diseased segment of bowel, he should be content with the ileocolostomy operation. It must be remembered that, should a subsequent resection become necessary, the technical maneuvers would be far less formidable. Under the circumstances I have enumerated, good surgical judgment calls for a safe two-stage procedure rather than a hazardous one-stage operation.

The Incision and Exploration

At present, our plan of procedure is as follows when operative intervention is indicated. Through a liberal right paramedian transrectus incision, the abdomen is entered. The full thickness of abdominal wall is covered on each side with thick moist pads which are not removed until the completion of the operation. The entire gastrointestinal tract is carefully examined for skip lesions. The surgeon should not fail to exclude skip lesions in the colon. In recent years, we have noted an increasing frequency of these complicating factors.

Placing the patient in moderate Trendelenburg position simplifies considerably the examination of the involved segment of ileum, especially with respect to the demonstration of fistulas between diseased bowel and sigmoid colon, or a loop of normal small intestine, or bladder. Greatly enlarged mesenteric lymph nodes are a constant finding, but the surgeon may encounter dense inflammatory masses binding diseased bowel to mesentery with firm retroperitoneal fixation. In my view, the disclosure of this form of extensive inflammation, the presence of internal fistulas especially with the sigmoid colon or rectosigmoid, and the preoperative existence of abdominal wall fecal fistulas all call for the operation of ileotransverse colostomy with exclusion. Hard experience has shown that primary resections undertaken under such circumstances will often present almost insurmountable technical difficulties, open up retroperitoneal areas to fulminating infections, result in breakdown of repaired fistulas in the colon, and cause an inexcusable considerable postoperative morbidity and mortality. The surgeon should examine the diseased area of bowel with great caution, scrupulously avoiding the separation of adherent loops where an internal fistula may be located. Inadvertent separation of two such loops confronts the surgeon with the problem of two openings in diseased bowel, which, of course, cannot be closed locally and must be treated by resection. This is to be avoided at all costs.

Ileocolic Resection

The operation of ileocolic resection for ileitis differs from that performed for right colon cancer with respect to the extent of removal of the colon and mesentery (Fig. 2). For ileitis, the colon is transected just distal to the ileocecal area, thus retaining the entire ascending colon.

Mobilization of the Right Colon

After incision of the lateral peritoneal fold, the ascending colon, cecum, and ileum are bluntly separated from the retroperitoneal areolar tissue. It is advisable to identify the right ureter and spermatic vessels, tracing these structures from above downward. Not infrequently, the inflamed small bowel mesentery may become fixed to these structures at the pelvic brim. Their identification above makes the dissection lower down much easier. The mobilized segments of bowel are now withdrawn from the abdomen. The site of transection of the ileum should be at least 6 to 8 inches proximal to the proximal end of the diseased segment. It is at this point that an opening is made in the mesentery to start the transection of the mesentery. By holding the mesentery toward a light for transillumination, an area free of vessels is quickly found. There is a popularly held misconception that it is important to remove all the enlarged mesenteric nodes when one is carrying out

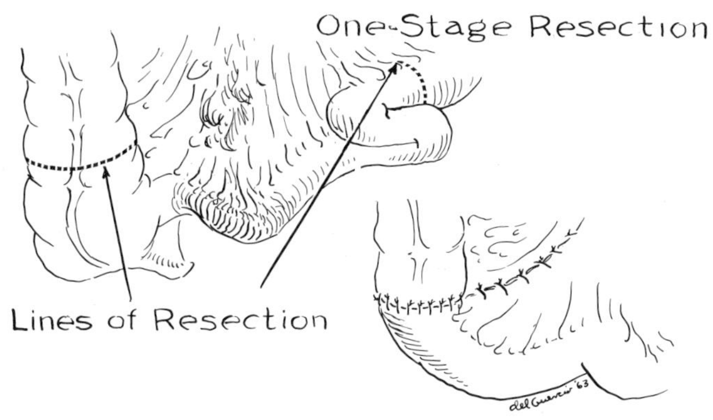

FIGURE 2. In the one-stage resection operation, the site of division of the colon is just distal to the ileocecal valve. This preserves the ascending colon for water absorption. The ileum should be divided well proximal to the site of disease. An end-to-end anastomosis is most desirable.

resection for ileitis. If this were true, the surgeon would frequently be compelled to go as far as the root of the mesentery, thus jeopardizing the integrity of the entire small bowel. The lymph node involvement in ileitis is secondary to the disease in the bowel, not vice versa. Witness the complete disappearance of all enlarged nodes after the ileocolostomy operation alone! The evidence is incontrovertible that the involved nodes have nothing to do with subsequent recurrences in the bowel.

Transection of the Ileum

Because of the great thickness of the mesentery of the ileum in this disease, any attempt to isolate individual blood vessels for ligation during the process of transection is fraught with considerable danger. Vessels may be easily torn, producing excessive bleeding, difficulty in applying clamps, and hematoma formation between the leaves of the mesentery. To obviate all these possibilities, I apply two Kelly clamps, starting at the initial opening in the mesentery, grasping about one-half inch of tissue and cutting between the clamps. This process is continued seriatim until the cecal area is reached. The vessels held in each clamp are ligated by transfixing sutures of No. 1 chromic catgut which are tied snugly as each clamp is removed. I have tried various methods of carrying out this difficult part of the operation, but have found this particular maneuver to be the simplest and most effective. The branches of the ileocolic vessels supplying the cecum and ascending colon are now clamped at right angles to the colon just distal to the ileocolic junction. After these have been ligated, the colon at the anticipated point of transection is cleared of bands, fat, and areolar tissue in order to expedite the end-to-end ileocolic anastomosis. It is not necessary to remove much of the mesentery of the diseased small bowel or of the ascending colon. This simplifies the operation considerably and assures a competent blood supply to the divided bowel ends.

Ileocolic Anastomosis

Short noncrushing rubber-covered clamps are now applied near the site of division of the ileum and the beginning of the ascending colon in such a way as to appose the cut edges of the respective mesenteries. This prevents any twisting of the two loops. Thin crushing clamps are applied an inch beyond each rubber-shod clamp, and the bowel (after establishment of a dirty field) is divided on each side. After removal of the specimen, the bowel ends are approximated for an end-to-end anastomosis. In spite of what appears to be a marked disparity in diameter between the colon and small bowel, an end-to-end union can usually be effected by a simple maneuver. Passing a traction suture through each pair of angles of colon and ileum elongates the contracted small bowel and simplifies the technique of the anastomosis. The inner layer consists of interrupted inverting sutures of 00 chromic catgut. I believe interrupted sutures obviate a shirring effect, minimize edema at the suture line, and probably avoid postoperative obstructive difficulties. The dirty field is discarded. An outer layer of 3–0 silk interrupted Cushing sutures completes the anastomosis. These stitches should be inserted in such a way as to prevent formation of a thick diaphragm. Entering the lumen of the bowel is to be avoided. The cut edges of the two mesenteries are brought together front and back with fine silk sutures so as to bury completely the raw edges. Because of the succulence of the mesenteric area incident to the disease itself, there may be considerable lymph drainage postoperatively. For this reason, I insert a Penrose drain through a right lower quadrant stab wound and place it in the retrocolic area. The operative incision is closed with buried figure-of-eight No. 30 stainless steel wire and silk for the skin.

Extent of Small Bowel Resection

The question has frequently been asked: How much of the small bowel can be removed in this disease without producing significant nutritional disturbances? This is extremely difficult to answer categorically, mainly because of the unpredictable response of the individual patient. One patient stands out startlingly as an example of one extreme. He was left with 3 feet of jejunum anastomosed to the distal transverse colon. Yet he gained 25 pounds, has three to four semiformed movements a day, and has remained well for more than a decade. On the other hand, another patient had 5 feet of small bowel excluded by ileotransverse colostomy. She suffers from watery diarrhea, has not gained weight, and appears chronically ill. There is no evidence whatsoever of recurrent disease. Certainly the surgeon should not hesitate to remove 3 or 4 feet of diseased ileum. It seems to me that postoperative diarrhea has been considerably ameliorated by anastomosing the ileum to the ascending colon.

The problem of diffuse jejunoileitis is an extremely difficult and complicated one. In my opinion, the finding of diffuse disease calls for termination of the operation. The possible exception is the disclosure of two or three strictured areas with large hammocks of dilated bowel between. Here I believe the surgeon is justified in performing localized resections of the strictures with end-to-end anastomoses. This, in effect, is a palliative procedure to lessen the severe symptoms of chronic obstruction. My experience with a number of these cases would lead me to say that this procedure is thoroughly justified.

Recurrent Ileitis

In the treatment of recurrent ileitis following the operation of ileotransverse colostomy with exclusion or, less commonly, ileosigmoidostomy, the surgeon is faced with the complex decision of the choice of operation when surgery becomes necessary. Unless the technical difficulties encountered are insurmountable, I would urge that the surgeon avoid another short-circuiting operation distal to the original one as the easiest way out of a complicated situation. These recurrences usually begin at the site of ileocolostomy and extend proximally in the ileum for varying distances. I would say that, in the majority of our cases, the diseased segment measures less than 6 inches and is resected. Skip lesions proximal to the obvious recurrence are not unusual and should be looked for and treated in the same way. If another short-circuiting procedure cannot be avoided, it should *never* be carried out in continuity with the original ileocolostomy, because the continuous loop of ileum between the first ileocolostomy and the new one will subsequently form a large hammock of dilated bowel, hanging down in the abdomen between the two anastomoses and producing an intestinal cesspool.

To obviate this, the ileum should be divided proximal to the diseased segment and both ends inverted in the same way as in the original procedure. The new distal ileocolostomy is fashioned as a side-to-side anastomosis. But I emphasize again that this kind of operation is not the most desirable, for the very good reason that more of the colon is thereby excluded from aiding the important function of water absorption. In the treatment of recurrent disease, for the past eight to ten years I have been employing what I believe to be a more physiological operation. When, at the time of exploration, usually through a right paramedian incision, the area of recurrence is demonstrated and considered resectable, the site of the original ileocolostomy is dissected away from contiguous adherent loops of bowel and mesentery. A dirty field is then established. A long noncrushing clamp is placed longitudinally over the transverse colon beyond the anastomotic site and another is applied to the ileal side. The anastomosis is divided on the colon side and the resulting opening in the colon is closed longitudinally in two layers, the inner one of fine chromic catgut and the outer one of interrupted fine silk.

The diseased segment of bowel is excised with its contiguous mesentery. Attention is directed to the terminal ileum excluded at the original operation. This portion of bowel will usually be found atrophic and contracted. An ileocecal resection is carried out, and an end-to-end anastomosis effected between the new terminal ileum and the beginning of the ascending colon, by the techniques described above. This operation restores to the patient the physiological function of the ascending colon, and the subsequent improvement in the symptoms has been a most gratifying feature of the surgical therapy of recurrent ileitis.

References

Crohn, B. B., Ginzburg, L., and Oppenheimer, G. D. Regional ileitis: a pathologic and clinical entity. *J.A.M.A.* 99:1323, October 15, 1932.

Garlock, J. H., Crohn, B. B., Klein, S. H., and Yarnis, H. An appraisal of the long-term results of surgical treatment of regional ileitis. *Gastroenterology* 19:3, November 1951.

Warren, S., and Sommers, S. C. Pathology of regional ileitis and ulcerative colitis. *J.A.M.A.* 154:189, January 16, 1954.

87. *Nonspecific Ulcerative Colitis*

JOHN H. GARLOCK

ULCERATIVE COLITIS is probably one of the most difficult problems in the whole gamut of inflammatory diseases of the gastrointestinal tract. It is true that only 20 to 25 per cent of patients afflicted with this illness become candidates for surgical therapy, but the problems posed by this group more than offset those that occur in the remaining 75 per cent. It is not in the province of this chapter to discuss the various pathological complications and the indications for surgery, but I venture to state that the major difficulties encountered are concerned mainly with the proper choice of the patient for operation, the timing of intervention, and the extent of surgery to be carried out. This calls for the most mature kind of judgment, based mainly on a repetitive experience with many patients.

In the treatment of this disease, various combinations of pathological findings require different surgical approaches. For instance, as therapy for the acute variety with marked toxicity and paralytic dilatation of the colon, the temporizing cecostomy originally suggested by Klein of our staff has much to commend it. The difficulty is the possible concomitant presence of a walled-off perforation. It must be remembered that nowadays practically every patient with ulcerative colitis has been on steroid therapy before coming to the surgeon. In the acute form of the disease, with previous intensive steroid therapy, it is extraordinarily difficult in most instances to make a preoperative diagnosis of bowel perforation. A cecostomy performed under such circumstances, while accomplishing decompression of the markedly distended bowel, could very well result in separation of the tenuous adhesions at the site of a walled-off perforation and cause general soiling of the peritoneal cavity.

There are those who scoff at the mere suggestion of a cecostomy in acute toxic dilatation of ulcerative colitis and who urge *total* colectomy as the procedure of choice. They claim immediate recovery and a low morbidity and mortality rate. From my observations, both at Mount Sinai Hospital and at various clinics in the United States and abroad, I would venture the opinion that these claims are far too sanguine. Admittedly, the operation of colectomy is frequently forced upon the surgeon when acute toxic dilatation is complicated by perforation. Simple closure of the perforation is inadvisable, and colectomy must be carried out in spite of the increased risk. But to categorize all such patients as candidates for only one form of approach constitutes a grave perversion of surgical judgment.

The choice of subtotal or total colectomy as the primary procedure is still being hotly debated in surgical circles. It is noteworthy that the younger group of surgeons favors the more extensive operation. So many factors are involved in the choice of one over the other that one assuredly cannot be dogmatic. For instance, a patient with chronic colitis presenting with exsanguinating hemorrhage should, in all probability, be treated by total colectomy in one stage, for the simple reason that the source of the bleeding may be in either the colon or the rectum, or in both. Similarly, a patient with chronic disease associated with hopeless involvement of the rectum (strictures, fistulas, extensive polyposis) may be subjected to the one-stage operation without additional undue risk. But, in my experience, these constitute the minority of the total group.

In 1939 I proposed the thesis that, after subtotal colectomy, the previously diseased rectal segment might, under observation, reach a degree of healing which would permit reanastomosis between the ileum and the rectum. Since then a number of patients have been treated in this fashion, with more than encouraging results. Now with Aylett's evidence that ileorectal anastomosis may be carried out as a primary procedure in the presence of active rectal disease, there is added incentive for employing total colectomy only in specific, well-defined circumstances. Removing the rectum at the first stage precludes any possibility of future reconnection. It is for these reasons that we favor, in the majority of patients, *subtotal* colectomy and ileostomy as the primary procedure.

The current technique of ileostomy and colectomy has been a gradual development during the past decade, and has been primarily concerned with the elimination of the numerous ileostomy complications so common in former years. These difficulties included prolapse, retraction, fistula formation, skin excoriation, wound infections, ileostomy dysfunction with associated severe electrolyte and fluid imbalances, early intestinal obstruction, and bag appliances that did not fit properly, because of a poorly placed stoma or scarring of the abdominal wall. It will be seen, therefore, that the primary consideration in the performance of the operation is the construction of an ileostomy stoma which will minimize these difficulties. From the technical standpoint, the colectomy is of lesser significance.

Technique

Placement of the Stoma

Prior to operation, it is advisable to mark out on the abdominal wall the contemplated site of the ileostomy stoma (Fig. 1). Certain desiderata should be met. Firstly, it should be located where the patient can take care of it with ease. Second, it should be fairly symmetrically placed for reasons of dress, especially in the female. Thirdly, it should not be placed in or near an abdominal scar or the umbilicus, because they make it difficult to achieve an accurate fixation of the flange of the ileostomy bag to the skin. Fourthly, the surgeon must take into consideration the

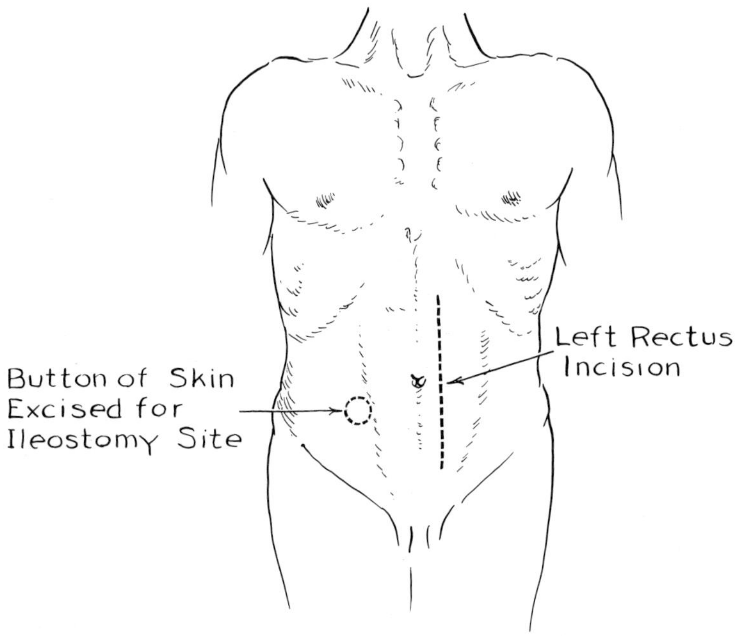

FIGURE 1. Buttonhole properly placed for ileostomy.

fact that there will be a weight gain of at least 30 pounds which will influence considerably the efficiency of the bag appliance. Finally, the stoma should not be located in the belt line. Experience has shown that the most desirable location is the right lower quadrant, about midway between the umbilicus and the anterior spine of the ileum.

The Incision and Exploration

Thorough relaxation of the abdominal wall makes for greater ease of performance of the operation and facilitates minimal handling of the small bowel, which is reflected in a smoother postoperative course. The abdominal incision is a long left rectus one about an inch to the left of the midline. Examination of the preoperative barium enema films will show the height of the splenic flexure, thus indicating the cephalad extent of the incision. Increased bleeding is always present, and hemostasis of the abdominal incision should be complete. Protective pads are placed on both sides of the incision and appropriate retractors are inserted. Examination of the colon and small bowel is now carried out, with especial attention to the presence or absence of terminal ileum involvement. The intestines are gently packed off to the left of the midline and held in this location by broad Deaver retractors.

Mobilization of the Right Colon

Mobilization of the colon is begun on the right side by incising the lateral peritoneal fold and bluntly freeing the terminal ileum, ascending colon, and hepatic flexure. It is advisable to ligate the small vessels in the outer edge of the peritoneal fold so as to leave a completely dry retrocolic area. The supplying vessels of the colon are ligated and divided under direct vision. This maneuver can be greatly simplified by holding the mesentery before a light for transillumination. It is not necessary to remove much mesentery, and the individual vessel isolation obviates mass ligation.

Mobilization of the Transverse Colon and the Splenic Flexure

Mobilization of the transverse colon is begun by entering the lesser sac on the right side. The right half of the gastrocolic ligament is divided between clamps and the transected vessels are snugly ligated. The transverse mesocolon is clearly delineated, permitting accurate individual ligation of the major vessels. The splenic flexure, which may prove troublesome, may be more easily mobilized after first freeing the descending colon. Therefore, the abdominal pads are removed and the small bowel is packed toward the right of the midline and held in this location by retractors. The lateral peritoneal attachment of the descending colon is incised, permitting blunt mobilization of this portion of bowel. The supplying vessels are ligated and divided under direct vision. Attention is now directed to the freeing of the splenic flexure (Fig. 2). This should be done carefully so as to avoid inadvertent tearing of the colon, which is frequently thinned out in this area. The splenic flexure ligaments are divided between clamps which are snugly ligated. This brings into view the rest of the transverse mesocolon, permitting accurate ligation of its remaining vessels.

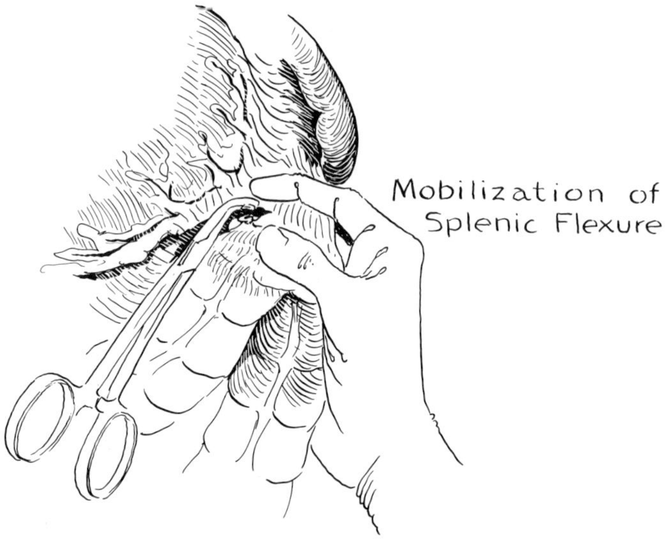

FIGURE 2. The mobilization of the colon should offer few difficulties. Transillumination of the mesentery permits accurate ligation of the vessels. The splenic flexure mobilization may present a technical problem. The technique is described in the text.

Mobilization of the Sigmoid Colon and Division of the Terminal Ileum

By placing the patient in mild Trendelenburg position, mobilization of the proximal two-thirds of the sigmoid colon is simplified. If a subtotal colectomy is to be done, the inferior mesenteric artery should be preserved to assure adequate nutrition to the lower sigmoid and rectum. The mesosigmoid is transected to the point of contemplated division of the sigmoid at about the junction of its middle and lower thirds. Accurate hemostasis is important here. Division of the terminal ileum can now be performed. This should be as close to the cecum as possible. Of course, the disclosure of any backwash or granulomatous ileitis necessitates removal of this diseased segment, also. After a temporary dirty field has been established, two small thin-bladed Payr clamps are placed across the bowel, which is divided between them. The clamp attached to the distal segment is left undisturbed and removed later with the specimen. A purse-string suture of 00 silk is placed in the proximal ileal segment just beneath the blades of the clamp. As the clamp is opened and withdrawn, the suture is tightened and tied snugly, inverting the cut edges of bowel. The suture ends are left long for subsequent use. The dirty field is discarded. The mobilized colon is then wrapped in a moist towel and withdrawn from the abdomen.

The Ileostomy

The next step is concerned with the withdrawal of the proximal ileum through the abdominal wall at the ileostomy site. The abdominal wall coverings on the right side are temporarily placed aside, exposing the marked-out site of the ileostomy. A circular incision is made at this point, approximating the size of the terminal ileum. The incision is deepened to the fascia, excising whatever fat is encountered in the process. All bleeding points are accurately ligated. The anterior rectus sheath fascia is now incised in a crisscross maneuver and the rectus muscle is bluntly separated in a vertical direction. It is sometimes necessary to ligate and divide the epigastric vessels. The withdrawal of the terminal ileum may be expedited by the following technique. Three or four clamps are placed on the edge of the parietal peritoneum on the right side of the main incision. This permits the assistant to elevate the abdominal wall. The surgeon, standing to the left of the patient, inserts his left index finger through the newly made opening for the ileostomy, thus pushing the parietal peritoneum into view. This is incised vertically for about 2 inches. A clamp inserted from without inward through the ileostomy incision grasps the ends of the purse-string suture closing the proximal ileal stump and is withdrawn, bringing with it the loop of ileum which will form the ileostomy. The ileostomy loop is so placed that the cut edge of its mesentery faces toward the pelvis. This cut edge is sutured to the opening in the peritoneum below the site of the ileostomy a distance of about 2 inches, using 0 chromic catgut interrupted stitches. This fixation of the mesentery is the major insurance against subsequent prolapse. The opening in the peritoneum at the site of the ileostomy should hug the bowel snugly. The withdrawn ileum should project beyond the skin surface about 2½ inches. We have found that plication of the terminal 12 to 18 inches of ileum is added insurance against postoperative ileostomy dysfunction. By this maneuver, the surgeon fixes the bowel in the position of his choice, thereby minimizing haphazard inflammatory adhesions which could produce partial obstruction. The plication is accomplished by apposing two successive loops of ileum, commencing at a point proximal to the emergence of the ileal loop from the abdomen, and suturing the opposed mesenteries together with fine silk sutures. About three pairs of such loops should suffice.

Wound Closure and Exteriorization of the Mobilized Colon

The towels covering the right side of the main incision are now replaced and repair of this wound is commenced. The mobilized colon wrapped in a towel is withdrawn at the lower angle of the incision, which is closed with buried figure-of-eight wire sutures and silk. I never bury ulcerative colitis bowel in the abdomen. The ablated end is always exteriorized for drainage purposes. This is a basic surgical principle in colitis surgery. After the main incision has been closed about the exteriorized lower sigmoid colon, a noncrushing clamp is applied to the bowel just above the skin surface, another clamp is placed proximal to this one, and the bowel is divided between them. The specimen is removed. This clamp remains in place for five or six days, assuring fixation of the loop to the abdominal wall.

Fashioning of the Ileostomy

By far the simplest and most effective method of fashioning the ileostomy is the technique described by Brooke (Fig. 3). The procedures recommended by both Crile and Turnbull are more complicated, and are not suitable for routine use. The Brooke method is simple and produces rapid maturation of the ileostomy stoma. The suture closing the end of bowel is removed and the bowel end is opened. It may be necessary to freshen its edges, and it is important to tie off all bleeding points. The full thickness of bowel is now everted completely so that the cut edge approximates the circular skin incision. The bowel edge is sutured to the skin incision, utilizing interrupted stitches of 3–0 chromic catgut. The completed ileostomy should project about 1 to 1½ inches. A plastic ileostomy bag is applied and held snugly in place with adhesive paste. A loose dressing over the main incision completes the procedure.

Segmental Colitis

Not infrequently in the variety of colitis classified as Crohn's disease of the colon, or granulomatous colitis, the rectum and sigmoid may be found to be normal both sigmoidoscopically and by barium enema examination. In the so-called right-sided colitis of the nongranulomatous type, the rectum and sigmoid are found to be normal, also. Under such circumstances, a different surgical approach is indicated. Instead of constructing an ileostomy, the surgeon may, after he removes the

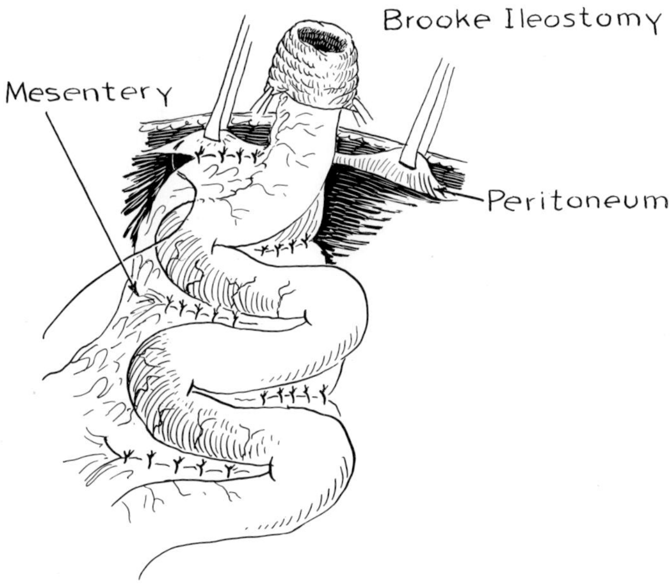

FIGURE 3. The proper fashioning of the ileostomy minimizes subsequent complications. Fixation of the cut mesentery, plication of the mesentery, and the Brooke eversion of the exteriorized ileum are important features.

diseased colon, anastomose the ileum to the lower sigmoid or rectosigmoid end-to-end. The technique of this anastomosis is the same as in anterior resection (see Chapter 91). However, two technical details should be stressed. Firstly, it is important to avoid any twisting of the ileal loop as it is approximated to the colon stump. Secondly, the mesentery of the ileum along its site of division should be anchored firmly to the posterior parietal peritoneum to prevent internal herniation of loops of bowel.

Staged Procedures

Because of hazards due to the poor condition of the patient, it is occasionally necessary to carry out this operation in two stages. At the first operation, through a left rectus incision, the terminal ileum is divided and its distal end is inverted by three layers of silk sutures and replaced in the abdomen. The lower sigmoid mesocolon is transected without dividing the superior hemorrhoidal vessels. A short noncrushing rubber-shod clamp is applied distally, and just proximal to it a DeMartel clamp. The bowel is then transected. An end-to-end anastomosis is carried out between the proximal ileal opening and the distal colon. The ileal mesentery is tacked down as described above. The proximal colon stump occluded by the DeMartel clamp is exteriorized through the upper end of the incision, which is closed snugly about it. The occluding clamp is removed in a few days to permit external drainage of diseased bowel contents.

When the patient's condition improves, as it usually does in the following three or four months, the colectomy is carried out through a right rectus exposure. The exteriorized colostomy is first freed from the left rectus scar. The technical details of the colectomy are the same as described above.

When subtotal colectomy and ileostomy has been performed, the final operation in the majority of patients will consist of an abdominoperineal resection of the remaining segment at a future time. If the criteria for a reconnection operation can be met, the operation will consist of an end-to-end anastomosis between the detached ileostomy and the upper rectum.

References

AYLETT, S. Total colectomy and ileo-rectal anastomosis in diffuse ulcerative colitis. *Brit. M. J.* 1:489, March 2, 1957.

BROOKE, B. N. *Ulcerative Colitis and Its Surgical Treatment.* London: E. & S. Livingstone, 1954.

GARLOCK, J. H. The surgical treatment of intractable ulcerative colitis. *Ann. Surg.* 113:2, January 1941.

GARLOCK, J. H., and LYONS, A. S. The role of surgery in the therapy of ulcerative colitis. *Gastroenterology* 26:709, May 1954.

GARLOCK, J. H., and KIRSCHNER, P. A. The prevention of ileostomy dysfunction. *Surgery* 40:678, October 1956.

88. *Ileostomy*

RUPERT B. TURNBULL, JR., AND
FRANK L. WEAKLEY

THE TECHNIQUES of ileostomy vary with the diseases or with the conditions under which surgery is done. Regardless of circumstances, however, a few standards are to be fulfilled concerning the ileal stoma. These are (1) proper placement, (2) adequate abdominal wall aperture for the ileum, (3) avoidance of tension, (4) fixation of the mesentery, and (5) use of the eversion stoma.

Location of the Stoma

The site should be marked before the abdomen is opened through a left paramedian incision. Placement will be correct if an ileostomy pouch disc is placed below the umbilical level and is moved medially (Fig. 1A) until the disc overrides the midline. The ileum traverses the belly of the rectus muscle and the stoma will be located at the summit of the infraumbilical fat roll. This spatial relation is especially important in patients who have become wasted from ulcerative colitis, as they eventually may gain from 30 to 40 pounds.

Do not bring the ileum through the abdominal wall at the *lateral rectus border*, because eventration and parastomal hernias may occur; moreover, the lateral border of the pouch disc will override the pararectus "furrow," and such overriding will cause leakage. *Midline placement* of the stoma is rarely successful; the stoma will reside in a "valley" when the patient gains weight. Stomas *near the anterior iliac spine, pubis, or inguinal ligament* are unmanageable because the ileostomy pouches fit poorly. Stomas placed *at the umbilical level or higher* are not successful because of the epigastric fat pad that falls over the pouch disc and produces ulceration.

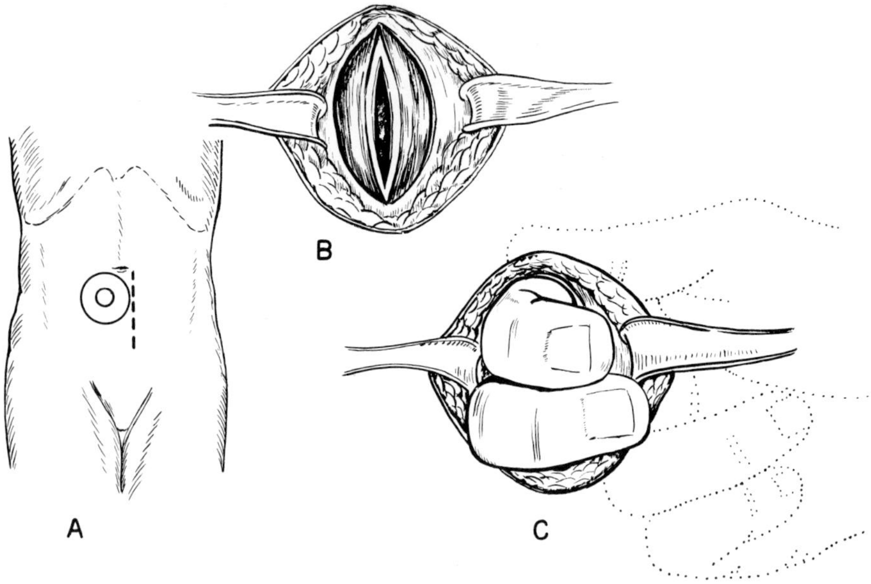

FIGURE 1. Location of the stoma; the abdominal wall aperture. (*A*) Disc below the umbilicus and overriding the midline. (*B*) Vertical rectus incision. (*C*) Two-finger width aperture.

Abdominal Wall Aperture

After a button of skin has been excised, the subcutaneous fat, the rectus sheath and muscle, and the peritoneum are split vertically so that two fingers can be inserted comfortably into the abdomen (Fig. 1B, C). The end of the ileum and its mesentery are then drawn through the abdominal wall for at least 2 inches. The ileum should lie without tension and exhibit no tendency to shorten or to retract. The mesentery is oriented within the abdominal wall with its free edge located superiorly.

Fixation of the Mesentery of the Ileum

The ileal mesentery should be fixed to the parietal peritoneum (Fig. 2) whenever possible, and particularly at the time of colectomy for ulcerative colitis. In some patients in whom this was not done, volvulus around the exit point of the stoma occurred, causing chronic recurrent obstruction and, finally, gangrene of the stoma.

The injection of saline solution under the peritoneum of the mesentery (Fig. 2A) allows the placing of silk sutures superficial to the underlying arterial pattern. A two-layer interrupted or continuous silk suture fixation is best. Superiorly, the

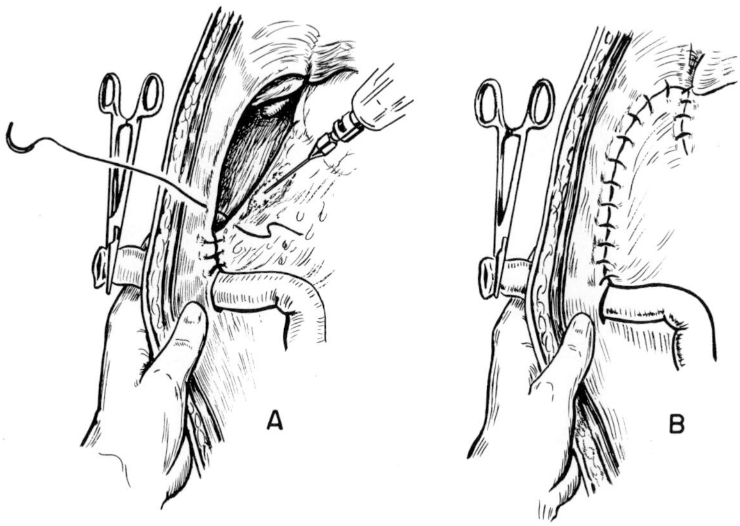

FIGURE 2. Fixation of the ileal mesentery to the free edge of the falciform ligament. (A) Subperitoneal injection of saline to avoid injuring vessels. (*B*) Suture completed.

round ligament can be used until there is room enough only for the duodenum (Fig. 2B). The abdomen is then closed and the skin edges are approximated with sutures.

External Construction of the Ileal Stoma

Eversion Technique

Since the mesentery is brought through the abdominal wall aperture, the protruding ileum often will be bowed. The first step is to correct this deformity by mass suture ligation of the mesentery at the level of the skin (Fig. 3A). Atraumatic 00 chromic catgut will best serve this purpose. Excess mesenteric fat is trimmed away (Fig. 3A) to avoid tension under the everted stoma. The end of the ileum is trimmed until it is apparent that, when everted, the finished stoma will be about one-half inch in length. Bleeding vessels in the cut edge are ligated with fine chromic catgut. The final eversion of the end of the ileum can then be effected by placing four quadrant sutures (Fig. 3B) between the end of the ileum and the subcuticular fascia. When traction is exerted on the sutures, eversion readily takes place, and interval sutures of 4–0 atraumatic chromic catgut are added to complete the eversion (Fig. 3C). The skin should not be pierced by sutures; mucosa of the ileum may readily grow in the suture holes and eventually secrete enough mucus to prevent the pouch from adhering to the skin around the base of the stoma.

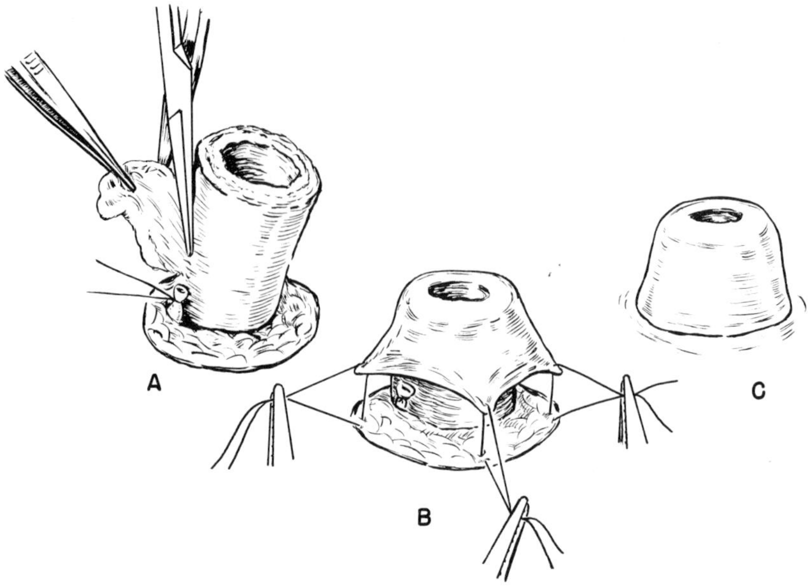

FIGURE 3.. Eversion of the stoma. (*A*) Ligation and excision of the mesentery. (*B*) Eversion effected by placing four quadrant sutures between the end of the ileostomy and the subcuticular fascia. (C) Completed eversion. The skin has not been pierced by sutures.

Mucosal Graft Technique

The mucosal graft technique, as shown in Figure 4, consists in stripping away the seromuscular layers so that the remaining mucosal-submucosal layers may be pulled down over the residual short stoma and be sutured to the subcuticular fascia as shown in Figure 3B. The mucosal graft stoma does not swell, is soft, and has a narrow diameter.

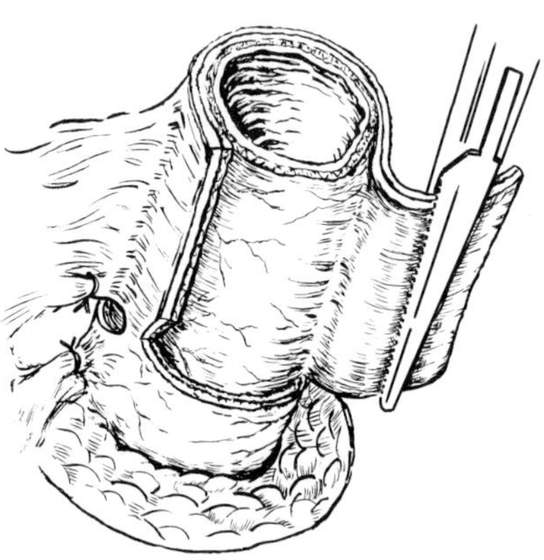

FIGURE 4. Mucosal graft technique. The seromuscular layers are stripped away and the mucosal-submucosal tube is everted and sutured to the subcuticular layer of the skin.

The mucosal graft technique should be utilized when (1) the ileum is edematous because of obstruction, and (2) the stoma is to be made from jejunum.

Obstructed Edematous Ileum. Here an ordinary eversion stoma, like that shown in Figure 3, would swell considerably, and in three weeks would not shrink sufficiently to accommodate the usual permanent appliances. Moreover, there would be some dysfunction due to the edema. In addition, attempts to evert the edematous ileum would create tension at the suture line at the base. The mucosal graft technique is useful for this condition.

Jejunal Stoma; Total Mucosal Graft. When the major part of the small intestine has been removed because of inflammatory disease, it becomes necessary to construct an external jejunal stoma. If the usual eversion technique is used for jejunostomy, the jejunum, being muscular and much more active than the ileum, inevitably retracts within the abdomen; the retracted stoma causes intestinal obstruction. A jejunal stoma made by the total mucosal graft technique obviates these problems. The jejunum is prepared as shown in Figure 3A. The seromuscular layers are superficially incised for one-half to three-fourths inch near the tip, and are stripped up with a gauze pledget to obtain a seromuscular cleavage plane, as shown in Figure 4. *All* the seromuscular layers are removed to the level of the skin, and the residual mucosal-submucosal tube is turned down over itself and sutured to the subcuticular fascia. The completed stoma is devoid of muscular layers other than the muscularis mucosae, and does not exhibit edema or peristalsis. Retraction does not occur, because the muscle layers have been removed.

Ileostomy in Children

In children, the ileal stoma may be constructed by any technique recommended in this chapter. The surgeon has but to remember that in children the abdominal wall is thin, and in the crying infant it offers little "holding power" to the stoma. Consequently, the new stoma is likely to prolapse; or, worse, adjacent loops of intestine may herniate. Figure 5 shows the important detail of placement of multiple fine (4–0 atraumatic chromic intestinal catgut) seromuscular sutures circumferentially to the subcuticular fascia. In the thin child, the peritoneum is pulled up into the wound and the seromuscular layers are fixed to it. One must take care to avoid puncturing the lumen of the bowel.

Loop Ileal Stoma

The loop type of ileal stoma may occasionally be indicated. The details of the technique are depicted in Figure 6. The laparotomy is best done in the left side of the abdomen. When the site for the stoma has been determined, a circular piece of skin slightly larger than the ileum must be excised. All layers (rectus, rectus

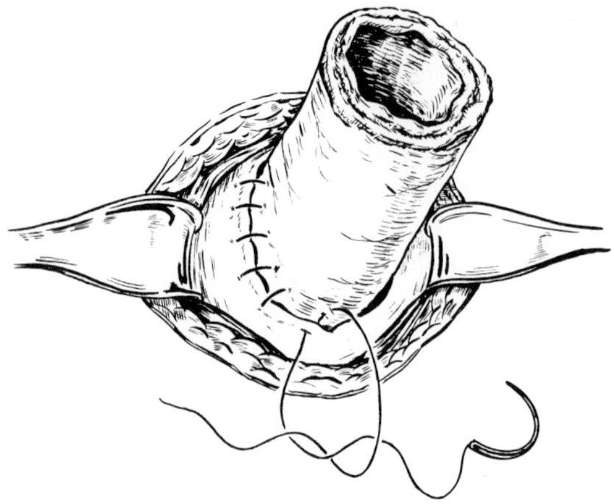

FIGURE 5. Ileostomy in children. Circumferential interrupted seromuscular sutures to the peritoneum.

fascia, peritoneum) are then split vertically. A loop of ileum is delivered through a generous two-finger width aperture in the abdominal wall (Fig. 6A).

In average-weight adults, a few fine chromic interrupted sutures will fix the mesentery to the subcutaneous fibrofat; but in thin adults or in children, the suture fixation technique illustrated in Figure 5 is best. The loop is opened transversely about halfway on the antimesenteric aspect (Fig. 6B) and everted, and the free ends are sutured with fine chromic catgut to the subcuticular fascia as shown

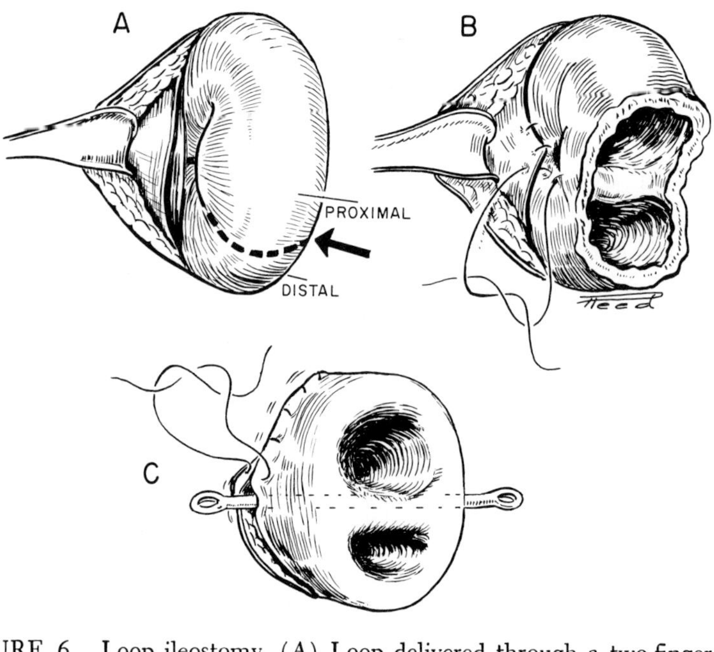

FIGURE 6. Loop ileostomy. (*A*) Loop delivered through a two-finger width vertical rectus aperture. (*B*) The loop is opened transversely. Insertion of interrupted sutures to the fascia. (*C*) The loop is everted and sutured to the subcuticular fascia. The proximal end is prominent.

in Figure 6C. The ileum is opened rather to the distal side of the loop so that the proximal or functional side will be most prominent (Fig. 6B, C).

Ileal Stoma in Obese Patients

In obese patients with a deep abdominal wall, the "end-loop" type of ileal stoma is the most satisfactory. An umbilical tape is passed around the ileum (Fig. 7A, B) at a distance from the end that is equal to the thickness of the abdominal wall, and the loop is pulled through a *generous* two-finger width aperture (Fig. 1C). The loop must protrude without any tension whatsoever. The stoma is fixed in the wound, opened, everted, and sutured to the subcuticular fascia as shown in Figure 6. If there is any tendency for the loop to sink, a short glass rod may be left under it for five days.

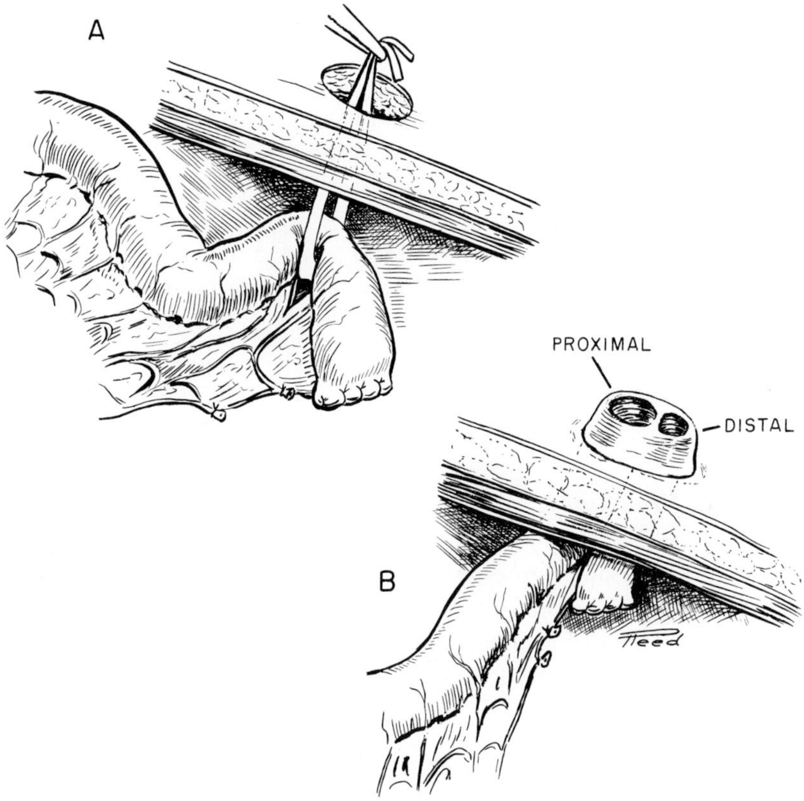

FIGURE 7. "End-loop" ileostomy in obese patients. (*A*) A loop of ileum with mesentery can be pulled through an obese abdominal wall. (*B*) Completed ileostomy. Loop opened transversely, everted, sutured to the subcuticular fascia. The distal end should be visible inside the abdomen.

Transplanting the Ileal Stoma Without Laparotomy

The ileal stoma must be transplanted to a new site when (1) an interparietal (parastomal) hernia becomes intolerable, (2) there is constant retraction or prolapse, or (3) the surgeon has placed the first stoma where it is impossible to have a satisfactorily fitting ileostomy pouch.

Method

After repeated trial applications with a pouch disc on the patient in various sitting and standing positions, a new stomal site is marked. First- and second-choice sites are marked by needle scratch and gentian violet. The stoma is mobilized by a circumferential incision made to include a one-fourth inch collar of skin. The stoma is kept under traction during the dissection until the peritoneal cavity is entered. The previously sutured mesentery is easily brought into view and is dissected free of the peritoneum until 6 to 8 inches of ileum and mesentery has been mobilized. Adjacent adherent loops of ileum are carefully separated as they are encountered. The end of the stoma is securely tied, leaving the tie long for later traction to the new site. The stoma is placed within the abdominal cavity, the surgeon's index finger is inserted, and by following the anterior wall inside the abdomen and dissecting adherent loops of bowel free of old scars, etc., the new stomal site is palpated. A disc of skin is excised; the rectus sheath, muscle, and peritoneum are split vertically, and the ileum is pulled through a new two-finger width aperture in the abdominal wall to form a new stoma. Fixation of the stoma or its mesentery to the subcutaneous fat or fascia is carried out as shown in Figure 6B, and an eversion maneuver is completed (Fig. 3). The deep abdominal wall layers of the vacated stoma site are closed with heavy through-and-through interrupted chromic catgut sutures, leaving the site for possible use in the future.

Conventional Ileostomy

In the event of failure of the foregoing techniques for the ileostomy, the old (non-eversion) conventional method may be utilized. The protruding ileum must be trimmed to within one-half inch of the skin. There is little dysfunction with a short stoma, the main problem being a skin stricture that may develop during the maturation phase.

References

Brooke, B. N. Management of ileostomy including its complications. *Lancet* 2:102, July 19, 1952.

CRILE, G., JR., and TURNBULL, R. B., JR. Mechanism and prevention of ileostomy dysfunction. *Ann. Surg.* 140:459, October 1954.

TURNBULL, R. B., JR. Management of ileostomy. *Am. J. Surg.* 86:617, November 1953.

TURNBULL, R. B., JR. Intestinal stomas. *S. Clin. North America* 38:1361, October 1958.

WARREN, R., and MCKITTRICK, L. S. Ileostomy for ulcerative colitis; technique, complications, and management. *Surg., Gynec. and Obst.* 93:555, November 1951.

89. *Diverticulitis*

JOHN H. GARLOCK

THE PATHOLOGICAL COMPLICATIONS of diverticulitis of the colon (usually confined to the sigmoid flexure) may be so varied that the surgeon must be conversant with a number of procedures, each of which might be applicable to a specific set of circumstances. In recent years there has developed a more aggressive approach to some of the types of diverticulitis which were previously accorded conservative management. This has been made possible by the advent of the intestinal antibiotics and a better understanding of the pathological variations of this disease.

In addition to appraising the extent of the disease, the surgeon should remember that most of these patients are obese and have foreshortened sigmoid mesenteries infiltrated with fat. This increases considerably the difficulties of the operative procedures. The concomitant presence of marked induration of the tissues due to long-standing chronic inflammation complicates the picture still further, and the surgeon is faced with technical difficulties of considerable magnitude.

Diverticulitis with Acute Perforation

In the acute episode with free perforation of a ruptured diverticulum, the patient presents himself with an acute abdominal emergency, not infrequently misdiagnosed as a perforated appendix (the so-called right-sided diverticulitis). How should this situation be handled? Surgical treatment will be influenced by a number of factors: viz., the duration of the acute episode, the general condition of the patient, the severity and extent of the peritonitis, the site of the perforation, and the degree of involvement of the sigmoid loop. Not infrequently, it is possible to invert the perforated diverticulum, drain the lower abdomen, and perform a transverse colostomy to divert the fecal stream. In a very ill patient, exteriorization of the involved sigmoid by the Mickulicz technique may be carried out expeditiously, with minimal surgical trauma, if the perforation cannot be visualized. If the patient is not desperately ill, the surgeon has another choice of procedure, namely, immediate resection of the diseased segment with the formation of a double-barreled

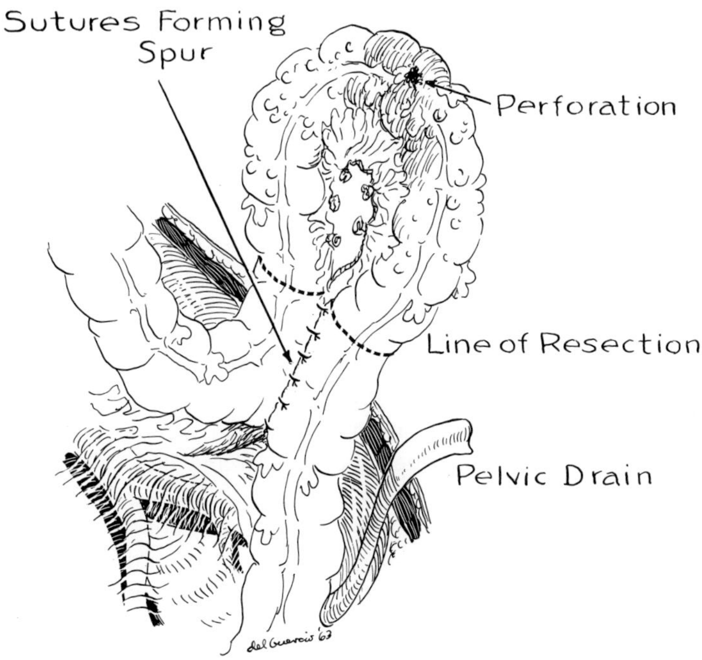

FIGURE 1. The operation of obstructive resection may on occasion be utilized in the emergency treatment of some of the acute complications of diverticulitis. It obviates the need for a proximal colostomy.

colostomy (Fig. 1). This is essentially the obstructive resection operation of Rankin. It can frequently be done without too much dissection of retroperitoneal areas, which should be avoided in the presence of a spreading peritonitis. This method of handling a difficult situation has been utilized frequently by both Gilchrist and Boyden.

In the past, the operative therapy for free perforation with gross soiling was followed by a high mortality. However, since the advent of antibiotics, the mortality figures have reached a more reasonable level. In all such cases, I believe that the pelvis and lower abdomen should be drained extensively and that aggressive antibiotic therapy should be given postoperatively.

Diverticulitis with Slow Perforation

A less acute form of diverticulitis, with slow perforation and fixation of the inflamed segment in the left lower quadrant, produces a palpable tumefaction in this region which may go on to the formation of a superficial abscess of the abdominal wall. It is inadvisable to undertake any operation for the eradication of the disease at this stage of the pathological process, and the surgeon should be content to wait out either the subsidence of the inflammation or the formation of a superficial abscess, which should be treated by simple incision and drainage. In a number of instances, I have noted complete resolution of the mass after the drainage of an abscess, with recovery and no further episodes of diverticulitis. More frequently, a fecal fistula will follow the drainage operation, and resection of the sigmoid will eventually become necessary.

Chronic Diverticulitis

Another variety of diverticulitis which was rarely subjected to operation is that encountered in the patient who experiences repeated mild attacks of sigmoid inflammation with a degree or two of fever, soreness in the left lower quadrant, tenderness on physical examination, and incapacity for two or three days, followed by complete recovery. In spite of adequate medical and dietary management, the attacks recur. The barium enema roentgenogram usually discloses nothing more than a few sigmoid diverticula with spasm. Our attitude toward this type of diverticulitis has become more aggressive in recent years, and rightly so. Removal of the sigmoid colon by the operation of anterior resection with a complementary tube cecostomy can be accomplished with a negligible mortality and complete symptomatic cure.

A further stage in the chronic variety of diverticulitis is characterized by (1) inflammation that produces marked thickening of all layers of the sigmoid colon, and (2) fixation of the organ to the left iliac fossa and pelvic cavity, with resultant extensive chronic inflammation of the parietal peritoneum and the underlying tissues. In this type of diverticulitis, it may be difficult to diagnose the concomitant presence of a carcinoma, both preoperatively by x-ray examination and at the operating table with the specimen in the surgeon's hand. For this reason alone, surgery is mandatory and the procedure should always be radical, with wide excision of mesentery and bowel. The possibility of a concomitant carcinoma has been variously estimated at from 1 per cent to 10 per cent of cases in reported series; in our own group, it has been found in about 4 per cent of cases. The opposite combination, the finding of diverticulosis with an obvious sigmoid carcinoma both preoperatively by x-ray examination and at laparotomy, usually poses no problem.

It is difficult to delineate the normal anatomical structures in this area, such as the left ureter and the iliac vessels, and the fat-infiltrated sigmoid mesocolon is foreshortened and twisted. Under such circumstances, the technical difficulties of a resection may indeed be very great. As a precautionary measure, it is advisable to catheterize the left ureter preoperatively to aid the surgeon in locating this structure during the operation. The separation of the colon and its mesentery must be carried out with great care and usually requires sharp dissection.

There has been considerable discussion concerning the amount of colon to be removed for this disease. In the vast majority of patients, the major inflammation is confined to the sigmoid loop, and its complete removal by the operation of anterior resection usually suffices. The distal site of transection is located at the rectosigmoid junction and it is not necessary to remove any part of the rectum. Mobilization of the rectum posteriorly brings the divided end out of the pelvis and expedites the technical maneuvers of the anastomosis. Not infrequently, the preoperative barium enema film discloses diverticula in the descending colon and scattered diverticula in the transverse colon. Is it, therefore, necessary to remove every portion of the large bowel which discloses such diverticula? I do not believe so. It must be remembered that the fecal content does not become solid until the left half of the colon is reached, and that the genesis of diverticulitis is the trapping of solid fecal material in the diverticula, not liquid feces. Therefore, when radical removal becomes necessary, the site of proximal transection need not be further back than the splenic flexure. Freeing of the splenic flexure from its ligamentous attachments permits the surgeon to approximate the distal end of the transverse colon to the rectosigmoid with ease. An important technical point to remember is to avoid making the anastomosis at the site of a diverticulum in the proximal segment. A fistula may form at this site postoperatively. The details of the anastomosis are the same as for anterior resection and are described in Chapter 91.

Many surgeons still favor a three-stage procedure for advanced chronic diverticulitis. This consists of a preliminary transverse colostomy, resection of the diseased segment of colon with end-to-end anastomosis and, finally, closure of the colostomy. The procedure entails a rather prolonged period of disability and hospitalization, but its safety commends it. In the absence of any possibility of carcinoma, the surgeon has the alternative of a two-stage procedure. This consists of a primary obstructive resection with the formation of a double-barreled colostomy and subsequent closure of the colostomy. Boyden champions this approach. My preference in recent years has been a radical primary resection with a complementary tube cecostomy. If a careful anastomosis is made between the two ends of *normal* bowel, there should be no higher incidence of suture line breakdown than with the operation for cancer. The obvious exception has been in those patients who were admitted with obstruction. Under these circumstances, the operation of obstructive resection should be favored. Or, if obstruction is complete, a preliminary transverse colostomy may be more desirable.

Complications

Probably the most important complication of diverticulitis is the formation of a sigmoidovesical fistula. With the passage of gas and fecal material into the bladder, a urinary tract infection ensues. The three-stage operation is indicated in such cases. A preliminary diversionary transverse colostomy decreases considerably the inflammatory reaction in the pelvis and bladder, thereby simplifying the technical details of the subsequent resection. The interval between the first and second stages varies, but the average is between one and three months. At the time of resection, the surgeon must clearly delineate the site of fixation of the sigmoid to the bladder, marking the location of the fistula. In most instances, the fistula will be located nearer the base of the bladder than the dome. With the patient in deep

Trendelenburg position and the intestines packed away toward the upper abdomen, it will be easier to clarify the anatomy of the parts and separate the colon from the bladder. The latter is then closed with an inner mucosal layer of interrupted fine chromic sutures and an outer layer of fine silk stitches. It may be possible to reflect a flap of pelvic peritoneum to cover the suture line for added protection. The diseased sigmoid is then resected as previously described. The indwelling bladder catheter should be maintained for five or six days after operation. Before closing the colostomy two or more weeks later, it is desirable to visualize the suture line by a barium enema examination. The demonstration of any sinus tracts leading from the anastomotic area calls for deferment of the colostomy closure until the local area presents a normal contour.

It has been suggested that, instead of the three-stage operation, it is frequently possible to correct these sigmoidovesical fistulas by the operation of obstructive resection with the formation of a double-barreled colostomy, i.e. a two-stage procedure. While I am sure this can be done occasionally, there is no doubt that the preliminary diversion of feces in the three-stage operation causes a substantial diminution in the pelvic inflammatory process and makes for an easier and safer later resection. Safety in the surgical therapy of diverticulitis is of paramount importance. A careful appraisal of each case should indicate whether a multiple- or single-stage operation should be undertaken. Antibiotics and surgical bravado cannot take the place of sound surgical judgment.

Finally, there is a complication of diverticulosis of the colon which, though fortunately uncommon, may tax the surgeon's judgment to the extreme. I refer to the elderly patient with extensive diverticulosis, usually involving the entire colon, who begins to bleed actively and soon becomes a subject for emergency therapy. Not too many years ago, the opinion was generally held that bleeding rarely, if ever, emanates from colonic diverticula, but subsequent experience has thoroughly disproved this concept. Erosion of sclerotic vessels at the rim or in the depths of a diverticulum can cause, not only sporadic minor bleeding episodes, but alarming hemorrhage of serious proportions. In the latter eventuality, the whole colon may be filled with liquid and clotted blood and it becomes impossible to pinpoint the source of the hemorrhage. In three patients in our own series, it was necessary to perform subtotal colectomy as an emergency procedure. In one instance, an open vessel was found in the hepatic flexure, and in the remaining two the site of bleeding was located in the sigmoid colon. It would seem that the surgeon should not wait too long before embarking on what might at first appear to be a hazardous undertaking.

References

Boyden, A. M. Two-stage (obstructive) resection of the sigmoid in selected cases of complicated diverticulitis. *Ann. Surg.* 154:210, December 1961.

Ranson, H. K. Diverticulitis of the colon. *Gastroenterology* 26:12, January 1954.

Smithwick, R. H. Surgical treatment of diverticulitis of sigmoid. *Am. J. Surg.* 99:192, February 1960.

90. *Cancer of the Colon*

NEIL W. SWINTON

IT IS OUR IMPRESSION, after having evaluated our experience and that of others, that there has been little increase in survival rates in the last decade in the treatment of cancer of the colon. What increase has occurred has been primarily the result of bringing larger numbers of patients to operation earlier than in the past. Improvements in the preoperative evaluation and preoperative preparation of patients, improved anesthesia, the availability of blood banks, and improvements in our ability to control infection with antibiotics, resulting in lower mortality rates, have been additional factors.

We are frequently impressed with the fact that patients still come to us with long-standing malignant disease of the large intestine, and that although they have sought medical advice early in the course of the disease, operation has been delayed because of inadequate examinations. It has long been our practice to emphasize the importance of sigmoidoscopic examinations, not only for evaluation of gastrointestinal symptoms but also as part of a routine physical examination. The most significant advance that will be made in the treatment of cancer of the large intestine will be the general adoption of this policy by all physicians interested in the diagnosis and treatment of pathological processes of the large intestine. Seventy per cent of large bowel cancers can be diagnosed with use of the ordinary 25 cm. sigmoidoscope.

The treatment of cancer of the colon and rectum is primarily surgical. Radiation has provided some palliation to certain patients, particularly in the relief of pain. The status of chemotherapy in the treatment of malignant disease of the large intestine is still experimental, although we have been encouraged recently with the results of treatment using intraarterial infusions in certain patients with metastatic lesions, particularly involving the liver, with the chemical compound 5-FUDR (5-fluoro-2′-deoxyuridine).

Over the years we have developed definite policies with regard to the surgical removal of malignant lesions of the colon. It is the purpose of this presentation to review some of these concepts.

Preoperative Care

Evaluation of the Patient

The first step in any successful operation for malignant disease of the colon is the preoperative evaluation of the patient. Since most of these patients are in the late fifties and sixties, and many in their seventies and eighties, a careful preoperative medical evaluation should be made. Blood volume should be returned to normal preoperatively. Anesthetic agents should be carefully selected. Other physical defects should be corrected or controlled when possible. Careful digital, sigmoidoscopic, and rectal examinations of the colon, and x-ray examination of the remainder of the gastrointestinal tract with due regard to the problem of retained barium, should be done as a part of the physical examination, not only to obtain all information concerning the lesion, but to determine the presence of other pathological change, particularly the presence of multiple lesions.

Preparation of the Intestine

Mechanical cleansing of the intestine with laxatives and irrigations is of the utmost importance. In recent years sterilization of the lumen of the intestine with sulfa drugs and antibiotics has also become essential. At present we use sulfathalidine, 2 grams every six hours, and Humatin, 1 gram every six hours, for an average of three days before the anticipated operation. Immediately before operation, the placing of a gastric tube and an indwelling Foley catheter is desirable. Arrangements should be made with the blood bank for one to three blood transfusions if they should be necessary at the time of surgery.

Cancer of the Cecum, Ascending Colon, and Hepatic Flexure

For all malignant lesions of the colon, the objective of the operation is the removal of the widest possible margin of lymph-bearing tissue and colon consistent with an adequate blood supply to the remaining colon and the general condition of the patient. For lesions of the right colon, a right hemicolectomy and ileotransverse colostomy is generally accepted as the operation of choice.

A generous right paramedian incision is made and the peritoneal cavity opened. The edges of the wound are carefully draped with moist pads and protected at all times to prevent contamination. The abdominal contents are methodically examined, including the retroperitoneal tissues, for the presence of metastases or other disease. The lesion itself is probably best examined last, and the size, extent, adherence, induration, and the degree of any perforation or associated infection are noted. When an operating table that will tilt laterally is available, the patient can be rotated and the small bowel and left colon can be packed into the left half of the abdomen without difficulty using moist pads.

The extent of the resection should now be considered. Umbilical tape surrounding the bowel may next be placed distally and proximally to the tumor, as advocated by Cole and others.

The right colic and right branch of the middle colic vessels are first ligated at the root of the mesentery. There will be instances in obese patients with a short mesentery in which this may not be practical. We do not do this preliminary ligation of the blood supply of the right colon routinely. Vessels can usually be easily identified and ligated individually through a small incision in the peritoneum on the medial side of the mesentery at its root (Fig. 1). The right colon and distal ileum are then retracted medially and the parietal peritoneum divided at its point of fusion with the visceral peritoneum. This will expose the ureter, the spermatic or ovarian vessels, the inferior vena cava, and the duodenum (Fig. 2). The duo-

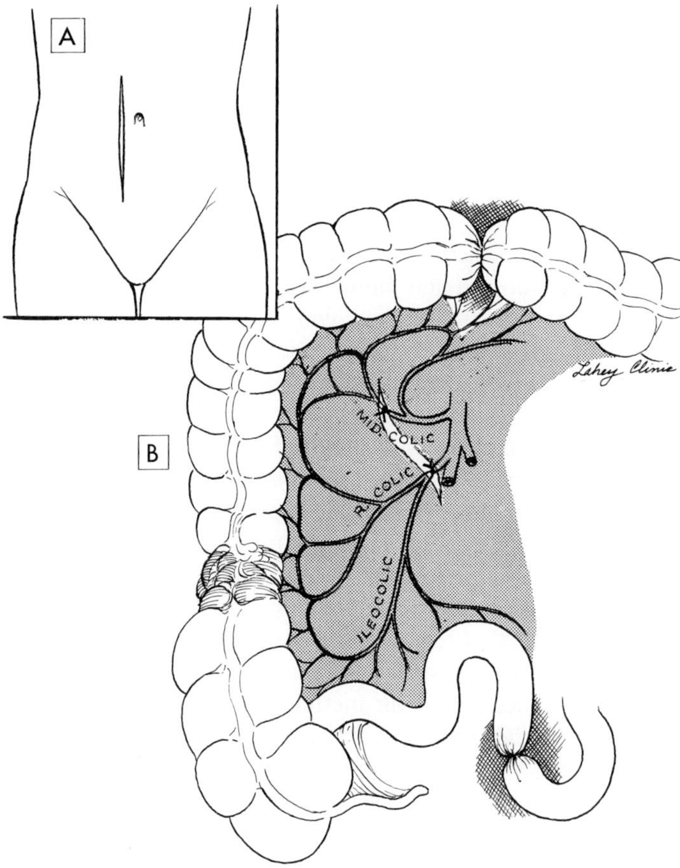

FIGURE 1. Cancer of the ascending colon. Preliminary ligation of the right colic and the right branch of the middle colic artery at the root of the mesentery. The lumen of the ileum and lumen of the transverse colon have been ligated with tapes.

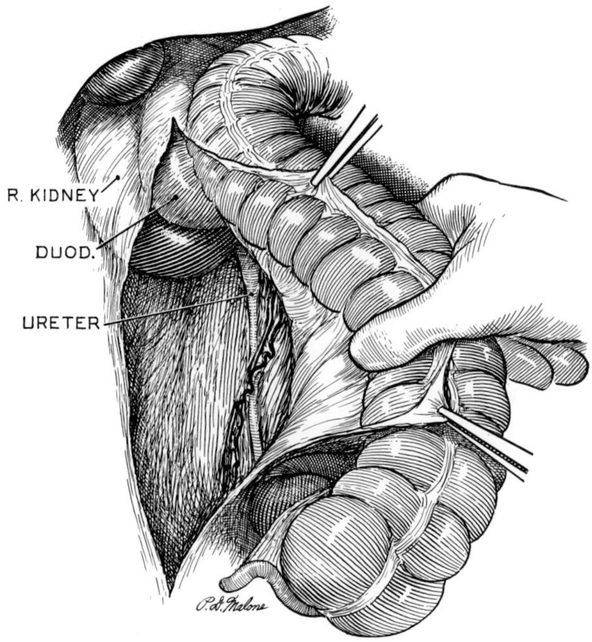

FIGURE 2. Division of the parietal peritoneum exposing underlying structures.

denum may be adherent to the undersurface of the ascending colon and must be separated with care.

The site of transection in the terminal ileum and the transverse colon is next selected. The main trunk and left branch of the middle colic artery supplying the distal segment of the transverse colon must be carefully preserved. The mesentery between the selected sites of resection is then serially clamped, cut, and ligated. Two Ochsner clamps are applied to the intestine at the selected sites and the bowel is divided with cautery (Fig. 3).

The specimen is given to an associate, preferably a pathologist, for immediate gross inspection of the open specimen and frozen section study if indicated. Not infrequently, multiple tumors or associated polyps will be discovered in this manner. When multiple lesions are found, it may be necessary to re-evaluate the extent of the resection to be performed. We do not believe it practical, because of the danger of contamination, to do colonoscopy or intraluminal observation of the remaining colon at the time of resection for cancer.

When the colon is first opened, a specimen is taken from the lumen for cultures and sensitivity studies. With our method of preparation, over 80 per cent of such cultures do not reveal pathogenic organisms. We do not routinely give antibiotics after operation. When a perforated lesion, a walled-off abscess, or other evidence of infection is present, however, antibiotics are administered immediately after operation. The final choice of the antibiotic will be determined by bacteriological studies made at the time of surgery. We must also remember that although antibiotics may sterilize the lumen, they will not destroy the virulent organisms so commonly found within the cancer.

Anastomosis between the ileum and transverse colon is next performed (Fig.

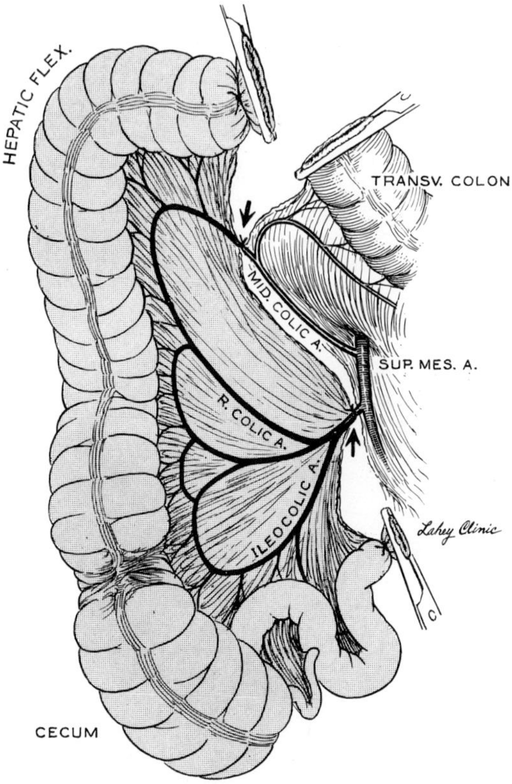

FIGURE 3. Terminal ileum, cecum, ascending colon, and right half of the transverse colon divided beyond tapes.

4). An inner layer of interrupted catgut sutures and an outer layer of interrupted fine silk are used. Any tissue injured by application of the clamps is excised before the sutures are placed. The bowel ends can be held in place with Allis clamps or traction sutures after the Ochsner clamps have been removed. We do not irrigate the open ends of the colon, but we carefully swab out the open lumen with moist saline sponges. We have not routinely utilized bichloride or any of the other solutions that have been advocated for the destruction of cancer cells in these regions. There must be no tension on the suture line.

On occasion there may be an appreciable disparity between the size of the lumen of the ileum and the lumen of the transverse colon. We prefer an end-to-end anastomosis whenever possible, but on occasion an end-to-side or side-to-side anastomosis may be desirable. One method of increasing the size of the lumen of the ileum is to cut the ileum longitudinally for 1 to 2 cm. on its antimesenteric border (Fig. 4D).

The rent in the mesentery is closed with continuous chromic catgut sutures, avoiding injury to the blood supply in the remaining mesentery.

The abdominal wall is closed in layers without drainage. The choice of suture material used in the abdominal wall apparently is not of great significance, provided the wound edges are approximated without tension and are clean. We prefer catgut to silk, or wire if the wound is under tension or if gross contamination has occurred.

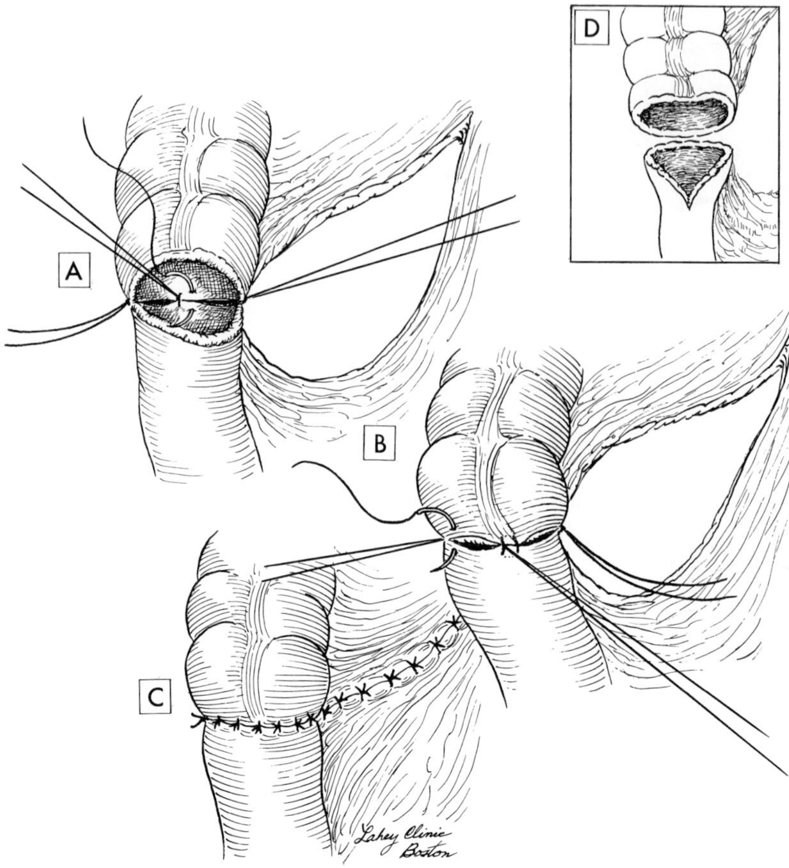

FIGURE 4. (*A, B, and C*) Anastomosis of the ileum to the transverse colon. (*D*) Method of enlarging the caliber of the bowel.

Cancer of the Transverse Colon

Opinions have differed somewhat concerning the extent of resections for cancer of the transverse colon. It has been our policy to perform a segmental resection when a long mesentery is present and an extensive resection can be done utilizing an end-to-end anastomosis without tension and without mobilizing the splenic and hepatic flexures. Many, however, advocate routine resection of both flexures as a more radical procedure for tumors in this region. No significant difference in survival rates has been noted. Technical details of resection of the transverse colon do not differ from those of resection for lesions of the right colon. A left paramedian incision is used, the gastrocolic ligament and the mesentery of the transverse colon are divided in separate layers, and the omentum is removed with the specimen. The middle colic vessels are ligated as close to their origins from the superior mesenteric as possible (Fig. 5).

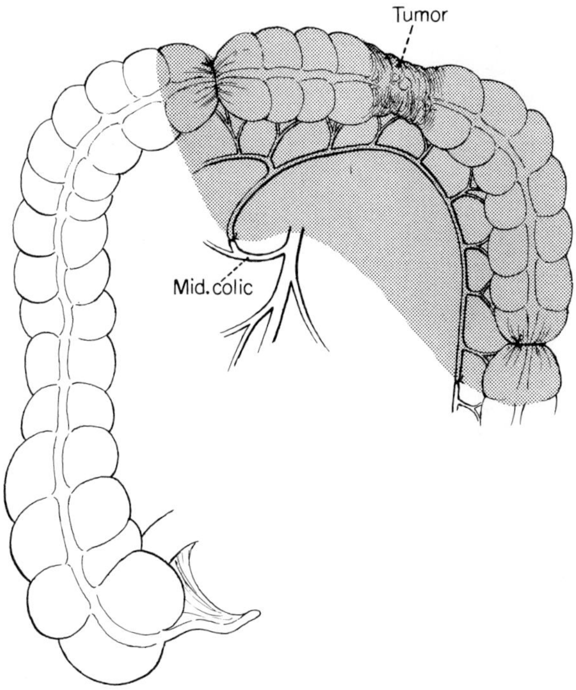

FIGURE 5. Resection of tumor of the left transverse colon.

The surgeon may have difficulty in freeing the splenic flexure. Tilting of the table and the patient to the right will facilitate the packing off of the small bowel. One helpful maneuver in obtaining the best possible exposure of the splenocolic ligament at the splenic flexure is to discontinue the division of the mesentery of the transverse colon and gastrocolic ligament 3 to 4 inches from the flexure, and then begin to divide the parietal peritoneum from the descending colon at about its midpart, proceeding proximally to the flexure. As the splenic flexure is reached, the area of the spleen can usually be easily brought into view by gentle traction on both the transverse colon and the descending colon (Fig. 6).

After the resection of the lesion and adjacent tissue, an end-to-end anastomosis is performed, as previously described.

Cancer of the Descending Colon and Upper Sigmoid

Cancers of the descending colon and upper sigmoid are resected in much the same manner as lesions in the right and transverse colon. Segmental resection may be adequate. In many instances, however, the splenic flexure must be mobilized and resected, or simply mobilized, to permit adequate removal of the colon and mesentery and allow a tension-free anastomosis.

The blood vessels supplying the left colon and sigmoid should be ligated at the junction of the inferior mesenteric artery and the aorta (Fig. 7). When this is done, the left colic artery will be divided. It must be remembered that in about

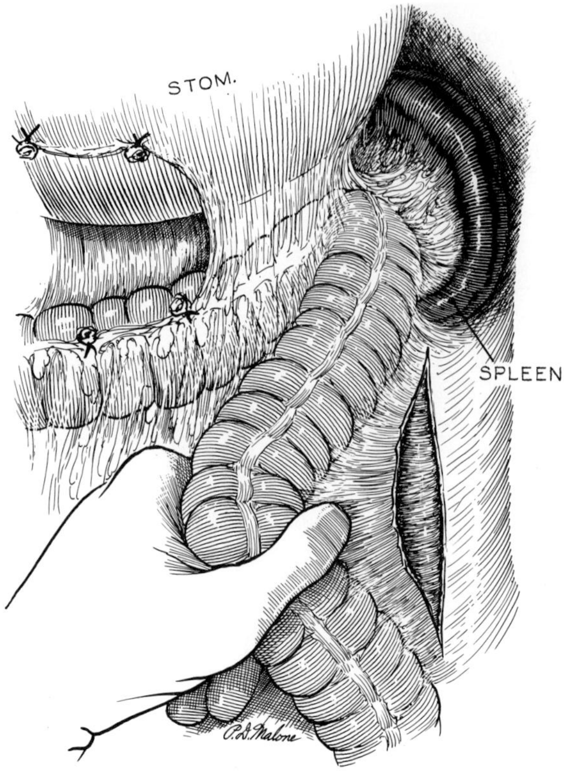

FIGURE 6. Method of freeing the splenic flexure.

20 per cent of patients the blood supply to the left colon and sigmoid will be inadequate when the left colic artery has been divided, because of absent blood supply or inadequate blood supply coming down from the middle colic artery through the marginal vessels. This possibility must always be considered, and in such situations the transverse colon should be brought down for anastomosis.

Cancer of the Lower Sigmoid and Rectum

Removal of cancer in the lower sigmoid and rectum has been discussed by other authors in this volume. A few observations, however, might be made on the removal of such tumors.

In recent years at the Lahey Clinic, the number of patients submitted to anterior resection for lesions in the low sigmoid and upper rectum has increased greatly. Our policy has been to do anterior resections for lesions in these areas if the descending colon can be anastomosed satisfactorily to the rectum, and the latter divided at least 8 cm. below the lower margin of the tumor, as measured by the surgeon at the time of operation, with the left colon and sigmoid on tension. This is a length of approximately 4 cm. as measured by the pathologist in the resected specimen. In women, because of the broader pelvis, lower anastomoses can, of course, be performed (Fig. 8).

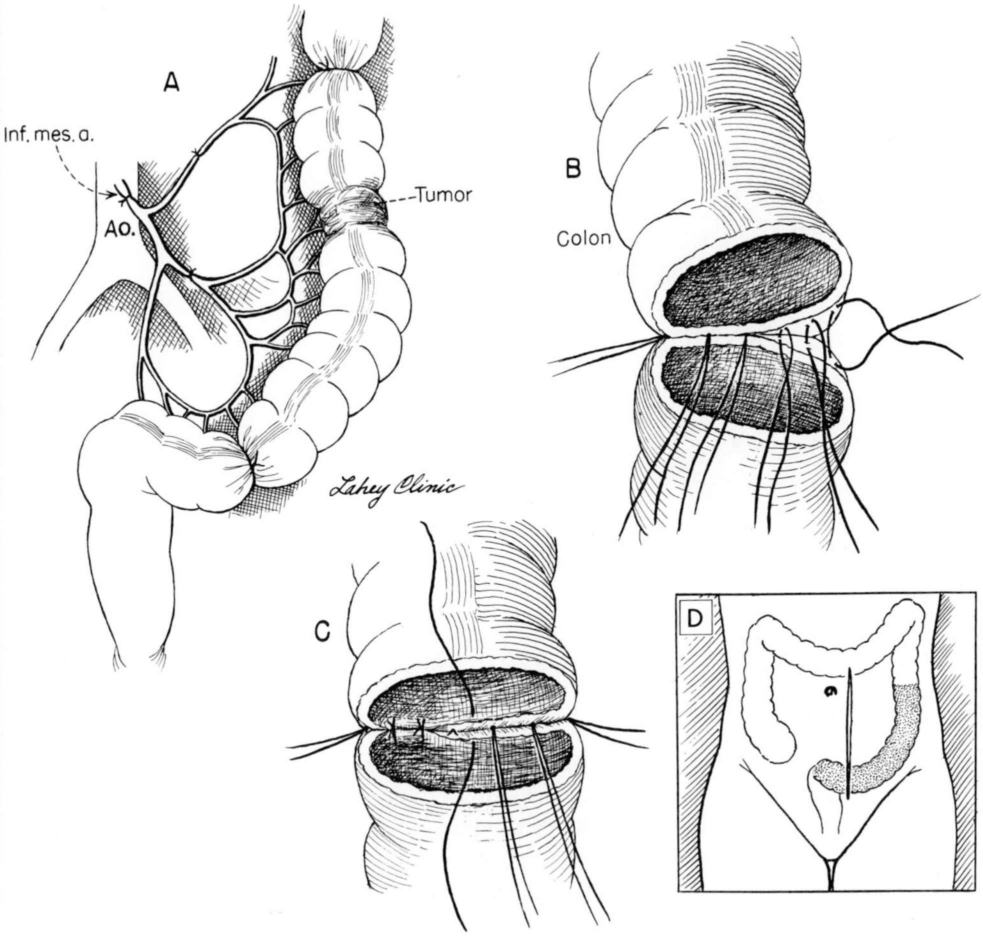

FIGURE 7. Resection of cancer of the sigmoid or upper rectum.

We have encountered a disquieting incidence of leaks and perforations at the site of, and adjacent to, the anastomosis. When this postoperative complication is noted and is disturbing, we immediately perform a transverse colostomy with complete diversion of the fecal stream. One should realize, however, that many of these leaks are small and heal spontaneously without difficulty. Mortality and survival rates following removal of lesions in these regions by anterior resection are among the best for locations in the large bowel. It must be appreciated, however, that this is largely explained by the careful selection of the patients who are submitted to this procedure. We do not routinely perform a cecostomy or transverse colostomy as an adjunct to this type of resection and anastomosis, but depend on intragastric suction for decompression in the majority of instances.

In cancer situated low in the rectum, a standard abdominoperineal resection is employed. We have had no experience with the "pull-through" type of operation for malignant disease, nor with the combined synchronous operation. Sur-

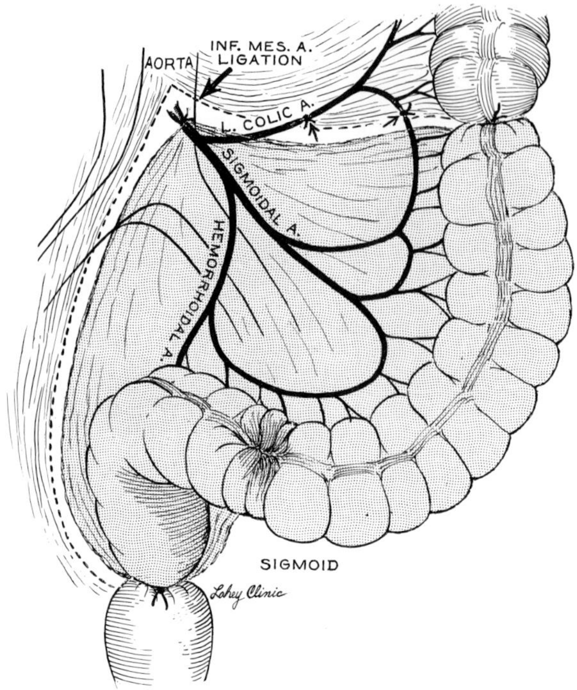

FIGURE 8. Anterior resection; preliminary ligation of the inferior mesenteric artery at its origin from the aorta.

vival rates following the pull-through operation are satisfactory. Because of the increased incidence of complications, inadequate bowel control, and the problem of a perineal colostomy, however, this procedure is best reserved for those few surgeons who have had an extensive experience with it.

The peritoneal floor is carefully closed intraabdominally. We do not ordinarily use massive packs in the perineal wounds. The wound is partially closed around a small cigarette drain, which is removed early in the convalescent period.

It is of paramount importance to have patients who have had an abdominoperineal resection adjust to the colostomy as rapidly as possible. We do not allow them to leave the hospital until they have been carefully instructed in a diet that will control their colostomy and in the use of colonic irrigation, usually on a two-day schedule, for adequate control of bowel function. We avoid appliances whenever possible.

ACKNOWLEDGMENT

The author is indebted to George J. Farha, M.D., former Fellow in Surgery at the Lahey Clinic, for his assistance in preparing this chapter.

91. *Anterior Resection for Carcinoma of the Lower Sigmoid, Rectosigmoid, and Upper Rectum*

JOHN H. GARLOCK

THE NOTABLE ADVANCES in the surgical therapy of cancer of the colon and rectum during the past decade are related to the adoption of measures to prevent cancer spread (by the manipulations of the surgeon himself) through the vascular system, into the bowel lumen with subsequent suture line implantations, and from the surface of the tumor to the abdominal cavity and the operative incision. Separately, these possibilities of cancer spread have been known for many years, but it remained for Cole to clarify the situation and to emphasize the need for preventive measures. In the operation of anterior resection, these measures may be carried out with relative ease.

There are many variants of this operation. Each surgeon develops for himself a fairly standardized technique and comes to believe that his particular method is the most desirable. However, each step in the operation must have a logical reason for its use, in terms of simplicity of performance, postoperative morbidity and mortality, and incidence of cancer recurrence; and modifications indicated by increasing experience should be adopted. The technique to be described was developed with these desiderata constantly in mind. One of the basic concepts of surgical technique, which unfortunately is frequently forgotten nowadays, is the utilization of technical steps which simplify rather than complicate the performance of a surgical procedure. One can become so lost in a maze of trivial technical details as to state publicly, as one prominent surgeon has done, that when one undertakes the operation of anterior resection, he should have no other commitments that day!

There is fairly general agreement that anterior resection is the procedure of choice for cancers of the lower sigmoid, rectosigmoid, and upper rectum. On the other hand, there is no unanimity of opinion that it is the preferred treatment for cancers of the middle and lower rectum, say, as low as 3 to 4 inches from the anal verge. The surgeon should not be bound by rigid criteria, but should be guided rather by conditions in the pelvis at the time of operation, the age and psychological make-up of the patient, the magnitude of the technical difficulties, and the histological report on the preoperative biopsy specimen, to mention a few factors. For example, one is frequently surprised at the time of operation to find a wide pelvis with a comfortable margin of safety distal to the tumor after mobilization of the rectum when preoperatively all indications pointed to a need for an abdominoperineal resection. In regard to the patient's age, it seems to me that every effort should be made to avoid a permanent colostomy in an elderly, decrepit patient, even though the risk of recurrence might be increased. A technical problem of considerable magnitude is encountered in laying down a satisfactory suture line when a low-lying tumor is buried in a narrow pelvis; in addition there is a greatly increased risk of local cancer cell implantation. Under such circumstances, an abdominoperineal resection would be in order. Finally, the finding of a highly malignant invasive tumor in the biopsy specimen calls for an operation of the most radical variety, with no sentiment for sparing the sphincter muscles.

Technique

The Incision and Exploration

The operation of anterior resection is greatly simplified by placing the patient in deep Trendelenburg position. Many anesthetists have a great fear of this position because of the pressure of abdominal contents on the diaphragm, with possible resultant anoxemia. Intubation usually obviates this possibility. The occasional patient with marked obesity or severe hypertension may react adversely to this position, if it is extreme, and must be watched carefully by both the anesthetist and the surgeon. The incision is midline in position, starting at the symphysis pubis and curving around to the left of the umbilicus. It should be liberal in extent. After protecting the abdominal incision with warm moist pads, the surgeon attains comfortable exposure by means of a properly placed self-retaining retractor. An orderly examination of the abdomen should then follow, commencing with the liver, then the preaortic area for enlarged nodes, the mesentery of the sigmoid, the cul-de-sac of Douglas and, finally, the tumor itself (gingerly) for local fixation, penetration, etc. The first step is the placing of a stout silk ligature tightly about the colon proximal to the tumor. For this purpose, heavy silk is more effective than umbilical tape. It may be possible to tie off the bowel distal to the tumor at this time, but usually this step is deferred until the rectum has been mobilized.

Mobilization of the Sigmoid

By drawing outward and downward on the sigmoid flexure, the inferior mesenteric vessels are brought into sharp relief. These are approached through an incision in the posterior peritoneum on the right side of the mesentery and are doubly ligated and divided under direct vision. Before doing so, it is advisable to free the mesosigmoid from peritoneal attachments in the left iliac fossa and identify the left ureter. Not infrequently, this ureter is pulled over toward the midline and may be accidentally included in the ligature placed about the inferior mesenteric artery. The site of division of this artery has been open to debate. I do not believe it is necessary to ligate it at its origin from the aorta. I usually choose a point just distal to the left colic branch. After continuing the incision in the posterior peritoneum downward on each side of the rectum and joining these extensions in front deep in the pelvis, large peritoneal flaps are bluntly dissected free from the pelvis, and the ureter on each side identified during the process (Fig. 1). These flaps are important in the subsequent pelvic repair and are fashioned more expeditiously at the beginning of the operation than later. Moreover, mobilization of the rectum is made easier.

Mobilization of the Rectum

At the level of the sacral promontory, blunt dissection of the rectum is begun from above downward, the plane of cleavage being in front of the presacral fascia and plexus. It is continued downward posteriorly and laterally with the gloved hand

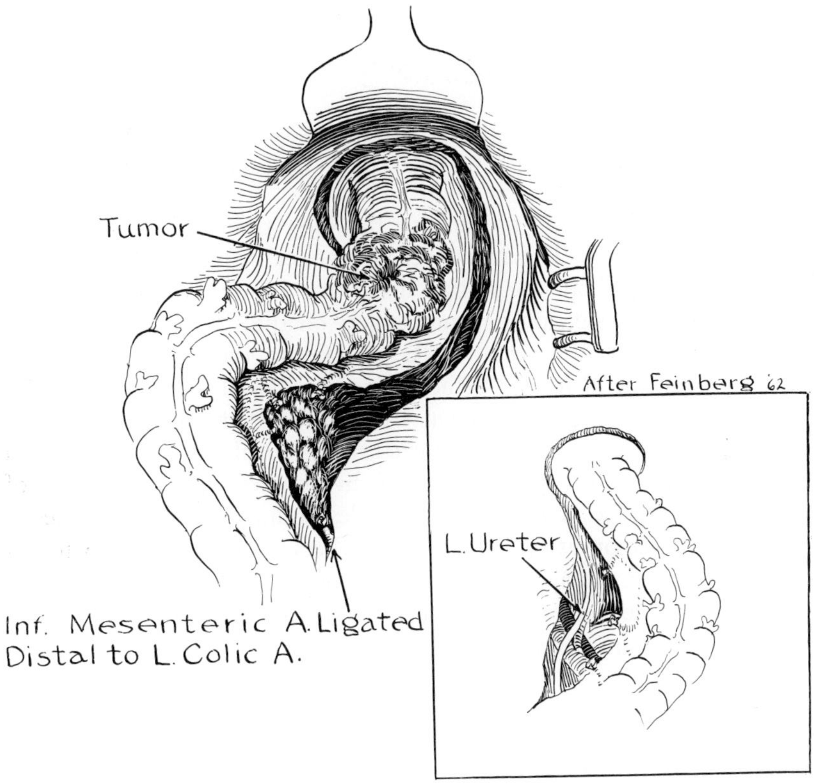

FIGURE 1. Anterolateral incision in the peritoneum. Mobilization of the peritoneum early in the operation preserves this layer to form the new pelvic diaphragm. Both ureters should be identified.

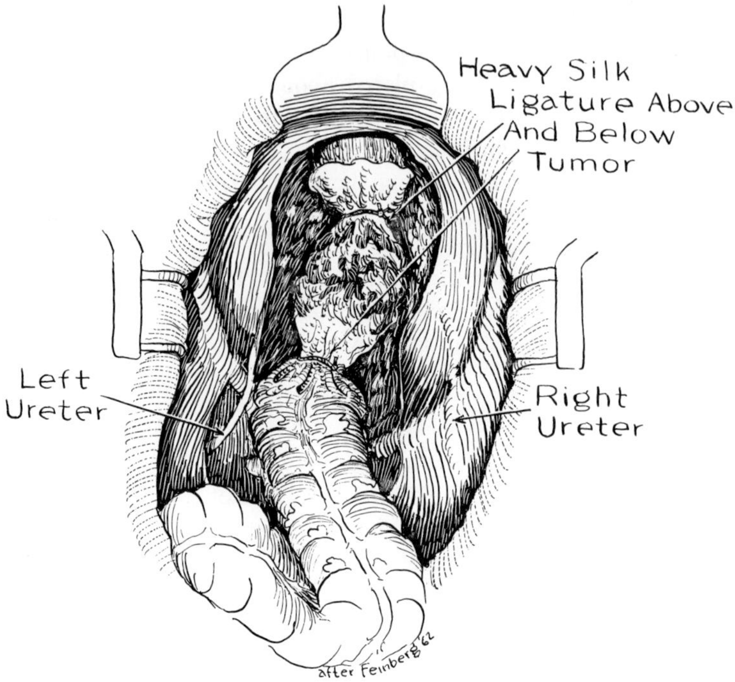

FIGURE 2. Heavy ligatures are tied about the bowel proximal and distal to the tumor. This maneuver minimizes intraluminal spread of dislodged cancer cells.

in such a way as to direct the pressure of the dissection away from the tumor-bearing area of the bowel. The maneuver is practically bloodless. The silk ligature is now tied snugly about the rectum distal to the tumor (Fig. 2).

The depth of the dissection depends largely on the site of the tumor. Rarely is it necessary to divide the rectal stalks containing the middle hemorrhoidal vessels. There should be *at least* 2 inches of normal bowel distal to the tumor at the eventual site of transection. Experience has shown that this desideratum must be met if local recurrence is to be minimized. Division of the upper mesosigmoid or lower left mesocolon follows. The site of division will depend on the site of the tumor and the degree of mobility of the descending colon. It may be necessary to mobilize the colon as far proximally as the splenic flexure in order to obtain adequate mobility. There must be no tension whatsoever at the subsequent suture line. The transection of the mesocolon should be at right angles to the direction of the bowel, and each vessel should be accurately ligated.

The Resection

We are now ready for the dirty field. The entire field is covered with moist towels and the retrorectal space is packed off with moist pads. It is beyond the intent of this chapter to detail the technique of clean and dirty fields in intestinal surgery. Suffice it to say that strict adherence to this facet of technique makes for a smoother postoperative course and almost complete elimination of infections. (I personally do not employ antibiotics routinely in the postoperative period, and I am convinced that reliance on them can be held largely responsible for the indifferent surgical technique observed in recent years.) At the site of expected transection of the rectum, a guide suture of silk is inserted on each side in the perirectal tissues (Fig. 3). A right-angle kidney clamp is placed across the rectum just proximal to this point and the rectum is gradually divided with a right-angle scissors. During this process, a sucker is inserted into the distal segment to minimize soiling, and the branches of the inferior and superior hemorrhoidal vessels are clamped. The latter are ligated with plain catgut until a dry edge of bowel is produced.

The next step is one that I believe to be especially important in the conduct of this operation. It is the mechanical cleansing of the distal rectal segment with copious amounts of warm solution to remove blood clot, fecal material and, above all, possible detached cancer cells. Cole has used numerous cancerocidal solutions locally, the latest hypochlorite solution, but the evidence so far is not convincing enough for me to abandon prolonged mechanical irrigation with suction. This maneuver can be expedited by spreading open the end of bowel with long Allis clamps strategically placed.

A noncrushing, short-bladed right-angle clamp is now applied to the proximal colon about 1 inch proximal to the site of transection, and the bowel is divided at this site (Fig. 4). This open end of proximal colon is now apposed to the open

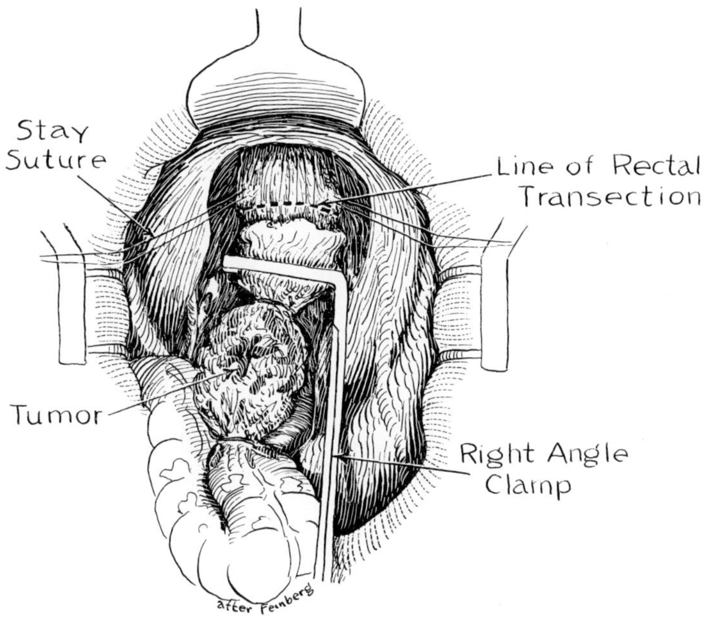

FIGURE 3. Stay sutures at each angle of the lower segment suspend this portion of the bowel for anastomosis. The rectum is cut across with a right-angle scissors. Bleeding vessels in the perirectal fat are carefully ligated.

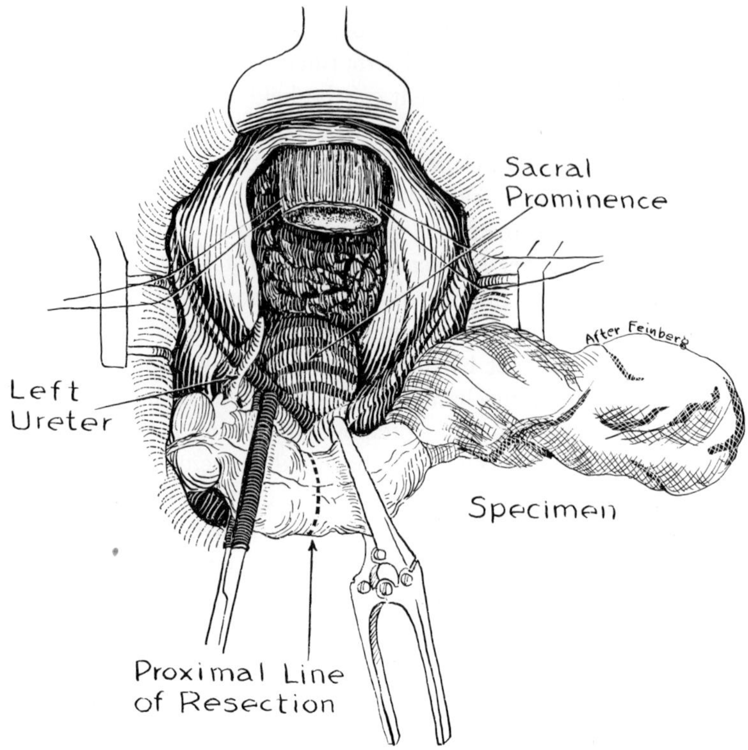

FIGURE 4. Proximal line of transection in the proximal sigmoid. The presacral area should be packed off with gauze pads to prevent soiling.

end of rectum so as to have the antimesenteric side lie anteriorly, and a two-layer anastomosis is begun (Fig. 5).

The Anastomosis

The first posterior layer consists of interrupted Cushing sutures of 3–0 silk approximating the perirectal fat and the posterior mesenteric side of the proximal colon. By placing two angle sutures of 00 chromic between the two loops, the apparent disparity in diameter between the two segments will be largely overcome. The mucosa-submucosa sutures of fine chromic catgut are interrupted Connell inverting stitches. The final anterior layer is composed of interrupted Cushing sutures of silk. In most instances, enough peritoneum is left on the distal segment to effect a peritoneum-to-peritoneum closure anteriorly.

I have been asked frequently how many sutures are necessary to attain an effective anastomosis at this site. In must be remembered that healing, especially posteriorly and laterally, is by granulation and secondary intention. The insertion of too many stitches not only compromises local blood supply but also adds an unnecessary amount of foreign material. Only as many sutures should be used as are needed to hold the tissues in position while healing takes place. I am convinced

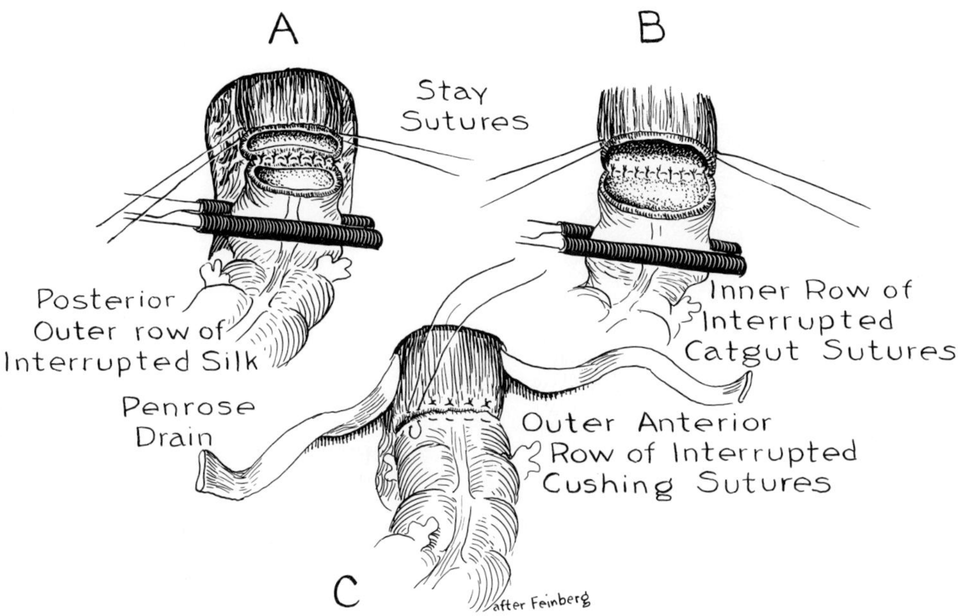

FIGURE 5. Details of the two-layer anastomosis. Interrupted sutures should be used and it is desirable to avoid too many.

that too many stitches, tied too snugly, impede the local processes of repair and increase the incidence of leakage. Twelve to fourteen outer layer stitches for the entire circumference should suffice. The mucosal stitches are placed about one-eighth inch apart.

The dirty field is now discarded and clean instruments and gloves are provided for the completion of the operation.

The Closure

Peritonealization of the operative area is now in order (Fig. 6). This begins at the stump of the inferior mesenteric vessels, which should be completely covered. The two peritoneal flaps are approximated so as to bury the anastomatic suture line beneath them and to eliminate all pockets. A Penrose cigarette drain is placed on each side of the rectum to the bottom of the pelvis. These are brought out through an opening at the lower end of the newly constructed peritoneal diaphragm through the lower angle of the abdominal incision. The abdomen is closed with buried figure-of-eight steel sutures and silk.

Complementary Cecostomy

I always add a complementary tube cecostomy through a small right McBurney incision (Fig. 7). It is used as a gas vent mainly, and adds vastly to the comfort of the patient postoperatively. It is probable that it affords some protection to the

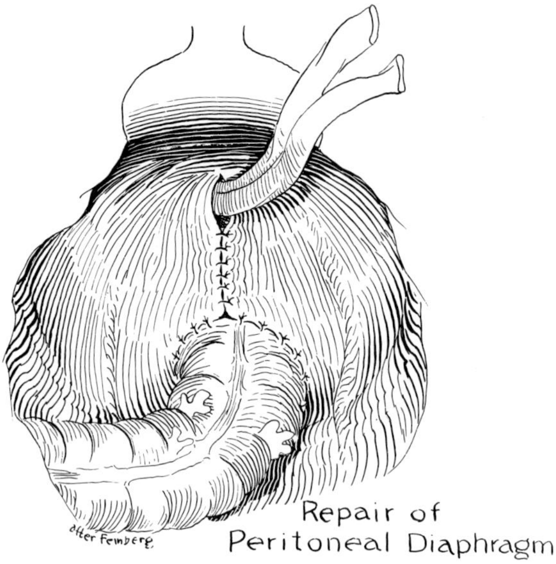

FIGURE 6. Reconstruction of the peritoneal diaphragm above the suture line. The Penrose drains extend to the bottom of the pelvis behind the rectum.

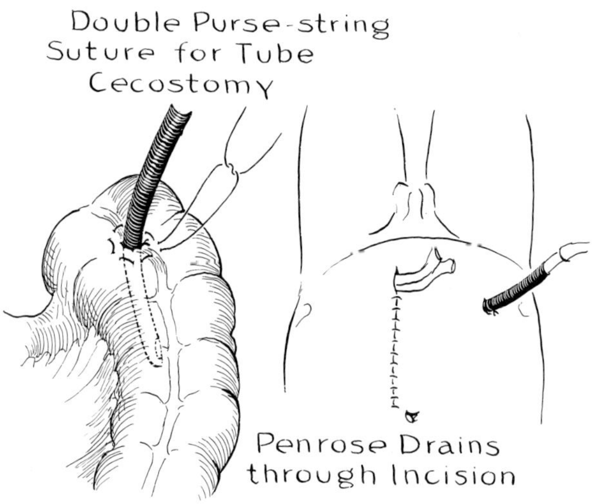

FIGURE 7. Complementary tube cecostomy through a small McBurney incision.

suture line, although it is not used primarily for that reason. The tube is removed after the first normal bowel movement. At no time has it been necessary to close a persistent cecal fistula.

References

GARLOCK, J. H., and GINZBURG, L. An appraisal of the operation of anterior resection for carcinoma of the rectum and rectosigmoid. *Surg., Gynec. and Obst.* 90:525, April 1950.

GARLOCK, J. H., and SELEY, G. The use of sulfanilamide in surgery of the colon and rectum. *Surgery* 5:787, June 1939.

DIXON, C. F. Anterior resection for carcinoma low in the sigmoid and the recto-sigmoid. *Surgery* 15:367, March 1944.

GOLIGHER, J. C., DUKES, C. E., and BUSSEY, H. J. R. Local recurrences after sphincter-saving excisions for carcinoma of rectum and rectosigmoid, *Brit. J. Surg.* 39:199, November 1951.

WHEELOCK, F. C., JR., TOLL, G., and MCKITTRICK, L. S. An evaluation of anterior resection of the rectum and low sigmoid. *New England J. Med.* 260:526, March 12, 1959.

92. *Synchronous Combined Abdominoperineal Excision of the Rectum*

JOHN C. GOLIGHER

THOUGH SPHINCTER–SAVING METHODS of resection have now an accepted place in the radical treatment of rectal cancer, probably the majority of patients suffering from this condition still require abdominoperineal excision. There are several ways of performing this operation. The classic Miles technique is perhaps the one most commonly used, the abdominal dissection being conducted in a fairly steep Trendelenburg tilt, and the patient subsequently turned onto the right or left side for the perineal dissection. Other surgeons prefer the lithotomy position for the perineal phase, and a popular modification of the latter plan in Britain is the use of a simultaneous lithotomy-Trendelenburg position (Lloyd-Davies, 1939), which allows two surgeons to operate synchronously from the abdominal and perineal aspects respectively. This is the technique that will be described in this chapter.

The advantages of the synchronous combined method are that it expedites the conduct of the operation, facilitates the removal of particularly adherent bulky growths, and allows easy closure of the pelvic peritoneum over an empty pelvis. For its successful performance, however, certain conditions are essential: (1) The legs must be supported on easily adjustable leg rests, such as Lloyd-Davies' (Fig. 1), and the sacrum on a well-padded, elevated sacral rest at the end of the table, such as my own (Fig. 1). (2) The external genitalia and urethral catheter must be drawn onto the front of the right thigh and held there by strapping so that they do not prolapse into the perineal operator's field. (3) Special attention must be devoted to the toweling of the patient, the arrangement of instrument tables (one over the patient's head for the abdominal operation, and one at the end of the table below the buttocks for the perineal surgeon), and lighting (Figs. 1 and 2). And (4) two *fully trained* surgeons must be available, nothing being more certain to discredit the method than the detailing of a junior assistant to carry out the perineal phase, for the anterior dissection from this aspect is often the most difficult part of the operation.

In the conduct of a synchronous combined excision the perineal operator naturally does not commence until the abdomen has been opened and the growth

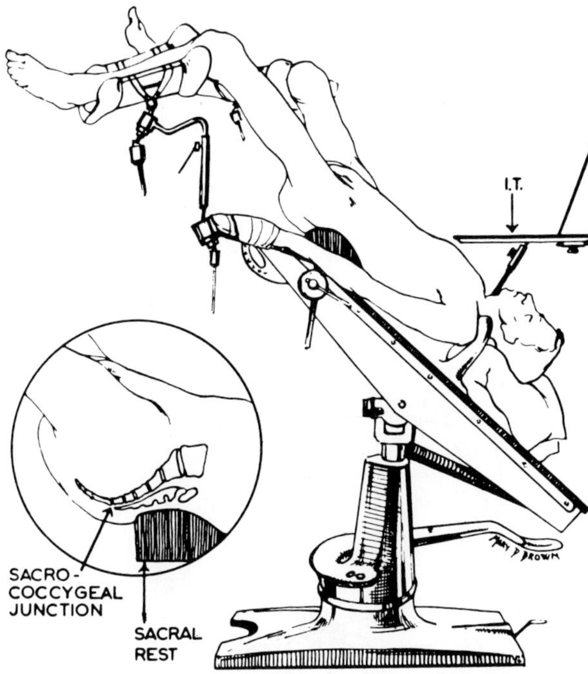

FIGURE 1. Lateral view of the patient in position for synchronous combined excision, with the legs supported on Lloyd-Davies leg rests and the sacrum on a special padded sacral rest (*insert*). Note that there is almost no flexion of the hips to embarrass the abdominal operator, the front of the thighs and the anterior abdominal wall being in almost the same plane. The instrument table (I.T.) for the abdominal surgeon is situated immediately above the patient's head. The head-down tilt shown is considerably steeper than that normally used. (From *Surgery of the Anus, Rectum, and Colon,* by J. C. Goligher, 1961, by kind permission of Cassell & Co., London.)

found to be operable. Thereafter the two phases proceed simultaneously, the relative proportions of the excision shared by the two surgeons varying according to the circumstances of the case. Usually the separation of the rectum from the sacrum and coccyx behind, and from the bladder, vesicles, and prostate in front, is accomplished by the abdominal operator; he also effects the division of the greater part or all of the lateral ligaments. But if the dissection from above is delayed by difficulties due to fixation of the growth, the perineal operator may extend his dissection a greater distance upward. In the account that follows the abdominal and perineal phases will be described separately.

Abdominal Dissection

Access to the abdominal cavity is obtained by a long, left, paramedian rectus-displacing incision extending from the pubis to at least 3 or 4 inches above the umbilicus. Once the decision is made to proceed with excision, a self-retaining retractor is inserted and the loops of small gut are turned out of the abdomen into

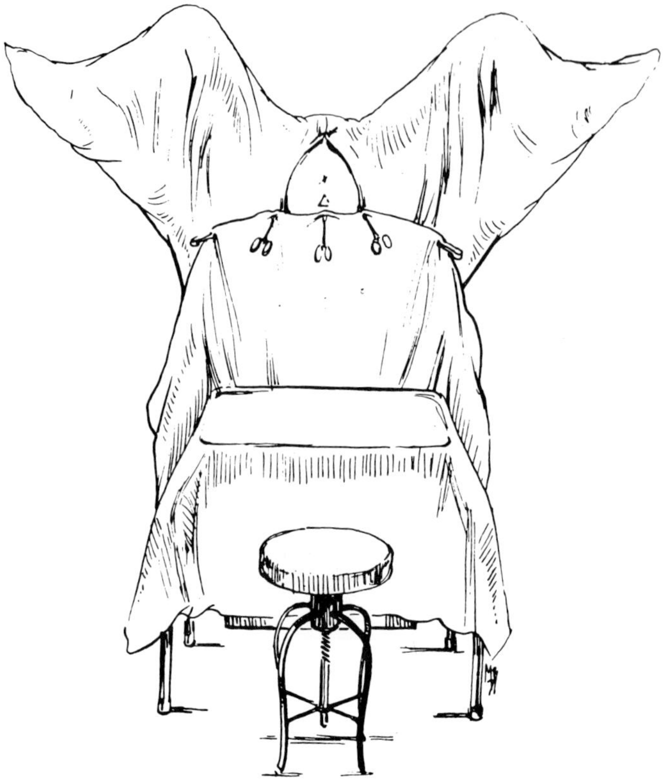

FIGURE 2. Perineal view of the toweled patient ready for synchronous combined excision. Note that the instrument table overlies the perineal operator's knees. Position of the coccyx outlined on the skin. (From *Surgery of the Anus, Rectum, and Colon* by J. C. Goligher, 1961, by kind permission of Cassell & Co., London.)

a plastic bag, in which they are retained throughout the operation. Before the dissection is begun, a tape is tied round the distal sigmoid to avoid upward intraluminal dissemination of exfoliated cancer cells from the primary growth in the rectum during subsequent manipulations. Similarly, to avoid intravenous dissemination into the portal circulation from the same cause, the first step in the actual excision is control of the inferior mesenteric vessels.

Ligation of the Inferior Mesenteric Vessels and Preparation of the Colon Stump for Colostomy

The adhesions of the peritoneum of the left iliac fossa to the outer side of the left mesocolon are separated by scissor dissection (Fig. 3). A cut is then made in the peritoneum on the left side of the base of the mesocolon, exposing the left ureter and spermatic vessels, which can be displaced laterally (Fig. 4). While the sigmoid colon and mesocolon are lifted upward, a plane of separation is developed between

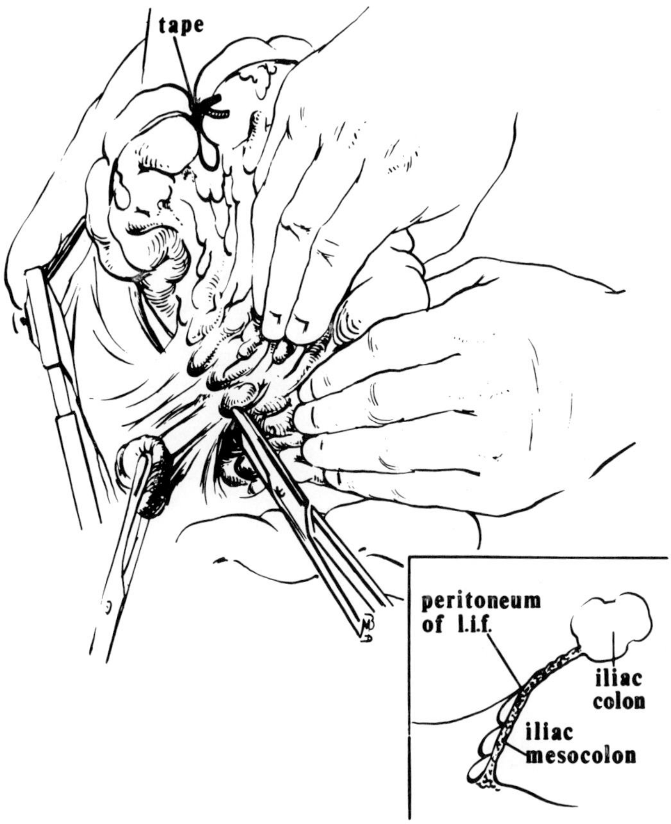

FIGURE 3. Separation of adhesions between the peritoneum of the left iliac fossa and the outer side of the iliac mesocolon by scissor dissection. Note the tape tied round the distal sigmoid to minimize intraluminal upward dissemination of exfoliated cancer cells from the growth. *Insert:* Diagrammatic section showing composition of these developmental adhesions. (The view shown in Figures 3 to 9 is that which the surgeon obtains when he is standing on the left side of the patient and looking into the pelvis.)

the left common iliac artery and the abdominal aorta posteriorly and the base of the mesocolon containing the superior hemorrhoidal and inferior mesenteric vessels anteriorly. The presacral nerve roots may be left on the aorta or carried forward with the inferior mesenteric vessels. The fingers are passed behind the latter to project under the peritoneum of the right leaf of the mesocolon. The latter is incised and the incision carried upward to expose the origin of the inferior mesenteric artery, which is doubly ligated and divided (Fig. 5). The inferior mesenteric vein is then displayed to the left of the artery and similarly tied and severed, care being taken that the left ureter is out of harm's way.

It only remains to divide the mesocolon obliquely from the point of ligation of the main vessels to the site on the sigmoid colon selected for the colostomy (Fig. 5) and to section the bowel between Cope's clamps.

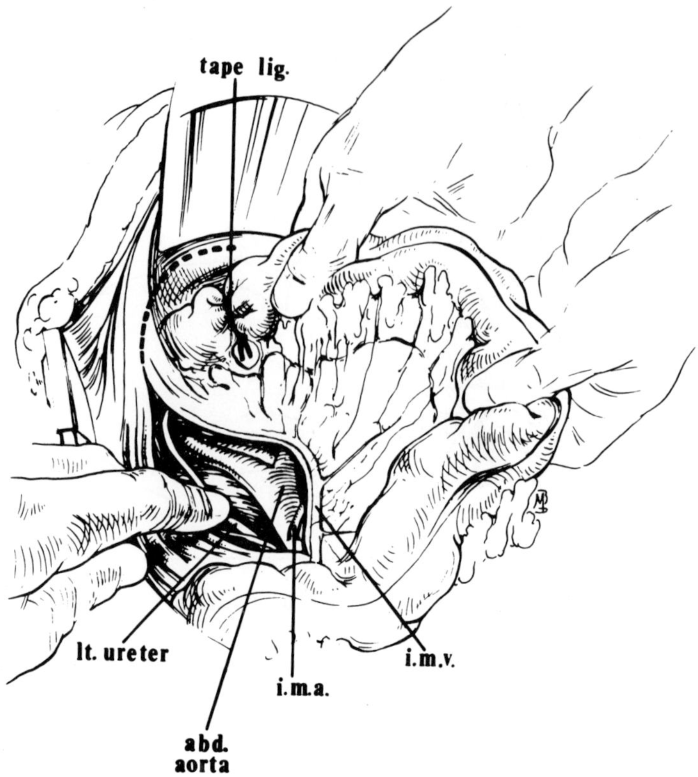

FIGURE 4. Peritoneal cut on the left side of the base of the mesocolon exposing the left ureter and spermatic vessels. Note the inferior mesenteric vessels being lifted away from the front of the aorta and the left common iliac artery by traction on the sigmoid loop.

Mobilization of the Rectum

The peritoneal cuts on either side of the base of the mesocolon are prolonged downward around the brim of the pelvis to meet anteriorly on the back of the bladder. These incisions are opened up to expose the ureters. The rectum is then drawn forward and the mesorectum stripped off the lower end of the abdominal aorta and the common iliac vessels. The presacral connective tissue is then opened up with scissors, and the hand is inserted between the rectum and the sacrum and coccyx, lifting the bowel out of the sacral concavity (Fig. 6).

Attention is now turned to the anterior dissection. The posterior edge of the cut in the peritoneum on the back of the dome of the bladder is seized with two or three long artery forceps, while a deep retractor lifts the anterior edge forward. By a combination of scissor and swab dissection a plane of cleavage is defined between the seminal vesicles and prostate anteriorly and the fascia of Denonvilliers posteriorly (Fig. 7).

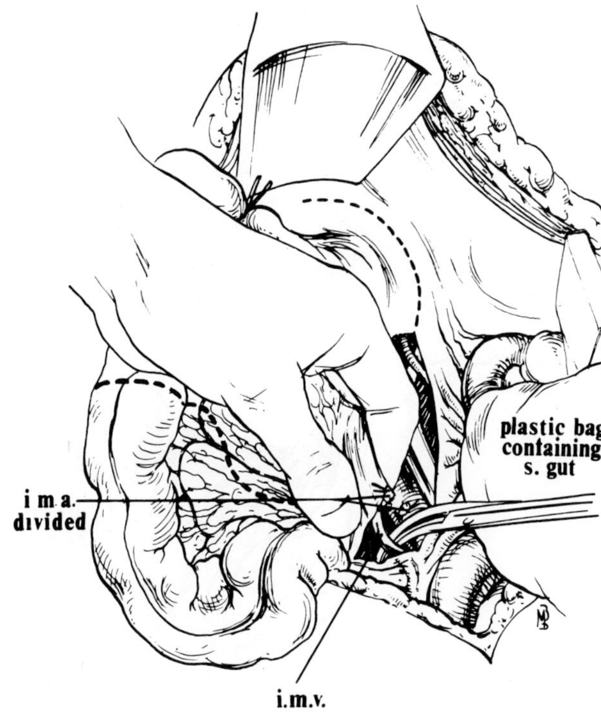

FIGURE 5. High ligation and division of the inferior mesenteric vessels. The artery has already been divided; the more laterally situated vein is being underrun. Note the dashed line on the mesocolon indicating the line of proposed section up to the site chosen for the colostomy, and also the plastic bag on the right containing the loops of small gut.

The rectum has now been freed behind and in front. It only remains for it to be mobilized by dividing the lateral ligament on either side. The ligament is defined first on one side between two fingers and cut with scissors close to the pelvic side wall, care being taken to retract the ureter out of danger in the process (Fig. 8). The same procedure is then carried out on the opposite ligament.

Closure of the Pelvic Peritoneum and Establishment of the Left Iliac Colostomy

By this stage the perineal operator will have completed his dissection so that the mobilized sigmoid and rectum can be withdrawn from below. The gap in the pelvic peritoneum is then easily closed in its anterior two-thirds by a continuous suture of fine chromic catgut (Fig. 9). Through the posterior third the iliac colon stump is drawn extraperitoneally to a separate small muscle-cutting incision in the left iliac region of the abdominal wall, and the pelvic peritoneum is sutured to the iliac mesocolon and colon at their point of exit (Fig. 10). Finally, after the main abdominal wound has been closed by suture in layers and sealed off with dressing

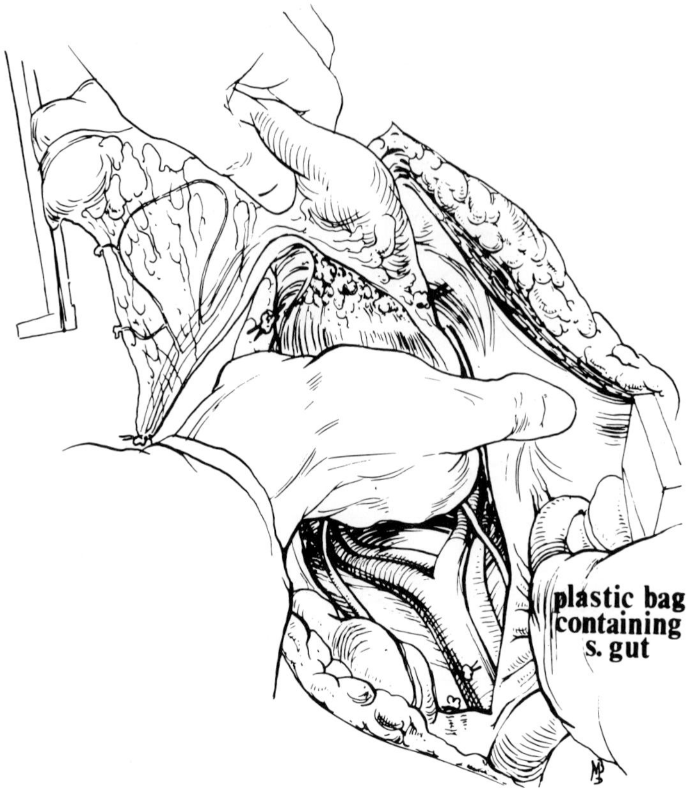

FIGURE 6. Lifting the rectum out of the sacral concavity.

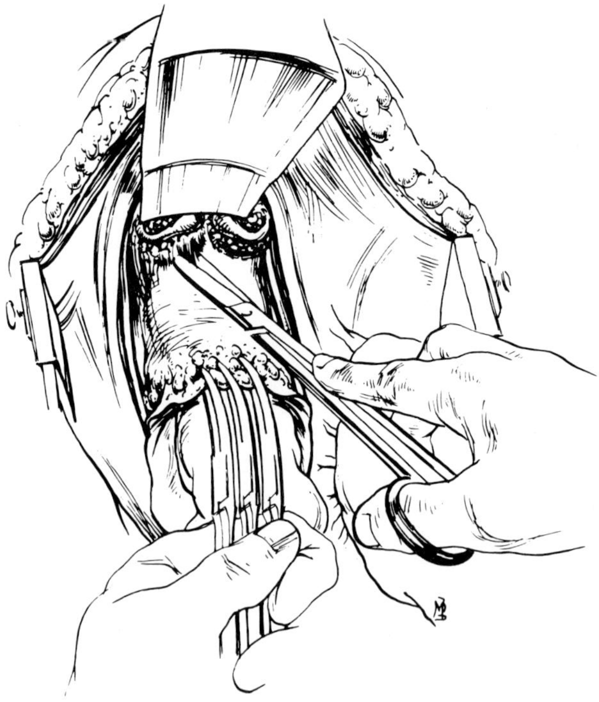

FIGURE 7. Starting the anterior dissection. The vasa deferentia and seminal vesicles are being dissected away from the fascia of Denonvilliers covering the front of the rectum.

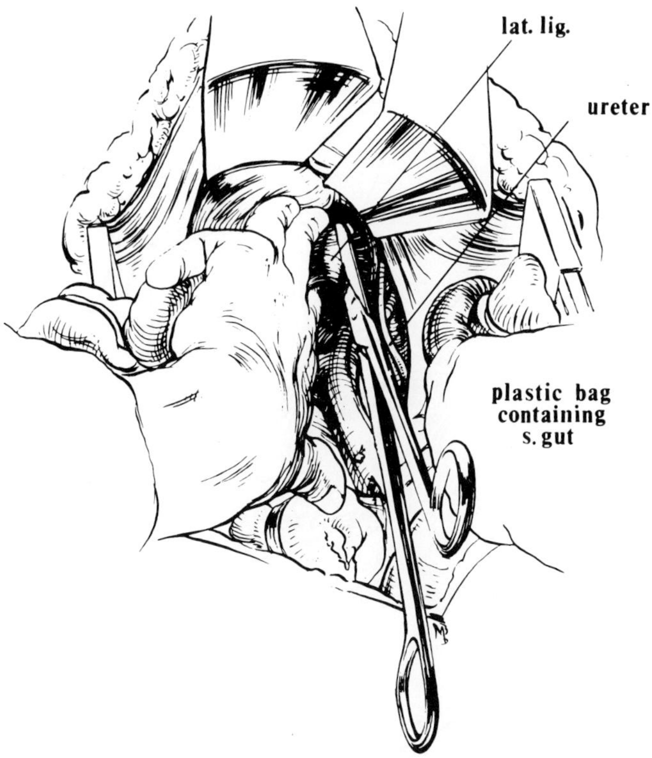

FIGURE 8. Division of the right lateral ligament. The ligament is defined between two fingers while the rectum is displaced to the opposite side, and the division is effected by long, heavy scissors. Note that the ureter is retracted out of harm's way.

and strapping, the clamp is removed from the colon and the end of the bowel is sutured to the skin as shown in Figure 10 (insert).

Perineal Dissection

Skin Incision and Detachment of the Coccyx

Before the operation is commenced, or indeed before the patient is toweled, the anus is closed by a purse-string suture of strong braided silk. An elliptical incision is now made, encompassing the anal region and extending backward in the midline over the coccyx (Fig. 11A). The posterior section of the wound is deepened first of all and the skin edges retracted laterally to expose the terminal coccygeal segments (Fig. 11B). While firm pressure is exerted by the surgeon's left thumb on the tip of the bone to flex it strongly forward and open up the sacrococcygeal and intercoccygeal joints on their posterior aspect, the scalpel is inserted into one of these joints and the bone disarticulated. Alternatively the coccyx may be re-

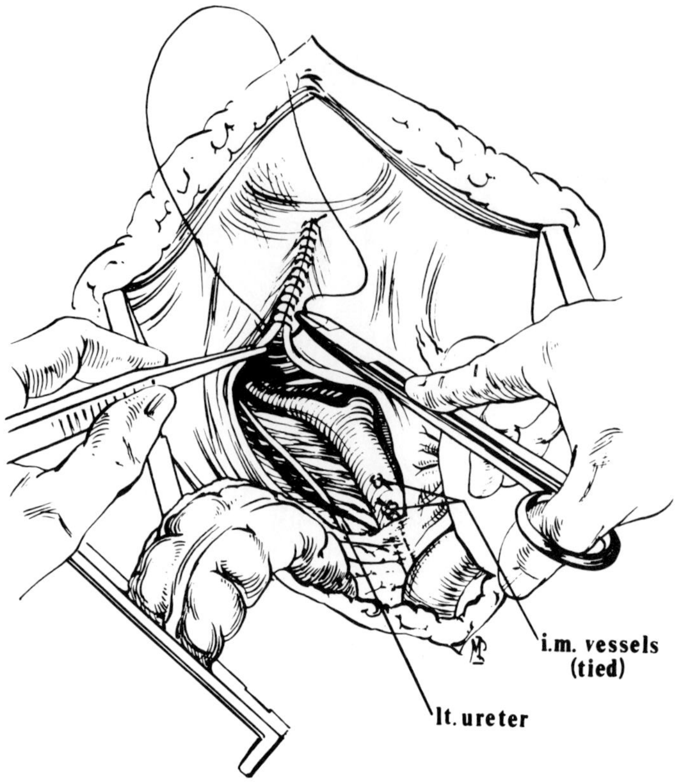

FIGURE 9. Suture of the pelvic peritoneum over the empty pelvis. Note the clamped sigmoid stump available for making the colostomy.

tained intact and the anococcygeal raphe divided instead just beyond the tip of the bone (Fig. 11C). The scalpel is now discarded and *henceforth throughout the perineal dissection all cutting is effected by scissors,* which are more controllable and accurate than a knife in a deep wound.

Division of the Posterior Parts of the Levators and the Fascia of Waldeyer

Through the gap created by detachment of the coccyx or division of the anococcygeal raphe, two fingers of the left hand are inserted forward alongside the rectum deep to the levator ani muscle (Fig. 12A). The subcutaneous and ischiorectal fat are divided down to the muscle, the branches of the inferior hemorrhoidal vessels being caught in the process, and finally the muscle itself is severed for 3 inches or so (Fig. 12B). The levator muscle on the other side is divided in the same manner. A self-retaining retractor is then inserted to separate the lateral edges of the wound. The mobilized end of the rectum is lifted forward, exposing the back of the bowel still covered by the white, tough fascia of Waldeyer. This is divided, exposing the

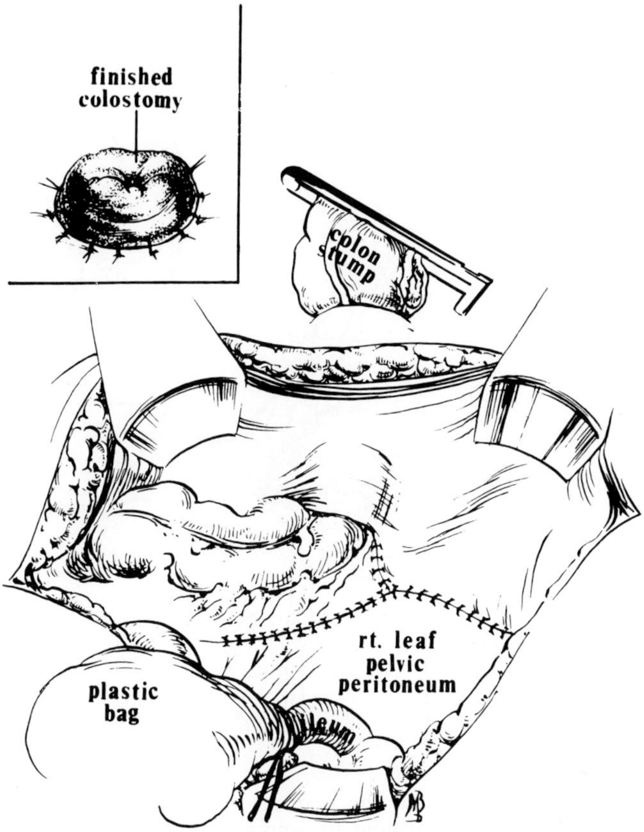

FIGURE 10. View from the right side of the patient showing the colon stump proceeding extraperitoneally to a separate wound in the left iliac region of the anterior abdominal wall. *Insert:* Completed colostomy, the end of the bowel being sutured to the skin.

perirectal fat (Fig. 13). A hand is then inserted into the presacral space to separate the rectum widely from the sacral concavity and to connect with the similar place of separation established by the abdominal operator on this aspect of the bowel (Fig. 14).

Anterior Dissection

The rectum is now drawn downward and backward by the assistant while the surgeon commences the anterior dissection. The portion of the wound in front of the anus is deepened onto the central point of the perineum, displaying the back of the transversus perinei muscles and urogenital diaphragm. The remaining portion of the levator muscle, mostly pubococcygeus and puborectalis, is then defined between fingers on one side and snipped through gradually to within one-third to

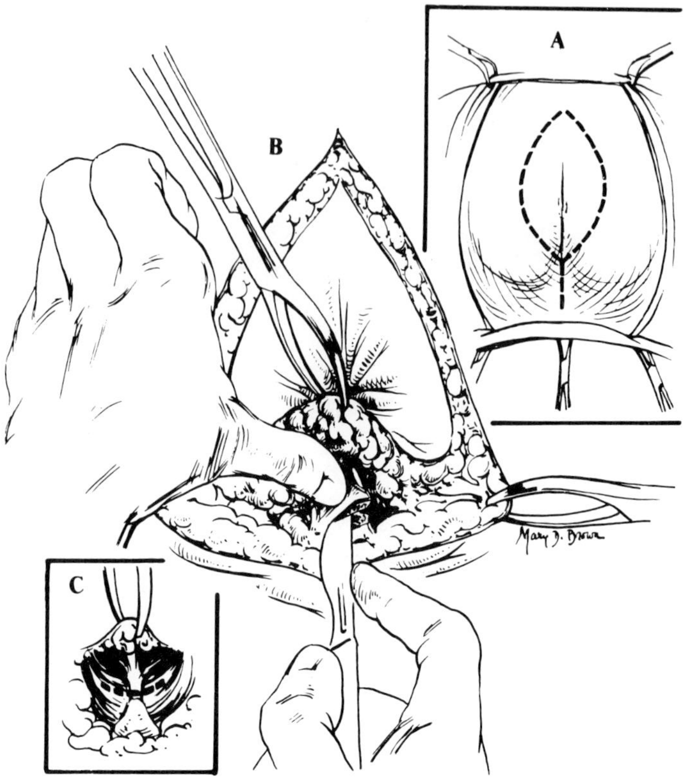

FIGURE 11. Commencement of the perineal dissection. (*A*) Incision. (*B*) Opening up the posterior part of the wound to expose the coccyx, which is being disarticulated. (*C*) Alternative method of incising the anococcygeal raphe just beyond the coccyx.

one-half inch of the midline (Fig. 15A, B). The same performance is repeated on the opposite side till all that remains to tether the anorectal junction at this level in front is a small band of muscular tissue in and immediately adjacent to the midline, consisting of rectourethralis and some medial fibers of the puborectalis. The division of this piece of muscle is perhaps the most dangerous part of the perineal dissection, because the membranous urethra and rectum lie very close together, so that either structure may be damaged if the correct plane is not struck. If the lateral edges of the back of the prostate are palpated by the tips of the fingers passed forward on either side of the rectum, the surgeon can gauge roughly the plane of this surface. His scissors should be in roughly the same plane as he divides the rectourethralis (Fig. 16).

Thereafter the rectum separates easily from the prostate, a fold of connective tissue requiring to be severed on either side as the separation proceeds (Fig. 17). When the seminal vesicles are reached contact is generally made with the abdominal operator's anterior plane of dissection. The lateral ligaments are then

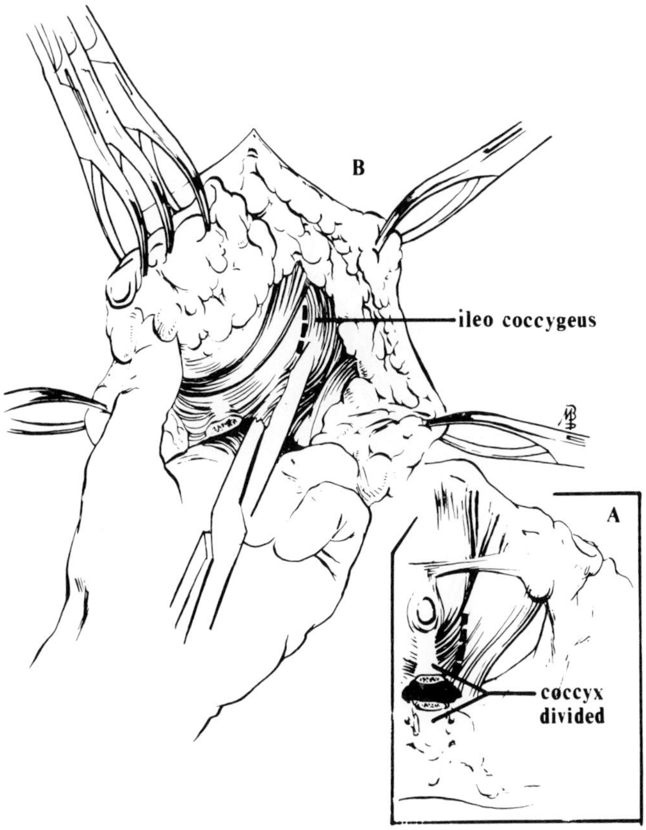

FIGURE 12. Division of the posterior (ileococcygeus) portion of the levator muscle. (*A*) Diagram showing the line of division extending forward from the site of section of the coccyx. (*B*) Fingers have been inserted forward into the pelvis alongside the rectum as a guide and the left muscle is being divided by scissors.

divided either from above or sometimes from below, and this completes the mobilization (Fig. 18). If the sigmoid colon has already been sectioned, the specimen can now be delivered down to the perineal operator.

Hemostasis and Closure of Wound

After careful hemostasis, the perineal wound is closed by a series of vertical mattress sutures of silk tightly round a centrally placed stout drainage tube leading to an underwater seal or suction motor. Alternatively, if there has been much bleeding or contamination the middle third of the perineal wound may be left open and drained by a corrugated rubber drain or packed with a naked gauze pack. It is only rarely that these latter methods are found necessary.

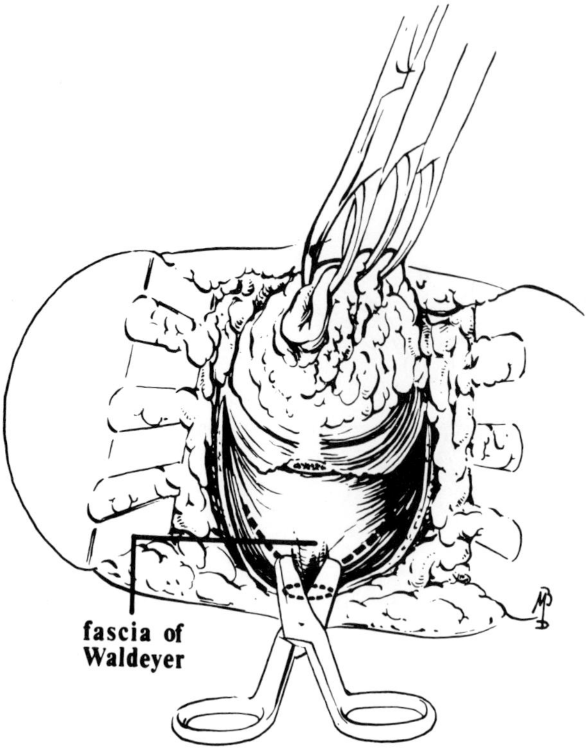

FIGURE 13. Cutting the fascia of Waldeyer exposed on lifting the rectum forward.

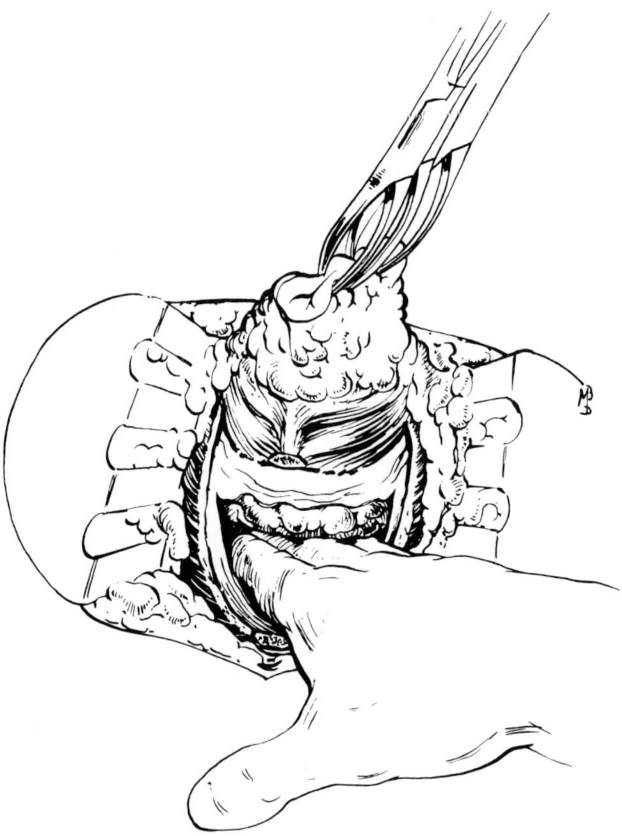

FIGURE 14. Separating the rectum from the sacrum. Note the lobules of perirectal fat bulging through the incision in the fascia of Waldeyer.

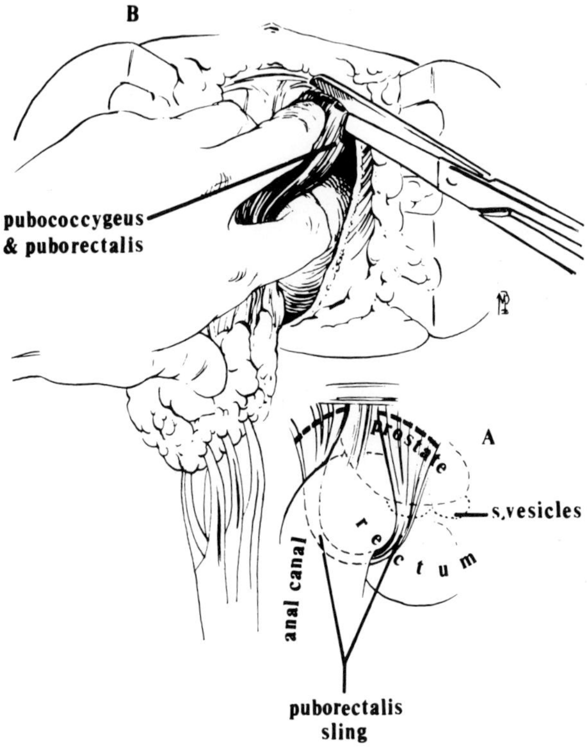

FIGURE 15. Division of the pubococcygeus and the puborectalis. (*A*) Diagram showing the relation of the puborectalis sling to the anorectal junction and prostate. (*B*) The left puborectalis and pubococcygeus have been defined between fingers and are being divided with scissors.

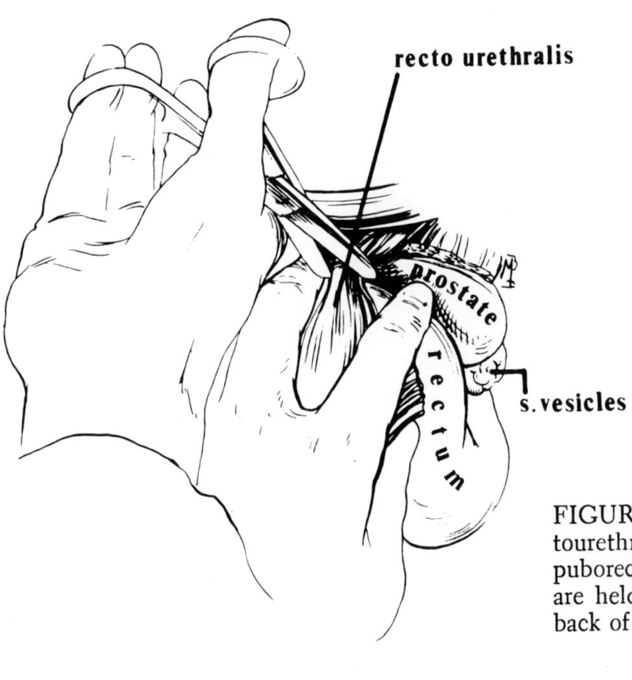

FIGURE 16. Division of the rectourethralis and remnants of the puborectalis. Note that the scissors are held in the same plane as the back of the prostate.

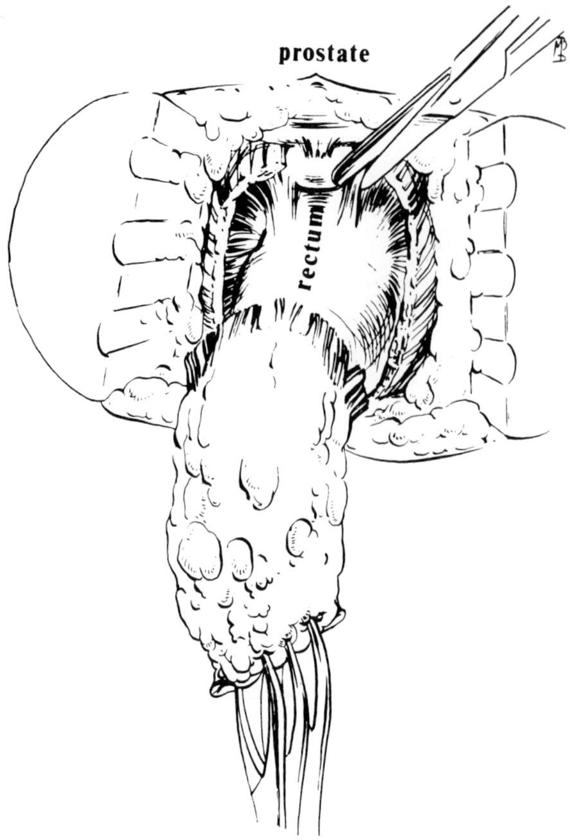

FIGURE 17. Separation of the rectum and the back of the prostate, a strand of connective tissue being divided on either side.

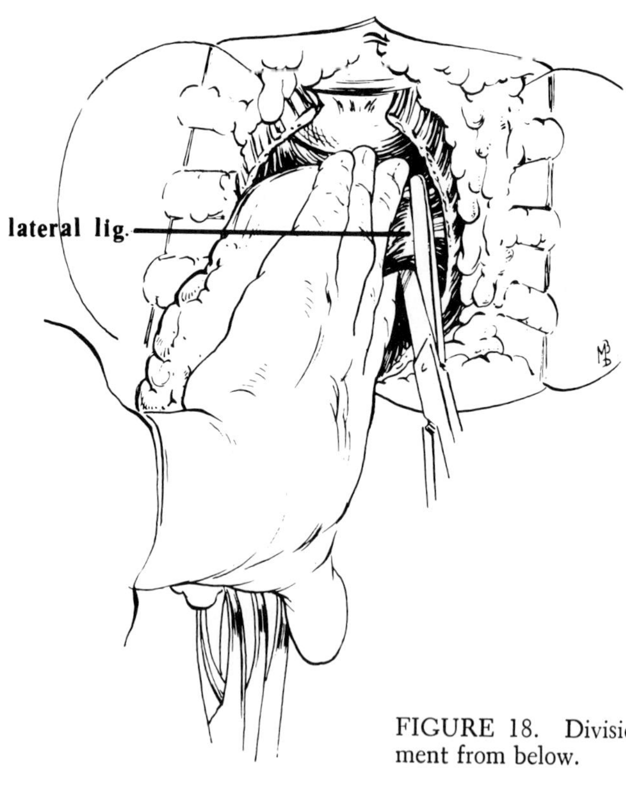

FIGURE 18. Division of the left lateral ligament from below.

Perineal Dissection in the Female

The operation in the female is usually easier than in the male because of the much simpler anterior dissection from below. It is a good plan to remove the posterior vaginal wall as a routine even when the growth is not adherent to it or even situated on the anterior aspect of the bowel (Fig. 19A, B). Subsequently the perineal wound is closed to within 1 inch of the vulva, and the drain is brought out from the pelvic cavity through the introitus to the vagina (Fig. 19C).

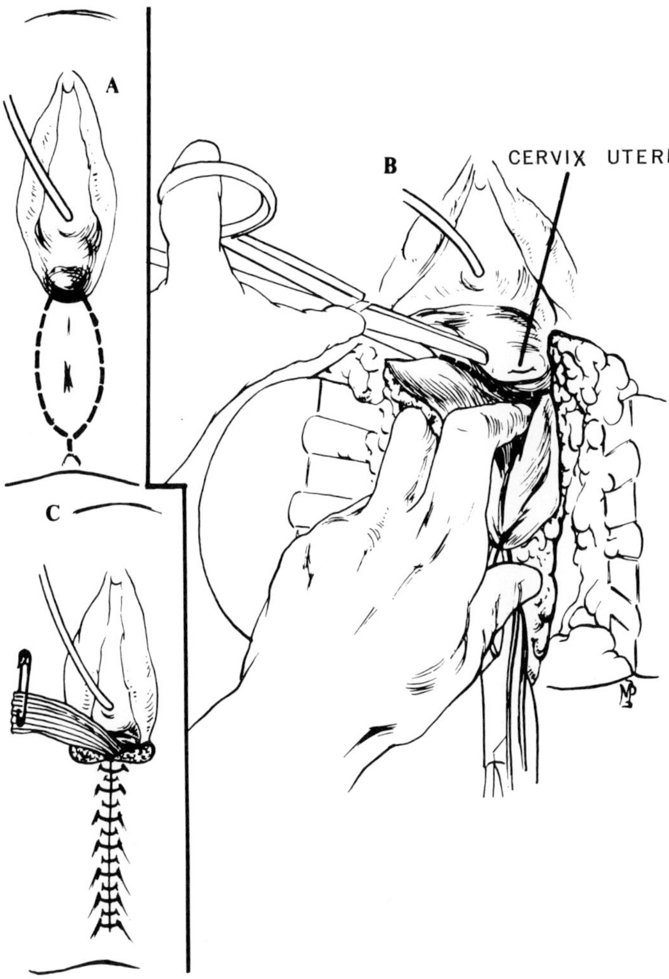

FIGURE 19. Perineal dissection in the female. (A) Outline of the incision usually employed, removing the posterior vaginal wall with the rectum. (B) The posterior vaginal wall has been divided on the left side up to the cervix and the line of proposed section on the right side is shown. (C) State of the wound at completion. The perineum is sutured almost to the vulva, and the pelvic drain is brought through the vaginal orifice.

References

Dukes, C. E. Discussion on major surgery in carcinoma of the rectum with or without colostomy, excluding the anal canal and including the rectosigmoid. *Proc. Roy. Soc. Med.* 50:1031, December 1957.

Goligher, J. C. Sacral rest for use in synchronous combined excision of rectum. *Lancet* 2:468, September 10, 1949.

Goligher, J. C. *Surgery of the Anus, Rectum and Colon.* London: Cassell and Company Ltd., 1961. P. 512.

Lloyd-Davies, O. V. Lithotomy-Trendelenburg position for resection of rectum and lower pelvic colon. *Lancet* 2:74, July 8, 1939.

Lloyd-Davies, O. V. Discussion on major surgery in carcinoma of rectum with or without colostomy, excluding the anal canal and including the rectosigmoid. *Proc. Roy. Soc. Med.* 50:1047, December 1957.

93. *Pull-Through Resection of the Rectum, with Delayed Anastomosis, for Cancer or Hirschsprung's Disease*

RUPERT B. TURNBULL, JR.

THE COMPLICATIONS following conventional pull-through procedures for cancer of the mid-rectum or Hirschsprung's disease are not to be minimized. Ischemic necrosis and retraction of the pulled-through segment, and abscess formation in the presacral space, are the most difficult complications to treat. Waugh and Turner in 1959 reported that 13.4 per cent of their patients had some degree of slough and retraction of the pulled-through colon, while in 20.9 per cent infection developed in the presacral space.

We believe that ischemic necrosis, retraction, and presacral infection are due to (1) the too frequent reliance on the sigmoid colon as the pulled-through segment, (2) insufficient external fixation of the exteriorized colonic segment, and (3) contamination of the presacral space by the immediate replacement of the colorectal anastomosis, as is done in Swenson's operation. The technique reported here insures the removal of the sigmoid colon (which occasionally is of doubtful viability after vascular mobilization), adequate and absolute fixation of the exteriorized colonic segment at the perineum, and a safe, delayed, perineal colorectal anastomosis after the incubation period of pelvic abscess is past, or the infection, if present, has been controlled. The delayed-anastomosis procedure was evolved by Turnbull and Cuthbertson in 1952 for adults having a Swenson pull-through resection for small cancers located in the mid-rectum. Since 1953, we have utilized the same technique in children undergoing resections for Hirschsprung's disease.

Technique

Abdominal Phase

The sigmoid colon is mobilized and its mesentery is stripped medially from the left ureter, iliac vessels, and aorta up to the third portion of the duodenum, where the

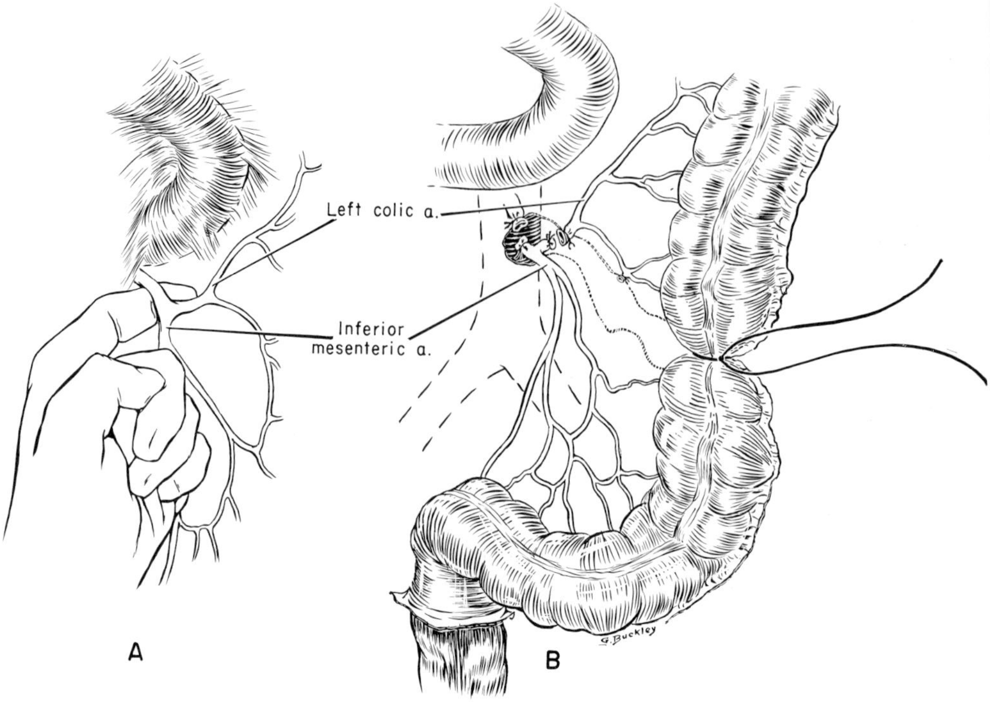

FIGURE 1. Arterial pattern of the left colon. (*A*) Inferior mesenteric artery and left colic artery isolated. (*B*) Division of the inferior mesenteric artery, the left colic artery, and the inferior mesenteric vein. Ligation of the descending colon with silk ligature. (Reproduced by permission of Hoeber Medical Division, Harper & Row, Publishers, Inc., from Allen and Barrows, *Abdominal Surgery.*)

inferior mesenteric artery, the left colic artery, and the inferior mesenteric vein are ligated and divided (Fig. 1A, B). The rectum is freed from its pelvic attachments as in the Miles operation, except that the distal dissection is carried down to the prostate and the levatores ani. In females, the vagina is freed from the anterior peritoneal reflection of the rectum to the level of the internal sphincter. Two stout braided-silk sutures are tied tightly around the rectum 2 inches below the neoplasm; another is placed just above it. First the lumen of the bowel is thoroughly washed with a cancerocidal solution. At this juncture, the pull-through operation requires that the entire left colon and splenic flexure mesentery be mobilized and be detached medially from the left kidney and the lower border of the pancreas above the ligament of Treitz. The inferior mesenteric vein is again divided, this time at the ligament of Treitz. The mid-sigmoid colon will now stretch to the mid-thigh. The junction of the sigmoid and descending colon is selected as the probable site for perineal resection of the left colon, and small arteries of the appendices epiploicae are cut in order to determine arterial flow. If arterial bleeding is not seen, larger mesenteric vessels are divided near the colon until a pulsing arterial flow is obvious. (*Note:* Distally, the blood from cut sigmoid arteries flows but does not pulsate.) A heavy black braided-silk suture with long ends is then tied around the colon as a marker (Fig. 1B). The bowel is not divided. Thus the presacral space is protected from unnecessary contamination during the perineal phase.

Perineal Phase

With the patient in an exaggerated lithotomy position (Fig. 2A), the anus is dilated; the lower rectal ampulla (below the silk suture) is cleansed thoroughly and repeatedly with tincture of benzalkonium chloride and soapy water. If the anus is rigid and unyielding, the lower band of the internal sphincter is divided through a short radial incision in the perianal skin of one of the posterior quadrants. The rectal mucosa above the dentate line is grasped with hemostats and is everted, and the rectum is completely severed by a circumferential incision through the mucosa about 1 cm. above the dentate line (Fig. 2B). The colorectal segment is gently pulled through the everted rectal stump until the long black-silk marker at the junction of the sigmoid and descending colon is in sight (Fig. 2C). The left colon now lies directly over the aorta, the rectum and sigmoid portions having

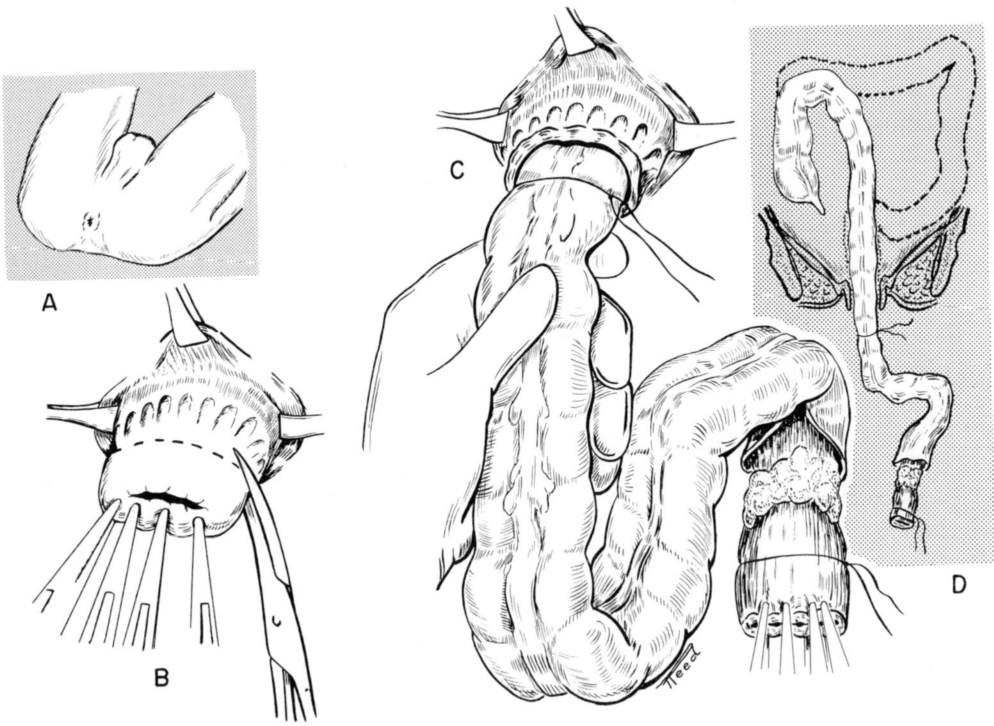

FIGURE 2. Details of the perineal phase of pull-through resection of the rectum. (A) Exaggerated lithotomy position. (*B*) Division of the everted rectum. (C) Pull-through of the colorectal segment. (*D*) Anatomical disposition of the left colon after the pull-through procedure.

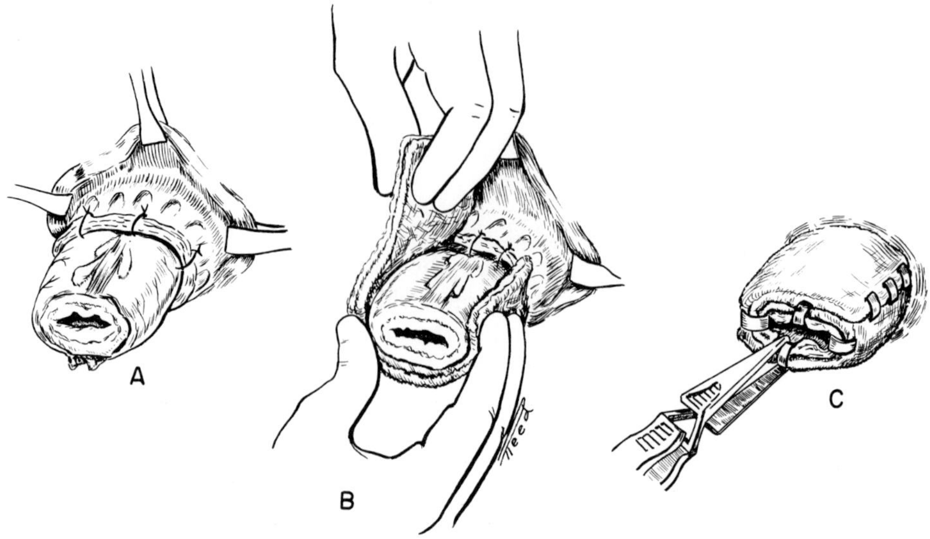

FIGURE 3. Completion of the perineal phase. (*A*) The completed resection: everted rectum sutured to pulled-through colon. (*B and C*) Application and fixation of the gauze stent.

been withdrawn (Fig. 2D). The mesentery lies posteriorly at the anus. The protruding colon is severed about 2 inches out from the anus; bleeding mesenteric vessels are ligated; and the short, everted rectal segment is sutured to the seromuscular layers of the protruding colon (Fig. 3A). The protruding colonic segment is wrapped in folded gauze, and is held in firm position by skin clips to prevent retraction (Fig. 3B, C). The end of the colon is clipped to the gauze wrapping.

Completion of the Abdominal Phase

The left colon mesentery is sutured to the preaortic tissues. The accumulated blood in the pelvis is removed by suction. The pelvic peritoneum is not reconstructed; it is left open to allow free drainage of blood and serum into the abdominal cavity. The abdomen is closed with interrupted, vertical, steel wire sutures.

Management of the Temporary Perineal Colostomy

During the first ten postoperative days, the colon is lavaged daily by enema through the perineal colostomy. Ointments are used on the skin to prevent irritation. By the twelfth day, there is firm union between the colon and the everted rectal stump, and posterior resection with anastomosis can be performed. If an abscess has developed in the presacral space, it can be drained through a paracoccygeal inci-

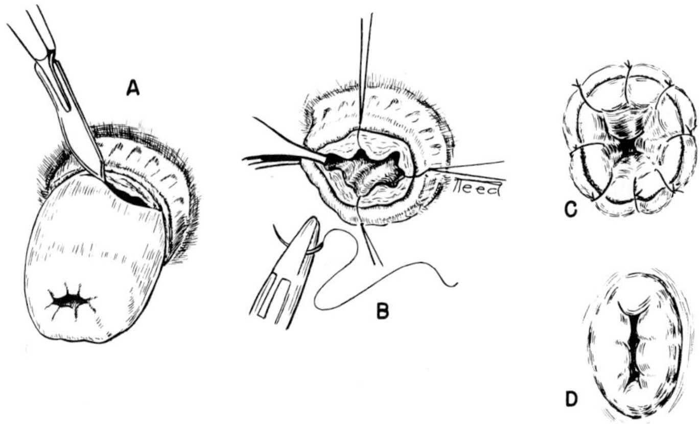

FIGURE 4. Perineal colorectal anastomosis (twelfth day). (*A*) Protruding colon being severed flush with the everted rectal stump. (*B*) Anastomosis with through-and-through sutures in quadrants. (*C*) The completed anastomosis. (*D*) The retracted anastomosis.

sion, and the space can be lavaged with a catheter until the abscess has healed. The perineal anastomosis may be delayed as long as is necessary.

Perineal Anastomosis

Figure 4 shows the details of the perineal colorectal anastomosis. With the patient in the left lateral position under caudal or general anesthesia the gauze collar is removed. Figure 4A shows the edematous colonic segment being cut off flush with the protecting everted rectal stump. An end-to-end anastomosis is made with 4–0 interrupted chromic catgut sutures through all layers. In adults, 1 cm. (or less) of mucosa-covered rectum above the dentate line must be preserved, since a segment longer than 1 cm. will not retract spontaneously after the anastomosis has been made. Figure 4B shows the placing of catgut sutures (by quadrants), Figure 4C the finished anastomosis, and Figure 4D the final spontaneous retraction that occurs within 24 hours. Figure 5 shows the retracted anastomosis in position.

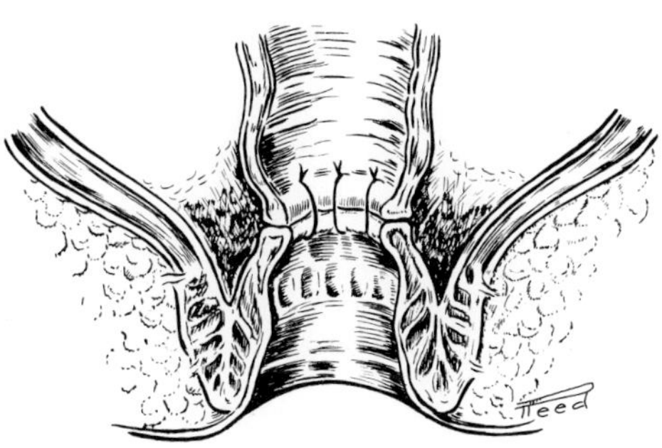

FIGURE 5. The finished (retracted) colorectal anastomosis.

Bowel Management

Although true continence is possible in young patients, the majority have many small movements. A one-quart daily enema will stop further movements until the anastomotic region becomes soft and sensitive.

References

MILES, W. E. Method of performing abdominoperineal excision for carcinoma of rectum and terminal portion of pelvic colon. *Lancet* 2:1812, December 19, 1908.

SWENSON, O., and BILL, A. H., JR. Resection of rectum and rectosigmoid with preservation of sphincter for benign spastic lesions producing megacolon; experimental study. *Surgery* 24:212, August 1948.

TURNBULL, R. B., JR., and CUTHBERTSON, A. Abdominorectal pull-through resection for cancer and for Hirschsprung's disease; delayed posterior colorectal anastomosis. *Cleveland Clin. Quart.* 28:109, April 1961.

WAUGH, J. M., and TURNER, J. C. Abdominoperineal resection with preservation of the anal sphincter, for carcinoma of the midrectum. In Turrell, R. (Ed.), *Diseases of the Colon and Anorectum*. Vol. 1. Philadelphia: W. B. Saunders, 1959. P. 515.

94. *Aganglionic Megacolon*

JOHN H. FISHER

THE LACK of myenteric ganglion cells in certain cases of megacolon was recognized at least sixty years ago, but it was not until fifteen years ago that Swenson suggested a rational operative method to correct the megacolon. His technique for removal of the aganglionic segment and restoration of intestinal continuity with a pull-through anastomosis has been widely accepted. Initial interest was centered in the management of older children having the complete syndrome of obstipation, a voluminous colon, and poor nutrition. With accumulation of experience, the challenge of diagnosis and management of the infant under 1 year of age was investigated, particularly after the high mortality in unrecognized cases was pointed out.

Rectal Biopsy

A reliable test is needed for the infant with Hirschsprung's disease since the barium enema may not be diagnostic. At birth the caliber of the colon is normal. The megacolon develops over a period of weeks or months in response to the partial mechanical obstruction caused by the aganglionosis in the distal colon. The rectal biopsy is a dependable method for choosing from the group of infants with gastrointestinal complaints those children with Hirschsprung's disease. The defect in the parasympathetic ganglion cells extends from the internal anal sphincter proximally and usually involves the rectum and sigmoid colon. Examination of a full-thickness specimen of the rectal wall establishes or rules out the diagnosis. Every histological section from normal colon contains ganglion cells in Auerbach's plexus in the "sandwich" layer between the longitudinal and circular muscle coats. The biopsy specimen diagnostic of Hirschsprung's disease has no ganglion cells in any of the sections, neither in the myenteric plexus nor in the submucosal plexus. Although a specimen of the submucosal plexus is more easily obtained, since general anesthesia is not necessary, it is less satisfactory for study than a full-thickness specimen, because the normal tissue has only a sparse scattering of ganglion cell in this area. Therefore, many sections must be studied to be sure that no ganglion cells are present. For the same reason a specimen from the anal sphincter is unsatisfactory.

Technique

To obtain adequate exposure of the rectal wall and relaxation of the anal sphincter, general anesthesia is used. The infant is hung by the legs with the buttocks resting on the table (Fig. 1A). The older child is placed in lithotomy position. The anal sphincter is gently dilated and the rectum cleaned of gross feces. The perineum is prepared and draped. A sponge is put into the rectal lumen above the biopsy site to prevent fecal material from running into the field. The biopsy site is chosen on the posterior rectal wall 1 cm. above the mucocutaneous margin in the infant and 2 to 3 cm. above this line in the older child. On the anterior wall a biopsy may create a rectovaginal fistula in the female or damage to the urethra in the male. Three traction sutures are placed in the rectal wall about the biopsy site, one on each side and the third where the upper end of the incision will end (Fig. 1B). With a scalpel and a small scissors, an ellipse of tissue measuring 5 to 10 mm. and including both layers of the muscle coats is excised (Fig. 1C, D, E). The defect in the rectal wall is closed in two layers with interrupted sutures, fine silk to the muscle layer and fine chromic catgut to the mucosa (Fig. 1F). No special postoperative precautions are necessary.

The tissue is fixed and stained in the routine manner, and the permanent sections are studied subsequently. Since the diagnosis of Hirschsprung's disease is made on the basis of the absence of ganglion cells, rapid or frozen sections are not adequate. However, the frozen section technique is essential at a later stage when one is choosing the site for colostomy or resection. After the diagnosis of Hirschsprung's disease has been made by biopsy, a colostomy may be done promptly, but it is better to defer resection until the biopsy site has healed.

Colostomy

The proper treatment for the infant weighing less than 10 kilograms (22 pounds) is elective colostomy. It has been found that resection of the aganglionic segment in the very young has a mortality in the range of 25 to 30 per cent.

The acutely obstructed infant should be decompressed by rectocolonic irrigations using copious amounts of saline, a soft rectal tube, and a rubber bulb syringe. Excessive mortality may be expected if the colostomy is done while the infant is acutely obstructed and particularly during an episode of enterocolitis. By deferring definitive resection until the child weighs over 11 kilograms (25 pounds), a mortality of less than 5 per cent may be expected.

A loop colostomy is performed over a glass rod. The incision in the abdominal wall is placed in the quadrant where the aganglionic segment is thought to end (Fig. 2A). Very often the extent of the lesion may be suspected from careful study of the barium enema films even though they may not be diagnostic. A gross

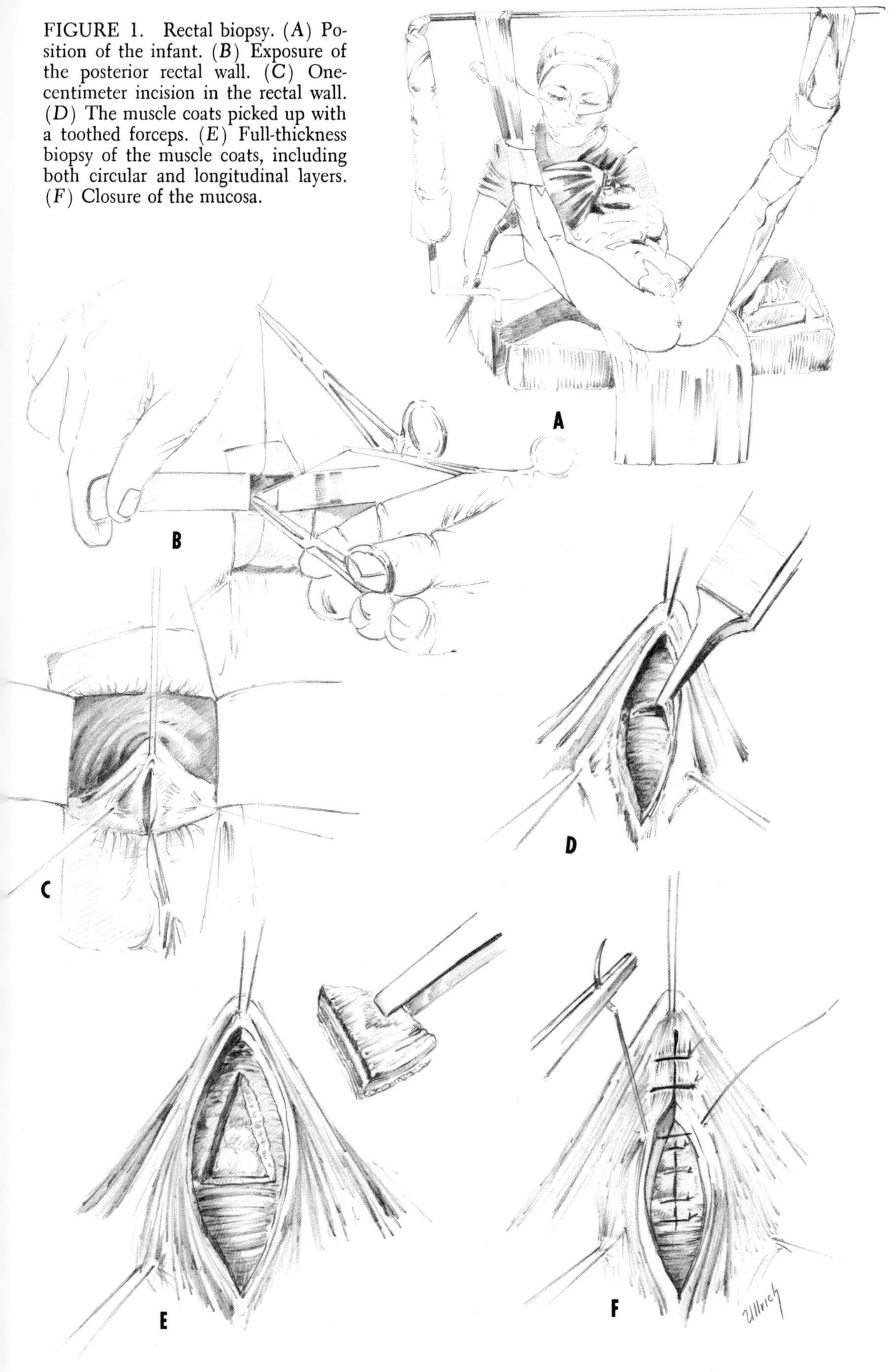

FIGURE 1. Rectal biopsy. (*A*) Position of the infant. (*B*) Exposure of the posterior rectal wall. (*C*) One-centimeter incision in the rectal wall. (*D*) The muscle coats picked up with a toothed forceps. (*E*) Full-thickness biopsy of the muscle coats, including both circular and longitudinal layers. (*F*) Closure of the mucosa.

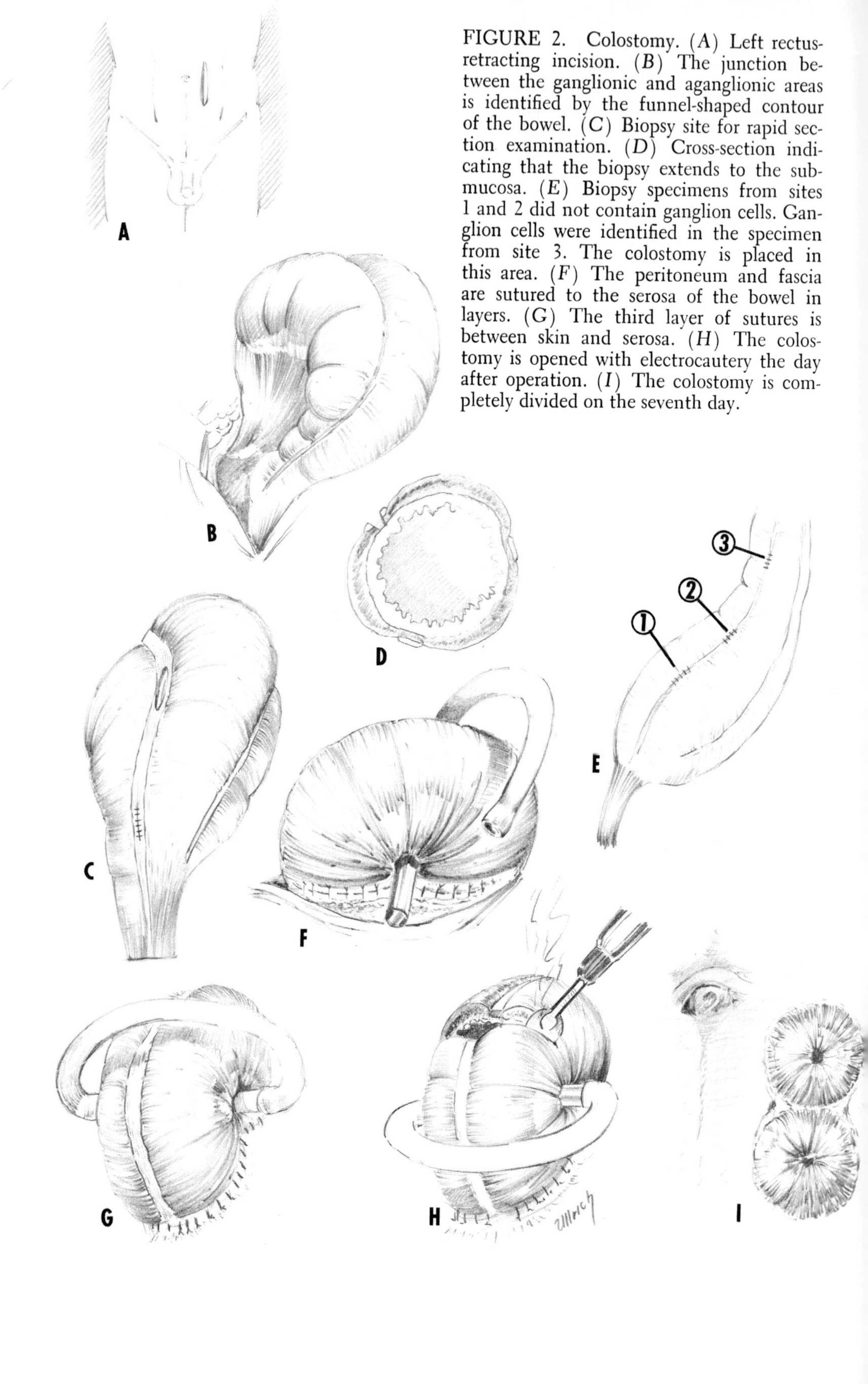

FIGURE 2. Colostomy. (*A*) Left rectus-retracting incision. (*B*) The junction between the ganglionic and aganglionic areas is identified by the funnel-shaped contour of the bowel. (*C*) Biopsy site for rapid section examination. (*D*) Cross-section indicating that the biopsy extends to the submucosa. (*E*) Biopsy specimens from sites 1 and 2 did not contain ganglion cells. Ganglion cells were identified in the specimen from site 3. The colostomy is placed in this area. (*F*) The peritoneum and fascia are sutured to the serosa of the bowel in layers. (*G*) The third layer of sutures is between skin and serosa. (*H*) The colostomy is opened with electrocautery the day after operation. (*I*) The colostomy is completely divided on the seventh day.

estimate is obtained by examining the bowel to find the area of transition from normal-appearing aganglionic colon below through a funnel-shaped segment to the ganglion-containing intestine proximally (Fig. 2B). In the ganglionic area the lumen is dilated and the wall thickened with hypertrophied muscle and edematous mucosa. Ideally, the colostomy should be placed in the most distal part of the ganglionic segment. At the definitive resection, the colostomy is excised with the aganglionic segment, and the ganglion-containing colon is connected to the lower rectum with a pull-through anastomosis. Error in selecting the colostomy site has unfortunate consequences. If the colostomy is placed in the aganglionic segment, it functions poorly; if it is placed well above the transitional zone, the sacrifice of colon is excessive. To be certain that the colostomy site contains ganglion cells, a 3 mm. by 5 mm. biopsy specimen containing both muscle layers is submitted to the pathologist for immediate examination (Fig. 2C, D). The defect in the muscle coats is closed with interrupted fine silk sutures. If no ganglion cells are found, another specimen is obtained from the colon proximally, and so on until an area is found where Auerbach's plexus does contain ganglion cells (Fig. 2E).

The performance of a loop colostomy in an infant differs from its performance in adults in that all the layers of the abdominal wall must be sutured to the seromuscular coats of the bowel (Fig. 2F, G). The crying infant increases intraabdominal pressure until loops of small intestine prolapse beside the colostomy unless the precaution of tacking each of the layers of the abdominal wall to the bowel wall has been taken. The glass rod should slip through the mesentery between the marginal vessel and the bowel wall. If the rod is below this vessel, considerable hemorrhage may occur when the colostomy is divided. The colostomy is opened by electrocautery the day after it is performed (Fig. 2H). On the seventh postoperative day, the colostomy is divided (Fig. 2I). Two Kocher clamps are left on the divided ends for six hours to crush the blood vessels in the bowel wall. No mucosal continuity between the colostomy ends is permitted. In our experience with loop colostomies before we divided them completely, fecal spillage occurred into the distal segment. Fecaliths formed and caused ulceration extending through the bowel wall.

The infant with the colostomy properly placed presents no particular problems. He should gain well with the usual dietary management. A colostomy bag is not applied. Rather, a diaper is wrapped around the waist as a band and changed at each feeding and as necessary. The child may be bathed in a tub and the skin washed with soap and water. The area about the colostomy is protected with zinc oxide ointment.

Temporary Ileostomy for Aganglionosis of the Entire Colon

The infant with aganglionosis of the entire colon is managed with loop ileostomy. Technical aspects are similar to the management of an infant with a colostomy. Unless the infant has severe enterocolitis, fluid loss from the ileostomy is not excessive and a regular formula without intravenous supplements is used. When the child has gained weight to 11.3 to 13.6 kilograms (25 to 30 pounds), the ileostomy is resected with the entire colon. The ileum is connected to the rectum 2 to 3 cm. from the mucocutaneous margin by a pull-through anastomosis. During the first weeks after operation, frequent liquid movements occur, leading to excoriation of the buttocks. However, the ileum develops a reservoir function. After one to two months, bowel movements occur two to three times each day and are semiformed.

Coloproctectomy

The Swenson operation for removal of the aganglionic segment in Hirschsprung's disease restores the continuity and voluntary control of the lower digestive tract by an exact anastomosis of the proximal, ganglion-containing segment to the rectum just above the anal sphincter. The proximal colon segment is pulled through the inverted rectum and a two-layer anastomosis is constructed just outside the anus. If the operation is to be successful, each step in the procedure must be meticulously performed, in an unhurried fashion and with exact attention to detail. Often a resection and pull-through anastomosis may require five to six hours. It is precisely this requirement of a time-consuming meticulous technique that probably stimulated others to devise less complicated procedures.

The diagnosis of aganglionic megacolon in the older infant or child is usually made by x-ray study of the colon by barium enema. Resection of the aganglionic segment is an elective procedure and not performed during a bout of acute intestinal obstruction or enterocolitis. Symptoms of acute obstruction are relieved by a large rectal tube passed well up into the colon and irrigated with saline. Even in the older child a temporary colostomy is indicated if the chronic obstruction has caused severe weight loss and anemia. A preoperative intravenous pyelogram will reveal the status of the urinary tract. No preoperative antibiotic or other bowel preparation is used.

Long procedures on children under general anesthesia require continuous monitoring of the body temperature. An esophageal probe connected to an electric thermometer is passed after the oroendotracheal tube is in place. Infants under 2 years of age tend to become hypothermic and are placed on an electric heating pad. Older children become hyperthermic as the colon is manipulated, and are therefore placed on a rubber blanket through which refrigerated fluid is circulated. A cutdown on the saphenous vein is performed to allow the administration of small quantities of whole blood according to the blood loss as estimated by weighing the gauze sponges. A Foley catheter is passed to decompress the bladder and identify the urethra during pelvic dissection. A modified lithotomy position permits simultaneous exposure of the abdomen and perineum. The infant is suspended by the feet and legs from a bar arched over the lower end of the table (Fig. 3A). The older child is flexed at the hips and knees, and the feet are taped to small slats extending out from the lower end of the mattress. The flexed knees are supported with adhesive plaster strips from the bar and padded laterally to protect the peroneal nerve. Only the abdomen is initially prepared and draped. The perineum is draped in a separate field from a second scrub nurse and table after the rectum has been mobilized and inverted out through the anus.

Technique

The Incision and Exploration. The abdomen is opened through a left rectus muscle-retracting incision extending from the pubis to the umbilicus or higher. If a colostomy is present, it is dissected free from the layers of the abdominal wall and excised (Fig. 3B, C). A von Petz stapling clamp is particularly useful during the various phases of this procedure to close temporarily the lumen of the divided bowel (Fig. 3D). After the abdomen has been opened, the colon is examined to determine the extent of the resection. In the majority of the cases the aganglionic lesion is limited to the rectum and sigmoid colon. This area will appear normal or slightly smaller than normal in caliber and contain only a small amount of feces. The bowel containing ganglion cells just proximal to the aganglionic segment is widely dilated and all the layers of the wall are thickened. The mucosa is edematous and often contains ulcers. The muscle coats are hypertrophied. The bands of the longitudinal muscles are widened and spread out over the surface of the colon. The mesentery is thickened and contains many enlarged lymph nodes. The blood vessels are enlarged to meet the demands of inflammation and hypertrophy. This characteristic dilatation and hypertrophy gradually returns to normal as the colon is examined more proximally. The site to begin the resection is chosen in the dilated colon 2 to 5 cm. from where the caliber begins to narrow into the aganglionic segment. A funnel-shaped deformity may be present in the transitional zone between the ganglionic and aganglionic segments. To make certain that ganglion cells are present at the proximal end of the resection, a piece of colon is excised and examined histologically. If no ganglion cells are identified in the myenteric plexus, a higher resection is made and again examined by frozen or rapid section. The resection is made as conservative as possible, particularly in the infant, to preserve the water-absorbing area and insure formed stools.

Mobilization of the Colon. The colon is mobilized to allow it to be pulled into the pelvis, by dividing the lateral peritoneal attachments. The splenic flexure may be taken down to obtain the necessary length (Fig. 3E). It is imperative that the mobilized segment have an excellent blood supply. This is obtained by dividing the mesenteric blood vessels near their origin and depending on retrograde flow through the arcades from more proximal vessels. To have the required length of left colon to reach through the pelvic floor, it is usually necessary to divide all the sigmoid branches of the inferior mesenteric vessels. If more mobilization is necessary, one or both branches of the left colic vessels may be divided near their origin. Adequacy of flow through the arcades and the marginal vessel may be estimated by placing a serrefine clamp on the artery that is to be divided and then observing the pulsations in the small arteries at the distal end of the mobilized segment. The veins and arteries are ligated separately by passing ligatures around the vessels before they are divided. Higher resections depend on blood supply

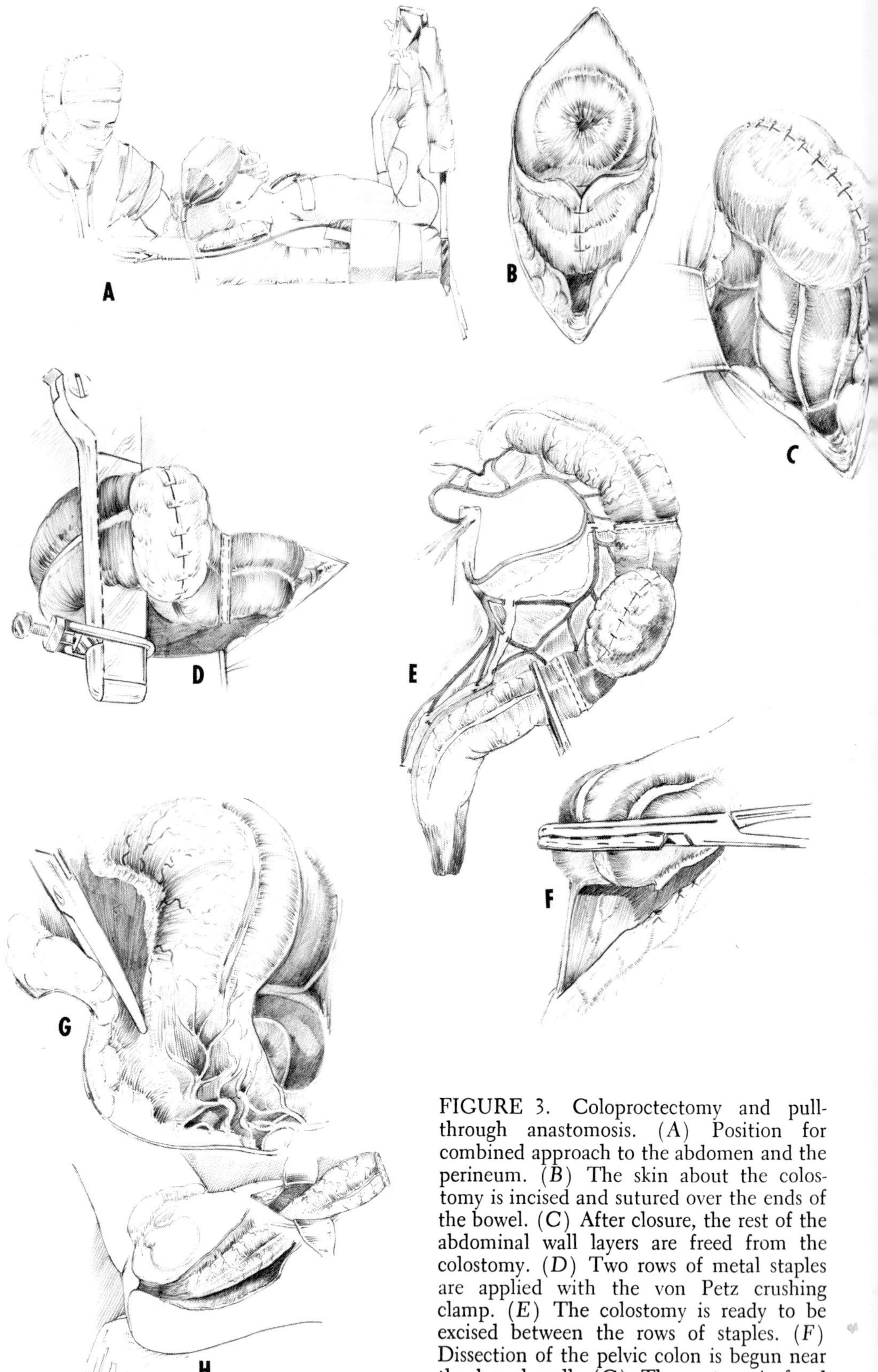

FIGURE 3. Coloproctectomy and pull-through anastomosis. (*A*) Position for combined approach to the abdomen and the perineum. (*B*) The skin about the colostomy is incised and sutured over the ends of the bowel. (*C*) After closure, the rest of the abdominal wall layers are freed from the colostomy. (*D*) Two rows of metal staples are applied with the von Petz crushing clamp. (*E*) The colostomy is ready to be excised between the rows of staples. (*F*) Dissection of the pelvic colon is begun near the bowel wall. (*G*) The rectum is freed by sharp dissection. (*H*) The dissection is continued to the levator ani muscles.

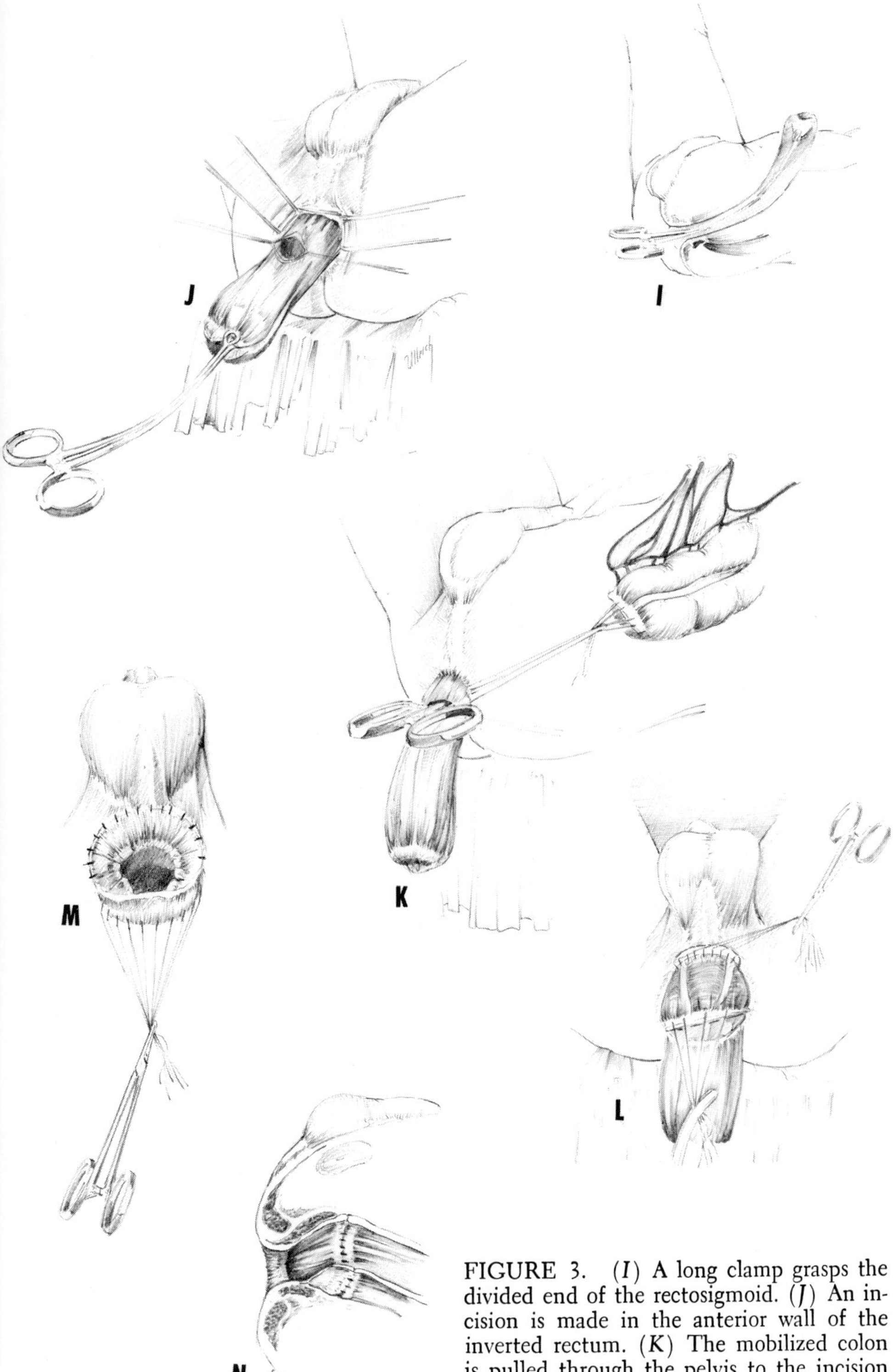

FIGURE 3. (*I*) A long clamp grasps the divided end of the rectosigmoid. (*J*) An incision is made in the anterior wall of the inverted rectum. (*K*) The mobilized colon is pulled through the pelvis to the incision in the rectum. (*L*) A row of silk sutures is placed between the muscle coats of the rectal wall and the seromuscular layer of the colon. (*M*) The second layer of the anastomosis is catgut in mucosa. (*N*) Relationship of the anastomosis to the pelvic floor.

from the middle colic vessels. If the resection extends to the transverse colon, the right colon may be mobilized and turned down into the pelvis for the pull-through anastomosis. In those rare infants with aganglionosis of the entire colon, the terminal ileum is mobilized by dividing one or two primary arcades.

MOBILIZATION OF THE RECTOSIGMOID AND THE RECTUM. The technique of dissection in the pelvis is modified to preserve the autonomic nerve supply to the bladder and genital apparatus. The rectosigmoid colon and the rectum are freed from surrounding areolar tissue and blood vessels by sharp dissection with the scissors directly on the muscle coats of the bowel wall (Fig. 3F, G). The superior hemorrhoidal as well as the middle hemorrhoidal vessels are divided at the bowel wall rather than near their origin. There is no blunt dissection with the fingers. Sharp dissection is tedious because there may be many small blood vessels to ligate, but impotence and bladder dysfunction are prevented by this method. The dissection about the rectum is continued almost to the level of the levator ani muscles (Fig. 3H).

TRANSECTION OF THE RECTOSIGMOID AND INVERSION OF THE RECTUM. The von Petz clamp is applied in the rectosigmoid region and the bowel divided between the two rows of staples. The surgeon then goes to the perineum, dilates the anus, and passes a long Kelly clamp into the rectum. The clamp is opened and the assistant inverts the divided end of the rectosigmoid into the clamp (Fig. 3I). The clamp is pulled out, inverting the rectum, through the anus. If the dissection in the pelvis is low enough, traction on the rectum will expose all the mucosa of the anal canal and rectum. If the dissection is insufficient, the rectum may be returned to the pelvis and mobilized another centimeter.

RESECTION OF THE AGANGLIONIC COLORECTUM AND THE COLORECTAL ANASTOMOSIS. The rectum is turned inside out through the anus. The rectal mucosa and perineum are prepared with aqueous solution of benzalkonium, and sterile drapes are applied. A 2 cm. transverse incision is made in the anterior rectal wall 1.5 to 2 cm. from the mucocutaneous margin in the anal canal (Fig. 3J). A long Kelly clamp is passed through this incision into the pelvis and abdomen. The assistant places two or three sutures on the divided end of the left colon and puts the sutures in the clamp. As the clamp is pulled out of the pelvis, the left colon is drawn down into the pelvis, through the inverted anal canal, and into the incision in the rectum (Fig. 3K). Interrupted 4–0 or 5–0 silk sutures are used to attach the muscle coats of the inverted rectum to the corresponding muscle layer of the left colon. The sutures are placed 2 to 3 mm. apart, tied, and used to maintain traction on the inverted anus (Fig. 3L). The transverse incision in the rectum is continued posteriorly and the first layer of the anastomosis completed. From 25 to 50 sutures are needed. The stapled end of the left colon is then excised just beyond the line of silk sutures, and for the first time contamination of the anastomosis is possible, from the lumen of the colon. Ten of the sutures anteriorly are cut near the knots, and the second layer of the anastomosis is begun. Interrupted 4–0 or 5–0 chromic catgut sutures attach the colon mucosa to the rectal mucosa and are tied so as to cover the silk knots (Fig. 3M). The catgut sutures are used to maintain traction on the inverted anus, and the silk sutures are cut a few at a time. When the catgut layer has been completed, the sutures are cut and the anal canal returns to its normal relationships. The anastomosis may be palpated 2 to 3 cm. from the anal verge (Fig. 3N).

THE CLOSURE. While the anastomosis on the perineum is being completed, a second operating team completes the abdominal portion of the operation. The pelvic peritoneum is not sutured to the colon since the colon is usually large and fills this space. However, the colon is sutured to the back of the abdominal cavity over the sacral promontory and the lumbar vertebrae to prevent prolapse of the

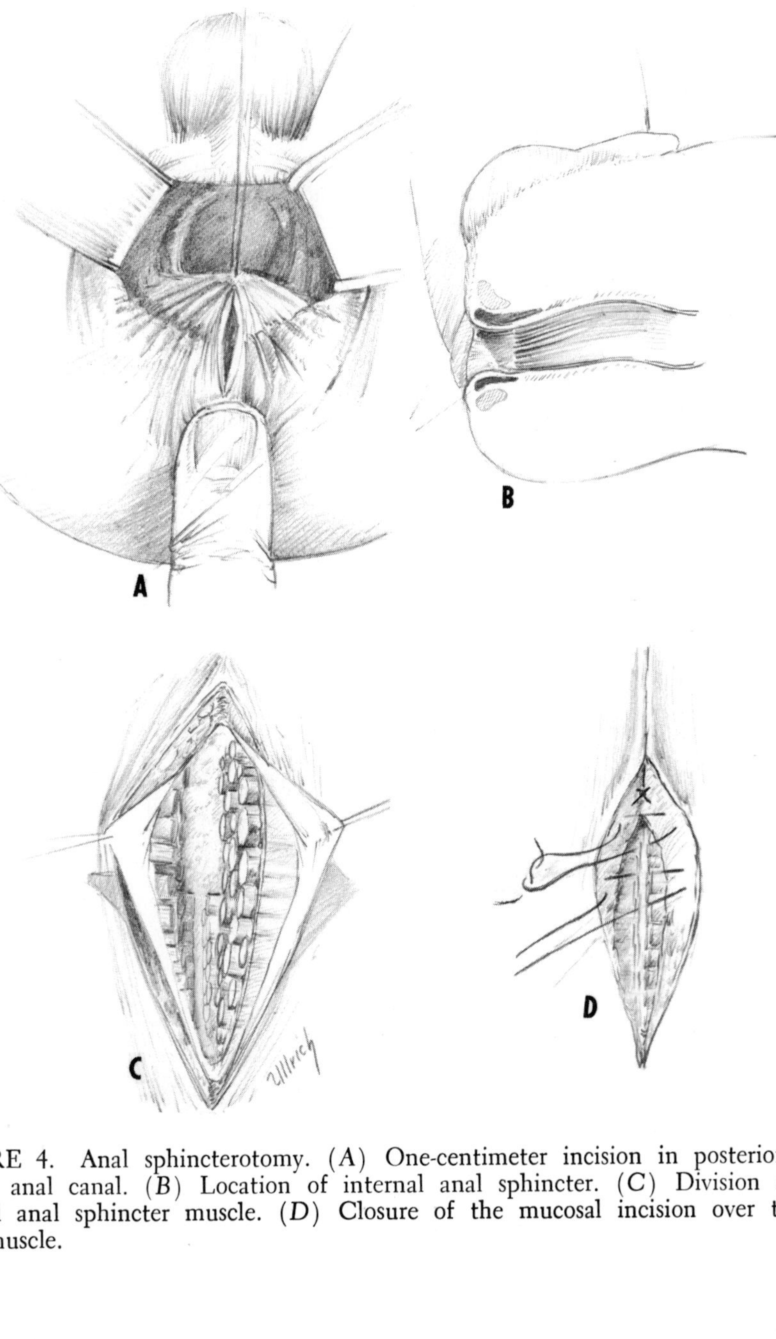

FIGURE 4. Anal sphincterotomy. (*A*) One-centimeter incision in posterior midline of anal canal. (*B*) Location of internal anal sphincter. (*C*) Division of the internal anal sphincter muscle. (*D*) Closure of the mucosal incision over the divided muscle.

small bowel. Inadvertent placement of the sutures in the blood supply to the colon will cause leaks in the anastomosis or more extensive necrosis. The abdominal wall is closed in layers with interrupted sutures of fine silk. The postoperative management is similar to that of an intestinal anastomosis.

Anal Sphincterotomy

Rarely, enterocolitis may continue after resection and pull-through anastomosis. A child with chronic enterocolitis has a distended tympanitic abdomen and has explosive, liquid bowel movements. Anorexia, weight loss, and a low-grade fever are characteristic. If colonic decompression with a large, soft rectal tube and saline irrigation is unsuccessful in relieving this condition, an anal sphincterotomy should be considered. With the patient in the lithotomy position and under general anesthesia with standard sterile technique, a 10 to 15 ml. incision is made in the posterior midline of the anal canal (Fig. 4A). The incision is centered over the mucocutaneous line and extends through the internal anal sphincter to the perirectal fascia. The external anal sphincter is preserved (Fig. 4B). Bleeding points are secured. The divided ends of the muscle are allowed to separate, but the incision in the skin and mucosa is closed with interrupted 4–0 chromic catgut sutures buried subcutaneously (Fig. 4C, D).

References

SWENSON, O., and BILL, A. H., JR. Resection of rectum and rectosigmoid with preservation of the sphincter for benign spastic lesions producing megacolon. *Surgery* 24:212, August 1948.

SWENSON, O., FISHER, J. H., and MACMAHON, H. E. Rectal biopsy as an aid in diagnosis of Hirschsprung's disease. *New England J. Med.* 253:632, October 13, 1955.

SWENSON, O., and FISHER, J. H. Treatment of Hirschsprung's disease with entire colon involved in aganglionic defect. *Arch. Surg.* 70:535, April 1955.

SWENSON, O. *Pediatric Surgery* (2d ed.). New York: Appleton-Century-Crofts, 1962. P. 388.

95. Clamp Technique for Closed Intestinal Anastomosis

REGINALD H. SMITHWICK

SOME TWENTY YEARS AGO, after many years of trial and error, the Smithwick clamp for the performance of closed intestinal anastomoses was perfected. It has been used by me and by a number of my associates and former residents over a long enough period and in a sufficient number of cases to demonstrate its value. A detailed description of the clamp with numerous illustrations of its use in all portions of the gastrointestinal tract has recently been published. Its use in the performance of gastrojejunostomy will be illustrated in this chapter. The reader is referred to the article just mentioned for the details of its use in other gastrointestinal procedures.

First, the important features of the clamp will be described, and its use in the three basic maneuvers which are involved in various gastrointestinal operations explained.

Features of the Clamp

The clamp consists of two wide, thin blades some 4 inches long (Fig. 1a). They approximate in a parallel fashion, permitting a secure grasp of the tissue, which is uniformly distributed. The clamp is closed manually and held in place by tightening the thumbscrew device to the point of increasing resistance. Thus, the tissue is not crushed. One blade has a narrow projecting ridge and the other a groove. At the tip of one blade is a wider, more prominent projection which inserts into a corresponding groove in the other blade to prevent scissoring (Fig. 1b). The ridge and groove construction makes for secure holding of tissue without crushing (Fig. 1c). The bowel is divided above the surface of the clamp with a dull red cautery, leaving sufficient tissue so that when it is charred dry and black a 1 mm. to 2 mm. layer of tissue remains (Fig. 1d). This char insures complete hemostasis. It also serves as a layer in which a basting suture is inserted in fashioning an anastomosis, or a continuous suture in turning in an end. The surface of the clamp contains grooves placed one-eighth inch apart over a distance of 3 inches (Fig. 1d). These permit the needle to be passed through the base of the char so that the suture line

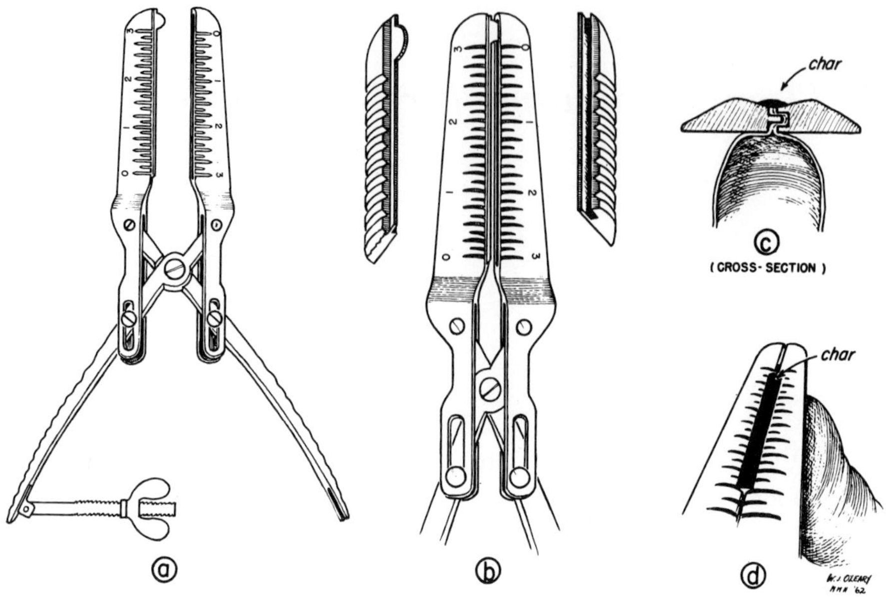

FIGURE 1. The Smithwick intestinal clamp. (Figures 1–5 are reproduced by permission from Smithwick, R. H., et al., *Am. J. Surg.* 104:613, 1962.)

will be secure and prevent leakage of gas or liquid after the clamp has been removed. Only when dealing with a distended bowel is a proximally placed, rubber-covered intestinal clamp necessary to prevent contamination.

The Basic Maneuvers in Intestinal Operations

There are three basic maneuvers which are employed in various intestinal operations: preparing an end of bowel for anastomosis, preparing the side of a loop of bowel, and turning in an end of bowel.

Preparing an End of Bowel for Anastomosis

The clamp is applied as illustrated in Figure 2, in such fashion that the mesentery is at right angles to the direction of the clamp. (This is shown most clearly in the lower half of the figure.) The thumbscrew is tightened as previously described (Fig. 2a). Two narrow clamps such as Kochers are placed above the surface of the Smithwick clamp. The middle clamp is removed, and the bowel is divided with a cautery (Fig. 2b, c). The basting suture is inserted as shown in Figure 2d and 2e. It is drawn back and forth as shown in Figure 2f, care being taken that the traction is parallel to the surface of the blades so as not to tear it out of the char. Actually, one should pull the baster back and forth after each inch of insertion, especially in large bowel or stomach. This makes it pull easily at the end and lessens the like-

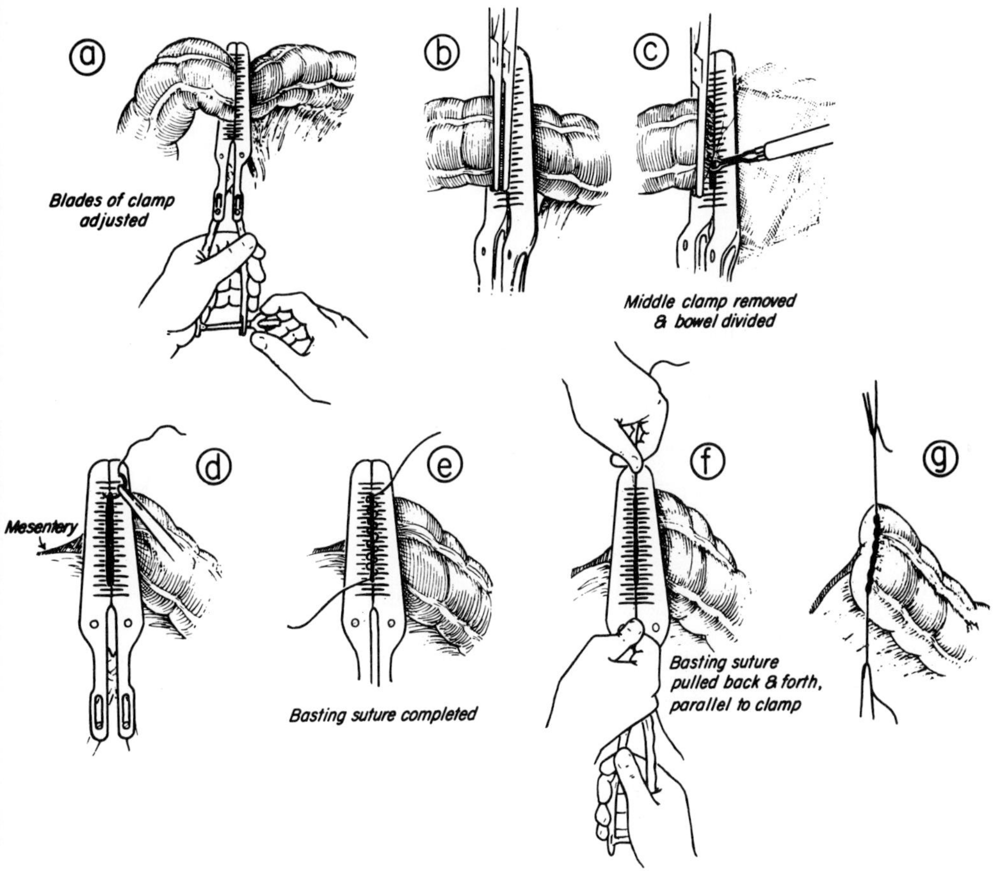

FIGURE 2. Preparing an end of bowel for anastomosis.

lihood of its breaking. The clamp must be held securely while the basting suture is being pulled. One should use 0 chromic, atraumatic catgut for the stomach and large bowel. Elsewhere, 00 catgut will suffice. After the basting suture is in place the clamp is removed. The end of bowel is now ready for anastomosis (Fig. 2g).

Preparing a Side of Bowel for Anastomosis

The steps one should take to prepare a side of bowel for anastomosis are illustrated by Figure 3. The bowel is grasped with one's fingers so as to emphasize the antimesenteric border and to insure that all layers of the intestine will be contained in a series of Allis clamps placed in a straight line (Fig. 3a, b). The Smithwick clamp is then applied as shown in Figure 3c. The Allis clamps are removed and a segment of bowel is removed with the cautery (Fig. 3d) and placed in a basin. It is then inverted, and the undersurface examined to be certain that a narrow strip of the full thickness of the mucosa is visible for almost the entire length of the ex-

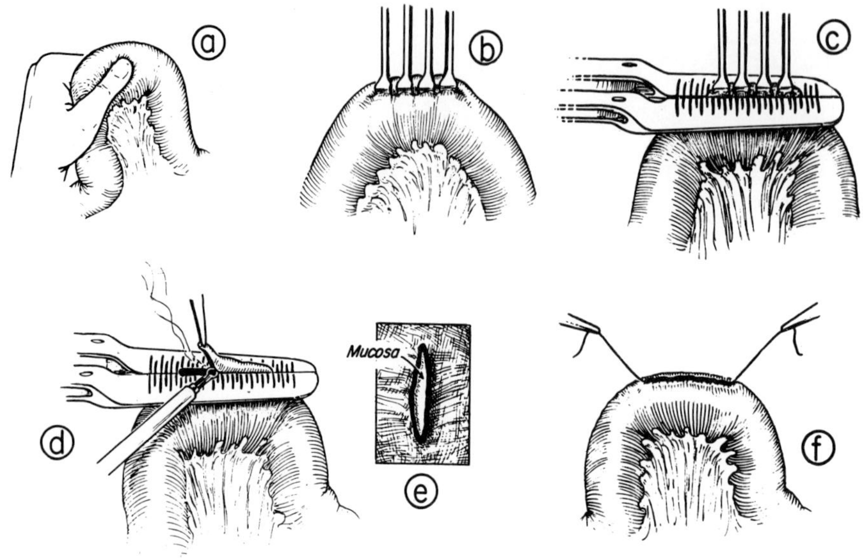

FIGURE 3. Preparing a side of bowel for anastomosis.

cised bit of intestine (Fig. 3e). The basting suture is then inserted exactly as previously described, and the side of bowel is ready for anastomosis (Fig. 3f).

Turning in an End of Bowel

Turning in an end is illustrated by Figure 4. The clamp is applied and the bowel divided as indicated in Figure 4a. By contrast with preparing an end of bowel for anastomosis, the clamp is applied so that it is in line with the direction of the mesentery. This is shown best in Figure 4c and 4d. A continuous rather than a basting suture is then inserted in the char (Fig. 4b). The clamp is removed and a second layer of interrupted or continuous sutures is inserted (Fig. 4c). The closed end is shown in Figure 4d.

In the rare circumstance that one wishes to turn in a side of bowel, the technique is similar to that used for preparing a side of bowel for anastomosis except that a continuous suture is placed in the char instead of a baster. A second suture line completes the closure.

Gastrojejunostomy

The technique for performing a gastrojejunstomy is illustrated by Figure 5. The end of the duodenum has been turned in as just described (Fig. 5a). If one wishes to do a Billroth I maneuver, a basting suture is placed in the duodenum instead. The stomach is divided as shown in Figure 5b. The lesser curvature side of the char is closed with a continuous suture. A basting suture is inserted in the greater

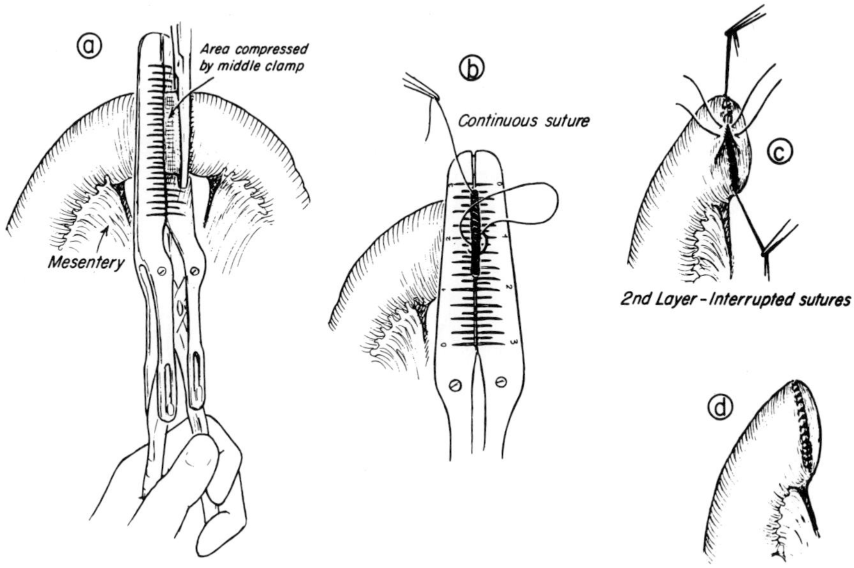

FIGURE 4. Turning in an end of bowel.

curvature portion over a length which will make the diameter of the anastomosis approximately that of the jejunum, or which will match the diameter of the duodenum if one is performing a gastroduodenostomy. The lesser curvature portion is turned in with a second layer of interrupted or continuous sutures (Fig. 5c). The side of the jejunal loop is then anastomosed to the distal curvature end of the stomach with a single layer of interrupted fine silk sutures closely placed in such fashion that the knots when tied will be on the outside (Fig. 5d, e, f). The basting suture is removed (Fig. 5g) and the anastomosis is complete (Fig. 5h).

Comments

Over a period of nearly twenty years, this technique for closed intestinal anastomoses has proved to be very satisfactory. It has been used in all portions of the gastrointestinal tract. As we have reported, it has been found to be associated with a significantly lower incidence of septic and hemorrhagic complications after gastric resections for ulcer or carcinoma than was the open technique. The incidence of septic complications following resection of the colon for carcinoma was also significantly lower with the closed technique. There were no recurrences in the suture line in the "closed" series of resections of the colon for carcinoma, in contrast to a 5 per cent incidence of recurrence at the suture line in a parallel "open" series. We believe that recurrences at the site of anastomosis are due to the incorporation of

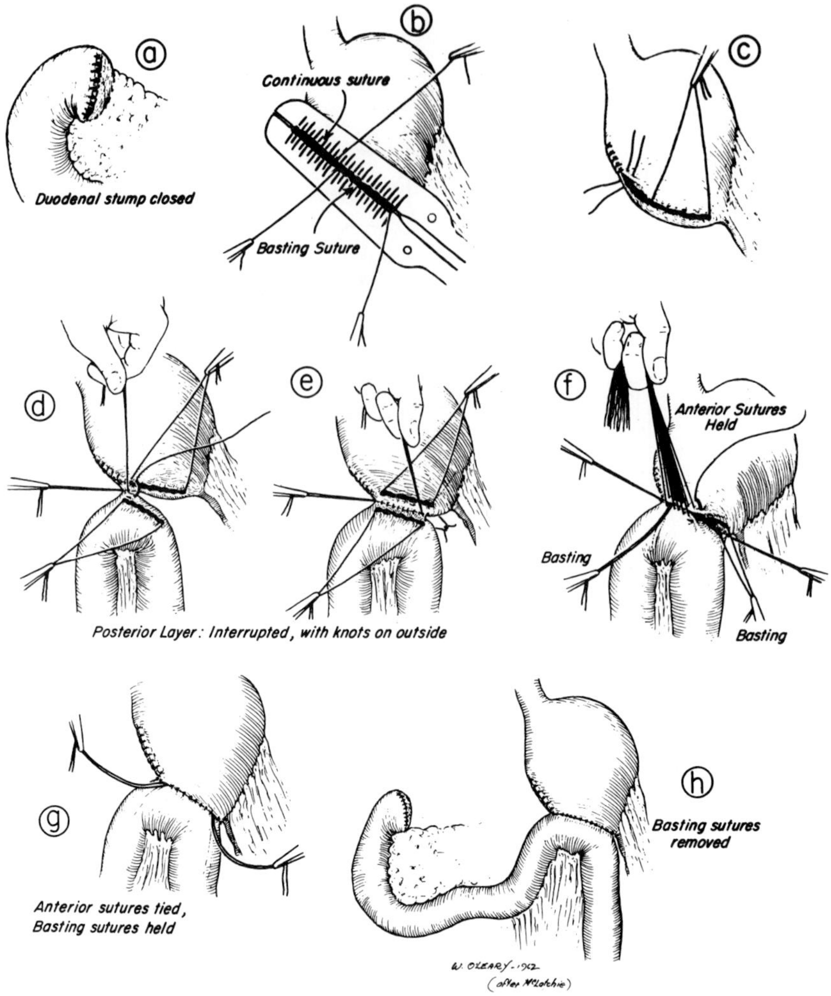

FIGURE 5. Gastrojejunostomy.

malignant cells into the suture line when the open technique is used. With our particular closed technique, the sutures do not penetrate the mucosa. They should include only serosa and enough muscularis for secure apposition. They do not have to be placed deeply enough to afford hemostasis since this is provided for by the turned-in dry, black char. The latter sloughs out completely and is not a satisfactory medium for the implantation of malignant cells which may be in the lumen of the bowel.

As with any special technique, the details of its use must be followed meticulously. It is urged that one practice this technique on autopsy material or in the animal laboratory before employing it in man. A single layer of interrupted nonabsorbable suture material has been found adequate for anastomoses in most situations if one is dealing with normal bowel. There is no objection to using two layers of sutures if one prefers. Two layers of sutures should always be used in anastomoses between the esophagus and other portions of the gastrointestinal tract and also when the proximal colon is anastomosed to the distal colon beneath the peritoneal reflection unless a proximal temporary colostomy is performed to protect the suture line. If properly used, this technique will be found to be simple, safe, and satisfactory.

Reference

SMITHWICK, R. H., HOWE, C. W., ROBERTSON, C. W., FARMER, D. A., and FULLER, C. H. The Smithwick gastrointestinal clamp. Closed ("aseptic") intestinal anastomosis. *Am. J. Surg.* 104:613, October 1962.

96. *Massive Rectal Prolapse*

CHARLES B. RIPSTEIN

SATISFACTORY REPAIR of massive rectal prolapse depends on an understanding of its cause. In all patients with such a prolapse, the rectum is mobile and can be displaced anteriorly (Figs. 1 and 2). In some patients this condition is due to a congenital mesorectum. In others there is no mesentery, but loose areolar tissue separates the rectum from the sacrum. Normally, an increase in intraabdominal pressure with straining pushes the rectum into the hollow of the sacrum. In massive prolapse, however, the rectum moves anteriorly, forming a straight tube, and the rectum intussuscepts caudally, the anterior wall of the rectum forming the greater part of the prolapse. It has become apparent to us that a pelvic floor defect anterior to the rectum is a variable factor; often it is nonexistent.

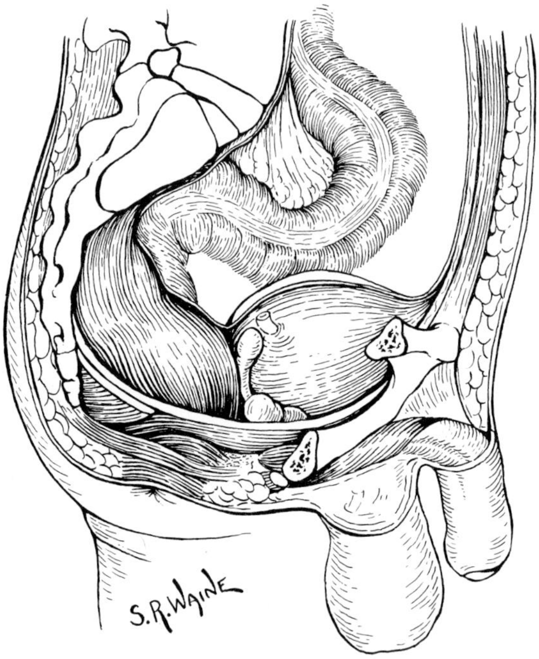

FIGURE 1. Normal position of the rectum in sagittal section. The rectum is retroperitoneal and curves posteriorly into the hollow of the sacrum. (Figures 1–3 are reproduced by permission from Ripstein, C. B., and Lantner, B., *Ann. Surg.* 157:259, February 1963.)

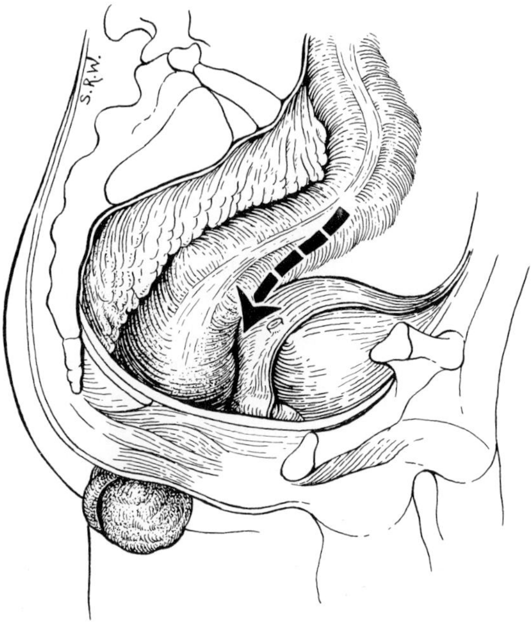

FIGURE 2. Prolapse of the rectum. The lower rectal segment is displaced anteriorly on a mesorectum. Intraabdominal pressure acts on the vertical axis of the bowel.

The basic techniques recommended for the surgical correction of massive rectal prolapse have undergone revision as experience has been gained in handling this problem. Moschovitz in 1912 advanced the concept that massive rectal prolapse was a sliding hernia through a defect in the anterior pelvic floor, and that the abnormally deep rectovesical pouch represented a hernial sac. That concept did not explain the occurrence of prolapse in persons with an intact pelvic floor, nor the fact that recurrences were frequent following operations which placed sole emphasis on a repair of such a defect.

A review of the literature reveals that a number of workers suggested that the mechanism of prolapse was associated with anomalies of the rectum itself. Bodenhamer in 1847, and Cooper and Edwards in 1892, described the vertical course of the rectum in patients with prolapse.

Until recently we felt that surgical correction of massive rectal prolapse required replacement of the displaced rectum into the hollow of the sacrum, removal of the hernial sac, and repair of a defect in the anterior pelvic floor. We have now reassessed our experience, and feel that the success in the repair is primarily due to proper and adequate posterior fixation of the rectum. An inadequate fixation will allow the prolapse to recur regardless of whether or not an anterior pelvic floor defect has been repaired.

Although at present we are using and recommending a simplified procedure involving posterior fixation of the rectum alone, the procedure earlier employed, which included repair of an anterior pelvic defect, will also be described. The results with either procedure have been excellent. The earlier employed procedure will be described first.

Technique of Correction of Massive Rectal Prolapse

Correction with Repair of an Anterior Pelvic Floor Defect

The patient is placed in Trendelenburg position. A left paramedian incision is made. The lateral peritoneal reflections are incised, and the rectum is freed from the hollow of the sacrum. The lateral peritoneal leaves are mobilized as in an abdominoperineal resection. Both ureters are identified, followed to the bladder, and then protected from injury. The peritoneum is incised anteriorly along the base of the bladder, and the excess peritoneum in the pouch of Douglas is excised. At this stage an anterior defect in the pelvic fascia, if present, can be demonstrated. Traction is placed on the rectum as it is pushed into the hollow of the sacrum, and the levator muscles are approximated in the midline, anterior to the rectum. This closure is reinforced by a V-shaped graft of fascia lata removed from the thigh, or by a similar-shaped piece of Teflon mesh. This prosthesis holds the rectum in the hollow of the sacrum. The apex of the prosthesis is sutured to the fascia at the base of the bladder, and the lateral edges to the levator muscles near their origins. The limbs of the V are brought around the rectum, crossed behind it, and sutured to the tissue overlying the sacrum. The edges of the defect in the graft or the mesh are sutured to the rectal wall (Fig. 3). The pelvic peritoneum is approximated over the prosthesis, obliterating the pouch of Douglas.

In the female, the graft or the mesh may be sutured to the cervix. If a hysterectomy is indicated, we prefer leaving the cervical stump to buttress the repaired pelvic floor in its anterior portion.

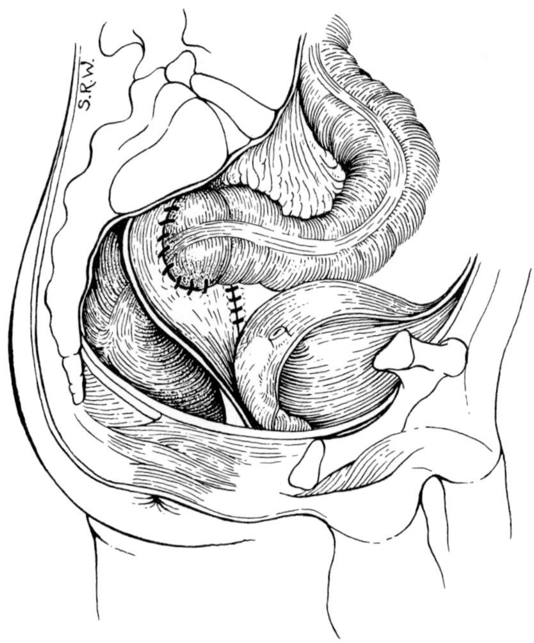

FIGURE 3. Repair of prolapse restores the posterior curve, and intraabdominal pressure forces the rectum into the hollow of the sacrum.

A high anterior resection of the sigmoid with end-to-end anastomosis is carried out if the length of the sigmoid and its mesentery presents a hazard from a potential volvulus. This is a more effective and safer method of removing excess bowel than the pull-through operation advocated by Altemeier and his co-workers. A catheter is placed in the hollow of the sacrum and brought out extraperitoneally through a lateral stab wound for suction drainage. The abdomen is closed in the usual manner.

This form of repair has been carried out in 45 patients over a 12-year period. There was one recurrence of the prolapse, three months following surgery. This patient refused reoperation, but rectal examination revealed that the fascial graft was not properly placed and the posterior curve of the rectum had therefore not been maintained. This must be considered a technical failure due to an inadequate operation. The remaining patients either are alive and well, or had experienced no recurrence by the time they died.

Correction without Repair of an Anterior Pelvic Floor Defect

A lower left rectus or transverse incision is made. The rectum is mobilized by incising the lateral peritoneal reflections and raising the bowel from the hollow of the sacrum by blunt dissection. The ureters are identified and protected from injury. The rectum and the rectosigmoid are then fixed to the hollow of the sacrum by suturing a 2 inches wide T-shaped sling of Teflon mesh around the bowel, to the presacral fascia and periosteum, approximately 2 inches below the promontory.

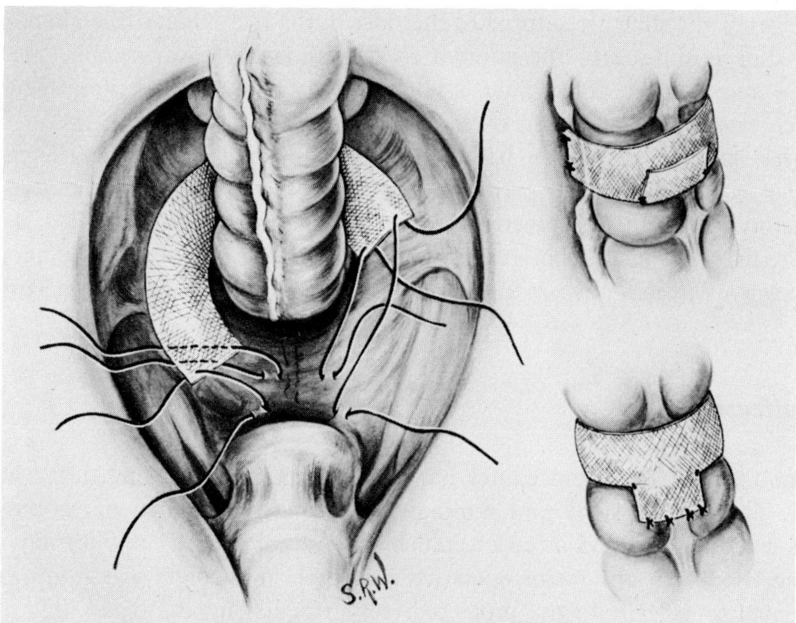

FIGURE 4. Simplified repair. Method of insertion of the T-shaped sling of Teflon mesh around the rectum. The sling is sutured to the presacral fascia and periosteum, to the sides of the rectum, and to the anterior rectal wall.

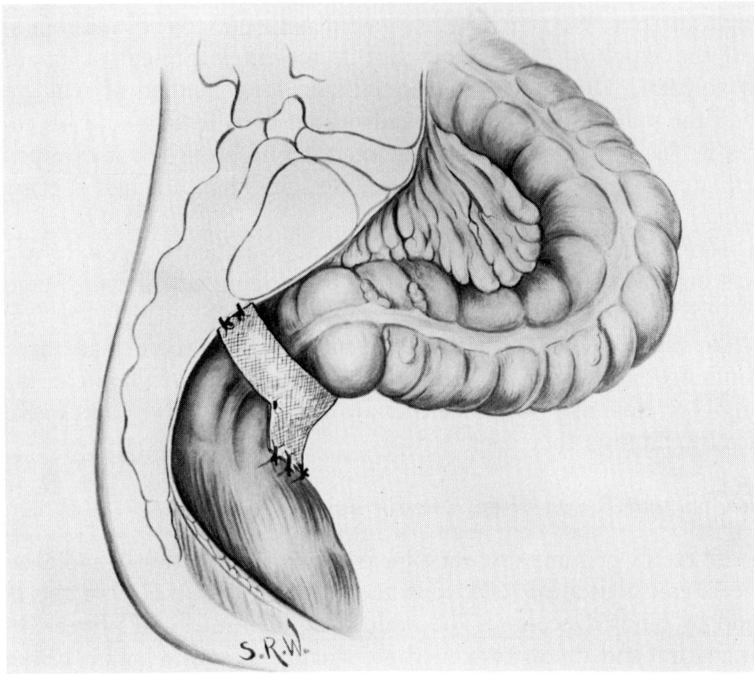

FIGURE 5. Simplified repair. Lateral view of the inserted sling of Teflon mesh.

The edges of the sling are sutured to the sides of the rectum, and the anterior limb of the sling is sutured to the anterior rectal wall below the peritoneal reflection (Figs. 4 and 5). The pelvic floor is not repaired. The lateral peritoneal incisions are then closed. The abdomen is closed in a standard fashion.

This simplified operation has been accomplished in 30 patients. There have been no recurrences over a period ranging from six months to three years. The satisfactory results of this procedure raise some doubt as to the need of a pelvic floor repair. The pelvic floor repair should probably be added to the procedure when such a defect is obvious in the patient with a long history of rectal prolapse.

Complications

The mortality of these procedures has been acceptably low (one death in each series). There was a significant morbidity following the original operation. Some of this was due to wound infection, phlebitis, and pulmonary complications which are associated with any major operative procedure in an older age group and are not related specifically to the prolapsed rectum or its surgical repair. The following complications were related directly to the pathology or to the procedure and have required specific measures.

1. Anal incontinence. A patulous sphincter ani is present in all long-standing

cases. In younger patients continence can be restored by exercises and by electrical stimulation of the sphincter muscle to improve sphincter tone. In older patients the sphincter may remain lax in spite of treatment and a secondary operation such as the Thiersch or gracilis sling operation may be necessary to regain continence. A secondary operation has been necessary in five patients, all in the older age group.

2. Urinary complications were frequent. Cystitis occurred in 10 patients. This was probably due to manipulation of the bladder or prostate and the inflammatory reaction around the graft in this area. Prolonged catheter drainage (seven days) has been necessary to avoid stasis and infection, especially in male patients. This problem has not occurred with the simplified operation.

3. Proctitis and perirectal inflammatory reaction are usually present for a few weeks after surgery and occasionally persist for several months. The graft can be palpated through the rectum and a good deal of induration and edema is often noted. This has cleared spontaneously but may produce temporary tenesmus and a mucoid rectal discharge.

4. Fecal impaction has occurred in patients in whom the sling has been too tight, producing an obstructing shelf. This complication can be avoided by making the sling loose enough to allow the insertion of a finger between the rectum and the underlying sacrum.

References

ALTEMEIER, W. A., GREENE, L., JR., and KEIRLE, A. The one stage perineal operation for prolapse of the rectum. In Mulholland, J. H., Ellison, E. H., and Friesen, S. R. (Eds.), *Current Surgical Management, II*. Philadelphia: W. B. Saunders, 1960.

MOSCHOVITZ, A. V. The pathogenesis, anatomy, and care of prolapse of the rectum. *Surg., Gynec. and Obst.* 15:7, July 1912.

RIPSTEIN, C. B. Treatment of massive rectal prolapse. *Am. J. Surg.* 83:68, January 1952.

RIPSTEIN, C. B., and LANTER, B. Etiology and surgical therapy of massive prolapse of the rectum. *Ann. Surg.* 157:259, February 1963.

XVI. THE PANCREAS AND SPLEEN

97. *Subtotal Pancreatectomies*

CHARLES G. CHILD, 3rd

PANCREATIC TUMORS and inflammations may be treated surgically by subtotal resection of the pancreas together with adjacent expendable organs. Malignant neoplasms of the duodenum, terminal common duct, and ampulla of Vater can be removed in this manner, and patients suffering one or another of these serious tumors either cured or provided substantial palliation. Occasionally gastrectomy or right colectomy is combined with pancreaticoduodenectomy for cancers primary in the stomach or colon which have extended to the stomach, duodenum, colon, and pancreas in a localized malignant mass.

The most widely known of these extensive operations is the Whipple procedure or pancreaticoduodenectomy (Fig. 1). "Radical" often modifies these terms. This adjective emphasizes that these operations are extensive, but erroneously suggests that they meet accepted criteria of radical operations for cancer. They do not, because regional lymphatic beds are not wholly removed, nor can primary tumors generally be excised together with substantial barriers of normal tissue. After one of these operations, the portal vein, superior mesenteric vein, hepatic artery, and superior mesenteric artery persist as essential structures which have often resided within millimeters of the primary neoplasm. Numerous organs are removed and extensive enteric reconstructions are required. These procedures, however, are local extirpations, not radical resections.

Conventional pancreaticoduodenectomy or a variety of distal pancreatectomies are performed for islet cell adenomas, cysts, cystadenomas, cystadenocarcinomas, fibrocalcific pancreatitis, and occasionally for serious injuries of the pancreas.

Subtotal Pancreatectomy for Pancreaticoduodenal Cancer (Whipple Procedure; Radical Pancreaticoduodenectomy)

So many well-known difficulties attend correct diagnosis of pancreaticoduodenal cancer that surgeons willing and trained to accept responsibility for patients with one of these tumors rarely approach operation armed with a precise diagnosis.

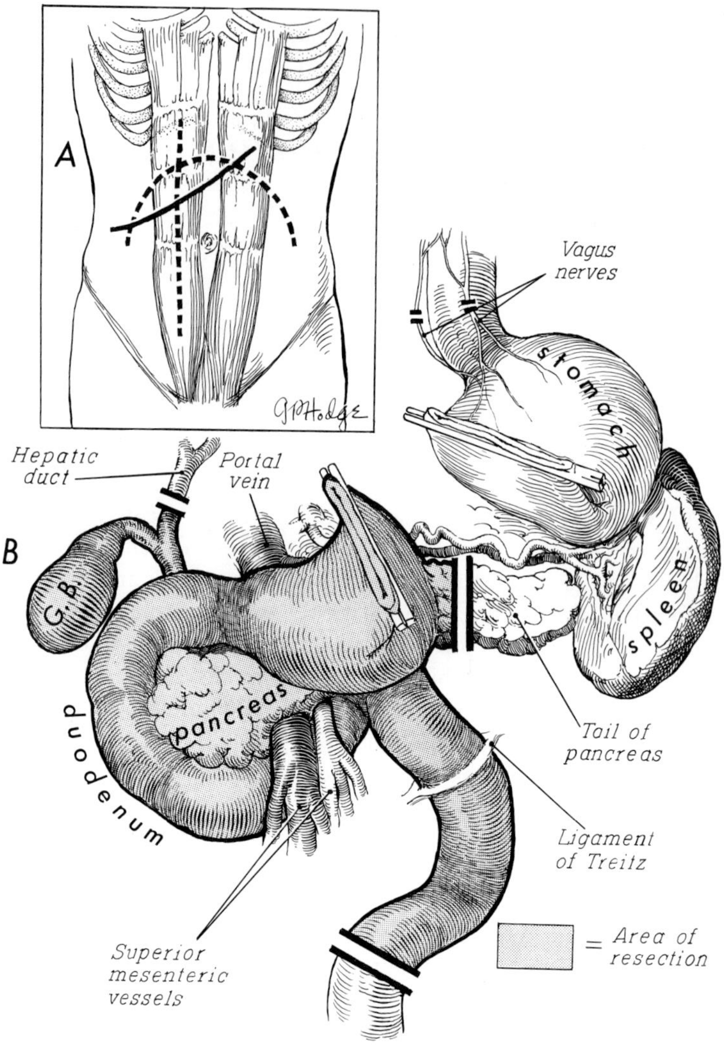

FIGURE 1. Extent of pancreaticoduodenectomy (Whipple procedure).

Indications for exploratory celiotomy may be clear or tenuous. For instance, sudden jaundice and stools consistently positive for blood strongly indicate ampullary cancer. Too often, however, the patient's history is vague, permitting little more than a tentative diagnosis of pancreaticoduodenal cancer. Even elaborate diagnostic studies give normal results or are inconclusive, and psychic disorders are often suspected until jaundice suddenly appears or widespread cancer is obvious to patient and physician alike. A decision to explore the patient's abdomen does not conclude the many difficulties encountered; positive or even tentative identification of a small cancer deep in the head of the pancreas is notoriously difficult. Most pancreaticoduodenectomies, therefore, are approached without confidence that a precise diagnosis will be reached at the operating table.

The Incision

Access to the peritoneal cavity is best gained through a long oblique incision extending from the left costal margin to the right flank. Such an incision offers ready access to the spleen, stomach, pancreas, duodenum, and upper jejunum. Pancreaticoduodenectomy can also be performed through a long right rectus incision or through an upper abdominal curvilinear transverse incision. The precise direction of the incision is less important than a generous length and the operator's familiarity with what needs to be accomplished through it.

The Exploration

After entering the abdomen, search is made for distant metastases in the liver, pelvis, regional lymph nodes, or on free peritoneal surfaces. If they are found, resection is usually abandoned and attention turned to palliative decompression of the biliary tract and stomach. Occasionally distant metastases are trivial and the primary tumor is clearly resectable. Here palliative pancreaticoduodenectomy should not be dismissed; relief of pain usually follows, and death due to metastasis is generally kinder when unassociated with a bulky pancreaticoduodenal cancer. Under these circumstances infallible rules of procedure are unavailable, since each case calls for individual judgment often based more upon surgical philosophy than science.

Metastases having been excluded, attention is directed toward visual and tactile exploration of the common duct, duodenum, pancreas, portal vein, and base of the mesocolon. A single objective is sought: differentiation of common duct stone or chronic pancreatitis from pancreaticoduodenal cancer. Surgical and cholangiographic exploration of the common duct usually excludes choledocholithiasis easily. Deciding whether an enlarged, edematous, and firm pancreas is the site of chronic pancreatitis or cancer may, however, be difficult. Direct or needle biopsy of the pancreas is notoriously unrewarding and even dangerous. If pancreaticoduodenectomy is not performed, pancreatotomy exposes patients to the risk of a pancreatic fistula and hemorrhage. Here a surgeon must usually trust his clinical acumen and capacity as a gross pathologist in deciding whether or not to proceed with pancreatic and duodenal resection. Frequently pancreaticoduodenal neoplasms will be resected without benefit of positive microscopic diagnosis of cancer.

In some jaundiced patients, however, Cattell's maneuver is helpful when a reasonable diagnosis of pancreatic cancer cannot be made. The common duct is drained by a T tube for three weeks. If common duct obstruction is benign, it subsides and pancreaticoduodenectomy is not required; if the obstruction is malignant, it persists and reoperation can be undertaken with reasonable assurance that the head of the pancreas harbors a malignant neoplasm.

Positive identification of ampullary tumors occasions special concerns most of which are resolved by remembering that very few of these lesions are benign; the majority are papillary adenocarcinomas. Whether duodenotomy for biopsy should be performed is an important question. Duodenotomy cannot be avoided where a stone impacted in the ampulla must be differentiated from ampullary cancer. In the majority of cases of ampullary tumor, however, opening the duodenum is unnecessary and even undesirable, because it exposes the patient to peritoneal implantation of viable tumor cells. Furthermore, rapid section of a small, friable ampullary tumor is difficult and unreliable. Most surgeons agree, therefore, that palpation of a discrete ampullary mass or infrapapillary ulcer warrants pancreaticoduodenectomy.

Some concept of the incidence of error in correctly identifying pancreaticoduodenal cancer may be derived from data from my personal experience with some 60 pancreaticoduodenectomies for these troublesome tumors. Three of these operations were performed unwittingly for benign disease—two for chronic pancreatitis of unknown cause, and one for chronic papillitis of the ampulla of Vater.

Decision Regarding Resectability

Convinced that the patient's abdomen is free of metastases, the surgeon will find three maneuvers helpful in arriving at a decision regarding resectability:

First, incision of the lateral duodenal peritoneum allows mobilization of the duodenum and head of the pancreas (Fig. 2). The space between the head of the pancreas anteriorly and the vena cava and aorta posteriorly is readily explored with the left index finger. Special care should be taken to extend this

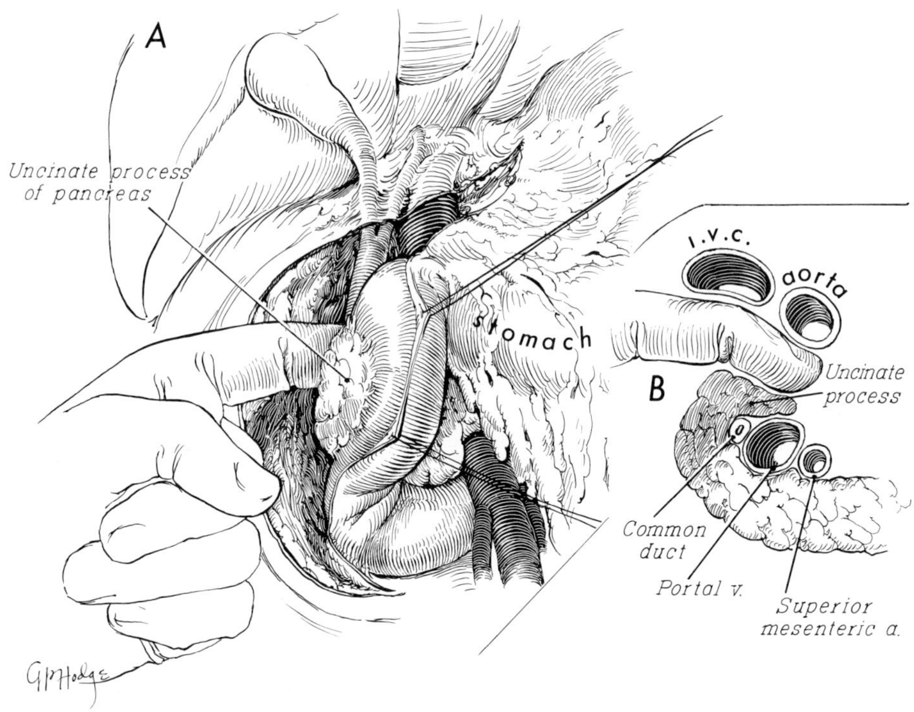

FIGURE 2. Mobilization of the duodenum and head of the pancreas.

tactile investigation as close to the origin of the superior mesenteric artery as possible. Tumor streaming posteriorly to invade the vena cava, aorta, and periaortic nodes is readily detected and contraindicates pancreaticoduodenectomy. Free mobilization of the duodenum and the head of the pancreas is encouraging and warrants the second step.

Second, by dividing the gastrohepatic ligament from the common duct to the midpoint of the lesser curvature of the stomach the hepatic artery is skeletonized (Fig. 3A). In this dissection one or more nodes are frequently encountered. If, on rapid section, they are positive for cancer, one surgical school insists that the operation be abandoned, because extension of cancer to these nodes precludes cure. Others, having faith in the palliative merits of pancreatectomy, are not deterred by one or two metastatic nodes in this area. After the structures of

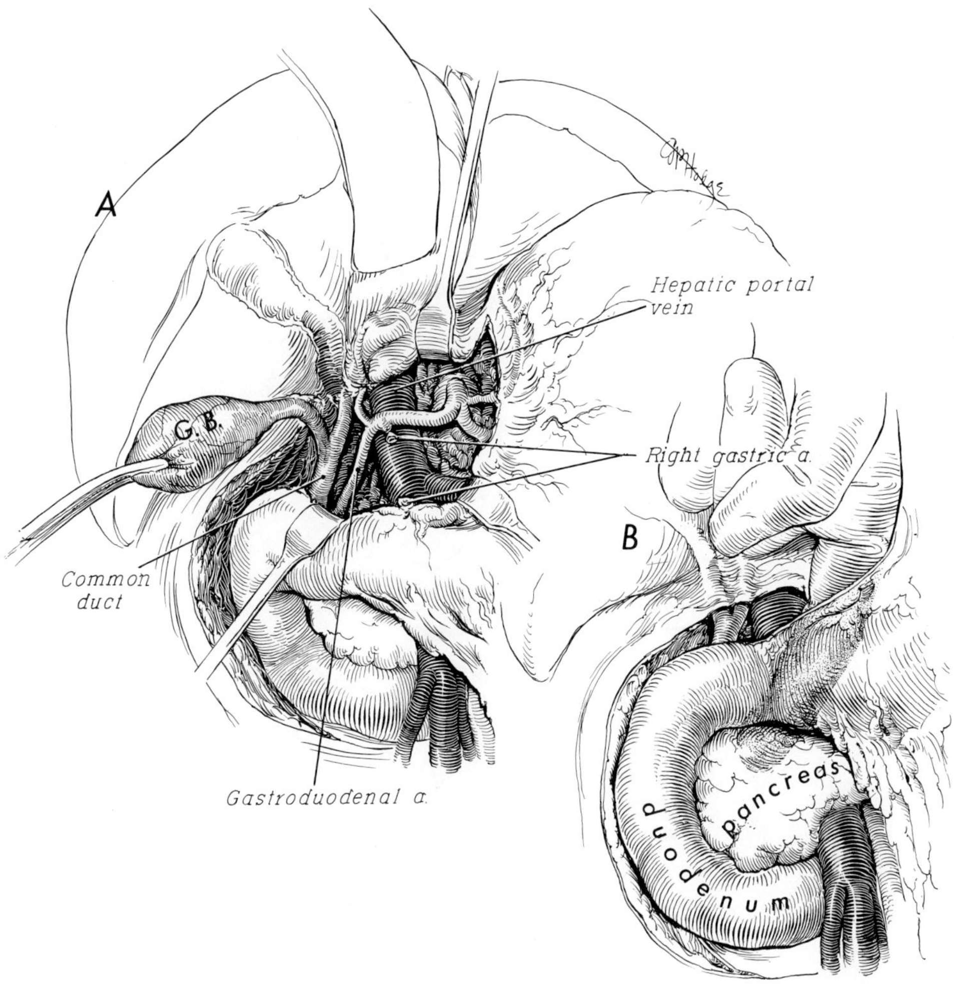

FIGURE 3. Mobilization of the distal stomach and pylorus, and identification of structures in the hepatoduodenal and hepatogastric ligaments.

the gastrohepatic ligament have been clearly placed on display, the left index finger is inserted between the body of the pancreas and the junction of the portal and superior mesenteric veins (Fig. 3B). Force must be avoided here lest tiny veins passing directly from the pancreas to the portal circulation be torn and troublesome hemorrhage started. If the gastrohepatic and retropancreatic spaces are free of tumor, the third step in determining local operability is undertaken.

Third, the stomach, colon, and the omentum are reflected superiorly, exposing the base of the mesocolon. This is incised transversely as far as the ligament of Treitz. The superior mesenteric vein, superior mesenteric artery, middle colic artery, and inferior pancreaticoduodenal artery are identified (Fig. 4A). Tumor invading these structures is a contraindication to pancreaticoduodenectomy. Freedom from tumor here may be further confirmed by inserting the index finger of the right hand between the body of the pancreas and the superior mesenteric vein (Fig. 4B). If this digital exploration is combined with a similar one from above, the tips of the index fingers meet easily and the body of the pancreas may literally be lifted a few millimeters away from the portal and superior mesenteric veins. Such mobility usually means that the tumor is confined to the head of the pancreas.

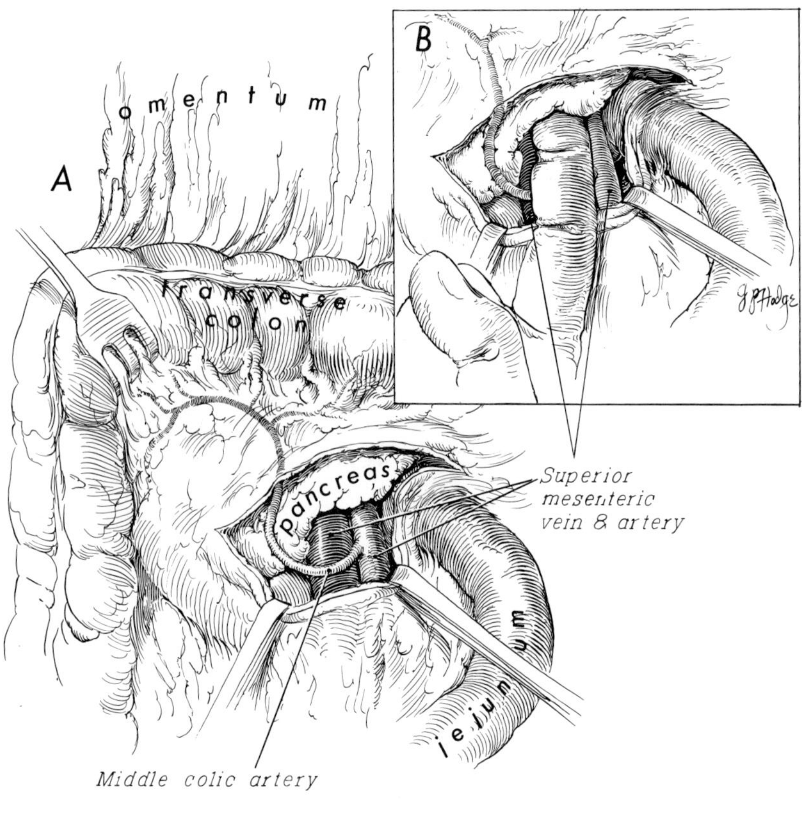

FIGURE 4. Exploration of the base of the mesocolon.

Successful completion of these three maneuvers almost guarantees that the particular tumor in question is locally operable. The only vital area remaining unexplored is the origin of the superior mesenteric artery. This defies precise investigation until the stomach and pancreas have been divided.

Up to this point no vital structure has been compromised. If local cancerous extensions are identified in the course of these maneuvers, the operation can easily be terminated.

Division of the Stomach and Pancreas

Locally destructive but not irreparable steps must now be taken. The stomach and pancreas are divided; the former at its midpoint, the latter at the junction of the body and tail (Fig. 5). Hemigastrectomy and vagotomy are important in preventing late gastrojejunal ulceration. Division of the pancreas through its tail provides a small stump which can be invaginated safely into the open end of the jejunum.

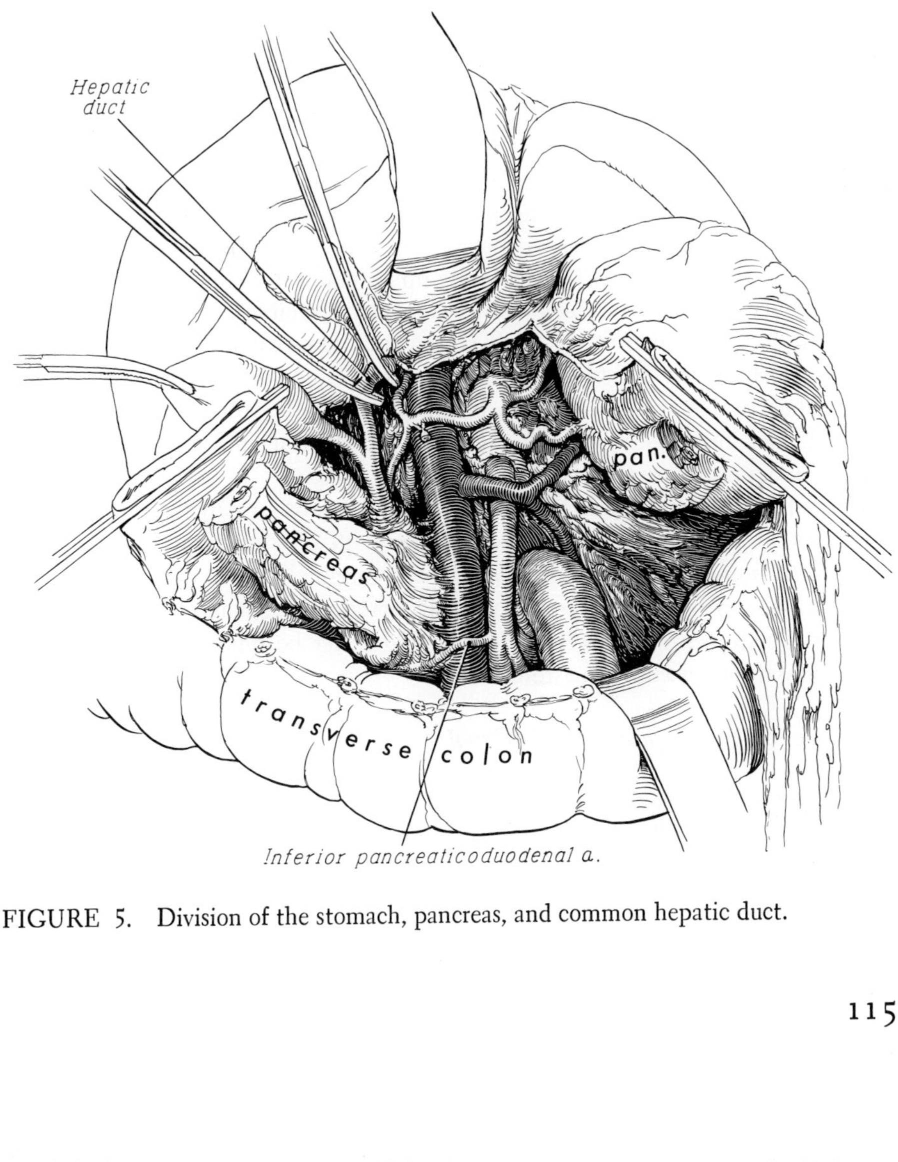

FIGURE 5. Division of the stomach, pancreas, and common hepatic duct.

Division of the stomach and pancreas allows reflection of the distal segments of these organs to the patient's right, thus exposing the portal venous groove of the pancreas. Here cautious sharp and blunt dissection frees the pancreatic head and uncinate process from the portal vein. Division of the inferior pancreaticoduodenal artery simplifies mobilization of the uncinate process from behind the portal vein. Dissection here is tedious and often exasperating because of small, short veins from the pancreas which empty directly into the portal and superior mesenteric veins. These should be divided between fine hemostats, because they bleed copiously if inadvertently torn from the portal vein.

Even at this point retreat from the operation is graceful should the portal vein and superior mesenteric artery be compromised by tumor; the spleen and the tail of the pancreas are removed and the stomach is sewed together again. Numerous efforts have been made to resect a portal vein invaded by tumor. The best of these is partial venous resection and closure; the poorest is an end-to-side anastomosis between the superior mesenteric vein and the vena cava. A complete portacaval shunt under these circumstances is inevitably followed by serious protein intolerance and ammonia intoxication. Intermediate steps such as venous autograft, resection of the right colon, or the Child two-stage resection of the portal vein have not achieved any very significant popularity. When these steps become necessary, hope of cure has been lost.

Division of the Common Hepatic Duct and Jejunum

The distal stomach, the gallbladder, the body, head, and uncinate process of the pancreas, and the duodenum having been mobilized, the common hepatic duct is divided about a centimeter or two below the junction of right and left hepatic ducts and attention promptly turned to the upper jejunum. This and its mesentery are divided about 6 to 10 cm. below the ligament of Treitz (Fig. 6). In effect this ligament is destroyed, permitting ready passage of the proximal jejunum and distal duodenum behind the superior mesenteric vessels. The surgical specimen is now free and the distal stomach, the head, body, and uncinate process of the pancreas, the gallbladder and common duct, the entire duodenum, and a few centimeters of the upper jejunum are removed together.

One of Dr. Allen O. Whipple's major contributions to pancreatectomy is his insistence that *all vessels should be ligated and all anastomoses should be performed with nonabsorbable suture material.* He originally recommended silk, but cotton, nylon, and fine steel wire are also appropriate. Catgut if used at all should only approximate mucosal layers. Catgut should never be relied upon for ligature of major vessels or for entire anastomoses.

Reconstruction of the Gastroenteric Canal

Reconstruction of the gastroenteric canal involves pancreaticojejunostomy, choledochojejunostomy, and gastrojejunostomy. Pancreatic and biliary are placed above gastric anastomoses lest Mann-Williamson ulcers in the gastrojejunostomy be encouraged. Extensive dissection in the base of the transverse mesocolon usually

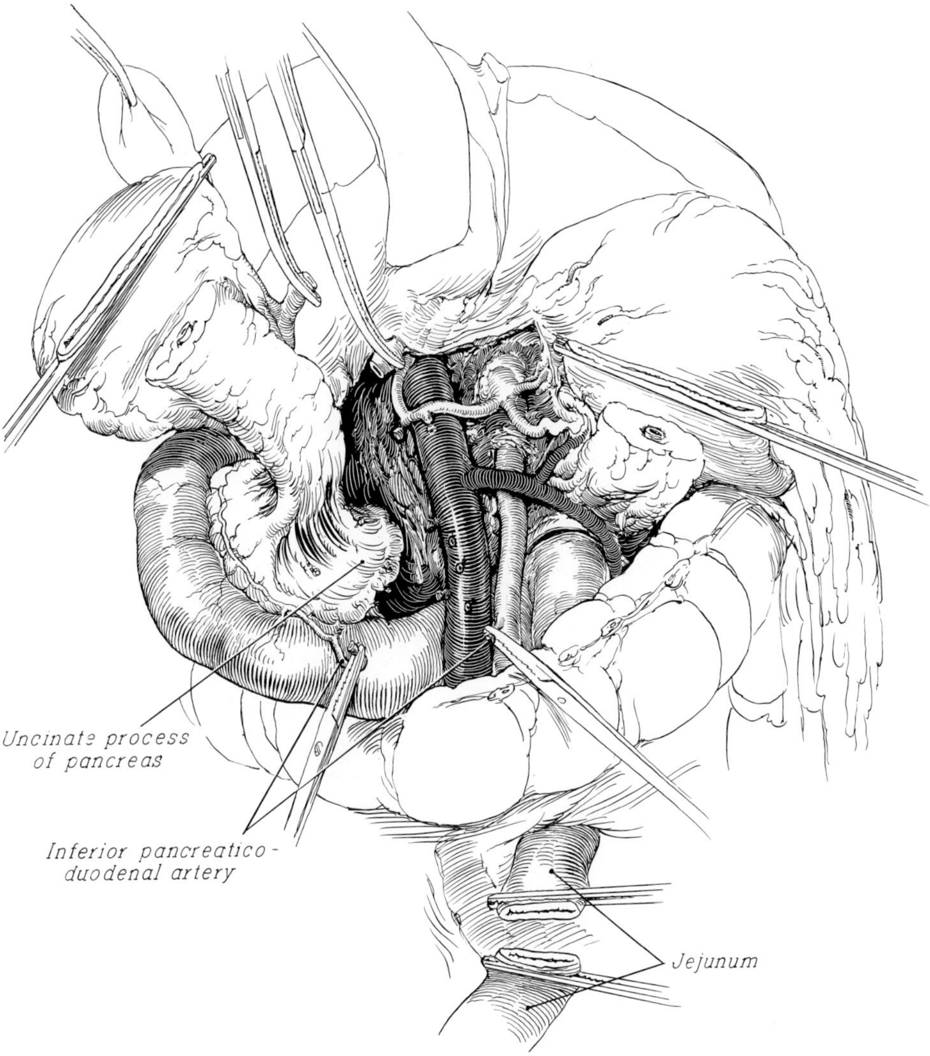

FIGURE 6. Division of the jejunum and inferior pancreaticoduodenal artery, and final mobilization of the entire specimen.

provides a wide rent in this structure which readily permits passage of the distal jejunum from the lower into the upper abdomen in the retrocolic position. Here biliary and pancreatic anastomoses are performed. Gastric drainage, however, is more easily secured anterior to the colon.

PANCREATICOJEJUNOSTOMY. Two techniques are available: end-to-end pancreaticojejunostomy (Fig. 7) or end-to-side pancreaticoductal anastomosis (Fig. 8). Few clear reasons indicate superiority of one of these anastomoses over the other. Both function and both are safe. Probably operators should acquire proficiency in both so that selection can be based upon the size of the pancreatic stump. If large,

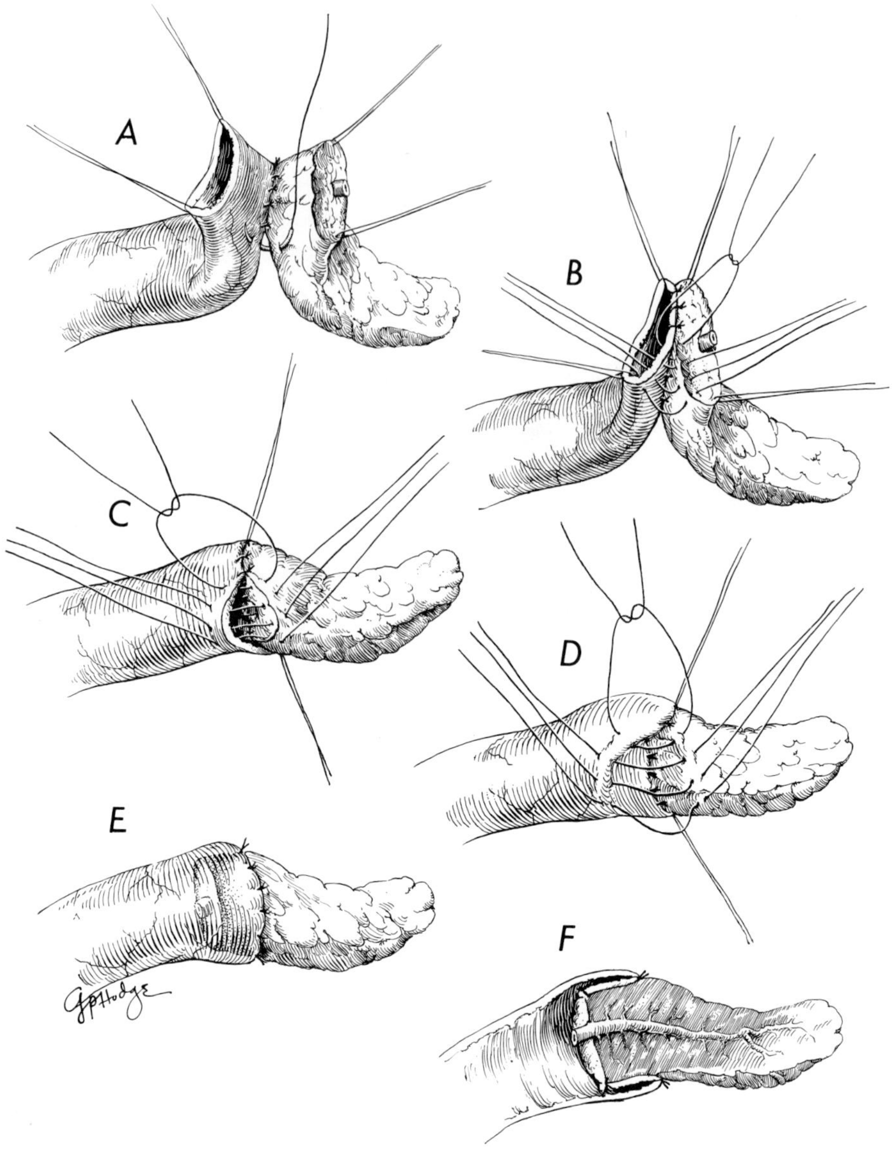

FIGURE 7. End-to-end pancreaticojejunostomy (invagination).

the stump is not invaginated easily into the open end of the jejunum and a ductal anastomosis should be employed. This, of course, requires end-to-end choledocho-jejunostomy (Fig. 8) rather than a biliary anastomosis in the end-to-side position (Fig. 9).

Choledochojejunostomy. This anastomosis is generally not difficult, since in the majority of patients with pancreaticoduodenal cancer the common hepatic duct is large and substantial. Standard varieties of these anastomoses are depicted

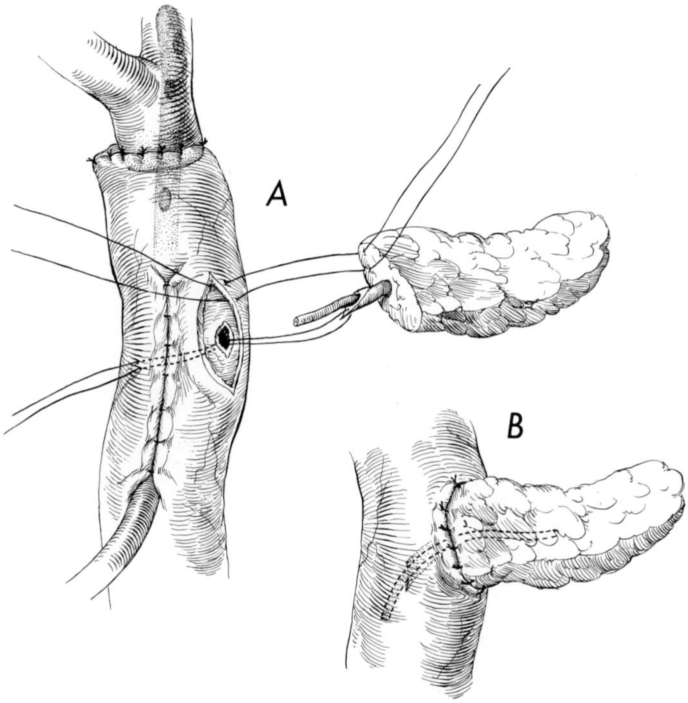

FIGURE 8. End-to-side pancreaticojejunostomy and end-to-end choledochojejunostomy.

in Figures 8 and 9. Each implies a double layer of nonabsorbable suture material and each is protected by a Witzel-type choledochostomy tube placed across the anastomosis.

Choledochojejunostomies should always be protected during early healing by some form of decompressive tube—either T tube or catheter. Leaks expose patients to bile peritonitis or choledochocutaneous fistulas.

Biliary enteric anastomosis must occasionally be performed if the common duct is normal. Small diameters and fragile walls support surgical anastomosis with the small bowel poorly. After unfortunate experiences with a variety of direct anastomoses, implantation has proved most successful (Fig. 10). Through a small stab wound the common duct is pulled within the lumen of the gut and anchored in place with two traction sutures. Reinforcement is secured by a row of serosal interrupted sutures of 5–0 silk. These anastomoses also are protected by a trans-anastomotic T tube or catheter during the early period of healing (Fig. 10).

Choledochoenteric anastomosis is the weakest link in pancreaticoduodenectomy. If jaundice, chills, and fever develop late in the postoperative course, recurrent cancer should never be assumed. Stricture at the site of choledochojejunostomy should be suspected and reoperation urged lest an occasional patient die unnecessarily of ascending cholangitis and hepatic sepsis.

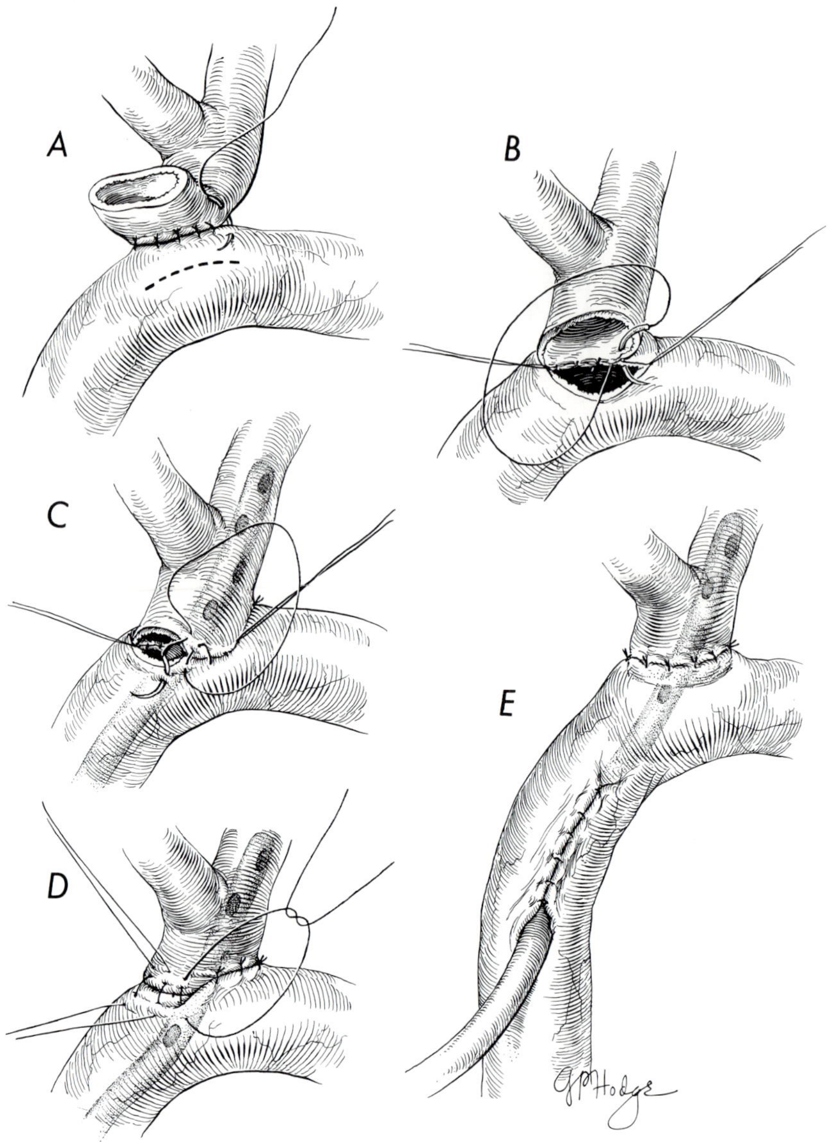

FIGURE 9. End-to-side choledochojejunostomy.

Gastrojejunostomy. This is the conventional type and usually is best fashioned anterior to the colon (Fig. 11).

Rent in Mesocolon. This is closed with a few interrupted sutures lest small bowel herniate into the upper abdomen and strangulate (Fig. 11).

Vagotomy. Both vagus nerves are divided to insure further that anastomotic ulceration will not mar the late postoperative course.

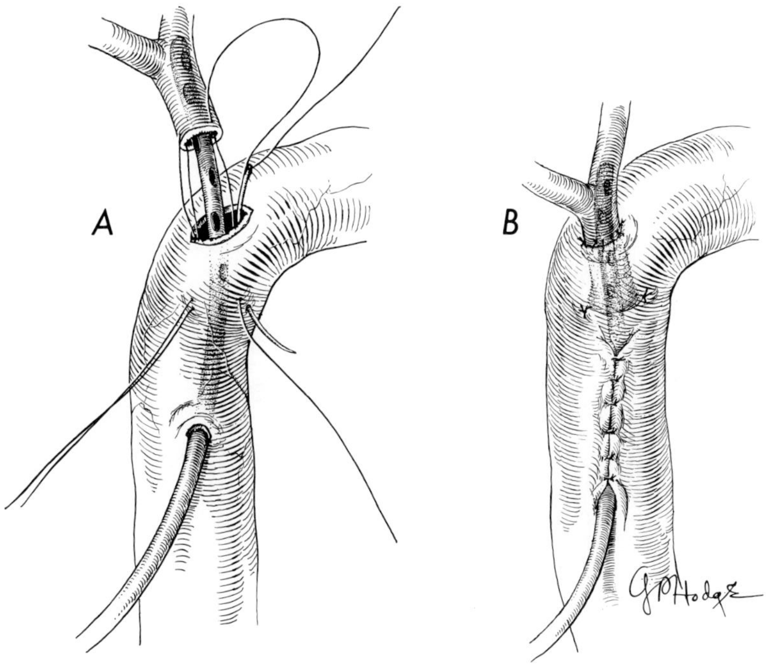

FIGURE 10. End-to-side implantation of a normal common duct into the jejunum.

Drainage

Three large cigarette drains are brought out through a generous stab wound in the right flank, one placed to the right gutter and one each to the choledochal and pancreatic anastomoses. The choledochal catheter is brought out through the abdominal wall through another stab wound. The abdominal wound is closed in layers (see last section of this chapter).

Subtotal Distal Pancreatectomy for Nonmalignant Disease of the Pancreas

Islet cell adenomas, cystadenomas (rarely cystadenocarcinomas), fibrocalcific pancreatitis, and traumatic pancreatitis may all require resection of generous segments of the distal pancreas without sacrifice of the duodenum or ampulla of Vater. There is compelling incentive to preserve these two structures if that is at all consistent with cure of the patient's primary disease. Not only is the duodenum an important digestive organ, but a normal common duct and ampulla of Vater are the only real insurances against ascending cholangitis and pyogenic hepatitis.

Two surgical objectives are sought in this form of subtotal pancreatectomy:

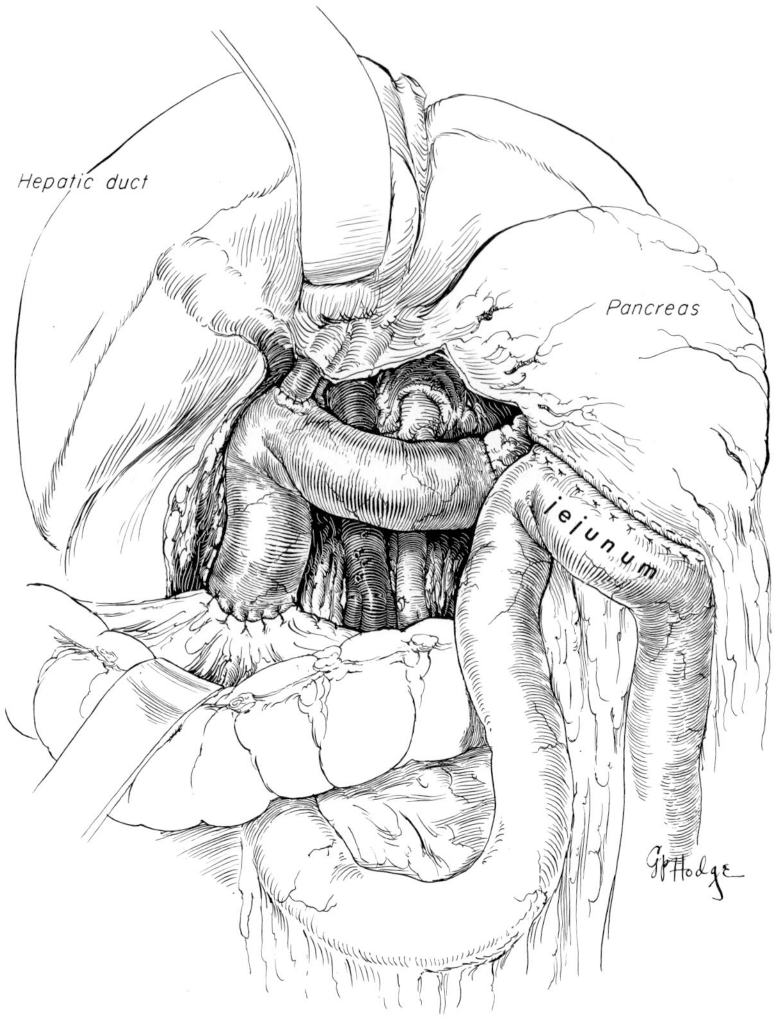

FIGURE 11. Gastroenteric reconstruction completed by antecolic gastrojejunostomy.

preservation of a cuff of normal pancreas 1 by 2 by 3 cm. within the lesser curvature of the duodenum and retention of either the superior or the inferior pancreaticoduodenal arteries.

Technique

The abdomen is entered best through a long oblique incision extending from the left costal margin to the right flank. Other conventional vertical or transverse incisions are acceptable, but do not offer as complete exposure of the pancreas as does the oblique incision.

Dissection is commenced by dividing the entire gastrocolic ligament, including the vascular colosplenic attachments. The stomach is reflected superiorly and the colon depressed inferiorly, thus exposing the entire pancreas (Fig. 12).

The spleen is freed from its peripheral vascular and peritoneal attachments, but its pedicle is not disturbed. If readily accessible, the splenic artery is ligated near the celiac axis (Fig. 12). Though not essential, this precaution may appreciably diminish blood loss as the spleen and pancreas are further mobilized.

After mobilization, both the spleen and the tail of the pancreas are reflected toward the patient's right side, thereby exposing the posterior body and portal venous groove of the pancreas (Fig. 13). Special care, particularly in pancreatitis, is necessary in freeing the body, head, and uncinate process of the pancreas from the superior mesenteric vessels. Sometimes this is impossible by usual methods, and dissection by knife becomes necessary. By sharp dissection, adherent pancreas is literally shaved from the portal and superior mesenteric vessels. Particular attention is paid to identification and preservation of the superior and inferior

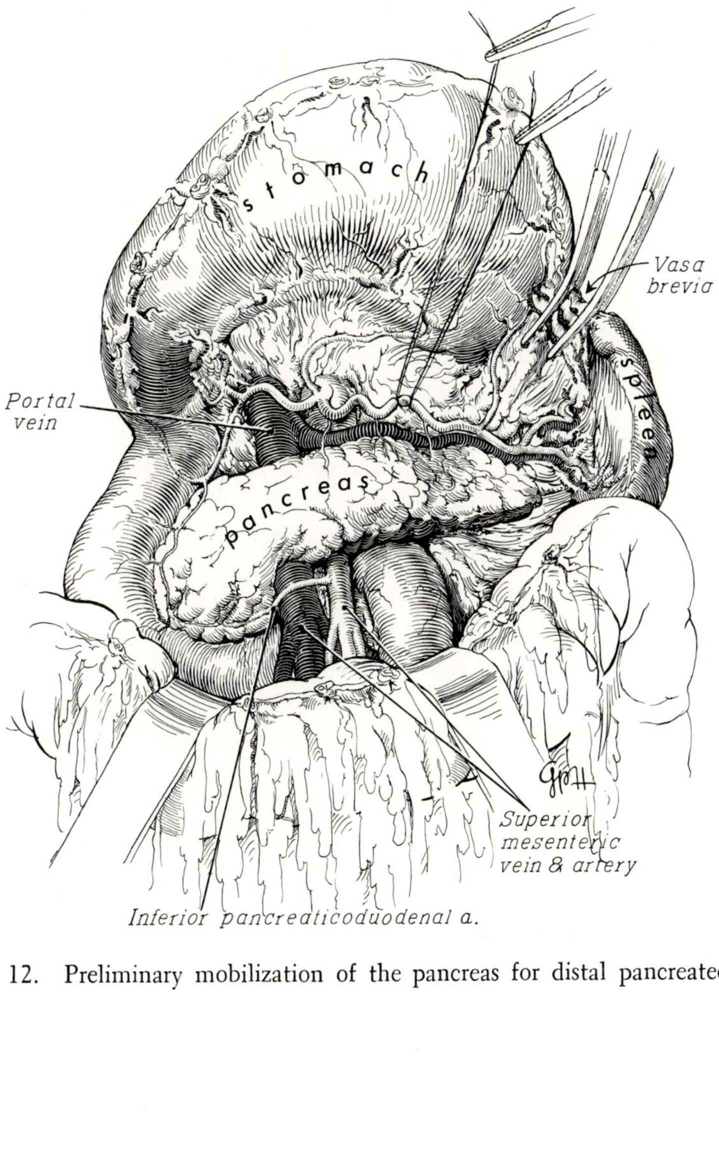

FIGURE 12. Preliminary mobilization of the pancreas for distal pancreatectomy.

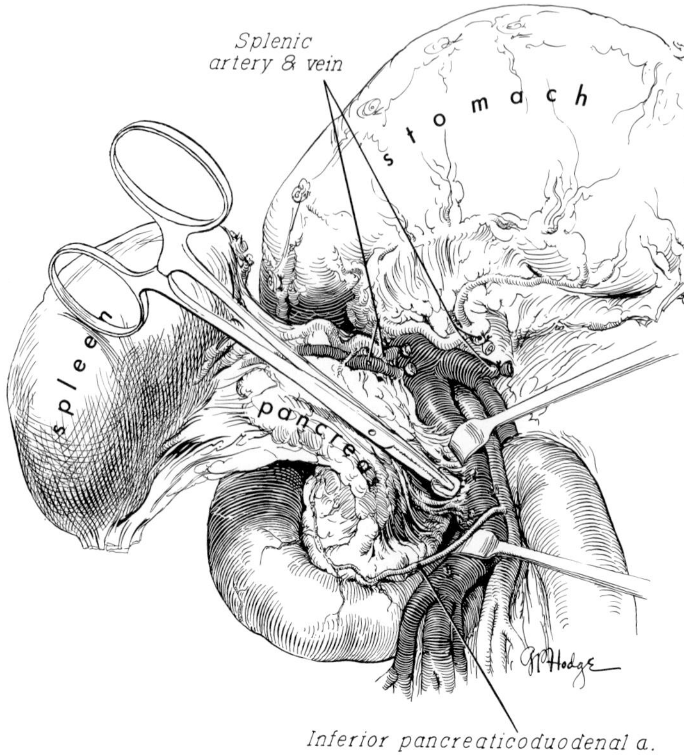

FIGURE 13. Mobilization of the spleen and the tail and body of the pancreas, and partial mobilization of the head and uncinate process of the pancreas.

pancreaticoduodenal arteries. If both of these vessels are divided, duodenal necrosis may defeat the major objective of this type of pancreatectomy: retention of the duodenum, lower common duct, and ampulla of Vater.

The mobilized spleen and pancreas are temporarily returned to their normal positions and separation of the pancreatic head from the lesser duodenal curve is commenced (Fig. 14). This is accomplished by sharp dissection between fine straight hemostats. During this dissection the position of the common bile duct is emphasized by intubating it with a woven silk catheter. A cuff of pancreas about 1 by 2 by 3 cm. is left undisturbed along the inner border of the duodenum (Fig. 14). This protects patients from the particularly capricious diabetes which follows total pancreatectomy.

Two cigarette drains are placed, one in the right gutter and one in the bed of the pancreas. These are brought out through a stab wound in the right flank. Further drainage may be achieved by a single drain placed in the splenic fossa and brought out in the left flank. A T tube is left in the common duct and brought out through a suitable, but separate, small stab wound.

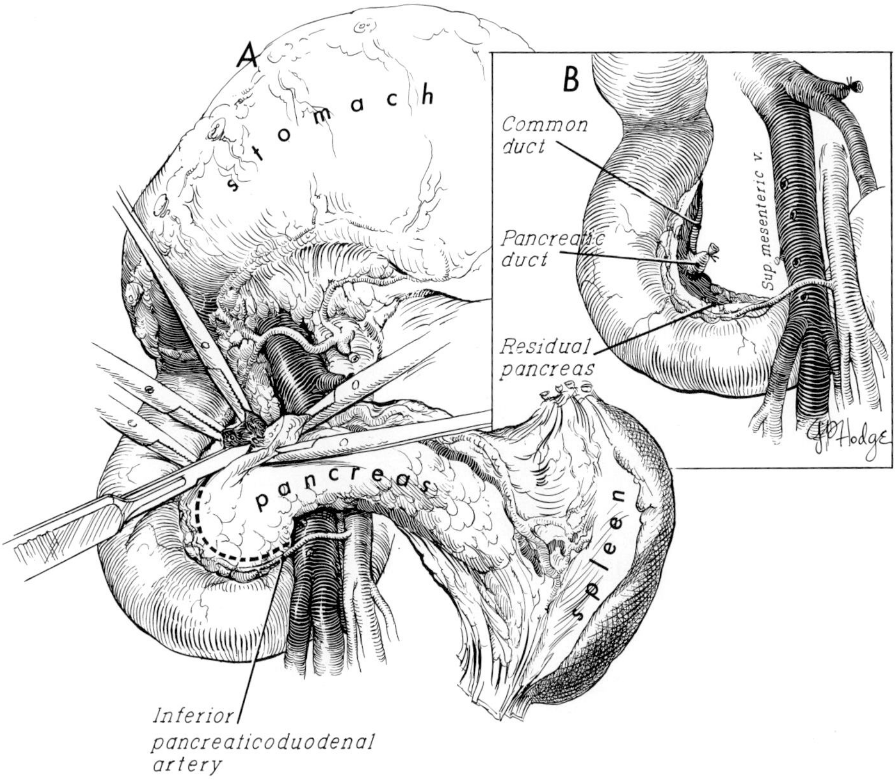

FIGURE 14. Separation of the head of the pancreas from the lesser curvature of the duodenum.

Closure of Abdominal Incisions Following Pancreatectomy

Most patients requiring pancreatectomy are debilitated, have often lost large amounts of weight, and are in negative nitrogen balance. They can ill afford postoperative dehiscence of their abdominal wound. Protection from this catastrophe can be provided by stay sutures of No. 28 stainless steel wire which include all layers of the abdominal wall except the skin and subcutaneous tissue. The posterior fascia and peritoneum may be closed with either continuous 0 chromicized catgut or interrupted fine steel sutures. Anterior fascia is approximated with No. 30 stainless steel wire or 00 cotton. Underlying viscera are protected from inadvertent inclusion in the through-and-through stays by holding these sutures taut during closure of the peritoneum and posterior fascia as well as while they are being tied. These should be tied snugly but not tight. If they are too tight, edema developing postoperatively may cause massive wound strangulation and defeat the very purpose

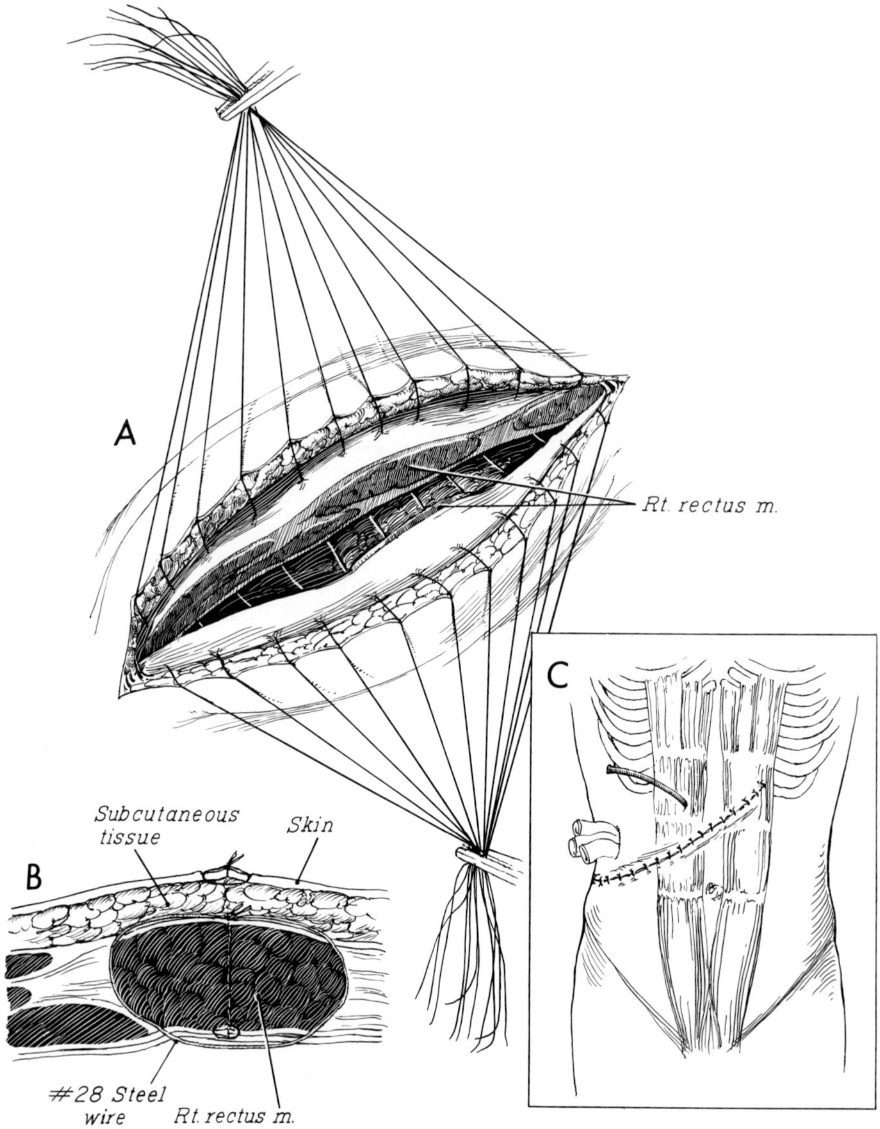

FIGURE 15. Abdominal closure employing buried through-and-through sutures.

of these sutures. Should wounds closed in this fashion become infected, they may be opened widely without risk of dehiscence. If stainless steel wire is used throughout, prolonged extrusion of suture material is avoided (Fig. 15).

References

DOUBILET, H., and MULHOLLAND, J. H. Surgical treatment of chronic pancreatitis. *J.A.M.A.* 175:177, January 21, 1961.

DuVal, M. K., Jr., and Enquist, I. F. The surgical treatment of chronic pancreatitis by pancreaticojejunostomy: an 8-year reappraisal. *Surgery* 50:965, December 1961.

Gillesby, W. J., and Puestow, C. B. Pancreaticojejunostomy for chronic relapsing pancreatitis: an evaluation. *Surgery* 50:859, November 1961.

Warren, K. W., and Cattell, R. B. Pancreatic surgery. *New England J. Med.* 261:280, 333, 387, August 6, 13, and 20, 1959.

Zollinger, R. M., Elliott, D. W., Endahl, G. L., Goswitz, J. T., Grant, G. N., and Taft, D. A. Origin of the ulcerogenic hormone in endocrine-induced ulcer. *Ann. Surg.* 156:570, October 1962.

98. *Pancreatic Resection*

MILTON R. PORTER

THE PANCREAS is in many ways a more difficult organ to manage surgically than other viscera. It is situated at a complex anatomical crossroad where its central position provides lymphatic drainage radially along several major routes (the splenic, hepatic, and superior mesenteric vessels). This makes it harder to design an operation which, in an orderly manner, removes primary, secondary, and tertiary nodal groups. Moreover, the intimate association of the pancreas with the major vessels of the epigastrium at once limits the extent of the procedure and dictates what must be removed. Thus, when a tumor spreads a short distance to involve the portal vein or the superior mesenteric artery it becomes incurable. Similarly, if the gland is removed, the need to excise the vessels which go with it makes removal of the spleen and duodenum necessary.

If only part of the gland is removed, or if the gland is incised, safe management of any draining pancreatic juice becomes a matter of primary importance since the enzymes, if allowed to remain in the abdomen, may wreak havoc. A first principle of pancreatic surgery is, therefore, the provision of adequate drainage. Secondly, since catgut is a protein substance which is rapidly digested by trypsin, it cannot be trusted as a ligature on major vessels or as a suture material for closing the abdomen. Silk, cotton, wire, or nylon is safer.

Technique of Total Pancreatectomy

Apart from the usual preparatory measures, it is well to be certain that candidates for pancreatic resection are not deficient in vitamin K if they are jaundiced; that there is a reasonable quantity of blood on call (the average pancreatectomy requires 1000 to 1500 cc. in the operating room); and that the patient understands in advance that he may be rendered diabetic.

The Incision

The operation is usually done through a bilateral subcostal incision with the incision longer on the right than on the left. In persons with unusually narrow costal angles, a vertical incision is made. The reasons for preferring transverse incisions in most patients are that they provide easier access to the lateral aspect of the duodenum without sacrificing good exposure of the spleen and the tail of the pancreas; they tend to run more nearly in the axis of the pancreas itself; they are relatively simple to make; and they are less apt to be complicated by weakness or intestinal obstruction postoperatively. In making the transverse incision it is well to keep it two fingerbreadths from the costal margin since this provides greater postoperative comfort and consequently better ventilation of the lung bases than would obtain otherwise.

Diagnosis in the Operating Room

One of the most difficult problems in pancreatic surgery is the differentiation between carcinoma of the head of the pancreas and chronic pancreatitis. This problem rarely occurs when the patient is jaundiced, but is more apt to come up because of a chance finding when the patient is being operated upon for other reasons. There is a small percentage of cases of carcinoma of the pancreas in which the tumor is very small and hidden in the midst of a virtually ligneous gland which is totally involved in fibrotic pancreatitis. In these instances, the diagnosis may elude discovery until the gland reaches the surgical pathology laboratory or autopsy table—no matter how great an effort is made to obtain a specimen of the growth for biopsy. Moreover, certain tumors in this area present the pathologist with a very difficult problem in identification on frozen section. It is well to remember that in the absence of *acute* inflammation and/or gallstones, solid, hard, noncystic masses in the head of the pancreas associated with obstructive jaundice and dilatation of the common bile duct are rarely due to pancreatitis and are *usually* carcinoma. Conversely, hard, noncystic masses involving a major part of the retroampullary part of the gland and unassociated with jaundice and dilatation of the biliary tree are *usually* pancreatitis. Small areas of induration in the head of the pancreas are *usually* benign, and because they are small they are more amenable to precisely placed biopsies (needle or knife) than larger masses.

Obviously, these generalizations, although helpful, will not serve to differentiate certain carcinomas from chronic pancreatitis. The surgeon must then decide whether to try to establish a diagnosis by doing frozen section biopsies. Each operator will quite properly be influenced by his own and his pathologist's experience in this field as well as by the clinical situation.

The policy in our clinic relative to biopsy can be briefly stated as follows:

1. All ampullary and small duodenal lesions are subject to biopsy through a duodenotomy. This must be done because benign growths occur in the area and gallstones impacted at the ampulla can exactly simulate tumors.

2. All inoperable tumors are diagnosed before the surgeon leaves the operating room, even if the job is time-consuming. This takes the matter out of the realm of doubt—an especially important point when a palliative procedure restores the patient to relatively good health for a long period and doubt is raised as to the diagnosis. A biopsy positive for carcinoma, on file, may then prevent a fruitless second laparotomy.

3. Frozen sections are made of lymph nodes peripheral to the proposed specimen to help establish operability.

4. Primary intrapancreatic growths are rarely subjected to biopsy when operable. (This does not necessarily apply when cystic tumors are present. They are managed differently.)

The arguments supporting these policies have been published previously. They include the following:

1. Representative sections from the pancreas are often hard to obtain because of confusion between tumor and surrounding pancreatitis.

2. Interpretation of frozen section biopsies of the pancreas may be difficult because some desmoplastic carcinomas closely resemble chronic pancreatitis.

3. The establishment of diagnosis by means of frozen section biopsies is often time-consuming and traumatic.

When a pancreatic biopsy is done, the operator should make great efforts to avoid the major pancreatic ducts and vessels, whose typical anatomy must be well fixed in mind. Hemorrhage when encountered is often profuse and difficult to control. Silk mattress sutures are more effective than clamping and tying. Chromic catgut should not be used, since it may digest rapidly in the presence of trypsin spilled by the gland. As previously explained, pancreatic wounds should be drained.

Assessment of Operability and Choice of Procedure

Briefly stated, the lesion is considered inoperable if there are distant metastases, invasion of the major blood vessels (especially the portal vein), or extension beyond the area of the usual pancreatectomy specimen. Experience with extended resections has proved the futility of developing a more radical block than that of a total pancreatectomy.

Apart from the usual exploration of the abdomen, special care should be used in searching for involved lymph nodes in the area of the root of the small bowel mesentery, the celiac axis, and the middle colic vessels. A surprisingly large number of patients are found to have metastases below the transverse mesocolon in the root of the small intestinal mesentery and no metastases above the pancreas. Suspicious nodes in these areas should be examined by frozen section; if they are involved, there is no point in resecting. Positive nodes in the areas to be included in the specimen are no contraindication to resection. There are usually large, rubbery, greenish nodes behind the common duct in these patients; they are much less apt to reveal metastases than are smaller, harder nodes from the area under discussion.

In assessing operability, the lesser sac is entered through the gastrocolic omentum, and a thoroughgoing mobilization of the duodenum and pancreatic head is done (Kocher maneuver). This not only reveals invasion of the lumbar gutter structures such as the vena cava, if such invasion exists, but also facilitates examination of the portal vein and superior mesenteric artery and their relationship to the tumor. The artery can be felt with the fingers behind the gland. If the tumor invades it or completely surrounds it posteriorly, the case is considered inoperable. The portal vein cannot be felt, but it lies anterior and to the right of the artery (i.e. closer to the operator); hence, if that area is involved in tumor it is best to check the vein more carefully. This is done from the anterior aspect of the gland. First, the superior mesenteric vein is found just above the mesocolon where it ducks beneath the pancreatic neck. It can be rapidly located by following the middle colic vein to the point where it enters the superior mesenteric. As soon as it goes beneath the pancreas, the superior mesenteric is joined by the splenic to form the portal, which emerges from beneath the superior border of the pancreas. There are almost never any tributaries to the anterior surfaces of these veins behind the pancreas, and instruments and fingers can be gently inserted anterior to the portal vein to assess tumor invasion. Some prefer to enter this passage from above; if this is done, division of the gastroduodenal artery may facilitate the approach.

If the portal vein is invaded, the case is inoperable. Operable tumors located in the pancreas, whatever their cell type, are treated by total pancreatectomy. Operable tumors confined to the duodenum or ampulla are treated by resection of the head of the pancreas.

As has been previously reported, a review of our clinic's experience has shown that duodenal and ampullary lesions are often cured by resection of the head of the pancreas. On the other hand, a study of the cases of carcinoma of the pancreas has brought to light three facts all of which are interpreted as reasons for doing total pancreatectomy. (1) Microscopic, intraglandular strands of tumor have often been cut through at the time of partial resection. (2) Scattered microscopic foci of carcinoma have been found in the tail of the gland after total resection for carcinoma of the head of the pancreas. (3) Postoperative management of the totally pancreatectomized patient is not nearly as difficult as had been thought. To these reasons can be added our admitted prejudice against partially resecting any gland harboring a carcinoma.

One is rarely called upon to resect a carcinoma which has arisen in the tail of the gland, since such growths are virtually always inoperable by the time they come to attention. Benign lesions and cystic lesions often require resection of the tail only.

The Resection

The gastrocolic omentum is opened and the short gastric vessels are divided and ligated.

The spleen is then mobilized from its posterolateral attachments. Its pedicle is divided and ligated and it is removed, thus reducing the bulk of the specimen and getting rid of an organ which often oozes blood from its posterior bare areas. The accompanying illustrations show the spleen attached in order to make the relations clear.

The tail of the pancreas and the splenic vessels are mobilized as one unit. One should never try to take the tail of the pancreas out and spare the splenic vessels. Too many tiny tributaries and branches would have to be managed, and saving the spleen is not worth the time or effort.

At this stage it is usually best to divide the stomach to provide better exposure for subsequent pancreatic mobilization. Resection of the stomach and part or all of the pancreas (which contributes the major share of alkali to the intestinal tract) predisposes to marginal ulceration in long-term survivors. For this reason it is preferable to remove all the antrum by dividing the stomach just above the incisura, rather than by dividing through the distal antrum as recommended by some. We have also recently added a complete subdiaphragmatic vagotomy to the operation. The dissection of the pancreatic tail then moves rapidly from left to right, and the point of origin of the splenic artery from the celiac axis is found and divided, care being taken to protect the axis itself and the hepatic artery.

The point of entry of the inferior mesenteric vein into the splenic varies rather widely. It is divided at the point where it enters the splenic. It sometimes enters the superior mesenteric; when it does, it is not disturbed. The splenic vein is divided just proximal to its junction with the portal (Fig. 1).

The gastroduodenal artery is then divided at its origin from the hepatic. The weight of the specimen and traction often tent the hepatic artery at this moment and invite damage to it. The anatomy should be clearly defined to prevent such damage. Lymph nodes which obscure the view may have to be cleaned away from the front surface of this vascular junction.

The common bile duct is then divided at a convenient level between clamps. Care must be taken not to divide it too close to the junction of the right and left

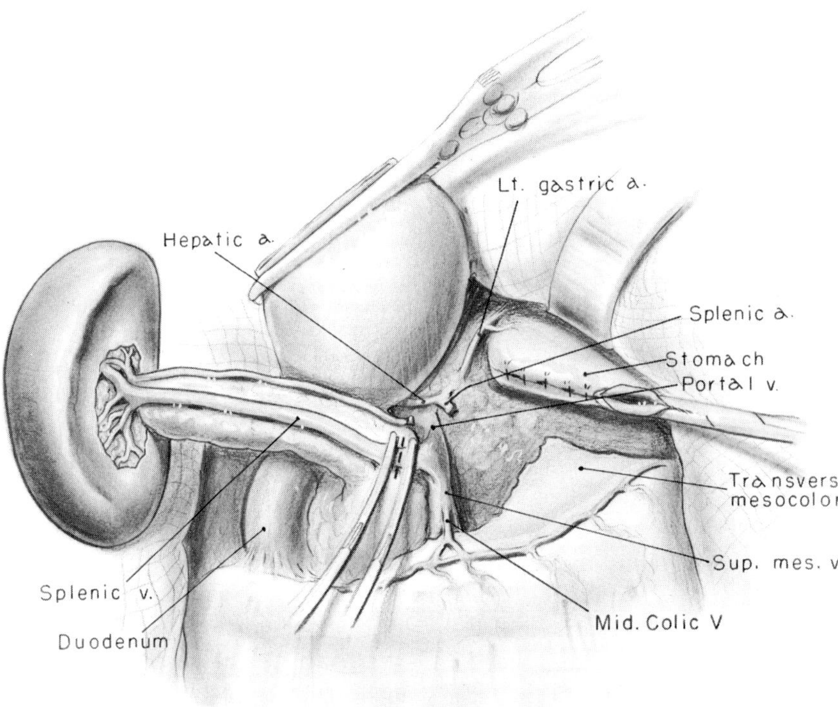

FIGURE 1. The splenic vein is clamped, cut, and ligated near its junction with the portal vein.

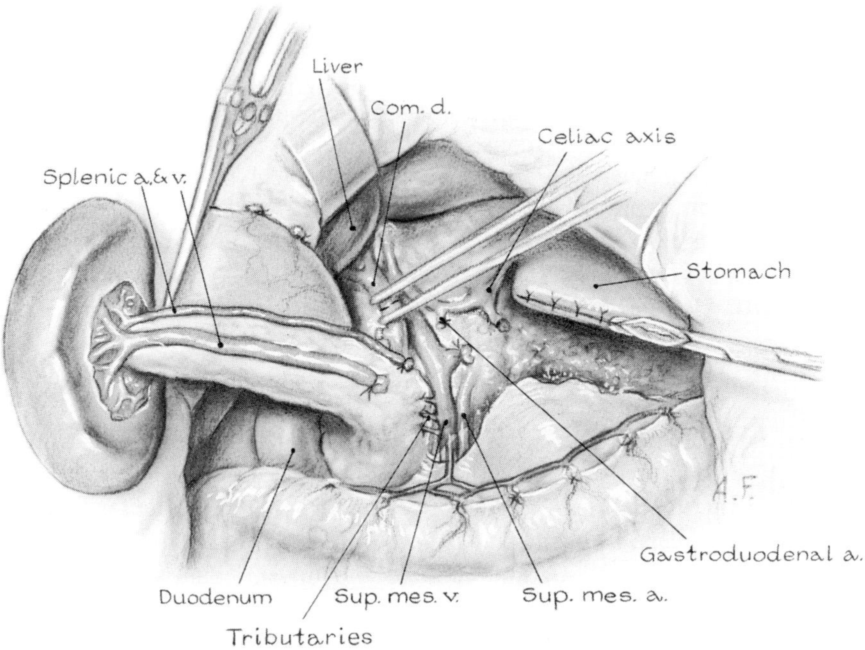

FIGURE 2. The common bile duct is clamped and cut.

hepatic ducts (Fig. 2). The gallbladder is removed. In the absence of an ampulla of Vater, the previously normal gallbladder is predisposed to develop cholecystitis and may subsequently need to be removed. Moreover, the cystic duct often implants at a low level, forcing cholecystectomy upon the operator.

The specimen now remains attached only by the bowel and vascular attachments. At this point it is best to free the bowel completely as it passes through the transverse mesocolon, by cutting the peritoneum around the circumference of the duodenum as it emerges from beneath the superior mesenteric vessels in the area of the duodenojejunal junction.

The left hand is then placed beneath the head of the pancreas and the specimen is folded to the patient's right and held by the operator's left thumb in front. The major tributaries from the uncinate process to the portal vein are gently "wiped into view" with "peanut" sponges, divided, and ligated. There are usually about four such tributaries, and they can be easily isolated and managed.

Occasionally at this point, with all bridges burned, the portal vein is found to be invaded. In this circumstance, we elect to cut through tumor to remove the specimen, leaving the vein undisturbed—such cases in our opinion being incurable. In the past it was decided to resect the portal vein in five patients. The vein ends were simply ligated and no anastomosis or shunt was done. All had uncomplicated postoperative courses but one, and he was found at autopsy to have a thrombosed hepatic artery. The other four died later of metastases. Since the retroperitoneal collateral circulation is adequate to manage the portal flow, we feel strongly that it is poor judgment to embark upon a portacaval shunt at this point.

The portal vein is retracted to the left with a vein retractor, and the dissection drops down one level to the bridge of tissue between the uncinate process and the superior mesenteric artery, which is defined by the left thumb anteriorly and the left forefinger behind the pancreas. Unlike the venous connections of the area, the arteries are not all easily demonstrated, and it has seemed easier and faster to divide the entire fibrofatty isthmus which contains them between serially placed clamps. Adson clamps are best for this purpose since they have fine curved points but are long enough to reach the area. Kelly clamps are too gross for this work. About nine pairs of clamps are needed. During this step the location of the superior mesenteric artery is constantly checked, using the left thumb and forefinger. This prevents damage to that vessel which, although palpable, is not usually clearly visible at this stage (Fig. 3). Figure 4 shows the anatomy of this area in cross-section.

It is always best to tie all clamps and tidy up the field before starting this step. Otherwise the wound will fill up with clamps and it is awkward to stop short of completion of the step. When the inferior pancreaticoduodenal artery is tied, often a bridge of tissue remains which binds the bowel to the vascular structures. This can best be defined by herniating some of the upper jejunum into the right upper quadrant beneath the mesenteric vessels. When the uppermost few vessels of the jejunal mesentery are divided the bowel slides easily into the subhepatic space where it can be divided to free the specimen (Fig 5). It is then anastomosed to the common hepatic duct.

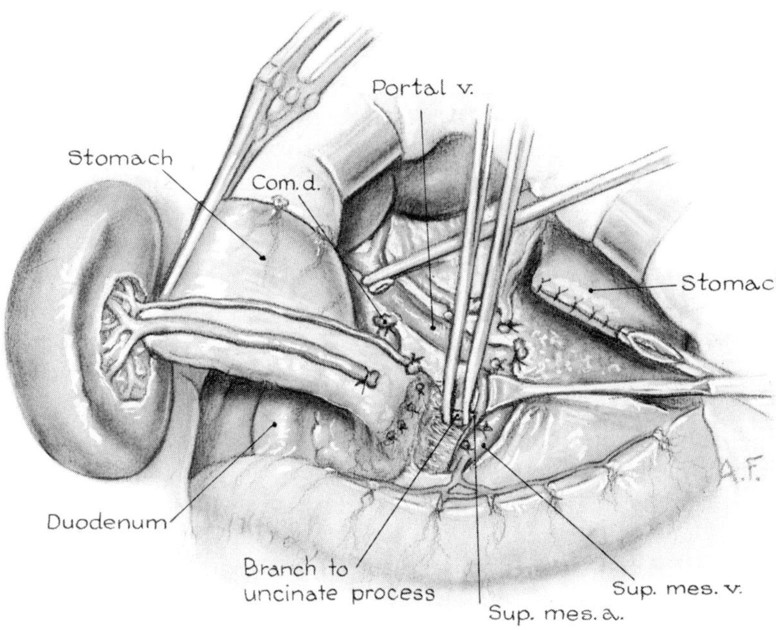

FIGURE 3. Dissection between the uncinate process and the superior mesenteric artery. The portal vein is retracted.

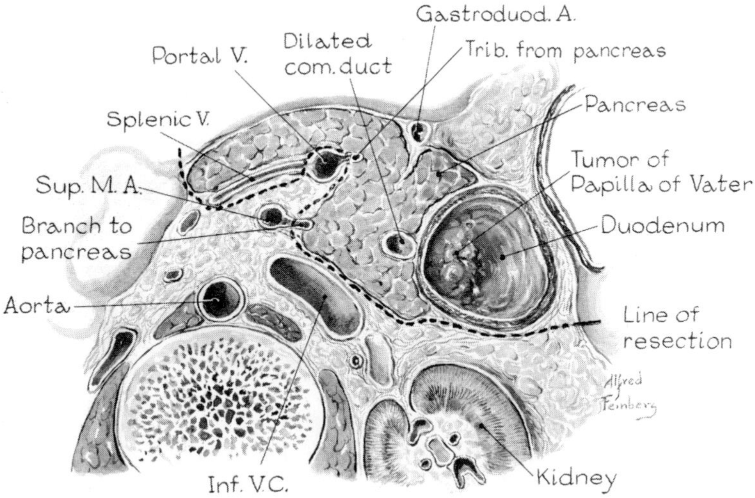

FIGURE 4. Cross-section diagram of the region of the head of the pancreas.

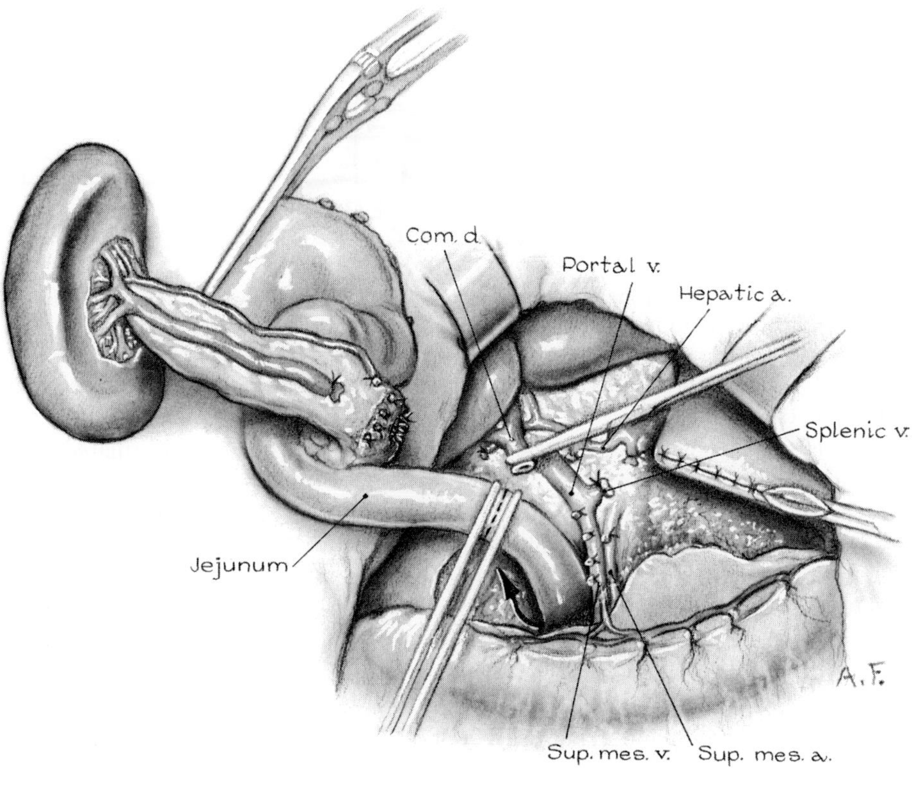

FIGURE 5. The jejunum is delivered through a rent in the mesocolon and divided.

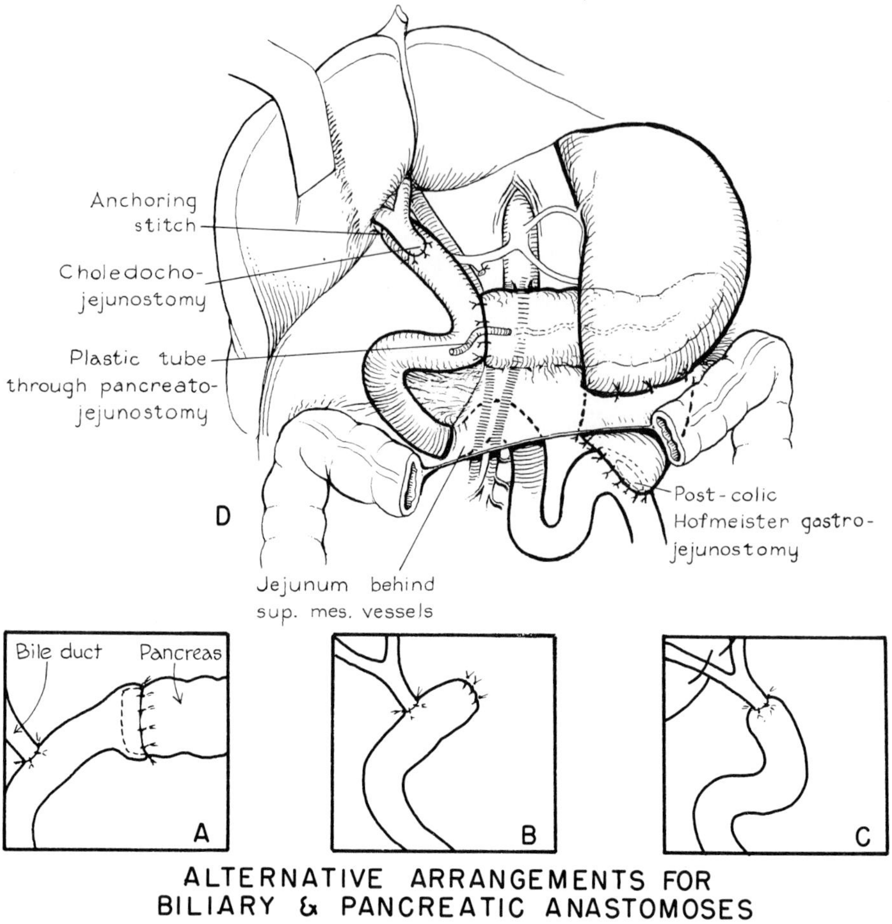

FIGURE 6. Biliary and pancreatic anastomoses. Unless the common bile duct is very large, it is better to put it into the side of the jejunal limb as in *A*, *B*, or *D*.

In many patients the diameter of the common hepatic duct may be as great as that of the jejunum, or even greater. In such cases an end-to-end anastomosis is done (Fig. 6C). Occasionally, however, the duct will not be very dilated, and in these patients it may be easier to close the end of the bowel and put the duct into the side of the jejunum as shown in Figure 6B and 6D. The arrangement in Figure 6B often proves less difficult technically.

In doing the choledochojejunostomy, 4–0 arterial silk mattress sutures are used as the outer layer, and the posterior row is placed while the common hepatic duct is still held in its clamp. The clamp is then cut off, insuring removal of all crushed tissue. The inner layer of 5–0 atraumatic chromic catgut is then put in as a continuous locked stitch through all layers. This insures an accurate mucosa-to-mucosa approximation and makes leakage less likely.

In the uncommon situations in which the duct is small or the tissues unusually friable, a T tube splint is used, but in the majority of instances it is not. It is interesting that in contrast to the patients with injured bile ducts upon whom plastic procedures are done (and in whom T tube splints are always used) late stenoses are rare. Recurrent tumor, however, has occluded the duct on occasion.

Some surgeons do not pull the small intestine up beneath the mesenteric vessels, but prefer to close the duodenojejunal junction as they close a duodenal stump and bring the jejunum in front of the colon to reach the duct. However, the more direct route recommended here seems to provide a more radical excision and requires one less suture line in the bowel. The mesocolon is reconstructed around the jejunum, and at a point about 14 inches below the choledochojejunostomy an antecolic or postcolic gastrojejunostomy is done according to any of the accepted techniques. The 14-inch distance insures against reflux of gastric content into the biliary tree, which sometimes predisposes to cholangitis.

The area of the biliary anastomosis is drained and the abdominal wound closed. The deeper layers may be closed with chromic catgut, but the external oblique and anterior rectus sheath are closed with figure-of-eight mattress sutures of No. 30 gauge stainless steel wire. When only part of the pancreas is removed and there is the possibility of leakage of pancreatic juice, it is especially important that all layers of the wound be closed with nonabsorbable suture material since catgut may be rapidly digested by the enzyme. For the same reason all intraabdominal ties and sutures are of silk.

A nasogastric tube is left in the stomach until there is evidence of return of peristaltic activity.

Technique of Partial Pancreatectomy (Head of the Pancreas)

When malignant tumors are confined to the duodenum and/or ampulla the operation of choice (after obtaining a positive biopsy) is resection of the head of the pancreas. This operation is done in the same manner as the total pancreatectomy except that the neck of the gland is divided and its tail and the spleen are left in. This requires an additional anastomosis between the tail of the pancreas and the jejunum.

There are two ways of doing this: end-to-end or end of pancreas to side of jejunum. Each method has to date resulted in a few late stenoses with resultant sprue, but ordinarily either method gives satisfactory results, and it seems hard to defend simply ligating and draining the cut end of the pancreas and not doing any anastomosis.

The end-to-end anastomosis is done by plugging the pancreatic stump into the jejunal lumen and holding it with silk sutures. No attempt is made to do a mucosa-to-mucosa anastomosis. When the end-to-side method is used, fine atraumatic catgut is used at the mucosal level, and silk sutures for the outer layer of the anastomosis. A short plastic catheter is left as a splint until the fine transfixion suture of chromic catgut which holds it dissolves and it is passed down the intestinal tract (Fig. 6D).

When a partial pancreatectomy is done and the tail of the gland remains in the abdomen a rubber tube drain is placed to the area of the pancreaticojejunostomy. It is held in exactly the correct position by a suture of 3–0 plain catgut. If profuse drainage occurs, a smaller tube can be suspended in it to provide sump drainage. There is rarely much drainage, and if it does occur it rapidly dries up.

Palliation

It is our opinion that pancreatic resection is too formidable a procedure to be employed for palliative purposes. If cure is impossible, cholecystojejunostomy is the preferred operation for biliary decompression since it is less apt to be obstructed by the expanding primary tumor. The likelihood of duodenal obstruction must always be considered and if it exists, or is impending, a gastrojejunostomy should be done. It is an unhappy situation to find that several months after having decompressed the biliary tree it is necessary to reoperate for duodenal obstruction. It is much wiser to anticipate the need and provide the solution at the first operation.

Pain, especially the characteristic backache, is not effectively managed by sympathectomy and is, we believe, best handled by narcotics. Unexpectedly, codeine and aspirin often seem to be more effective than Demerol or morphine.

Since most of these patients have complete obstruction of the alkaline pancreatic juice, they are prone to develop benign peptic ulcers of the duodenum and even hemorrhage from them. For this reason and especially because epigastric distress is difficult to interpret in such patients, the use of an antacid is recommended.

Postoperative Problems

Deepening Jaundice

When a biliary tree which has been completely obstructed for many weeks is suddenly decompressed it is usually found to contain light-yellow, watery bile. Within a few minutes it may become somewhat sanguineous in appearance or even grossly bloody. Occasionally the fluid which runs from the common duct or gallbladder may seem to contain more blood than bile, and the hemorrhage on a few occasions may reach alarming proportions. It has, in our experience, always stopped. The discharge seems to be analogous to the bleeding from the kidneys which occurs when long-standing urinary obstruction is suddenly relieved. The release of the dammed-up bile produces oozing from the walls of the bile passages. When this occurs jaundice may not improve or may even deepen for a few days, but within four or five days steady improvement is noted. Fortunately, this complication is not frequent, but it has been seen after both palliative cholecystojejunostomies and pancreatic resections. We have not felt it necessary to try to arrange for a slow release of the pressure.

Diabetes Following Total Pancreatectomy

Total pancreatectomy leaves the patient with a relatively mild type of diabetes which in the average case requires only about 30 units of insulin a day to control it. In only one instance in our clinic's experience has the diabetes been difficult to control. In general the management of total pancreatectomy patients is like the management of a mild diabetic who has had a gastrectomy.

The urine must be examined every six hours and standard insulin given as indicated. It is dangerous to try to switch to the long-acting type of insulin preparations until the patient's appetite and food intake have stabilized at reasonably normal levels. Chlorpropamide and tolbutamide are useless since their action depends upon the presence of pancreatic tissue.

Enzyme Replacement

The absence of pancreatic juice is compensated for by giving three pancreatin tablets (N.F.) with each meal. More may be used if evidence of greater need exists. Pancreatin powder (N.F.) is, if anything, more effective than the tablets but it is malodorous and unpleasant. Three teaspoonfuls are taken in any liquid (fruit juice is often preferred).

Sprue and/or Diabetes Following Partial Pancreatectomy

A few patients who have had the head of the pancreas resected with a pancreaticojejunostomy will develop sprue and/or diabetes after having been asymptomatic for 18 or more months. They lose weight and strength and give the impression of being patients whose tumors are metastasizing. Actually they may have developed stenosis of the pancreaticojejunostomies with the late development of sprue. The diabetes seems to be due to the loss of islets because of fibrosis in the remaining tail of the gland. Care must be taken to rule out sprue and diabetes in such patients, since these disorders might otherwise go unrecognized and the patients be thought to be dying of metastases. Proper treatment rapidly restores them to normal health.

Reference

Porter, M. R. Carcinoma of the pancreatico-duodenal area, operability and choice of procedure. *Ann. Surg.* 148:711, October 1958.

99. *Chronic Relapsing Pancreatitis*

KENNETH W. WARREN

LACK OF PRECISE KNOWLEDGE of the cause of chronic relapsing pancreatitis and of the factors responsible for progression of this fascinating and bewildering disease have combined to complicate the choice of a surgical procedure in its management. The wide variation in the pathological manifestations of the condition and the numerous complications, which frequently involve adjacent abdominal viscera, demand individualization in the selection of a suitable surgical procedure. Unfortunately, many theoretical concepts regarding the cause of chronic relapsing pancreatitis have led to the advocacy of certain operations which have limited value as therapy. Thus, confusion in this field of surgery is rampant.

Historically, the initial operations employed in the treatment of chronic relapsing pancreatitis were directed toward the biliary tract, stomach, or the sympathetic or parasympathetic nerves, or both, supplying the pancreatic region. The results, for the most part, were unsatisfactory, especially in cases of far-advanced disease. Because of these failures and as a result of increasing experience in pancreatic surgery, more direct operations were performed upon the pancreas for chronic relapsing pancreatitis. These direct procedures increased our knowledge of the basic pathology and led, in turn, to a more rational choice of a surgical maneuver in a particular circumstance. As experience accumulated in the surgical management of this disease at the Lahey Clinic, a wide choice of operations was correlated with the broad spectrum of the disease, as reflected by the clinical and gross pathological manifestations. The surgical procedures currently employed include (1) drainage—internal or external—of pancreatic cysts or abscesses; (2) sphincterotomy and retrograde dilatation of the ducts of Wirsung and Santorini; (3) transpancreatic exploration and manipulation of the ducts of Wirsung and Santorini; (4) anastomosis of the duct of Wirsung to a segment of the gastrointestinal tract; (5) distal pancreatectomy; (6) pancreatoduodenectomy; (7) total pancreatectomy, and (8) combined direct procedures.

Factors Determining the Choice of Surgical Procedure

Cumulative experience—including careful evaluation of the gross pathological changes involving the pancreas and adjacent organs at the time of abdominal exploration—retrograde and transductal pancreatography, careful dissection of the resected segments of the pancreas or the entire pancreas, and autopsy material all indicate that the central problem in chronic relapsing pancreatitis is interference with the flow of external pancreatic secretion into the duodenum. This obstruction occurs much more frequently within the pancreas than at the sphincter of Oddi. In many instances there is probably more than one point of obstruction, and on rare occasions innumerable points of obstruction may be present.

In no field of major abdominal surgery is there less justification for a rigid preconception regarding the surgical procedure to be employed in a given case than in chronic relapsing pancreatitis. The key to surgical therapy is careful evaluation of the nature and extent of the pathological changes as they involve the pancreas and the adjacent anatomical structures and individualization in the application of one or more surgical procedures aimed at overcoming the intrapancreatic obstruction. This principle is particularly pertinent when the patient is desperately ill and when the pancreatitis is accompanied by edema of the gland and surrounding structures. Prolonged and major manipulation of the edematous pancreas is an invitation to acute pancreatitis after operation. In contrast, the pancreas which is fibrotic and calcific will tolerate an inordinate amount of manipulation without significant postoperative reaction.

Drainage of Pancreatic Cysts or Abscesses

Of the patients with far-advanced chronic relapsing pancreatitis who come to the Lahey Clinic, approximately 25 per cent have associated pancreatic cysts. In most instances these are retention cysts and result from intrapancreatic obstruction, but pseudocysts which may or may not communicate with the pancreatic ductal system are observed. The cysts may be treated by external drainage, internal anastomosis to the posterior wall of the stomach or to a defunctionalized segment of the jejunum, distal pancreatectomy when the cyst is confined to the distal segment of the gland and is of the retention type, pancreatoduodenectomy when multiple cystic areas result from multiple points of obstruction in the head of the pancreas, and occasionally by sphincterotomy (as advocated by Doubilet) when a pseudocyst communicates with the main pancreatic duct. In a small group of cases it has been possible to drain a retention cyst in the head of the pancreas by sphincterotomy and retrograde manipulation through the duct of Wirsung. This is accomplished by thrusting the tip of the small Bakes dilator into the cyst through the duct of Wirsung. Following dilatation of the opening created in this fashion, a small catheter of polyethylene tubing may be inserted into the cystic cavity; the proximal segment of the tube is left in the lumen of the duodenum and the tubing will be passed within a few weeks.

Pancreatic abscesses and peripancreatic and chronic collections may be drained externally (Fig. 1a and b). It is important to remember that in many instances the peripancreatic necrosis extends retroperitoneally and may extend into the mediastinum, into the left or the right colonic gutter, and into the pelvis. These

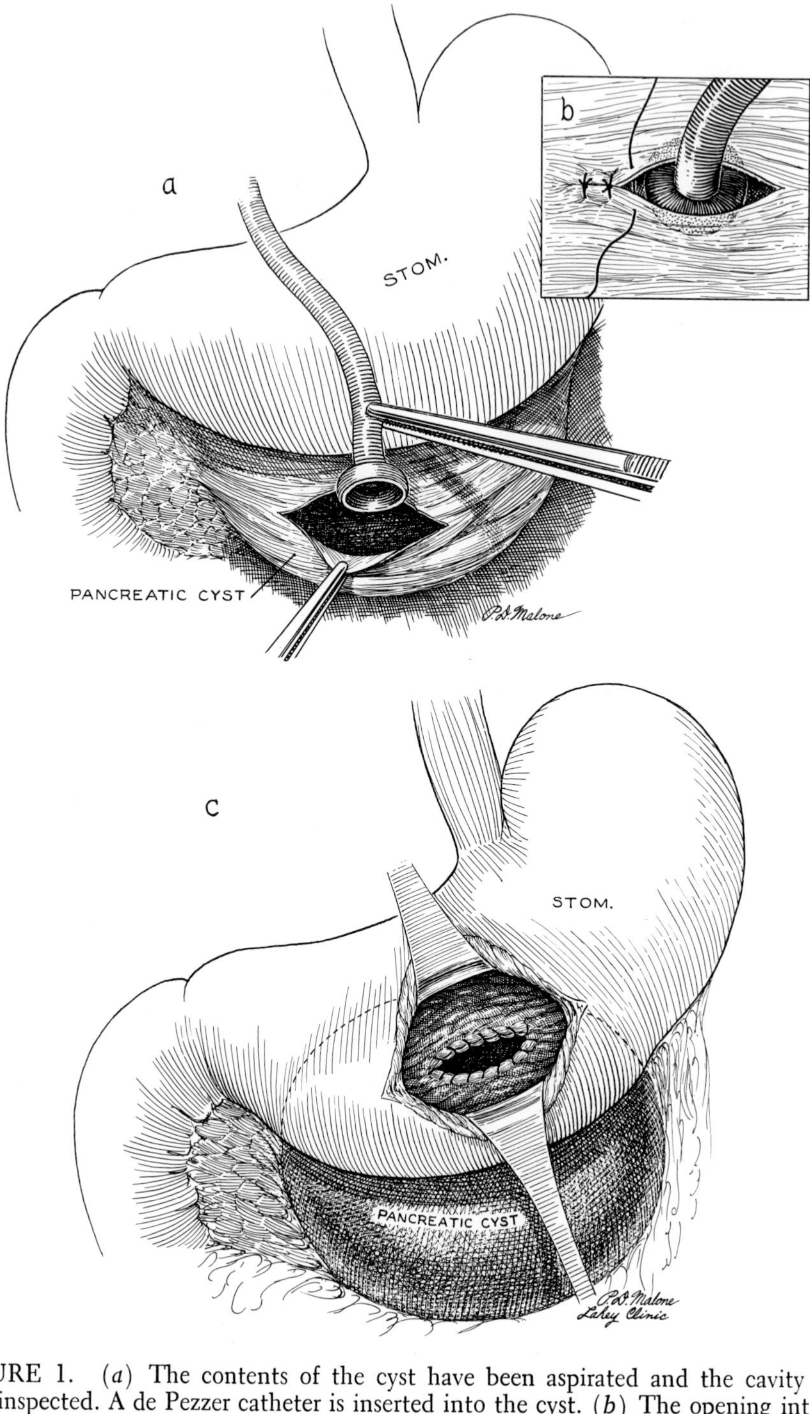

FIGURE 1. (*a*) The contents of the cyst have been aspirated and the cavity carefully inspected. A de Pezzer catheter is inserted into the cyst. (*b*) The opening into the cyst wall is closed around the catheter with interrupted sutures. The other end of the catheter is brought out through a stab wound. (*c*) Transgastric internal drainage of pancreatic cyst. The cyst has been exposed by dividing the gastrocolic ligament. Firm adherence of the posterior wall of the stomach to the anterior surface of the cyst is demonstrated. An incision is made in the anterior wall of the stomach. A trocar and cannula are inserted into the cyst through the adherent posterior gastric wall and the fluid contents removed. The opening is enlarged sufficiently to permit inspection of the cystic cavity. If no neoplastic elements are found, the edge of the opening into the cyst is encircled with a continuous interlocking catgut suture. The opening in the anterior gastric wall (not shown in the figure) is closed with a Connell suture of chromic catgut, reinforced with interrupted silk sutures.

areas of necrosis must be thoroughly drained. Frequently the location and extent of the pancreatic necrosis are obvious, but in other instances a diligent search must be made for isolated intraperitoneal collections. In determining areas of extension of retroperitoneal necrosis we have found it helpful to press on the suspected portion of parietal peritoneum while inspecting the primary site of the abscess. Such pressure may cause the escape of turbid or purulent material and may indicate the opening of the sinus which leads to the cavity.

External drainage of pancreatic cysts associated with chronic relapsing pancreatitis is reserved for the patient who is desperately ill or for cysts that are exceedingly small or in an unusual location, for example, the posterior aspect of the head of the pancreas or the uncinate process. Internal drainage is more commonly employed (Fig. 1c). If the cyst is large and is adherent to the posterior wall of the stomach, one should not be reluctant to drain the cyst by performing an anterior gastrotomy and by anastomosing the posterior wall of the stomach, which is densely adherent, to the cyst, followed by closure of the gastrotomy. If this method is to be employed, the cyst should be aspirated with an 18 gauge needle on a large syringe in order to confirm the diagnosis and to avoid the possibility of opening an abdominal aneurysm. This is especially true in the management of posttraumatic cysts. Such aspiration may also indicate the most appropriate place to open the cyst and thereby avoid injury to one of the major pancreatic arteries or to the splenic vein. Following this aspiration a trocar is used to deflate the cyst. The cyst is then opened widely to permit adequate inspection, thorough evacuation of the contents, and determination of the presence or absence of other locules or neoplastic elements. The stoma between the cyst and the stomach should be at least 3 or 4 cm. in diameter to allow free egress of the cystic contents into the stomach and to permit any food or gastric contents which may enter the cyst to flow freely back into the stomach. The cystic cavities usually collapse rapidly, the walls become adherent, and the communication between the cyst and the stomach disappears. It is equally urgent to use interlocking continuous sutures surrounding the stoma between the cyst and the posterior wall of the stomach to assure adequate hemostasis and to prevent leakage of the gastric or pancreatic contents into the peritoneal cavity.

Sphincterotomy and Retrograde Dilatation of the Pancreatic Ducts

Sphincterotomy in the management of chronic relapsing pancreatitis gave satisfactory results in approximately 50 per cent of cases. This procedure was then extended to involve transduodenal exploration, manipulation, extraction of pancreatic calculi, and intubation of the pancreatic ducts in an attempt to improve the flow of pancreatic secretions into the duodenum (Fig. 2). The technical considerations in the execution of this procedure involve (1) mobilization of the hepatic flexure of the colon, and (2) the generous mobilization of the entire duodenum

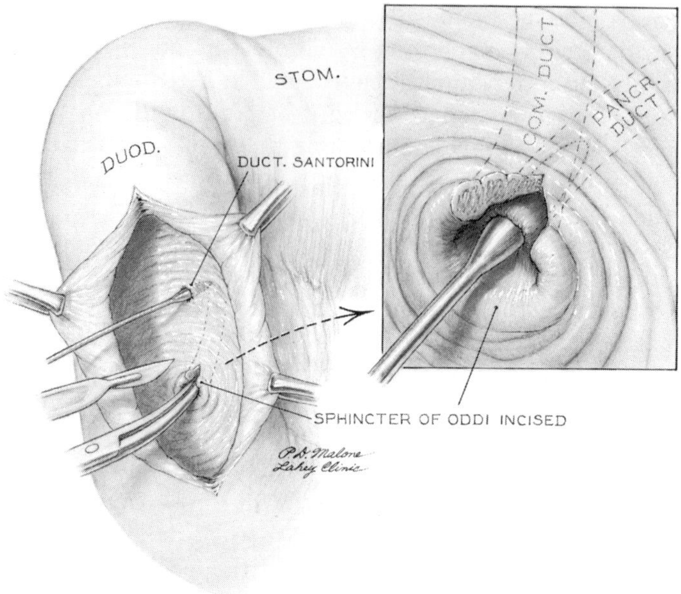

FIGURE 2. Transduodenal sphincterotomy and exploration of the pancreatic ducts. A duodenotomy has been made in the longitudinal axis, exposing the papilla of Vater. Division of the sphincter of Oddi is done after a curved or right-angle hemostat has been inserted into the ampulla of Vater from below. The tip of a 2 mm. Bakes dilator is shown entering the duct of Santorini (a lacrimal duct probe may be used). *Insert:* The sphincterotomy permits identification of the ostium of the duct of Wirsung, shown here with a Bakes dilator being inserted into the main pancreatic duct. Obstruction at or near the opening of the duct of Santorini or Wirsung is relieved by incising the ostium, probing and dilating the stenosed segment of the duct, and removing obstructing pancreatic calculi when present.

and head of the pancreas. This maneuver is facilitated by continuing the dissection close to the duodenum, staying in the cleavage plane and carrying the dissection to the left beyond the abdominal aorta, superiorly to the level of the common hepatic duct immediately superior to the duodenum, and anteriorly to the duodenojejunal junction. This wide mobilization permits adequate inspection and palpation of the duodenum, the head of the pancreas, and ultimately of the papilla of Vater.

Following this mobilization the level of the papilla of Vater is identified by palpation of the mesial wall of the duodenum where it is adherent to the head of the pancreas. The antimesenteric border of the duodenum is grasped gently with Babcock forceps opposite the site of the papilla of Vater and a duodenotomy is performed. The papilla of Vater is identified by direct vision or by palpation with the index finger. Following identification of the major papilla, three sutures of 0 silk on an atraumatic needle are placed circumferentially around the base of the papilla, taking exquisite care not to encroach upon the region of the ostium of the duct of Wirsung, which is at the 5 o'clock position on the circumference of the sphincter of Oddi. It should be borne in mind that the pancreatic duct may open on the summit of the papilla beyond the sphincter or a few millimeters distal to the papilla. With the three traction sutures in place, the papilla of Vater is elevated so that the manipulation may be carried out.

It has been a striking and surprising experience to find that a lacrimal duct probe of appropriate size, when inserted into the ostium of the papilla of Vater, goes into the duct of Wirsung more often than into the common bile duct. In 13 per cent of cases the opening of the duct of Wirsung is either on the summit of the papilla or 1 or 2 mm. inferior to the base of the papilla. In 3 per cent of cases the duct of Santorini is the major pancreatic duct, opening separately approximately 2 cm. proximal to the major papilla, and the obstruction occurs at the ostium or within the duct of Santorini.

If the papilla cannot be identified, choledochostomy is performed and a Bakes dilator is inserted distally into the common bile duct until the papilla of Vater is identified. An opening is made in the duodenum opposite the papilla.

Following the identification of the papilla, a search is made for the ostium of the duct of Wirsung. Pressure on the duct of Wirsung in the body of the pancreas may cause the escape of pancreatic secretion and identify the ostium. If the duct of Wirsung is not identified by gentle probing of the ampulla of Vater with a lacrimal duct probe, a sphincterotomy is performed at the 11 o'clock position on the circumference of the papilla of Vater. The incision is extended for 1 cm. Following the sphincterotomy the ostium of the duct of Wirsung is identified by direct vision. The ostium may be identified more readily by compressing the duct of Wirsung in the region of the body or the neck of the pancreas. If the opening cannot be found, secretin is administered intravenously, and within 45 to 90 seconds the flow of pancreatic juice is usually apparent. A lacrimal duct probe is inserted into the pancreatic duct. The most frequent site of obstruction within the duct is within a few millimeters of the ostium or at the junction of the duct of Santorini and duct of Wirsung.

Following the identification of the duct of Wirsung a catheter or a segment of polyethylene tubing of appropriate size is inserted into the duct and a pancreatogram is obtained. The pancreatogram is valuable in delineating the size and the course of the duct of Wirsung, in identifying sites of partial or complete obstruction of the duct, in demonstrating pancreatic cysts or pseudocysts, and rarely in demonstrating a fistula or a peripancreatic sinus. Despite the value of the pancreatogram, it is not essential for evaluating the gross pathological manifestations, determining the points of obstruction within the pancreas, or choosing an appropriate surgical procedure. If facilities are available, it is a helpful adjunct in the surgical management of this condition.

After the pancreatogram has been obtained, the duct of Wirsung is manipulated with graduated lacrimal duct probes or the common silver probe. The points of obstruction, when encountered, are frequently overcome. Following the dilatation of the strictured segment, the escape of turbid, chalky fluid signifies that stagnant pancreatic secretion is flowing through the duct. It may be necessary to intubate such a duct in order to keep this segment open.

Transpancreatic Exploration and Manipulation of the Pancreatic Ducts

When there is more than one point of obstruction in the pancreatic duct it may be necessary to combine retrograde manipulation with transpancreatic incision of the duct of Wirsung in the neck or body of the gland. If the duct cannot be cleared in this fashion, it may be widely incised. Numerous areas of constriction may be incised and dilated. If the points of obstruction can be completely overcome, we prefer to intubate the duct of Wirsung through the duodenotomy and leave a segment of catheter or of polyethylene tubing within the lumen of the duodenum. Occasionally we prefer to use a small, long-limbed T tube positioned so that one limb traverses the sphincter of Oddi and this tip of the tube rests in the lumen of the duodenum. The other limb of the T tube rests in the pancreatic duct. The external limb of the T tube may be brought out through the parietes or through the posterior and anterior walls of the stomach and then through the parietes. If the latter method is employed, it is necessary to approximate the opening in the posterior wall of the stomach to the opening in the pancreatic duct, and to approximate the anterior wall of the stomach, where the T tube emerges, to the parietal peritoneum. This method has the advantage of creating at least a temporary and perhaps a permanent anastomosis between the duct of Wirsung and the stomach. It is a modification of the ingenious method of anastomosing the duct of Wirsung to the posterior wall of the stomach, after distal pancreatectomy, that was described by Rodney Smith. This principle is exceedingly appealing and has considerable flexibility in its application.

Anastomosis of the Duct of Wirsung to the Gastrointestinal Tract

If retrograde dilatation of the duct of Wirsung is not successful, the duct of Wirsung in the neck and body of the gland may be opened and this segment of the pancreatic duct anastomosed to the stomach or to a defunctionalized loop of jejunum (Fig. 3).

In many instances it is possible to make a longitudinal opening 1 cm. in length into the duct of Wirsung, and through this opening clear the duct of small calculi that may be present and dilate the opening of the duct into the duodenum. A pancreatogram is obtained. Decompression of the duct by anastomosis to stomach or jejunum is then performed.

For advanced cases with numerous stones within the ductal system, it is preferable to make a large longitudinal opening, as advocated by Puestow, and anastomose the entire length of the opening to a defunctionalized loop of jejunum. However, even with this generous incision it is frequently impossible to clear the proximal portion of the duct. I prefer to do an endothelial mucosal anastomosis regardless of the size of the opening of the duct.

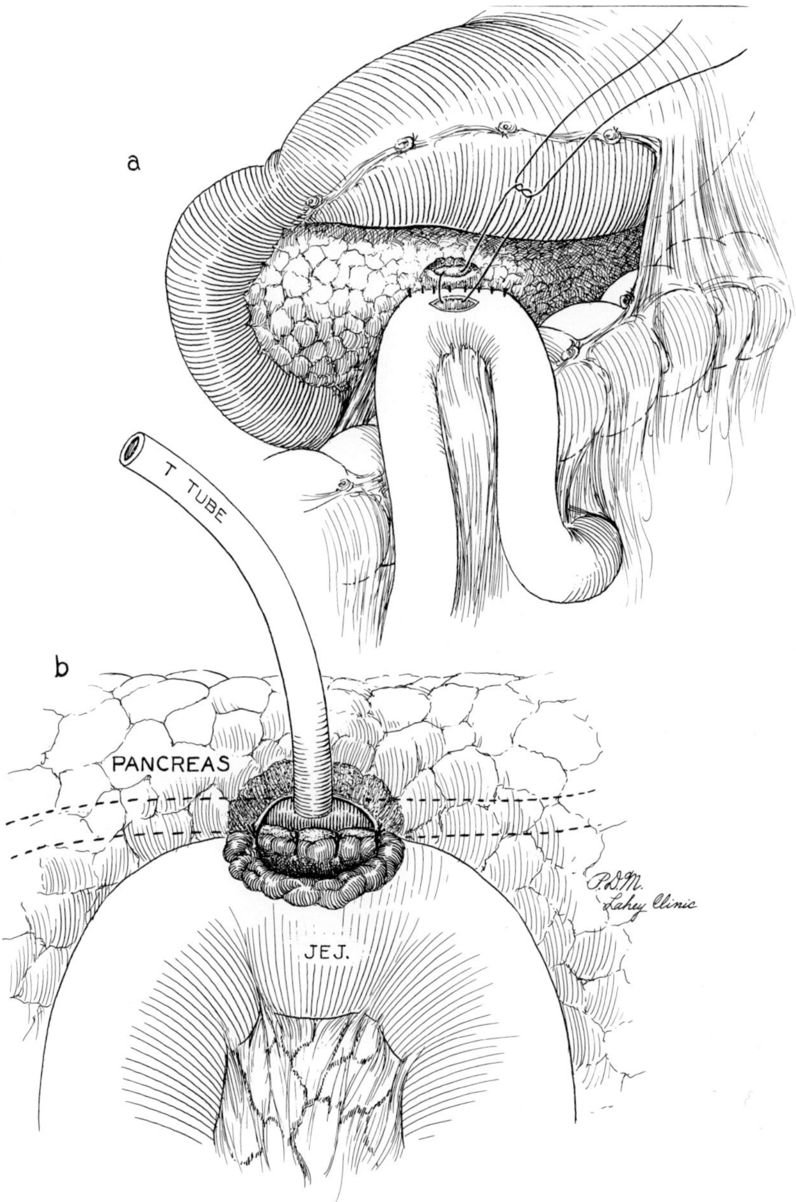

FIGURE 3. Anastomosis of the duct of Wirsung to a segment of the gastrointestinal tract (stomach or jejunum). The duct of Wirsung may be decompressed by anastomosis of the duct to the posterior wall of the stomach or to a loop of jejunum, as shown in (*a*). (The loop is defunctionalized by a Roux en Y jejunojejunostomy.) When a T tube is employed, the external limb is brought through the anterior wall of the stomach or jejunum, and thence through a stab wound in the anterior abdominal wall (*b*). This technique permits future pancreatography and affords a method of removing the T tube without reoperation.

Distal Pancreatectomy

Distal pancreatectomy (Fig. 4) is indicated when the pathological changes associated with chronic relapsing pancreatitis are confined to the distal segment of the gland. This localization may occur spontaneously but is most commonly observed following blunt trauma to the abdomen. When trauma is responsible for the chronic pancreatitis, the duct of Wirsung has usually been severed in the region of the neck of the pancreas. A cyst may or may not be present. Under these circumstances, when distal pancreatectomy is feasible it is the operation of choice.

Distal pancreatectomy is facilitated by a generous division of the gastrocolic omentum, by mobilization of the spleen and preliminary division of the vasa brevia between the spleen and the greater curvature of the stomach. It is customary in the Lahey Clinic to ligate the splenic artery superior to the tail of the pancreas

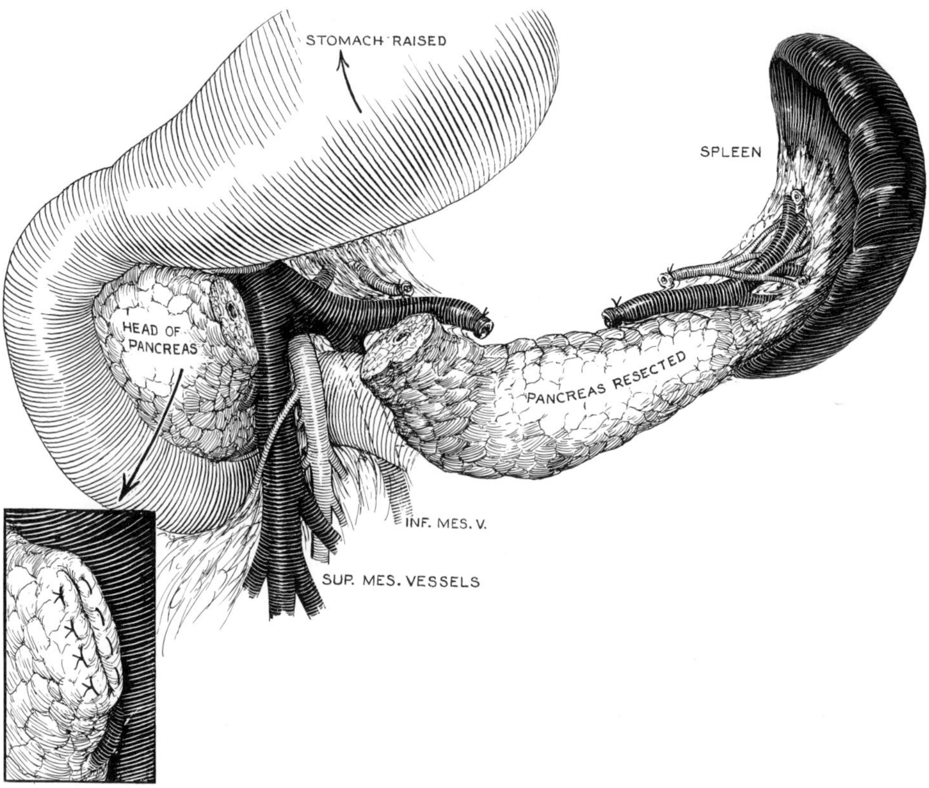

FIGURE 4. Diagram of the limits of distal pancreatectomy with splenectomy. The insert shows closure of the pancreatic neck. The duct of Wirsung and the neck of the pancreas may be anastomosed to the posterior wall of the stomach or to a defunctionalized loop of jejunum. This anastomosis should always be performed if obstruction of the proximal portion of the duct of Wirsung is present.

before the spleen is mobilized. The peritoneum overlying the inferior border of the pancreas is incised. I prefer to elevate the neck of the pancreas from the superior mesenteric and portal veins before mobilizing the spleen and distal pancreas. The spleen is then mobilized by incising the parietal peritoneum in the lateral splenic fossa. The spleen and the body and tail of the pancreas are elevated, along with the splenic vein. This maneuver obviates the possibility of injuring the portal vein during the posterior dissection at the junction of the splenic and superior mesenteric veins. The neck of the pancreas is divided after the superior and inferior longitudinal pancreatic arteries have been transfixed with a silk ligature. A long segment of polyethylene tubing of appropriate size is inserted into the divided duct of Wirsung in the neck of the pancreas. A Kirschner wire is inserted into the opposite end of the polyethylene tube and the tubing is passed through the posterior wall of the stomach, out the anterior gastric wall, and then through the abdominal wall. The duct of Wirsung at the point of division at the neck is snugged up to the posterior wall of the stomach by interrupted sutures of fine silk, and the anterior wall of the stomach is approximated to the parietal peritoneum in a similar fashion where the polyethylene tubing emerges. This procedure, originally described by Rodney Smith, is also applicable to the management of the duct of Wirsung following distal pancreatectomy when proximal obstruction of the duct persists.

Pancreatoduodenectomy

When multiple points of obstruction are present within the proximal pancreatic ductal system, it may be wise or necessary to remove the head of the pancreas in the management of far-advanced chronic pancreatitis. Eighty-five per cent of a group of patients so treated at the Lahey Clinic had had previous operations for pancreatitis, and one-third had had a sphincterotomy. The incidence of pancreatolithiasis, alcoholic abuse, narcotic addiction, pancreatic cysts, diabetes mellitus, and exocrine deficiency was high in this group. Frequently, the head of the pancreas was enlarged and cystic, and the cystic cavities were filled with pancreatic stones. This procedure should not be done for early chronic relapsing pancreatitis, nor should it be attempted in the presence of severe peripancreatic inflammation.

Technique

When this procedure is elected, the hepatic flexure of the colon is mobilized and retracted inferiorly, the entire duodenum and head of the pancreas are mobilized to the left, beyond the abdominal aorta (Fig. 5). With the gastrocolic omentum generously opened, the neck of the pancreas is elevated from the superior mesenteric and portal veins. This maneuver should be done with great care because the gland is frequently densely adherent to these venous structures in this type of pancreatitis. With diligence and patience, it is almost always possible to elevate the neck of the pancreas. I prefer to follow the course of the superior mesenteric vein, beginning at the inferior border of the neck of the gland. Instead of finger dissec-

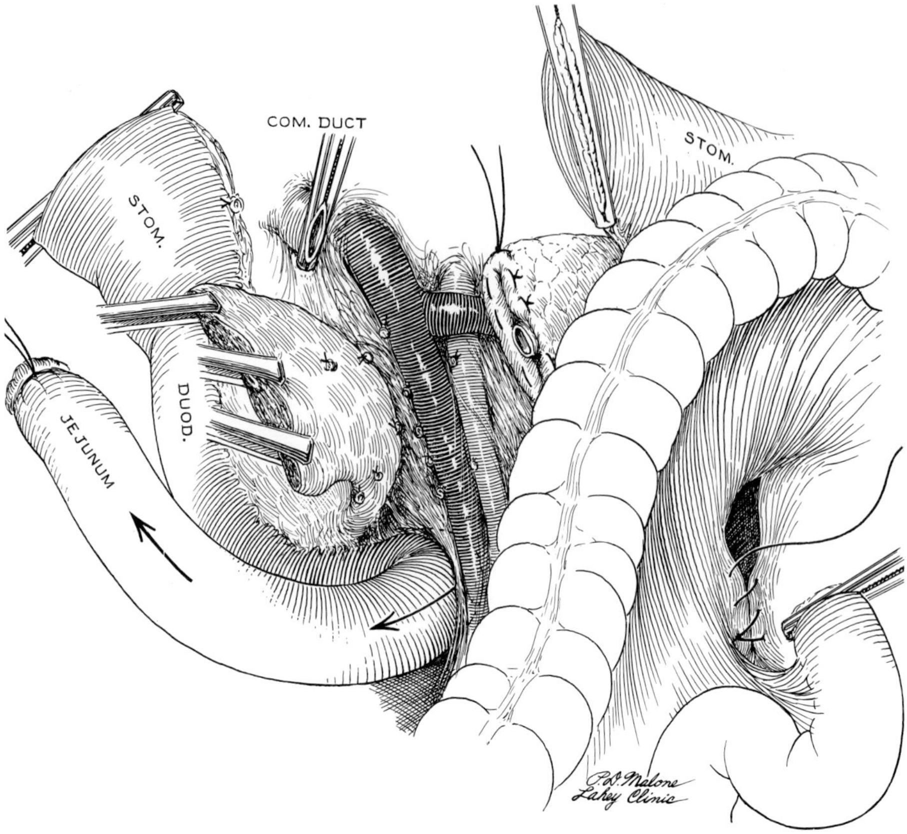

FIGURE 5. Mobilization of the head of the pancreas. The stomach, common bile duct, and proximal portion of the jejunum have been divided, and the neck of the pancreas has been severed at the level of the superior mesenteric and portal veins. The pancreatic stump has been prepared for subsequent anastomosis of the duct of Wirsung to the proximal jejunum. The entire specimen will be removed by dividing the short arteries and veins which supply the duodenum and the uncinate process of the pancreas.

tion, which is so commonly employed, a small gauze pledget, secured in a right-angle ductal forceps clamp, is used as a dissecting instrument. With the lower part of the retropancreatic superior mesenteric vein visualized, the neck of the gland is completely separated from the superior mesenteric and portal veins. The point of the clamp will emerge at the level of the superior pancreatic node, which frequently overrides the hepatic artery.

When the gland has been separated from these venous structures, a small Penrose drain is used to encircle the neck of the pancreas for later manipulation of this segment. If the neck of the gland can be elevated from the venous structures, the procedure can usually be carried out with safety. Once this has been determined to be possible, the stomach is divided, removing at least 50 or 60 per cent of this organ. The von Petz clamp is used for dividing the stomach, and the gastric remnant which ultimately will be anastomosed to the jejunum is displaced into the left upper quadrant of the abdominal cavity.

The gastroduodenal artery is identified immediately superior to the neck of the pancreas and is divided between silk ligatures. Pulsation of the hepatic artery along the mesial aspect of the common duct is always assured before the gastroduodenal artery is divided. The common duct is then mobilized in the supraduodenal area, great care being taken not to injure the portal vein, which usually runs posteriorly and slightly medial to the common bile duct. Occasionally the portal vein will run directly behind the common bile duct, or in rare instances will appear in the anomalous position to the right and posterior to the common duct. The common duct is then divided between clamps.

The fourth portion of the duodenum is mobilized in every dimension until the ligament of Treitz is encountered. The peritoneum at this level is incised circumferentially, thus exposing the proximal jejunum. By this method of dissection the proximal jejunum can be withdrawn beneath the superior mesenteric vessels and divided at an appropriate point a few inches beyond the ligament of Treitz. This maneuver obviates the necessity of dividing the jejunum to the left of the mesenteric veins and then mobilizing the duodenojejunal junction from the left to the right by dividing the mesenteric vessels in this area. Either method can be employed, but mobilization and division of the proximal jejunum from the right side of the mesenteric vessels are extremely helpful.

Once the jejunum is divided, the pancreas is divided between the paired sutures at a point overlying the portal vein. The large venous trunk, and particularly the inferior venous trunk, is dissected and divided between clamps. If this trunk is large, a transfixion suture is employed as a ligature. The uncinate process is then gently separated from the right lateral wall of the superior mesenteric and portal veins. Several small veins may be observed in this location and may be divided between paired clamps and ligated with fine silk. With the jejunum, common duct, and neck of the pancreas divided, and with the mesial aspect of the uncinate mobilized from the superior mesenteric and portal veins, the specimen can be removed by applying right-angle forceps to the series of mesenteric veins which supplies both the uncinate and the duodenum. These arteries and veins usually are very short and are best controlled by transfixion ligatures. After removal of the specimen, all bleeding points along the superior mesenteric artery and portal vein are secured because the subsequent reconstruction will obscure this field.

Reconstruction. There is a wide variety of methods applicable to reconstruction of the digestive tract following pancreatoduodenectomy. We employ one of two methods. The most commonly used is closure of the proximal jejunum, permitting the closed end of the jejunum to retract to the left of the mesenteric vessels. The opening at the level of the ligament of Treitz is then closed with a continuous suture of fine catgut. The pancreaticojejunostomy is then started by approximating the segment of jejunum to the posterior substance of the neck of the pancreas with interrupted mattress sutures of fine silk. The duct of Wirsung is anastomosed directly to an appropriate opening in the jejunum with interrupted sutures of fine silk. A soft rubber catheter or polyethylene tube is employed as a stent when the duct is small. If the duct is large, no stent is used. The importance of careful ductal to jejunal mucosa anastomosis between the pancreas and the jejunum cannot be overemphasized. The duct can be anastomosed in this manner regardless of its size. The anastomosis is then completed by inserting a row of interrupted sutures of fine silk, approximating the anterior surface of the divided neck of the pancreas to the jejunum.

The common duct is anastomosed about 5 cm. distal to the pancreaticojejunostomy with two interrupted rows of fine silk. Recently I have preferred to employ a T tube stent with an opening made in the common hepatic duct. The T tube employed in this fashion has several advantages. It will remain in place until it is deliberately removed. It will minimize the intrabiliary pressure and will reduce the intraluminal tension within the segment of jejunum which is anastomosed to the common duct and to the pancreas. The end of the T tube which rests in the lumen of the jejunum is deliberately placed proximally so that the tip of the T tube rests near the anastomosis of the pancreaticojejunostomy. If a fistula develops, the T tube can be converted to a sump drain, thus minimizing the amount of leakage at the pancreaticojejunal anastomosis.

A gastrojejunostomy is then performed approximately 16 inches distal to the hepaticojejunostomy. This long interval between the hepaticojejunostomy and the gastrojejunostomy minimizes the reflux of gastric contents into the biliary tract. The gastrojejunostomy is usually fashioned after the manner of Hofmeister, but the type of reconstruction is not of major consequence. It is of considerable consequence, however, to be sure that a significant amount of the stomach is removed or that the bilateral vagotomy is performed, because the incidence of jejunal ulcer when a simple antrectomy is performed has been unreasonably high.

Comments

Pancreatoduodenectomy has been performed in 63 patients with chronic relapsing pancreatitis. There have been but two postoperative deaths. When one considers that this procedure is employed only for far-advanced pancreatitis and usually only after other lesser procedures have failed, it is encouraging to note that approximately 65 per cent of these patients have obtained good results. It is obvious that the longer the follow-up the greater will be the number of patients who return with recurrent pancreatitis or with various complications related to the primary disease or to the nature of the operation. Much of the remote morbidity and mortality following this procedure is the result primarily of the persistent use of alcohol and narcotics. Pancreatoduodenectomy has definite merit but it is not to be undertaken lightly. It should be reserved for those patients in whom lesser procedures offer little prospect of relief of symptoms, and should never be utilized for the sake of sheer technical accomplishment.

Total Pancreatectomy

A very small number of patients with far-advanced chronic relapsing pancreatitis require total pancreatectomy, but the physiological consequences of this operation are such that it should be avoided if possible. We have utilized this procedure in six cases with no deaths, but despite the low mortality it has a very limited place in the management of pancreatitis.

Total pancreatectomy, technically speaking, is a combination of distal pancreatectomy and pancreatoduodenectomy. Since the determination of the procedure which should be employed is most frequently facilitated by a thorough mobilization of the duodenum and the head of the pancreas, this maneuver is performed initially. The next step is the elevation of the neck of the pancreas from the superior mesenteric and portal veins. Once this elevation has been accomplished, a fine Penrose drain is passed around the neck of the pancreas in order to identify the level of the superior mesenteric and portal veins, and also subsequently to elevate the neck of the pancreas from these structures when the splenic vein is to be divided. Attention is then directed toward the mobilization of the spleen and distal pancreas. The splenic artery is divided along the superior border of the tail of the pancreas and ligated with 0 silk. The vasa brevia vessels are divided between clamps and ligated. The peritoneum lateral to the spleen is incised. The splenic flexure of the colon is mobilized, and the spleen and the tail and body of the pancreas, along with the splenic vein, are mobilized to the level of the neck of the pancreas. At this point the splenic vein joins the superior mesenteric vein to form the portal vein. The inferior mesenteric vein may enter at any level, either directly into the splenic vein or at the junction of the splenic and superior mesenteric veins, or occasionally, into the portal vein. It is best to divide this vein unless it enters the superior mesenteric vein before it joins the portal vein. The superior and inferior longitudinal pancreatic arteries are ligated with a transfixion suture of silk at the point where the neck of the pancreas has been elevated from the superior mesenteric and portal veins. The splenic vein is divided between clamps just before it joins the superior mesenteric vein.

The remainder of the operation is identical with pancreatoduodenectomy. The stomach is divided at the appropriate level; the common duct is divided between clamps; the proximal jejunum is divided; the head and uncinate process of the pancreas are dissected from the right lateral margin of the portal vein. The vessels from the superior mesenteric artery and the accompanying veins, which supply the uncinate process and the duodenum, are divided between paired clamps and the specimen is removed. Following removal of the specimen, the common hepatic duct is anastomosed to the proximal jejunum and the gastric remnant is anastomosed approximately 16 inches distally after the manner of Hofmeister. Both the splenic fossa and the right upper quadrant of the abdomen are drained with sump drains. It is necessary to remove at least 60 per cent of the stomach, or to perform a lesser resection and do a bilateral subdiaphragmatic vagotomy in order to prevent jejunal ulcer.

Combined Procedures

It is occasionally necessary to do combined procedures in the treatment of chronic pancreatitis, since multiple points of obstruction may be present within the gland and radical resection of a segment will not relieve all of the points of obstruction.

These combined procedures may involve a transduodenal retrograde manipulation of the pancreatic ducts, in addition to transpancreatic exploration of the ducts, and perhaps anastomosis of the duct of Wirsung and the body of the gland to an isolated segment of jejunum or to the stomach. Occasionally, a distal pancreatectomy with retrograde anastomosis is necessary. We have also employed distal pancreatectomy and proximal transduodenal retrograde dilatation and manipulation of the pancreatic ducts.

Conclusion

Because of the complicated pathology of chronic relapsing pancreatitis with the frequency of multiple areas of partial or complete obstruction of the ductal system, no single operative maneuver is applicable to all cases. The operation must be individualized and it must be tailored to fit the precise pathology in a given case. Consideration must be given to the local pathological alterations and to the general condition of the patient. It must be realized that occasionally the initial operation will be designed to relieve the major pathology and to get the patient in condition for a definitive procedure. The central requirement in the surgical management of chronic relapsing pancreatitis is to overcome the obstruction to the outflow of the exocrine pancreatic secretions.

In view of the large number of patients suffering from chronic relapsing pancreatitis who are addicted to alcohol and narcotics, the results frequently are discouraging, but with careful evaluation of each case and with individualization in the choice of surgical procedure most of these patients can be helped.

References

CATTELL, R. B., and WARREN, K. W. *Surgery of the Pancreas.* Philadelphia: W. B. Saunders, 1953.

DOUBILET, H., and MULHOLLAND, J. H. Eight-year study of pancreatitis and sphincterotomy. *J.A.M.A.* 160:521, February 18, 1956.

WARREN, K. W. Pathologic considerations as a guide to the choice of surgical procedures in the management of chronic relapsing pancreatitis. *Gastroenterology* 36:224, February 1959.

WARREN, K. W. Surgery of pancreatic disease. *Modern Trends in Gastro-Enterology.* London: Butterworths, 1961. P. 264.

WARREN, K. W., and VEIDENHEIMER, M. Pathological considerations in the choice of operation for chronic relapsing pancreatitis. *New England J. Med.* 266:323, February 15, 1962.

100. *Cystointestinal Anastomoses for Cysts of the Pancreas*

MAURICE P. MERCADIER

Cystoduodenostomy

Cystoduodenal anastomosis is a simple and safe method to provide drainage of cystic or pseudocystic collections formed in the duodenal region. It can be used to evacuate cystic or pseudocystic collections which develop either within the pancreatic parenchyma or in its neighborhood, particularly when the major pancreatic ducts are not involved and the cystic fluid has no outlet through those channels. In that situation a sphincterotomy would not be effective. Operative roentgenographic studies after the injection of a contrast medium into the cystic cavity and the pancreatic ducts have shown that this type of collection not infrequently is dissociated from the duct of Wirsung.

Of all types of cystogastrointestinal anastomoses, the cystoduodenal anastomosis is based on the most logical anatomical and physiological considerations, for it provides a communication between the pancreatic cyst and the duodenum, the normal recipient of pancreatic secretion.

To fulfill its purpose best, the anastomosis should be located at the most dependent part of the cyst. Although this does not prevent reflux of food, it avoids stasis in the cavity by permitting thorough drainage. For this reason, cystoduodenostomy is indicated only when the cyst has developed in the vicinity of and above the inferior portion of the duodenum. In practice, the anastomosis is usually placed in the descending portion of the duodenum, under or above the ampulla of Vater, according to the location of the cyst. When the cystic collection is adjacent to the third portion of the duodenum, that is the choice site of anastomosis.

It has been stated that cystoduodenostomy entails a number of operative and postoperative risks. The operative risks include possible injury of the duodenopancreatic vascular system or the common duct. There is no denying the risk of injury to the blood vessels, in view of the rich vasculature of the pancreas, with blood vessels running between the border of the pancreas and the descending portion of the duodenum (Fig. 1). Hemostasis can be assured by making the incision in the duodenum under visual control and by using transfixion sutures. The risk

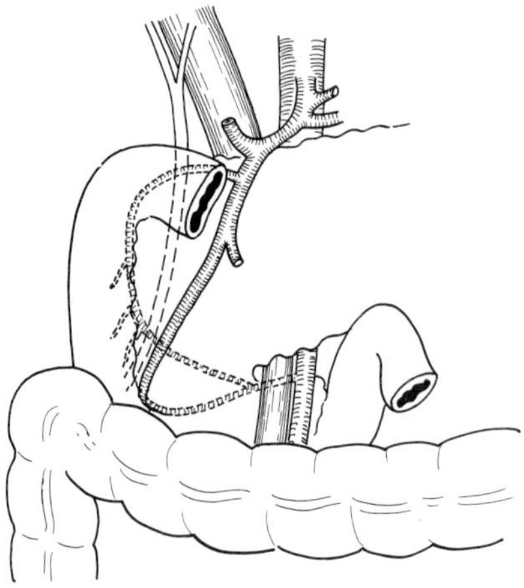

FIGURE 1. Diagram showing blood vessels in the neighborhood of the duodenum.

of injuring the lower part of the common bile duct is more theoretical than real, because in the majority of cases the cystic mass displaces it backward. Nevertheless, the precise position of the common duct in relation to the cyst, and the site of its opening into the duodenum, must be ascertained by preoperative or operative cholangiograms, with films taken in anteroposterior and lateral positions.

Postoperative risks include the consequences of reflux of food into the cystic cavity. Such reflux has been declared responsible for suppuration and abscess of the pancreas, hemorrhage resulting from inflammation of the cystic walls, and pancreatic necrosis. We have never experienced any of these problems. In our opinion, these complications are not due to the reflux of food but to its remaining in the cystic cavity, which can be avoided by placing the anastomosis at the dependent part of the cyst.

With the foregoing considerations in mind, we have made it a rule to take the following precautions: (1) to ascertain the precise position of the cyst in relation to the duodenum; (2) to make a transduodenal approach through an incision in the outer aspect of the descending portion of the duodenum; (3) to localize the papilla and catheterize the common bile duct with a rigid catheter; (4) to incise the inner aspect of the second portion of the duodenum away from the papilla, and nearer to the anterior than to the posterior wall to avoid the common duct.

Technique

A long paramedian incision is made from the costal margin to a point well below the umbilicus. Careful scrutiny and palpation of the cyst, the pancreas, the biliary ducts, and the liver follow.

Operative roentgenograms are made of the pancreatic cyst, the pancreatic duct system, the biliary ducts, and the site of the choledochoduodenal opening. First, under manometric control, the contrast medium is injected into the biliary tract by puncture of either the fundus of the gallbladder or the common bile duct above the duodenum. This reveals the morphology of the common duct, its junction with the duodenum, and the presence of biliary lithiasis. After radiomanometry of the biliary system, cystography is done by injecting the same substance into the cystic cavity either directly by puncturing its outer surface or indirectly by transduodenal puncture. The exploration is completed by injecting the contrast substance directly into the isthmic segment of the duct of Wirsung if the latter is enlarged. These various maneuvers, employed singly or in combination, enable the surgeon (1) to precisely determine the position of the cyst in relation to the duct of Wirsung; (2) to note how the common duct is affected by the cyst; (3) to know whether or not a communication exists between the cyst and the duct of Wirsung; (4) to detect defects of the biliary and pancreatic tracts requiring therapeutic measures; and (5) to appreciate the distance between the cystic cavity and the duodenal lumen, and the thickness of the parenchyma to be incised.

Operative pancreatography is unnecessary when injection of the contrast medium into the cystic cavity brings out the pancreatic ducts. In that situation, it is obvious that the cyst communicates with the pancreatic duct and surgical treatment will consist, not in cystoduodenostomy, but in draining the ducts, which may or may not be accomplished by sphincterotomy employing Doubilet's technique.

In all cases in which it has been demonstrated that the cystic cavity does not communicate with the pancreatic duct system and a cystoduodenostomy is indicated, the first move is to depress the hepatic flexure of the colon and to mobilize the duodenum by the Kocher maneuver (Fig. 2). The duodenum is pushed far to the left, toward the aorta, to provide full exposure of the head of the pancreas, which encloses the cyst. An incision is made through the outer wall of the descending portion of the duodenum. The papilla is identified, and the common duct found by inserting a rigid catheter either through a supraduodenal choledochotomy or from below through the opening on the papilla (Fig. 3).

Only at this stage can a communication be established between the duodenum and the cavity. The incision in the mucosa is made by electrocautery at a distance from the common duct. One identifies and ligates the parietal vessels with "points appuyés." The cyst is then collapsed by puncturing it with the tip of a bistoury, and the opening is gradually enlarged upward and downward under

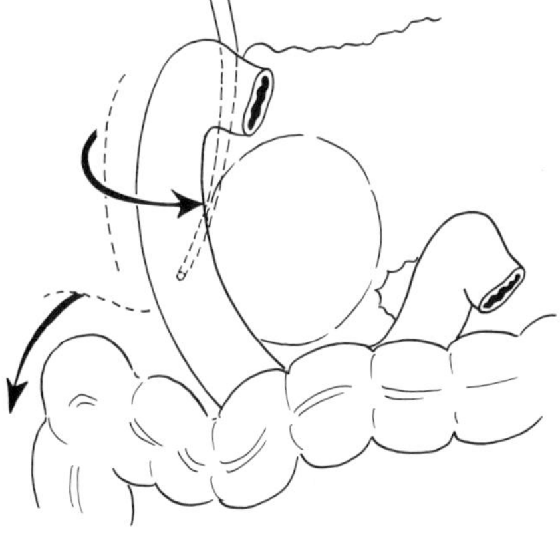

FIGURE 2. Mobilization of the hepatic flexure of the colon and of the duodenum.

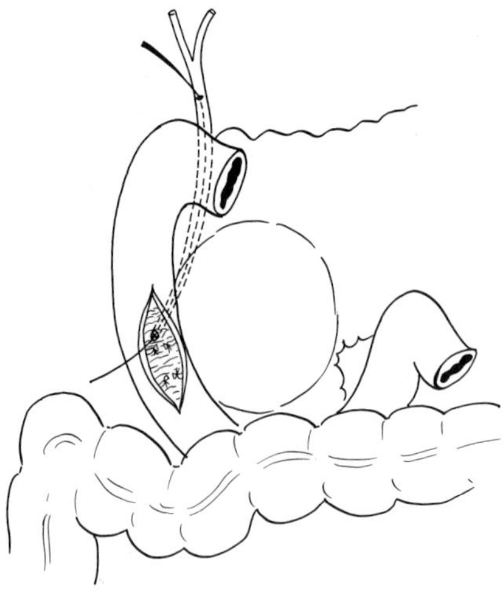

FIGURE 3. Incision in the outer wall of the duodenum, ligation of vessels in the internal wall, and insertion of a catheter through the common bile duct.

direct visual control (Fig. 4). When the opening has reached two to three fingerbreadths, the cystic and duodenal walls are united with either interrupted or continuous sutures of 0 chromic catgut (Fig. 5). When a thick cystic covering or a thick wall of tissue separates the cystic cavity from the duodenal lumen, this method is hazardous. In that case, the risk of injury to the blood vessels can be reduced by incising the anterior surface of the cyst as well as the duodenum, so that both lumens are under visual control. After the cystic covering has been incised, a strong forceps, such as a Kelly, is inserted into the cystic cavity, pressing the opposite wall of the cyst toward the duodenum. The duodenum is then incised at the site of the bulge raised by the forceps (Fig. 6). The small breach thus provided is progressively enlarged upward and downward. Hemostasis is assured by "points appuyés." When the orifice has been made large enough, the cystic and duodenal walls are united with interrupted or continuous sutures of chromic catgut and the external longitudinal duodenotomy is closed with interrupted sutures of 3–0 silk.

In all cases the operation is followed by the establishment of drainage from

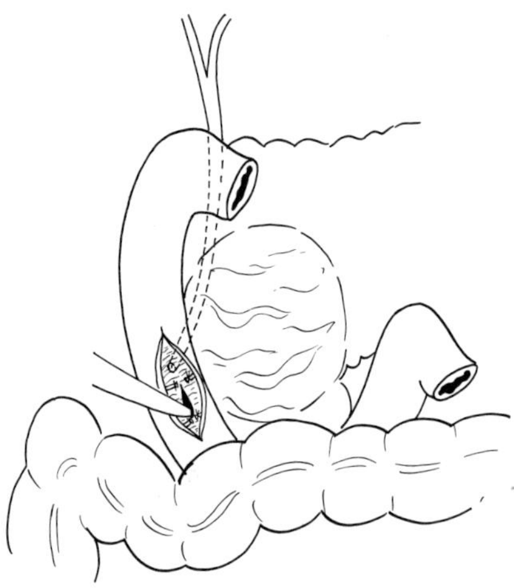

FIGURE 4. Incision through the inner wall of the duodenum into the cyst by electrocautery.

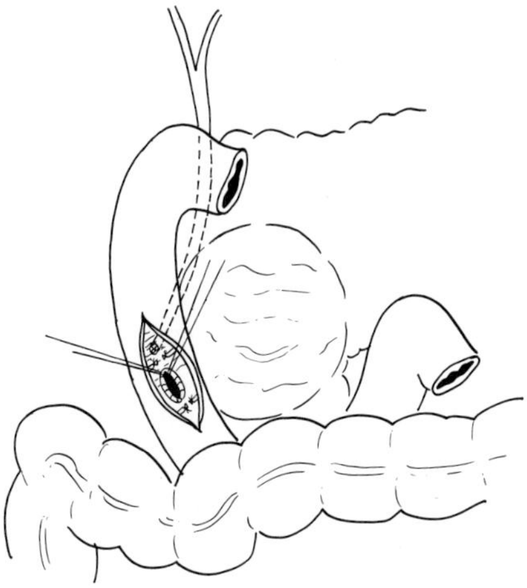

FIGURE 5. Suture of the edges of the incised cyst to the duodenal wall.

two points: (1) from the gallbladder or common duct area to insure drainage of the biliary system, avoiding leakage of bile if the gallbladder or the common duct has been punctured for radiomanometry; (2) from the retroduodenopancreatic space opened by Kocher's maneuver. In the past, we drained the cystic cavity with an ordinary drain, or with a T tube drain, which was exteriorized after being passed through a small opening in the outer duodenal wall. We have abandoned that practice because it is not really necessary.

Sometimes the pseudocyst is associated with other pancreatic pathology. There may be a scarring of the sphincter of Oddi, requiring sphincterotomy and drainage of the duct of Wirsung. More often, however, we have found the terminal part of the duct of Wirsung obstructed by lithiasis, or periductal fibrosis. In that situation, we proceed with a decompression wirsungojejunostomy, using a Y-shaped jejunal loop. Unfortunately such lesions, being usually due to chronic pancreatitis, are bound to recur.

In summary, transduodenal cystoduodenostomy is a simple and safe method.

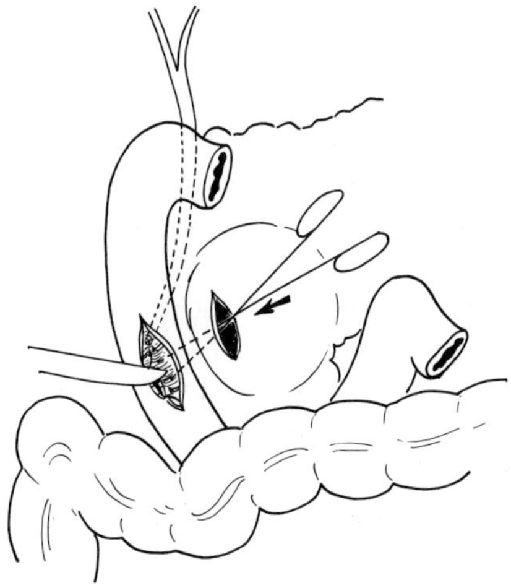

FIGURE 6. Incision of the cyst wall over the end of a Kelly forceps.

Its purpose is to provide internal evacuation of cystic or pseudocystic collections of the head of the pancreas lying close to the duodenum. The prognosis depends on the cause of the cyst. When the latter is secondary to acute hemorrhagic necrotic pancreatitis, the prognosis is favorable; it is more guarded when the cyst is due to chronic calcifying or noncalcifying pancreatitis.

Wirsungojejunostomy

Cattell and Warren proposed a surgical procedure involving an anastomosis between the duct of Wirsung and a jejunal loop for the relief of pancreatic secretion retention and all its attendant symptoms in cases of carcinoma of the head of the pancreas. We have now extended the indications of the operation to include all those affections localized in the head which result in retention of pancreatic secretion, distention of the ductal system, and pancreatic pain. We apply this method both to cancer and to calcifying and noncalcifying pancreatic fibrosis.

In certain situations when the cyst is firmly adherent to the posterior wall of the stomach and cannot be readily or safely exposed to allow a wirsungojejunostomy, a cystogastrostomy is performed by exploring the cyst through the posterior wall of the stomach. The opening should be dependent and large, and the edges of the stomach and cyst are approximated with interrupted sutures.

Technique

Starting from an anastomosis to a jejunal loop in the form of a reversed U, completed or not by jejunojejunostomy at the bottom of the loop, we fashion a wirsungojejunostomy in the form of a Y (Fig. 7). The use of a loop of jejunum as a bypass collateral to the digestive tract, following the technique of Roux of Lausanne, has much to recommend it (Fig. 8). Reflux of food into the pancreatic canal is prevented by the antiperistaltic position of the loop, and the consequences of fistula formation are reduced to those following the loss of pancreatic juice, while the food follows its normal course.

The various steps in the Roux technique are as follows:

1. Find the distended duct of Wirsung on the vertebral aspect of the pancreas. The duct is superficial, nearer the superior than the inferior border. Puncture the duct to collect a specimen of pancreatic juice for an analysis of its enzymes, and for the injection of the contrast medium to obtain roentgenograms of the ductal system and its opening into the duodenum.
2. Make a transverse incision, about 6 to 8 cm. long, over the isthmic segment of the duct.
3. Section the jejunum at a distance of 30 to 40 cm. from the duodenojejunal junction after ligating the vascular arcades of the jejunal segment to be divided.
4. Pull up the efferent segment of the divided jejunal loop, bringing it through an avascular area in the midportion of the transverse mesocolon. The

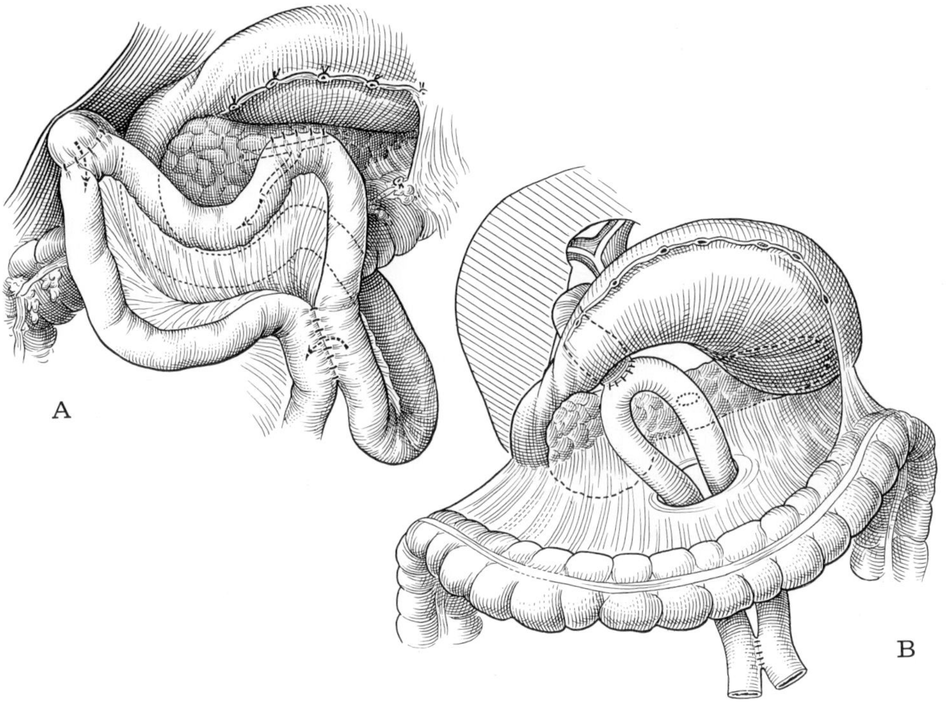

FIGURE 7. Wirsungojejunostomy (side-to-side) and jejunojejunostomy. Cholecystojejunostomy employed when obstruction is due to carcinoma. (*A*) Antecolic anastomoses. (*B*) Retrocolic anastomoses. The illustration does not show suture of the jejunum to the opening in the mesocolon.

jejunal segment thus brought up passes behind the transverse colon, the gastrocolic ligament, and the stomach, to emerge above the lesser curvature of the stomach.

5. Make an end-to-side anastomosis between the open end of the jejunal loop and the opening made in the pancreatic parenchyma and the duct of Wirsung.

6. Attach the jejunal loop to the mesocolic opening.

7. Re-establish the continuity of the digestive tract by an end-to-side anastomosis between the cut efferent loop of jejunum and the opening already made in the convex portion of the second jejunal loop. The jejunojejunostomy is located about 30 cm. from the wirsungojejunostomy, directly under the transverse mesocolon.

8. Close all incisions previously made in the mesentery.

All anastomoses are made in one layer with interrupted stitches, using either 3–0 silk or 0 linen. On the intestinal wall, the sutures include the seromuscularis, the submucosa, and the edge of the mucosa. On the pancreas, they include the whole of the sclerotic pancreatic tissue, taking support in the edge of the wall of the duct of Wirsung.

In patients with cancer or with fibrosis of the head, biliary retention will sooner or later follow pancreatic secretion retention. For this reason it is necessary to provide drainage for the biliary as well as the pancreatic system. This is done

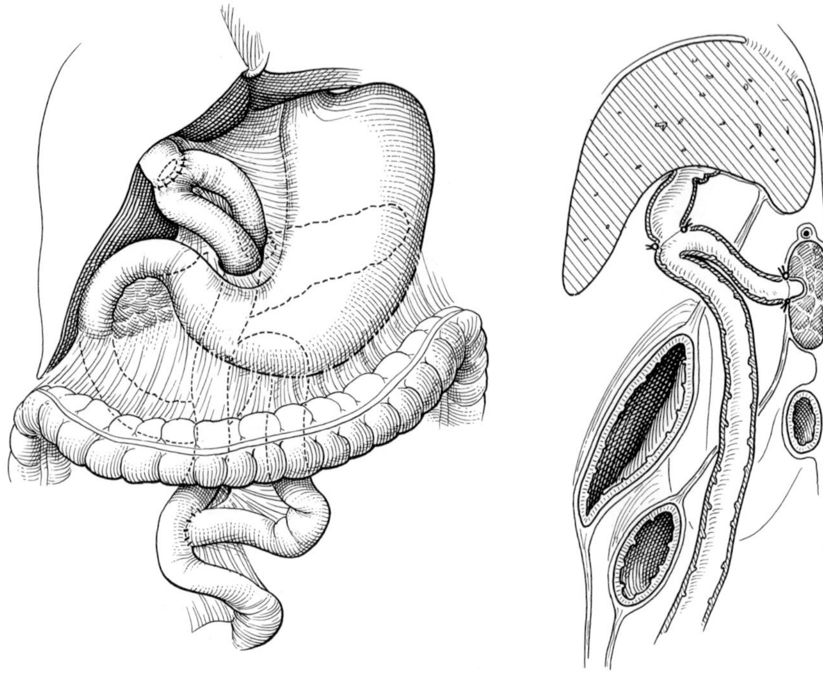

FIGURE 8. Wirsungojejunostomy (end-to-side) and jejunojejunostomy. Cholecystojejunostomy employed when obstruction is due to carcinoma.

by anastomosing the mounted jejunal loop either to the common bile duct, if the latter is sufficiently dilated above the pancreas, or to the fundus of the gallbladder (Fig. 8). Here again, the suturing is done in one layer with interrupted sutures of 3–0 silk or 0 linen.

In a series of over 150 cases, we have not observed fistula formation. The immediate results of pancreatic and biliary decompression are always satisfactory. The pain disappears promptly. Appetite returns and the patient begins to regain weight. Unfortunately the pathogenetic factors in pancreatic and biliary duct retention of secretion are still present. In patients with cancer, the remission lasts only a few months. In those with progressive pancreatic fibrosis it may continue for some years; eventually, however, the pancreas is destroyed. For this reason, this operation must be considered only as palliative.

References

MADDEN, J. L. *Atlas of Techniques in Surgery*. New York: Appleton-Century-Crofts, 1958. P. 454.

MERCADIER, M. P. Cystoduodenal anastomosis for cephalic cyst of the pancreas. *Ann. Surg.* 153:81, January 1961.

101. Surgery of Hypoglycemia

MILTON R. PORTER

IN FEW OPERATIONS is the differential diagnosis of such pivotal importance to the surgeon as in treatment of hypoglycemia. A high percentage of the patients explored for islet cell tumors reveal no lesion to the surgeon; consequently, he is obliged to do a "blind resection." In a Columbia-Presbyterian Hospital series that we reported in 1956, 28.8 per cent of the patients who had islet adenomas were "normal" when explored, but when subjected to empiric resection were found to have tumors. Obviously, the surgeon in such a situation has to feel secure about the diagnosis.

Conn and Seltzer in 1955, and others, have written about the differential diagnosis. Suffice it to say here that hepatic, pituitary, or adrenal disease sufficiently advanced to cause significant hypoglycemia is easily recognized if thought of and searched for. The harder and commoner problem is to differentiate between the various forms of functional hypoglycemia and that due to functioning islet tumors. Fortunately, we now have what may be a valuable and reliable test to help in this situation. Fajans et al. in 1961 published a description of the use of intravenously administered sodium tolbutamide in patients with various types of hypoglycemia. The tolbutamide apparently stimulates the islets of Langerhans to produce insulin, thereby driving the blood sugar down. The point is made that although the glucose level falls in all subjects, it stays at extremely low levels in persons with insulin-producing tumors for three hours or more, whereas in functional hypoglycemia a return to normal occurs earlier. If this test proves to have a high degree of reliability it will be invaluable. In the meantime it is necessary to employ the usual clinical criteria.

We recommend that the patient be studied in the hospital, where attacks can be observed and described by trained personnel, immediate blood sugar determinations can be done, and glucose infusions are easily given. Dr. Allen Whipple stressed the importance of the symptom complex which is now called the "Whipple triad": namely, (1) attacks of nervous or gastrointestinal disturbances coming on in the fasting state associated with (2) hypoglycemia with readings (blood sugar) below 50 mg. per cent, and (3) relief of symptoms by the ingestion of glucose.

Few patients who have tumors fail to exhibit the triad, but it is also true that some who have the triad do not have islet tumors. This latter group can be divided into three categories: (1) persons who have large sarcoma-like tumors associated with hypoglycemia—of which increasing numbers are being reported; (2) children —about whom more is said later in this chapter; (3) persons who may exhibit a perfect triad on one occasion but do not have a continuing, uniform pattern of attacks—a highly important finding. Patients in this third group should not be operated upon on the basis of one episode of hypoglycemia. If they have an islet tumor the syndrome will reappear and a little restraint on the part of the surgeon will enable him to be certain that the hypoglycemia is continuing in the typical repetitive manner. Once the diagnosis has been clearly established, however, further delay is pointless and may be dangerous.

Surgical Pathology

In most series of functioning islet cell tumors reported, the majority of patients are in the 35 to 60 age group. Such tumors, however, are certainly not uncommon in the third decade. The sex incidence is about even.

It is important to realize that these tumors can occur in any part of the gland and may be found in ectopic situations. When ectopic they are usually near the pancreas, in the duodenal, gastric, or jejunal walls, or in the jejunal mesentery.

There is no evidence that islet adenomas are premalignant lesions. Approximately 8 per cent of the functioning islet tumors prove to be malignant. As is the case with other endocrine tumors, the usual criteria of malignancy, such as blood vessel and capsular invasion, are unreliable when applied to islet cell growths.

Typically, benign functioning islet cell tumors are from 1 cm. to 2 cm. in diameter; if larger than 3 cm. in diameter, they should be suspected of being malignant. At the other extreme, functioning tumors as small as 3 mm. in diameter have been reported, emphasizing the difficulty of finding them. The bluish color of the typical adenoma is not invariably found. The tumor may be the same color as the surrounding pancreas.

Eighteen per cent of the patients in our reported Columbia-Presbyterian series had multiple tumors. Adenomatosis, or the occurrence of innumerable islet cell tumors, is found in a very small percentage of cases and may be part of the more complex syndrome of endocrine adenomatosis described by Wermer in 1954. Although many tumors may be palpable in the pancreas of a patient with adenomatosis, the majority are too small to be found without a microscope or at least a magnifying glass.

Hyperplasia of the islets of Langerhans has been much talked about and has occasionally been credited with causing clinical hyperinsulinism. In the series of *adult* patients operated upon at Columbia-Presbyterian Hospital, however, resection of non-tumor-bearing pancreas has not helped any patient who had a typical Whipple triad. It is an error, therefore, when exploring an *adult* for hypoglycemia, to assume that the finding of hyperplasia excuses the operator from further efforts to find a true neoplasm.

The Operative Procedure

These patients present no special problem for the anesthetist and are treated as any other candidate for major upper abdominal surgery except that they are given an infusion of 10 per cent dextrose in water. The infusion is started very early in the morning to prevent an attack of hypoglycemia. Obviously, it is desirable to arrange these cases as the first to be done in the morning schedule.

Some have advocated the use of steroids in the preparation of patients for operation, feeling that an "idiopathic postoperative hyperthermia" of major proportions may be avoided. Our experience leads us to believe that this unusual complication may be treated if and when it occurs by intravenous hydrocortisone, and therefore its preoperative use is not suggested. Fortunately, islet adenomas do not liberate excessive quantities of insulin when handled, as pheochromocytomas liberate epinephrine; therefore, no analogous problem occurs during operation.

The single most difficult problem in operating upon hypoglycemic patients is finding the tumor. The patient is often very obese and harbors in his pancreas an adenoma which may be only a few millimeters in diameter. As has been stated, in more than one-fourth of the patients in our Columbia-Presbyterian series who had tumors, nothing could be found until part or all of the gland was given to the pathologist.

It is therefore of paramount importance that the gland be most carefully inspected at laparotomy. Running the hand over the anterior surface of the organ is not enough. The peritoneum must be incised along the entire length of the tail of the gland and along the lateral edge of the duodenum, permitting complete mobilization of the pancreas from the structures posterior to it. The fingers are inserted behind the gland, and with the thumb on the anterior surface every centimeter of the substance of the organ is carefully studied (Fig. 1). *If this is not done, one cannot claim to have adequately explored for an islet adenoma.* Failure to cut the peritoneum and thus permit accurate palpation is one of the commonest causes of failure to find the tumor. The patient must then have another laparotomy or ultimately die of hypoglycemia.

Often a characteristic lesion is easily found on the anterior surface of the gland and quickly removed. It is an error, however, to remove such a lesion and close the abdomen without thoroughly mobilizing the gland as just described, because one or more other adenomas will be present in nearly one-fifth of cases. The operator should have all adenomas subjected to frozen section examination by the pathologist in the operating suite—not in order to see whether the lesion is benign or malignant, but to see whether it is an islet cell tumor at all. Lymph nodes and lobulations of normal pancreatic tissue may each exactly simulate the gross appearance of adenomas.

When an adenoma is found it is dissected out of the pancreas with a small margin of surrounding tissue. The technique used is much the same as that used in cutting through thyroid tissue. For the most part, it is safe and convenient to cut between clamps and to tie with silk or cotton (never catgut, since leaking en-

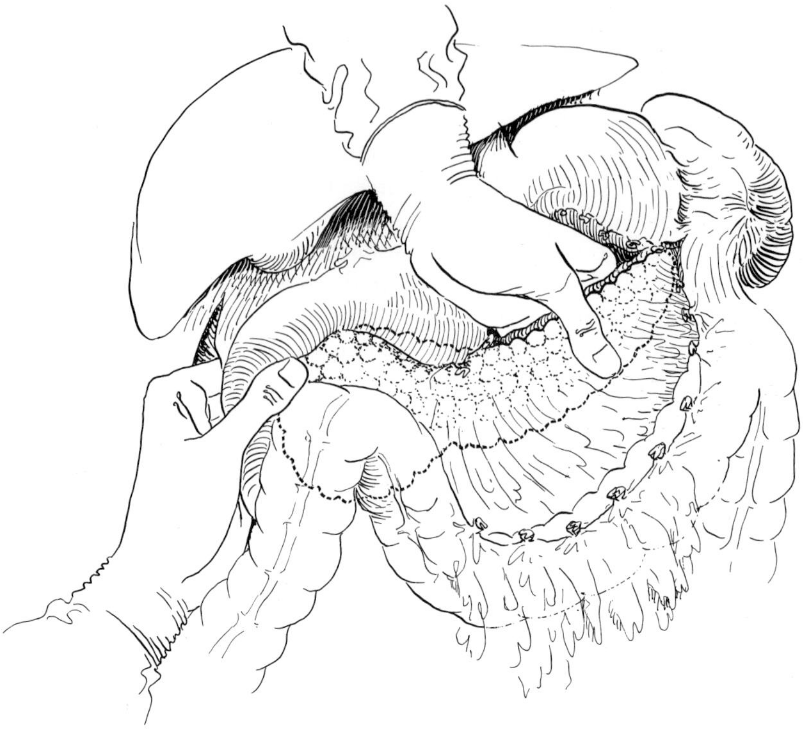

FIGURE 1. Palpation of the pancreas. Careful inspection must accompany the palpation.

zymes might dissolve it rapidly, with a resultant secondary hemorrhage). Such wounds should always be drained. A small fenestrated rubber tube is more efficient in this situation than the Penrose drain.

In those adult patients in whom exploration, however carefully done, reveals nothing, it is recommended that the spleen and tail of the pancreas as far to the right as the portal vein be removed (Fig. 2). The specimen is then given to an experienced surgical pathologist who very carefully slices it every few millimeters, looking for a tumor (Fig. 2, insert). Anything suspicious is examined microscopically. If nothing is found, most of the head of the gland is removed, leaving enough gland along the duodenum to protect the blood supply of the duodenum and common bile duct (Fig. 2). This fragment is similarly examined for tumor, and if none is found a pancreatoduodenectomy is completed and all the indicated anastomoses are done. The technical details are the same as those described in Chapter 98.

This radical approach stems from the experience at Columbia-Presbyterian Hospital which suggests that in properly studied patients, in whom operation is indicated, it is safer to keep on until the adenoma is found than to stop and have to operate again. The removal of non-tumor-bearing gland is of no use if the diagnosis of islet adenoma is correct; and if the diagnosis of islet adenoma is not

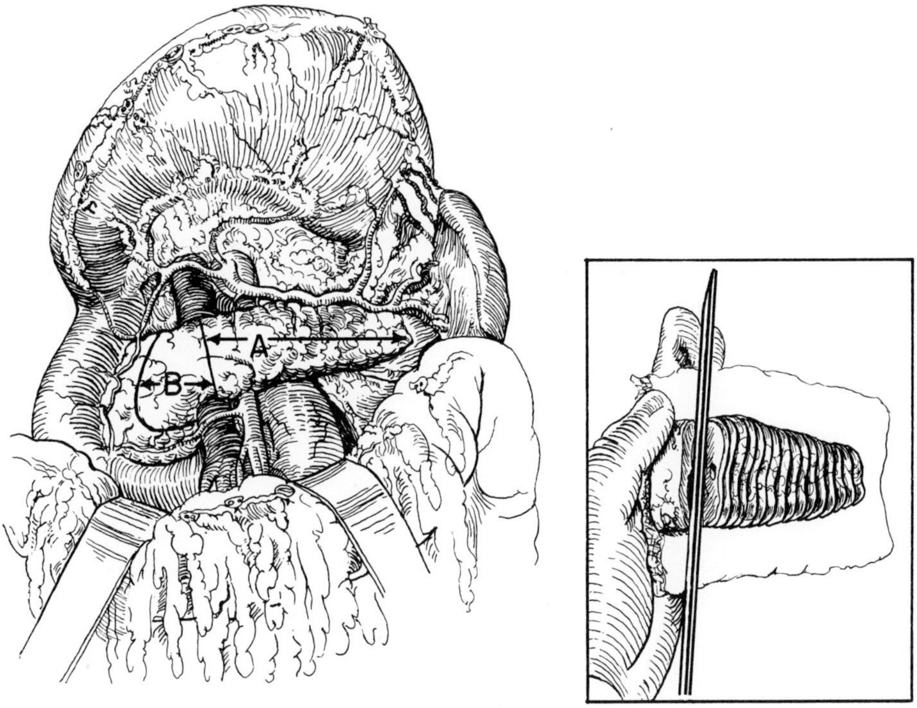

FIGURE 2. Segment of the pancreas first excised (A) and segment secondarily removed (B). The blood supply of the duodenum and the common bile duct is protected. *Insert:* Slicing of the specimen. The specimen is usually sliced on a cork board.

correct, no operation at all is indicated. One cannot, on the basis of our experience, take refuge in the thought that a negative exploration rules out the possibility of a tumor. It is essential that an agreement as to how the problem will be managed be made preoperatively with the surgical pathologist so that he understands the role he is to play.

Hypoglycemia in Children

Functioning islet cell adenomas do occur in the first decade but they are exceedingly rare. Various other types of hypoglycemia are relatively common, and some are peculiar to childhood.

The "idiopathic spontaneously occurring hypoglycemia in infants" described by McQuarrie in 1954 is probably the most important insofar as confusion with islet cell tumors is concerned. Some of the conditions included in this group have been found to be leucine-sensitive hypoglycemias and it is possible that in the future more if not all of these infantile hypoglycemias, previously regarded as idiopathic, will be explained.

The point of paramount importance for the surgeon to bear in mind is that an infant or child who would obviously qualify for exploration for islet tumors if he were an adult should not be operated upon until he has been carefully studied by a pediatrician, who in many instances will elect to treat the child with cortisone. Presumably a child patient harboring a functioning islet cell adenoma would not be able to get along without steroids and would ultimately be explored.

At such an exploration, if no tumor were found, only the tail of the pancreas would be removed. *Unlike the adult patients,* the resection of non-tumor-bearing pancreas has helped hypoglycemic children, and the more radical policy recommended for adults should *not* be applied to pediatric patients.

Postoperative Complications

Diabetes

Many patients whose functioning islet cell tumors have been removed develop transient mild diabetes postoperatively. This rarely lasts beyond 10 days. It should be watched for and treated with standard insulin according to the patient's needs as demonstrated by periodic urine analysis. The use of longer-acting insulin is contraindicated since the patient's requirements are constantly changing in the short period in question.

Fistulas

Whenever the pancreas is incised a fistula may develop. Fortunately, it does not happen often. There is no immediate danger if the drainage provided is adequate and if nonabsorbable ligatures and sutures have been used in the wound.

In our experience no paste or ointment is as efficient in protecting the skin from digestion by activated enzymes as is the use of an efficient sump type of suction drain which never lets the pancreatic juice reach the skin. If a tube drain has been used in the first place, a second smaller tube can be suspended in it and attached to suction if the need arises.

Unless a major duct has been lacerated, such fistulas usually dry up in a few weeks. If they do not, the tract is allowed to become mature or fibrous and is then implanted into the back of the stomach.

References

Conn, J. W., and Seltzer, H. S. Spontaneous hypoglycemia. *Am. J. Med.* 19:460, September 1955.

Fajans, S. S., Schneider, J. M., Schteingart, D. E., and Conn, J. W. The diagnostic value of sodium tolbutamide in hypoglycemic states. *J. Clin. Endocrinol. and Metab.* 21:371, April 1961.

Lowbeer, L. Hypoglycemia-producing extrapancreatic neoplasms. *Am. J. Clin. Path.* 35:233, March 1961.

Porter, M. R., and Frantz, V. K. Tumors associated with hypoglycemia–pancreatic and extrapancreatic. *Am. J. Med.* 21:944, December 1956.

Wermer, P. Genetic aspects of adenomatosis of endocrine glands. *Am. J. Med.* 16:363, March 1954.

102. *Splenectomy*

CORNELIUS E. SEDGWICK

TO NARRATE in detail the indications and contraindications for splenectomy is not within the scope of this chapter. It is important, however, to have a basic understanding of the reasons for removal of a particular spleen and the results that can be expected.

Certain indications for splenectomy are classified as surgical. They are definite, involve only the spleen, and are handled on the surgical service. They include splenic tumors, the "wandering" spleen, and the ruptured spleen. The second group of indications for splenectomy are medical and are not always definite. They are the concern of the internist as well as the surgeon. These indications involve not only the spleen but other organs as well, the reticuloendothelial system, the circulating blood, and the bone marrow. The medical indications for splenectomy do not lend themselves well to textbook discussions, and didactic statements must not be made. The most definite are familial hemolytic anemia, thrombocytopenic purpura, acquired hemolytic anemia, and splenomegaly with hypersplenism. As emphasized by Norcross, these indications are constantly undergoing a process of revision. Each year additions are made to the list of well-established reasons for surgical removal of the spleen, and occasionally new forms of treatment tend to lessen the advisability of splenectomy in some diseases. Indeed, only the rare surgeon who has confined his interest to the hematological problems associated with splenic disease will be competent to decide whether splenectomy should or should not be performed. The problem is complex and the opinions among even those best informed are changing constantly. It is wise for the general surgeon to be guided by his medical confreres when the advisability of removing the spleen of a patient with a particular blood dyscrasia is in doubt.

Elective Splenectomy

To perform a safe, well-planned splenectomy, the surgeon must utilize every advantage at his command. This means anesthesia with complete relaxation, good lighting, adequate assistants, and a generous incision. A gastric tube to keep the stomach deflated is of utmost importance. The patient should be placed on the operating table with the left side slightly elevated.

The Incision and the Exploration

No one incision is best for all cases. A long, left rectus muscle-splitting or paramedian muscle-retracting incision from the costal margin to well below the umbilicus is satisfactory for the usual patient who has a narrow or average costal angle. I prefer this incision particularly for those with a moderately enlarged spleen, as found in hemolytic anemia or thrombocytopenic purpura. However, in a patient who has a wide costal margin, or a patient who has congestive splenomegaly with the possibility of perisplenitis, and a tremendously enlarged spleen adherent to the diaphragm, or a patient in whom bleeding from portal hypertension is suspected, a long transverse or subcostal incision, extending from the midline well back to the lumbar muscles, is of greater technical assistance. If the spleen is extremely large and a splenorenal shunt for portal hypertension is to follow splenectomy, an abdominothoracic incision, extending the abdominal incision through the eighth interspace, gives adequate exposure and facilitates performance of the operation. If the abdomen is opened through an inadequate incision, the danger of tearing or rupturing a vessel, with troublesome hemorrhage, is always present. Revision or enlargement of an incision may transform what appears to be a difficult operation into a simple and safe procedure.

As in performing any laparotomy, on opening the abdominal cavity the surgeon does a thorough exploration. In performing elective splenectomy, however, especially when associated with a blood dyscrasia, particular care should be taken to ascertain the presence of any accessory spleens. These are usually found near the hilum of the spleen along the gastrosplenic ligament, or along the anterior-superior border of the pancreas. Also, because many of these patients may have an associated jaundice, care is taken to examine the extrabiliary tract.

Mobilization of the Spleen

After the abdomen has been explored and the decision made to proceed with removal of the spleen, the operator determines the mobility of the spleen. In some cases this may be extremely simple, and the spleen may be delivered into the wound. In other instances removal may be difficult because of the size of the spleen, because of adhesions running from the capsule of the spleen to the diaphragm, or because of the habitus of a particular patient with a short splenorenal ligament—in such cases the spleen may be so high up under the diaphragm that mobilization may become a problem. A large spleen may be simpler to mobilize than a small one. As the spleen enlarges, it protrudes farther caudad and toward the midline and may be more easily retracted into the wound. A very small spleen, situated high up under the diaphragm, with a short splenorenal ligament, may be extremely difficult to bring into adequate view. I prefer to determine the mobility of the spleen before any definitive dissection is performed, so that if hemorrhage becomes a problem during the procedure, I have some idea how I can rapidly mobilize the spleen.

Ligation of Vessels, Section of Ligaments, and Removal of the Spleen

In elective splenectomy, whether or not the spleen is mobile, I open the lesser sac and ligate the splenic artery along the superior border of the pancreas (Fig. 1). This conserves blood and allows the spleen to shrink and become smaller. When opening the lesser sac I divide as many of the short gastric vessels along the fundus of the stomach as possible. Frequently, with this exposure, the superior short gastric vessels cannot be safely ligated and divided. They are better handled later in the procedure when the spleen is delivered into the wound. Any attachments to the splenic flexure of the colon are divided and mobilization of the spleen is begun. The spleen is retracted downward and to the right. The splenorenal ligament is divided and an avascular plane is entered (Fig. 2). As dissection proceeds in this fascial plane, the hilus of the spleen, the splenic vessels, and the tail of the pancreas are mobilized into the wound.

In patients who have enlarged spleens with perisplenitis and in those with

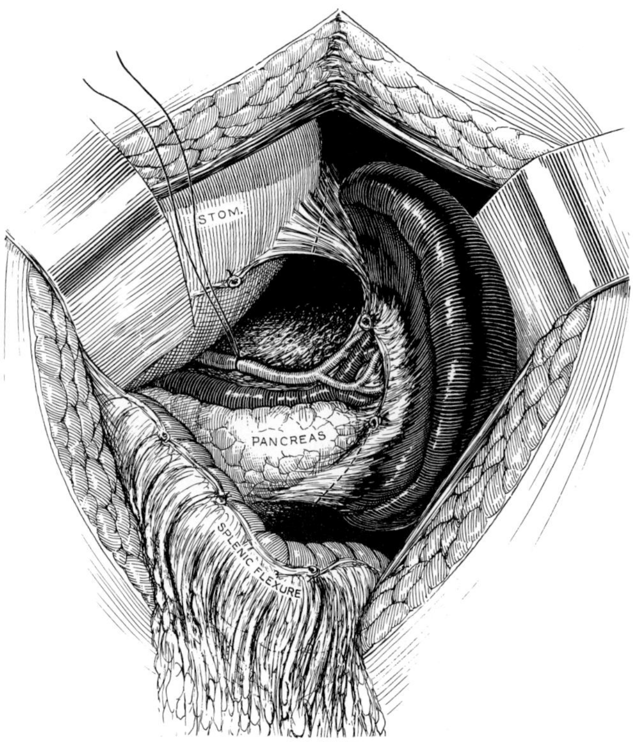

FIGURE 1. Lesser sac exposed. Splenic artery ligated in continuity. The remaining superior short gastric vessels are ligated from behind after the spleen has been further mobilized.

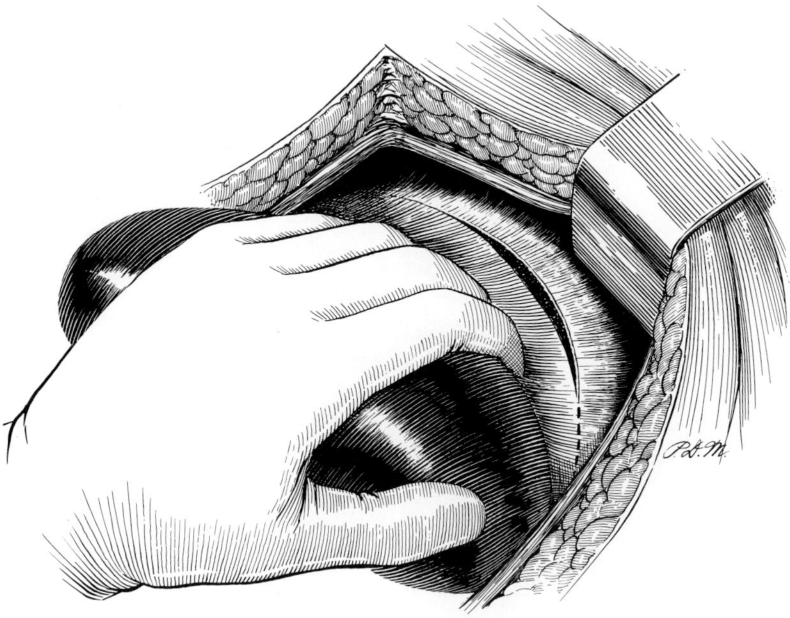

FIGURE 2. Splenorenal ligament incised so that the spleen may be retracted into the wound.

portal hypertension, there may be many dense, vascular adhesions between the spleen and the diaphragm. These can be divided quickly and a large pack placed up beneath the diaphragm for hemostasis. The spleen is then well mobilized into the surgical field and the vessels can be seen in the hilum posteriorly. The surgeon has complete control of the splenic pedicle, and if an accident occurs to the vessels, hemorrhage can easily be controlled. The remaining short gastric vessels are divided and the stomach is packed back into the abdomen. A point that deserves emphasis is that a hilar dissection of the vessels should be performed with individual ligation of the vessels in the hilum of the spleen, taking great care not to injure the pancreas (Fig. 3). The splenic artery is doubly ligated. The remaining vessels are divided and the spleen is removed.

Usually, when the pack that has been placed up under the diaphragm is removed, there is little or no bleeding. If any bleeders are present, they can be clamped and ligated easily because of the excellent exposure.

Comments

In a study of 220 cases, we found that the number of complications after splenectomy was quite high. Hemorrhage should not occur if sufficient care has been taken to assure hemostasis. Thrombosis and particularly pyelophlebitis are unusual, even though there may be an excessive rise in platelets after removal of the spleen. Subdiaphragmatic abscesses, however, are probably more frequent after splenectomy

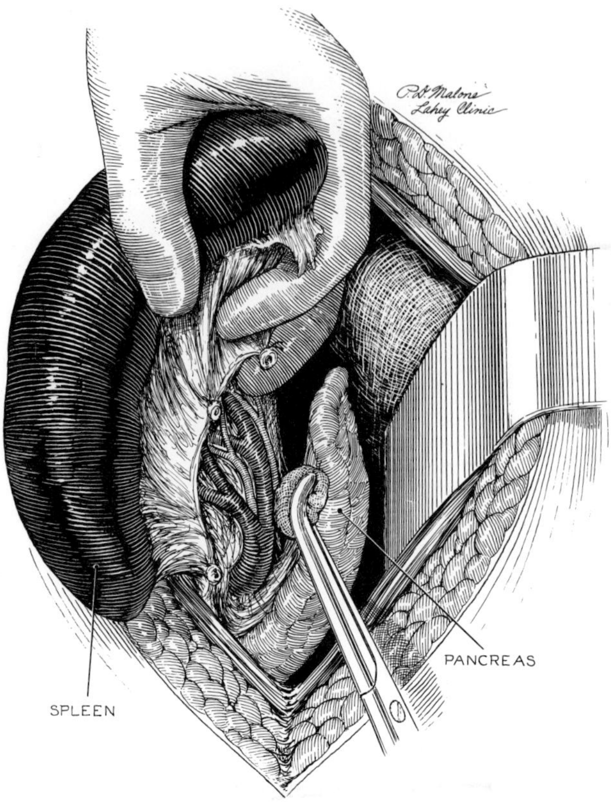

FIGURE 3. Hilar dissection of the splenic vessels from behind. Care is taken to avoid injury to the tail of the pancreas.

than after other abdominal procedures. The frequency of their occurrence can be reduced by taking care not to injure pancreatic tissue when the vessels in the hilum are ligated, and by instituting drainage in all cases.

Emergency Splenectomy

By far the most common indication for splenectomy is the ruptured spleen. The spleen frequently is abnormally large—for example, that found secondary to malaria. Ruptured spleen may be caused by direct external violence such as a stab or gunshot wound. The diagnosis of ruptured spleen is usually apparent if there is a history of trauma, and if signs and symptoms of blood loss, such as shock, are present. The amount of blood loss is not necessarily reflected by the hematocrit reading. Vasoconstriction may compensate for blood loss, and the hematocrit may vary little from normal. A better laboratory diagnostic aid is a rapidly rising white blood cell count to 40,000 or 50,000 in a few hours, because of peritoneal irritation.

The surgeon should be aware that the rupture may be intracapsular rather than into the free abdominal cavity. The patient may weather the initial injury and show little clinical evidence of severe trauma, while an intracapsular hematoma of the spleen develops. Later, this may rupture into the free abdominal cavity, producing all the signs and symptoms of perforation and hemorrhage. When splenic rupture is suspected, the patient should be hospitalized and carefully studied. Blood replacement and surgery should be available at a moment's notice.

I prefer a high, long, left rectus muscle-splitting incision for a ruptured spleen. This usually provides good exposure in case other abdominal parietes have been injured and require surgical attention. If this incision is inadequate, however, as soon as the peritoneum has been opened and the diagnosis confirmed, the incision should be extended transversely to the left, which allows better access to the spleen. Frequently, when the abdomen is opened, the peritoneal cavity is filled with blood and gastric and intestinal contents. The incision must be large enough

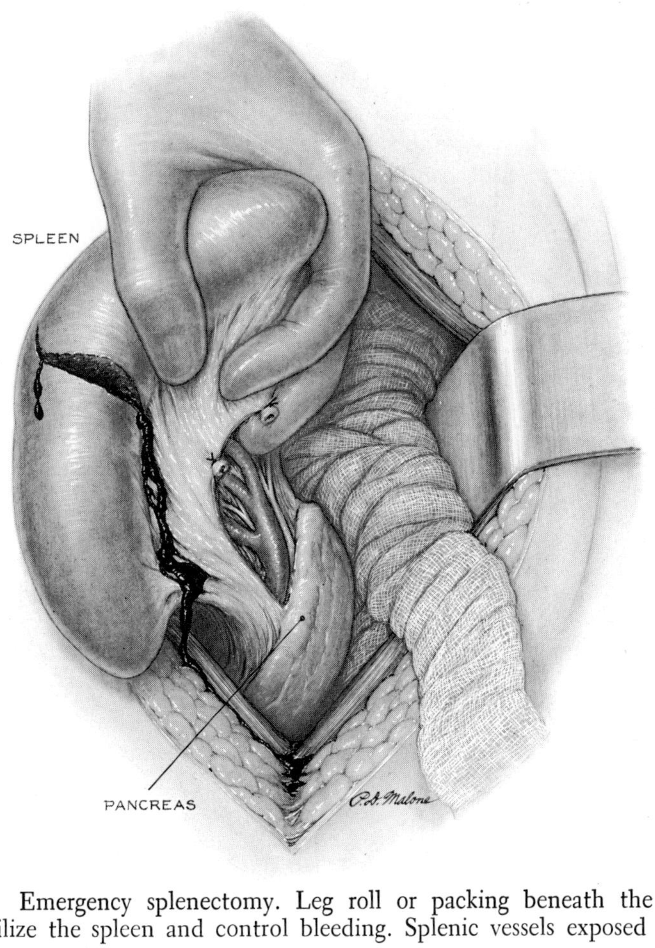

FIGURE 4. Emergency splenectomy. Leg roll or packing beneath the diaphragm to help mobilize the spleen and control bleeding. Splenic vessels exposed and ligated posteriorly.

to permit rapid exploration of the abdomen; all of the trauma should be quickly noted and evaluated.

If splenectomy is indicated, the technique is different from that described for elective splenectomy. It is too time-consuming and difficult in the presence of massive hemorrhage to open the lesser sac and to locate and ligate the splenic artery at its origin. It should be remembered that the splenic vessels are much more accessible from behind (Fig. 4). With the surgeon on the right side, the left hand is quickly introduced over the spleen and the spleen is retracted downward and to the right. The posterior leaf of the splenorenal ligament is divided and the spleen retracted anteriorly. Bleeding may occur from the vessels between the spleen and the diaphragm. As the spleen is retracted downward and to the right, a packing in the form of a long leg roll is placed beneath the diaphragm. As this packing is inserted, the spleen is gradually displaced downward and anteriorly and the vessels entering the spleen from behind are readily seen and can easily be ligated and divided. Care should be taken not to injure the stomach. When the hemorrhage is controlled, the attachments to the stomach and colon can be divided more leisurely and the spleen removed. The packing is then removed from beneath the diaphragm and any persistent bleeding is controlled. Once the spleen has been delivered into the wound, if massive hemorrhage persists, a rubber-shod clamp can be placed across the splenic vessels and tail of the pancreas for temporary control. When this situation has become stabilized, a more careful hilar dissection with individual ligations of vessels can be performed.

References

NORCROSS, J. W. Indications for splenectomy. *S. Clin. North America* 38:831, June 1958.

SEDGWICK, C. E., and HUME, A. H. Elective splenectomy: an analysis of 220 operations. *Ann. Surg.* 151:163, February 1960.

XVII. THE ADRENAL GLANDS

103. *Adrenalectomy*

HAROLD A. ZINTEL

THE ALL–IMPORTANT, very friable adrenal glands are tucked away deep in the abdomen in a well-protected place, much as the pituitary gland is tucked away in the cranial cavity. The adrenal glands are difficult to expose. Even at postmortem examination, when evisceration is not resorted to, it is usually difficult to visualize the glands and their position in relation to other structures. A knowledge of the relationship of the adrenal glands to the structures surrounding them, and of the blood supply of these glands, is most important for understanding nuances of surgical technique. The detailed anatomy of the adrenal glands and their relationship to other organs is poorly or incorrectly shown in present-day books of anatomy. Their structure, position, blood supply, and relationship to other organs will be described briefly here. The observations that follow are based on the exposure of some 600 adrenal glands at operations for hypertension, tumors of the glands, and disseminated carcinoma.

Anatomy and Anatomical Relations of the Adrenal Glands

The adrenal glands are situated in the posterior abdominal wall behind the peritoneum and in a layer of fat of varying thickness—the preperitoneal fat and periadrenal fat. When they are approached through the abdominal cavity, their general position can be described as being along the medial edges of the superior ends of the posterolateral gutters of the abdominal cavity. The most medial portion of the right adrenal gland lies within 5 to 10 mm. of the inferior vena cava, and the left adrenal gland lies within 1 to 2 cm. of the lateral border of the aorta (Fig. 1). The alternate name, suprarenal gland, indicates that these glands lie cephalad (and slightly medial) to the upper pole of the kidney. They are buried in capsules of fat which, like the fatty capsule of the kidney, are encased anteriorly and laterally by Gerota's fascia (Fig. 2). The fat separates the adrenal gland from the kidney by several millimeters. If the fat is peeled from Glisson's capsule of the kidney, the adrenal gland is not immediately evident. The fat is more resistant than fat in most other areas of the body, probably because it is the site of an arborization of

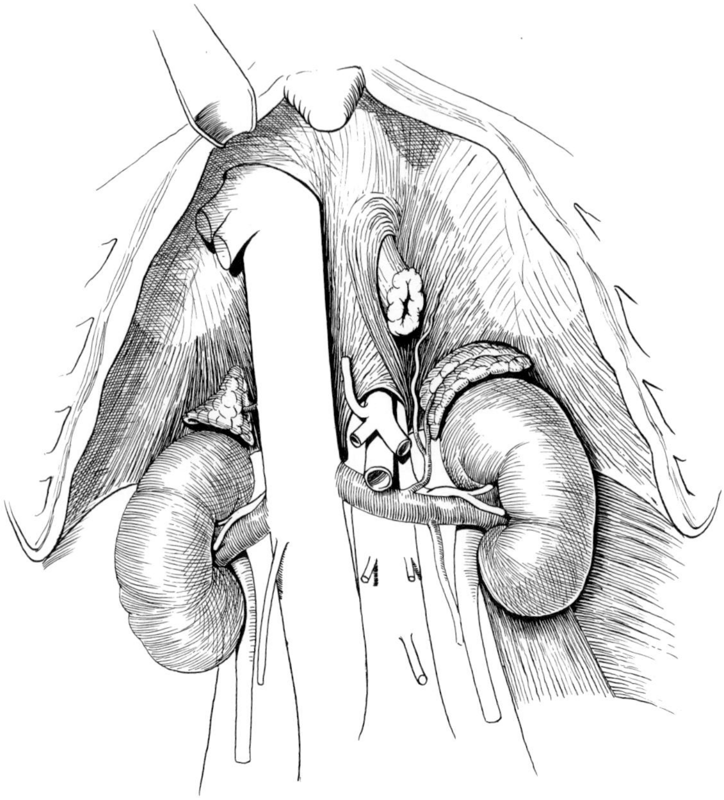

FIGURE 1. Relationships of the adrenal glands along the posterior abdominal wall to the attachments of the diaphragm, to the kidneys, to the major vessels, and to the esophagus. The fact that the two glands are rather different in shape is well demonstrated.

many small arteries and arterioles. Occasionally, branches of these same vessels also enter the upper pole of the kidney. With the patient in the supine position one finds, posterior to the adrenal gland, the fatty capsule just described and the lower portion of the tented diaphragm. The adrenal glands are situated at or slightly superior to the attachment of the diaphragm to the posterior wall. Posterior to the diaphragm, of course, are the pleural surfaces of the sulci. Posterior to these are the layers of the chest wall (Fig. 2).

Superior to the adrenal glands on either side are the tenting diaphragm and the posterior portions of the liver. Anterior to the left adrenal gland are the posterior edge of the liver, the fundic portion of the stomach very near the cardia, the gastrocolic ligament, and the splenic flexure of the colon. And slightly caudad, but still anterior, lie the tail of the pancreas, the spleen, and the major splenic arteries and veins. These latter structures occasionally lie almost directly over the adrenal gland. On the right side, the center of the mass of the liver lies almost directly anterior to the adrenal gland. The right gland lies posterior and a little superior to the position of the gallbladder and the cystic duct. It is necessary to retract and

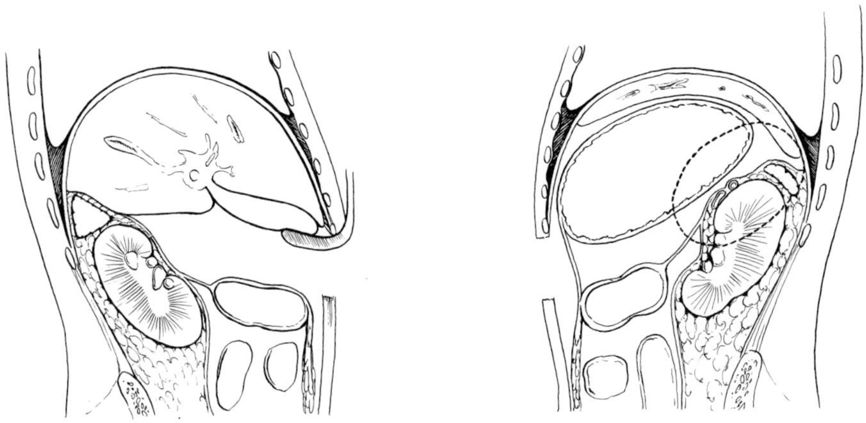

FIGURE 2. Sagittal sections through the right (*A*) and left (*B*) adrenal glands. The adrenal glands are surrounded and separated from the kidney by a capsule of fat. Posterior to the adrenals are the diaphragm, pleural sulci, and posterior chest walls. Superior to the glands is the liver. Inferior is the upper pole of the kidney. On the right side (*A*) the anterior abdominal approach is along the inferior surface of the liver to the adrenal gland, just posterior to the liver. On the left side (*B*) the stomach, gastrocolic ligament, and colon are anterior to the gland. Also, part or all of the tail of the pancreas, splenic vessels, and spleen may be anterior to the gland.

elevate the liver to gain access to the right adrenal gland, regardless of whether the anterior abdominal or lateral flank approach is used.

The vascularity of the adrenal gland is very great. It is a sinusoidal gland and, in this respect, is somewhat similar in structure to the spleen and liver. Although the gland normally weighs only 6 or 7 grams, continuous venous bleeding from the gland itself can be protracted and extensive. The gland is also very friable. Unlike any other organ of the body, it receives its arterial blood supply through innumerable arterioles which penetrate the cortical surface of the gland. These very small arteries gain access to the gland almost entirely at the periphery of the relatively flat gland (Fig. 3). Comparatively few of these tiny little vessels penetrate the

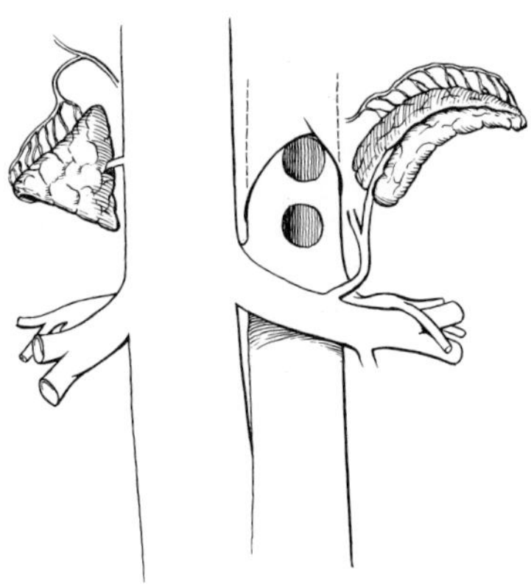

FIGURE 3. The comparative shapes of the right and left glands and their relationships to the vena cava on the left, the aorta on the right, and the renal vessels are shown. Also one of the usual three to five arterial trunks to each gland is shown with its many arteriolar branches perforating primarily the periphery of the gland. The openings in the aorta represent the origin of the celiac axis (*above*) and the superior mesenteric artery (*below*).

anterior and posterior surfaces of the gland. Merklin and Michels (1958) state that "the adrenal blood supply varies to such an extent that it is never the same in any two bodies or in any two sides" of a given body. Anywhere from 4 to 30 tiny branches entering the gland may be derived from each of the three to five arterial trunks supplying the adrenal gland. The main trunks of these arteries may vary in size from slightly less than a millimeter to approximately a millimeter and a half in diameter. Most frequently the major arteries are described as superior marginal, middle and inferior adrenal arteries, arising from the inferior phrenic arteries, the aorta, and the renal arteries respectively.

Venous drainage occurs almost invariably through a single vein. Normally this vein is about 3 mm. in diameter. When two veins emerge from the surface of the gland, they join into one within a few millimeters.

The left adrenal gland with its vein resembles in shape a very thick leaf with a stem vein (in reverse) and a stem—the vein. The anterior surface of the gland is corrugated longitudinally by one or two furrows. The furrows are always present in the left gland, but are rarely obvious in the right gland. After uncovering carefully the anterior surface of the left adrenal gland, one can follow the corrugations or valleys medially direct to the renal vein (Fig. 3). The vein from the left gland usually joins the vein from the diaphragm, and the confluence of these two, after a course of 2 to 5 cm., joins the left renal vein. The greatest thickness of the elongated, flat left adrenal is barely one-sixth or one-eighth of its total length. Its width varies from approximately one-half to one-fourth of its total length.

The right adrenal gland, when viewed from its anterior surface, has the outline of a triangle. Actually the view would be of the base of an inverted pyramid. The thickness of the right gland may represent one-third or one-half of its greatest length. The usual single vein emerges from the side of the triangular base, which parallels the wall of the vena cava. As previously mentioned, the right gland rarely exhibits a corrugation or valley. The vein is extremely thin-walled and runs transversely, traversing the fatty envelope for a distance of usually one-quarter to three-eighths of an inch to join, almost at a right angle, the relatively thin-walled inferior vena cava.

Approaches to the Adrenals

There are four obvious approaches to the adrenal glands. The most practical approach in most patients is the abdominal. This approach allows inspection and palpation of both adrenal glands as well as palpation of the entire abdominal aorta, along which most aberrant adrenal tissue is found. The lateral subcostal approach provides the most direct approach to either the right or the left gland only. It is used for the removal of a tumor demonstrated by x-ray examination in a very seriously ill patient. The lateral subcostal does not allow inspection of the opposite adrenal gland, a search for aberrant adrenal tissue, or inspection of both ovaries.

The posterior approach through a vertical incision along the lateral border of the sacrospinalis muscles is very difficult. In unusual circumstances, the adrenal gland can be exposed through the chest cavity by incising the diaphragm.

Abdominal Approach

In addition to allowing inspection of both adrenal glands and a search for aberrant tissue, the abdominal approach permits inspection of the ovaries. Lesions of the ovaries sometimes simulate adrenal disease. This same approach is also used for bilateral total adrenalectomy and bilateral oophrectomy in the treatment of patients in the advanced stages of carcinoma of the breast. A vertical incision is the preferred type (Fig. 4). The incision should extend well up into the angle beside the xyphoid process and the costal margin. The xyphoid process may be excised to provide more exposure. The incision may be made along the midline, circumventing the umbilicus, or it may be a paramedian rectus incision in the left rectus sheath. The latter allows a two-layer instead of a one-layer fascial closure. This incision circumvents the umbilicus and extends 4 to 5 cm. below the umbilicus. In obese and short, stocky individuals, a transverse incision curving upward toward the xyphoid process is used. Such an incision, when long enough, allows exploration from the dome of the diaphragm well into the depths of the pelvis. The upward curve eliminates the necessity for the right-angle extensions of the straight transverse incision which some surgeons have advocated for adrenalectomy.

Exposing the Right Gland

After the abdomen has been entered, the right adrenal gland, being the more accessible of the two glands, is usually explored first. However, if there is x-ray evidence of a functioning pheochromocytoma on the left side, such a tumor is attacked first. The first step is to do a Kocher maneuver, usually reflecting the duo-

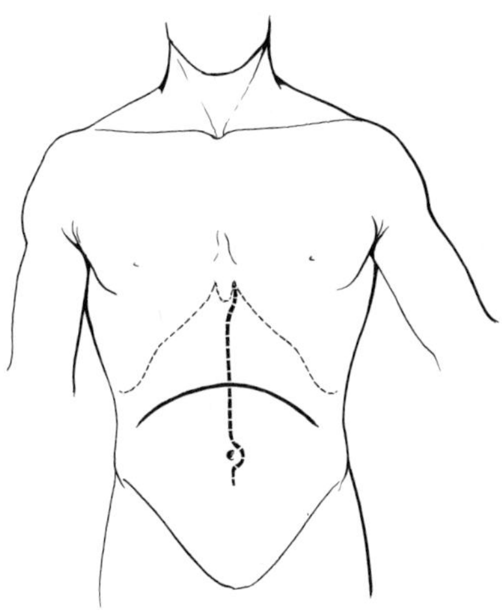

FIGURE 4. The dashed vertical incision is the preferred incision. Whether a midline, as shown, or paramedian incision is used makes no significant difference. For short, obese individuals the transverse curved incision is most desirable.

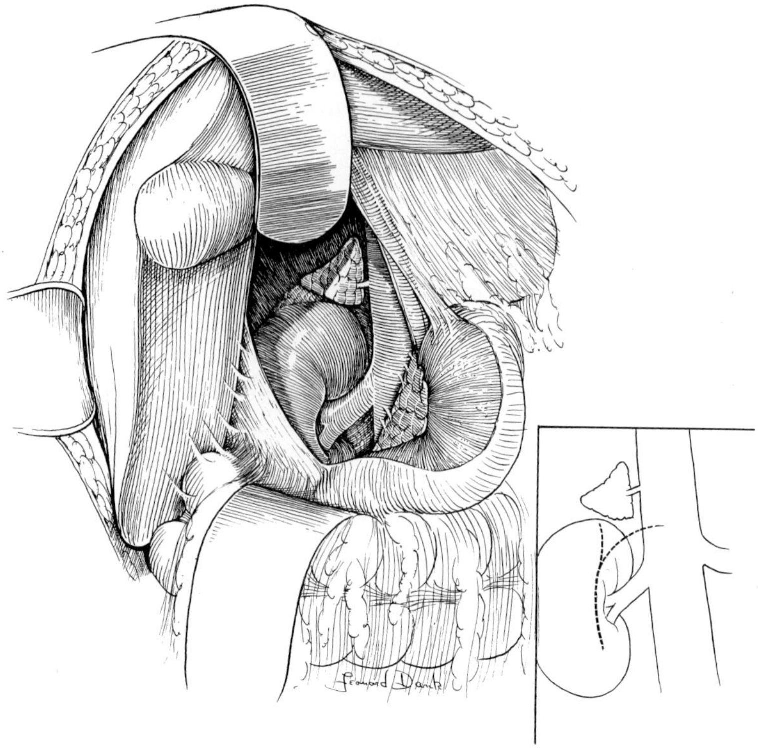

FIGURE 5. In the inset the curved dashed line indicates the peritoneal incision for the Kocher maneuver. A slight extension of the incision as shown allows further separation of the peritoneum by traction. Firm traction on the inferior surface of the liver allows sufficient elevation of gallbladder, cystic duct, and liver for visualization of the right adrenal gland. Traction applied downward–inferiorly on the upper pole of the kidney–usually brings the adrenal gland area more directly into view. The perirenal and periadrenal fat is not included in the diagram.

denal loop well over toward the left side and exposing a bit of the posterior surface of the head of the pancreas, as shown in Figure 5. In exposing the right adrenal area, it may be necessary to divide peritoneal reflections or adhesions between the colon and the undersurface of the liver. In very obese individuals it may be advantageous to detach and reflect inferiorly the hepatic flexure of the colon, as in the performance of a right hemicolectomy.

With a large, medium-wide retractor, the liver, gallbladder, and cystic duct are retracted cephalad and anteriorly, to expose the space behind the liver and the upper portion of the right posterolateral abdominal gutter. The colon and the transverse mesocolon are retracted caudad and to the right. The peritoneal surface lateral to the peritoneal incision used in the Kocher maneuver is then extended upward a centimeter or two, roughly parallel and approximately a centimeter lateral to the lateral edge of the inferior vena cava. The retroperitoneal, perinephric, and periadrenal fat is thus exposed. If the inferior vena cava is not well visualized after performance of the Kocher maneuver, the fat and the areolar tissue over the anterior surface of the vena cava are elevated with long, smooth forceps and the tissue is divided with long, curved scissors until the anterior surface of the vena cava is exposed. It is advisable to continue this dissection downward as well as upward. One should expose the right renal vein to prevent injury to this structure. Uncovering the vena cava superiorly exposes the short, thin-walled adrenal vein emerging from the lateral wall of the cava. Once these landmarks have been established, one can palpate the position of the upper pole of the kidney. The anterior edge of the adrenal gland is then exposed by both sharp and blunt dissection along a transverse plane 3 to 5 mm. superior to the tip of the upper pole of the kidney. This plane is several millimeters inferior to the adrenal vein and several centimeters above the plane of the inferior surface of the liver. The color of the gland is a cadmium yellow, which is a slightly more intense yellow than that of the surrounding fat.

Having exposed and positively identified a small area of the adrenal cortex, one then separates with the scissors the anterior edge of the periphery of the gland from the fat exactly at the surface of the gland. In doing so, one is usually able to divide the numerous tiny arterioles without any significant bleeding. Only occasionally does one divide an adrenal vessel that requires clamping and ligation in the periadrenal fat. No attempt is made to find the arterial trunks leading to the gland, because the trunks are very small and their origin is most uncertain in any particular person. Once the anterior edge of the periphery of the gland has been separated, the entire anterior and posterior flat surfaces are uncovered by blunt dissection. This is done with the finger or the tip of the closed scissors, with very little danger of producing any significant bleeding. Silver clips are placed on the short, thin-walled vein. If one attempts to place clamps and ligatures on this vein, occasionally a tear in the side of the vena cava will result. Since the venous pressure in the vena cava is 5 mm. of mercury or less, a well-placed clip or two is all that is required. The vein is divided. Finally the posterior superior edge of the periphery of the gland is separated from the fat with scissors—again cutting at the surface of the cortex.

An opening caused by separation of the adrenal vein as it joins the vena cava, or a small tear in the inferior vena cava, can be successfully repaired with carefully placed running sutures of 6–0 arterial silk. When this complication occurs, the first thing to do is to place a pad over the vena cava and support both with a finger. Then make your plans. Be sure to have two suction tips and two wall suction tubes ready. By the time everything is ready, including the arterial silk sutures, it may be your good fortune to find that the caval rent has stopped bleeding. Then all one has to do is reinforce the area with sutures. Such a complication is to be avoided, of course, since repair of such a lesion is difficult deep within the abdomen regardless of the approach used. The use of silver clips on the right adrenal vein will eliminate this complication.

Exposing the Left Gland

In approaching the left adrenal gland there are three main avenues one can use with an abdominal incision. The first is a direct approach between the diaphragm and the fundus of the stomach (occasionally through the gastrohepatic ligament). The second approach is through the lesser peritoneal cavity via the gastrocolic ligament. The third is through the left side of the transverse mesocolon and the lesser peritoneal cavity.

In a very asthenic person it is sometimes possible, when using the first approach, simply to retract downward and medially the fundus of the stomach and the spleen. A retractor elevates the costal margin and the left lobe of the liver. Occasionally the left lobe of the liver is detached from the diaphragm and folded medially. The spleen and stomach are best retracted by the surgeon's or the assistant's hand, over an abdominal pad. The danger of tearing the splenic capsule if a retractor is used, even over an abdominal pad, is obvious. If the spleen is adherent to the lateral abdominal wall, it can be freed by sharp dissection; similarly, peritoneal reflections can be divided by sharp dissection, usually without bleeding. Unfortunately, in a great many patients this first avenue of approach is not practical.

If one is unable to approach the adrenal area from above and laterally to the fundus of the stomach, one should take a look at the gastrohepatic ligament. In a very few persons it is quite long and very thin and will afford enough room to expose or remove an adrenal gland by this avenue. Any of the major vessels in the left half of the gastrohepatic ligament may be divided without fear of embarrassing the blood supply to the esophagus or the stomach, providing the remaining blood supply to the stomach is intact.

In using the second approach, through the lesser peritoneal cavity, one separates the avascular attachment of the posterior surface of the omentum to the colon, as in gastric resection for carcinoma. The fundic portion of the stomach is held upward against the left lobe of the liver, and the midportion of the stomach is held more or less medially with retractors. Occasionally in very obese individuals it is expedient to detach the colon so that the left half of the transverse colon, the splenic flexure, and a portion of the descending colon can be retracted further downward and medially. This step of the procedure is adequately presented in descriptions of resection of tumors in the region of the splenic flexure of the colon in standard texts.

In the third approach, entrance is gained through the lesser peritoneal cavity by way of the transverse mesocolon. In the left side of the mesocolon is a rather large avascular area, where a liberal incision can be made.

With any of these approaches to the left adrenal gland through the abdominal cavity the operator must assure himself by direct vision that he has adequate exposure of the upper pole of the kidney. An incision is made in the peritoneal surface and Gerota's fascia superior to the upper pole with the scissors after picking up the peritoneum with long, smooth forceps. This opening, exposing the upper portion of the perirenal fatty capsule and the periadrenal fatty capsule, is enlarged by simply inserting the fingers and further separating the peritoneum. Isolation of the left gland from the surrounding fatty tissue is accomplished in the same manner as separation of the right adrenal gland, namely, by cutting exactly at the surface of the cortical capsule around the periphery of the gland, in an effort to avoid any arterial bleeding, and then separating the anterior and posterior surfaces by blunt dissection with the finger. On the left side the very convenient corrugations or furrows that resemble the stem veins of leaves lead directly to the characteristic single vein draining the adrenal gland. Since the left adrenal vein is quite long in comparison with the right adrenal vein, it can easily be clamped and ligated. Chromic 00 catgut is used.

Subtotal Resection of the Adrenal

Usually when a tumor is found, it is necessary to excise the entire gland. If the adrenal tissue has not been completely destroyed, it is frequently so friable around the surface of the tumor that salvage of a portion of the gland is impossible. There are, however, occasions when subtotal adrenalectomy is indicated. With the shape of the gland in mind, right or left, the arterial filaments of the inferior edge can be divided along the distal half or two-thirds of the gland. Then by blunt dissection the entire anterior surface can be exposed, enabling one to judge the size of the gland and the remnant to be left in place. A mattress suture can then be passed through the complete thickness of the gland over the corrugations, ligating the central vein at the point of intended division of the gland. The remaining distal portion of the gland can be separated with the scissors. There will be a small amount of back bleeding. This usually stops spontaneously in several minutes and does not require application of Gelfoam. The application of clamps and additional sutures are to be avoided because of the great friability of the gland.

Aberrant Adrenal Tissue

Adrenal tumors, in addition to being bilateral in roughly 10 per cent of patients, may also be found in aberrant adrenal tissue. Because of the possibility of multiple tumors in normal and/or aberrant adrenal tissue, the areas where aberrant tissue occurs must be explored if the patient's condition permits. In looking for functioning adrenal tissue of the organ or body of Zuckerkandl, it is necessary first to locate the bifurcation of the aorta by palpation and then to demonstrate the bifurcation and the proximal courses of the common iliac vessels. A 4 or 5 cm. vertical incision is made in the peritoneal surface over the aorta from the inferior mesenteric artery to the bifurcation and the upper portions of the common iliac vessels. By blunt dissection it is possible to separate the fat and areolar tissue in this area and to demonstrate the anterior surface of the aorta at the bifurcation, the undersurface or the crotch of the bifurcation itself, and the upper portions of the iliacs.

Usually palpation indicates whether or not tumors exist along the course of the abdominal aorta. In very obese persons, it may be necessary to expose the aorta, or sections of it, to be sure that no tumors are present. The celiac axis area, a quite common site of aberrant adrenal tissue, can be investigated by following the hepatic artery retrograde to the axis and aorta.

Accessory adrenal medullary tissue arises from the paraganglia of the sympathetic system, which are found around the aorta and the urogenital system. These ganglia increase in size during infancy and decrease thereafter. The greatest mass of these paraganglia is the organ of Zuckerkandl over the lower aorta.

Lateral, Subcostal, or Flank Approach

For the lateral, subcostal, or flank approach, a transverse incision is made. This approach provides the most direct and the easiest access to either the right or the left adrenal gland. The incision begins at the lateral border of the rectus sheath, continues horizontally to a point 1.5 cm. below the lowest point of the costal margin on the ipsilateral side, then follows the twelfth rib at a distance of 1.5 cm., and ends at the sacrospinalis muscle. This incision must be carried well into the costovertebral angle.

The positioning on the operating table is most important for success of the lateral approach. For an operation on the left side, the patient is placed in the right lateral decubitus position with the right leg flexed; the left is separated from the right with a pillow and is almost fully extended. The patient's position on the table is adjusted so that the break in the operating table and the kidney rest are centered at a point just 3 inches cephalad to the lowest portion of the costal margin (Fig. 6). In other words, the break and the rest are superior to the lowest costal

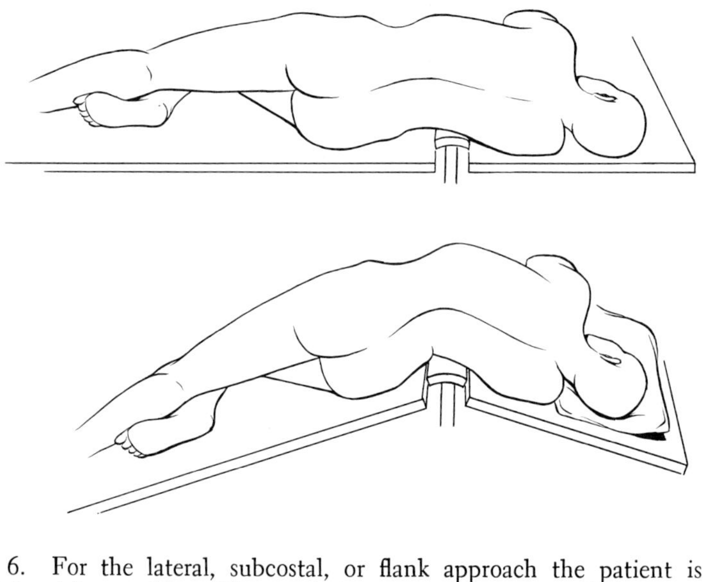

FIGURE 6. For the lateral, subcostal, or flank approach the patient is placed in the lateral decubitus position. The trunk is at approximately a 90-degree angle to the surface of the table. The trunk leans very slightly—several degrees—backward toward the operator. The break in the table and the kidney rest are centered 3 inches cephalad to the lowest point of the costal margin. Not shown are the adhesive straps used to maintain the position of the patient.

margin. The angle of the transverse axis of the body should be slightly less than 90 degrees and the patient should be leaning slightly toward the operator, who stands at the patient's back. Any change toward the prone position on the table will lessen the exposure considerably. The proper position is maintained by means of 2-inch or 3-inch adhesive tape straps. One or two straps are placed over the left shoulder, crossing the arm just above the elbow. Similarly, the hips are held in position by two crossing straps passed over the prominence of the hip region. Both ends of all the straps are fastened to the undersurface of the mobile top of the operating table. If the adhesive straps are fastened to the operating table stand and not to the mobile top, they will be torn loose as the table is flexed and the kidney rest raised.

After division of the skin and subcutaneous tissues, the external and internal oblique muscles are divided in the line of the incision. One set of intercostal vessels and nerves—or perhaps two—is divided and ligated with 3–0 plain catgut. As the dissection progresses the anesthetist gradually increases the break in the table and the height of the kidney rest. (A sudden combined break in the table and elevation of the kidney rest will produce severe circulatory disturbance in some patients.) The external fascial covering of the transversus abdominis muscle is then carefully incised along the direction of the muscle fibers. Posterolaterally, over the perirenal fat, the lumbar fascia (formed by the aponeuroses of the transversus abdominis, internal oblique, and external oblique muscles) is incised to the lateral border of the sacrospinalis muscle and the quadratus lumborum muscle. With the aid of the finger and a thick laparotomy pad (8 inches by 8 inches) the fibers of the thin transversus abdominis muscle are separated. Once this is done, the peritoneum is carefully peeled away from the area of the entire incision for a distance of 2 inches cephalad and 2 inches caudad of the incision. This is a most important maneuver which allows very satisfactory retraction and very satisfactory exposure. Through the separated, intact thin envelope of peritoneum on the left side can be seen loops of small bowel, the stomach, the left lobe of the liver, and the lower edge of the spleen. On the right side, usually all one sees is the liver beneath the peritoneum. No harm will come of opening the peritoneal cavity, but management of the retracted abdominal contents is much simpler when the peritoneal layer is intact.

The next step is to identify the lateral surfaces or fascial coverings of the erector spinae muscle bundle and the quadratus lumborum muscle. Just anterior to this will be found the perinephric fat surrounded by Gerota's fascia. A longitudinal incision is made in Gerota's fascia surrounding the perirenal fat. By blunt dissection along its lateral aspect and upper pole, the kidney can be partially separated, with its envelope of fat, from the surrounding fascia. This separation provides great mobility to the kidney.

The exposure of the kidney by this method is so very satisfactory that I do not understand why most urologists insist upon removing a portion or all of the twelfth rib for kidney surgery. Any procedure involving an intercostal incision or removal of part or all of a rib is associated with more pain than is a simple flank or subcostal incision. If additional exposure is needed, the upper pole of the kidney can be rotated—upper pole anterior—and then be retracted caudad and medially with a broad retractor over an abdominal pad. The liver, the tail of the pancreas, the splenic vessels, and the spleen, enclosed by the peritoneal layer, are retracted cephalad and anteriorly. The next maneuver is to expose a small area of the lower edge of the cortex of the adrenal and proceed as described in the exposure in the abdominal approach.

Reference

Merklin, R. J., and Michels, N. A. The variant renal and suprarenal blood supply with data on the inferior phrenic, ureteral and gonadal arteries. *J. Internat. Coll. Surgeons* 29:41, January 1958.

104. *Transabdominal Adrenalectomy*

JOHN K. LATTIMER

FOR THE REMOVAL of the adrenal gland in cases of tumor, an anterior abdominal incision is preferable, especially in operations for pheochromocytoma, in which multiple tumors may be found. In the average broad-chested person, a transverse incision can be made across the upper abdomen, with a slight convexity upward toward the sternum (Fig. 1). A sandbag under the spine just beneath the incision will help to open up the incision more adequately. In very young children, in whom the chest and abdomen are very slender, an upper midline incision may be preferable (Fig. 2). If this incision is made long enough, there is no trouble in finding the tumor in either side of the abdomen. When necessary, a T extension of the incision can be made in the line of one of the dermatomes at the appropriate level in the upper abdomen. If a radical dissection must be performed, this T-shaped incision can be continued up between the ribs and into the chest

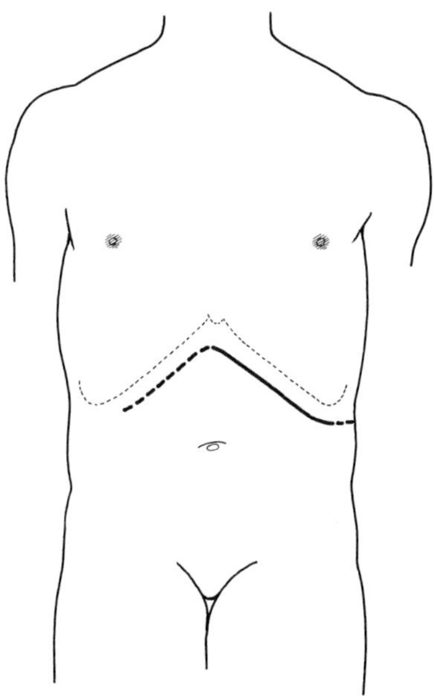

FIGURE 1. A transverse upper abdominal incision is preferred for persons with normal or broad chests. The incision can be extended across the midline if the opposite side is involved, and also around under the ribs on either side if necessary. A large enough incision makes all adrenal glands available. The multiplicity of pheochromocytomas makes it highly desirable to use this approach.

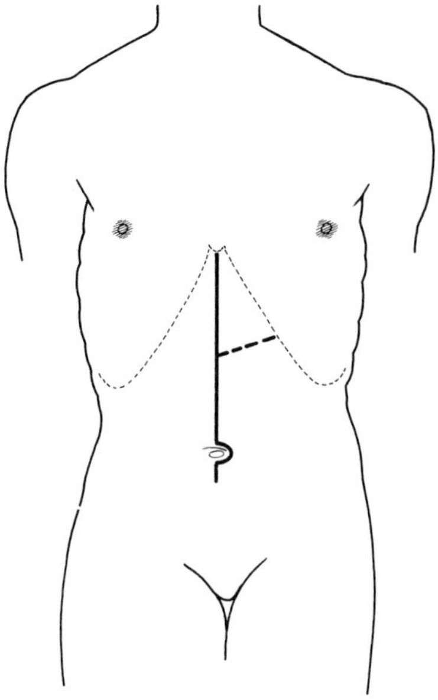

FIGURE 2. In patients with a very short sternum and asthenic habitus, a midline incision reaching up to and even splitting the xyphoid can be made to approach the adrenal glands. For additional exposure the incision can be carried downward, or a T-shaped extension can be made to either side.

cavity on either side, allowing further division of the diaphragm and better exposure of the area of the adrenal. This is not usually necessary, however.

By palpation, the tumor can be located above the adrenal gland on the appropriate side, even if its location is not known from previous pneumograms and other x-ray studies. A careful search for multiple foci must be made, remembering that pheochromocytomas are more likely to be multiple in children and often occur along the para-aortic ganglia up and down the midline. After the tumor has been located, an incision can be made in the parietal peritoneum lateral to the colon on the appropriate side, and the colon reflected medially (Fig. 3). This exposes the

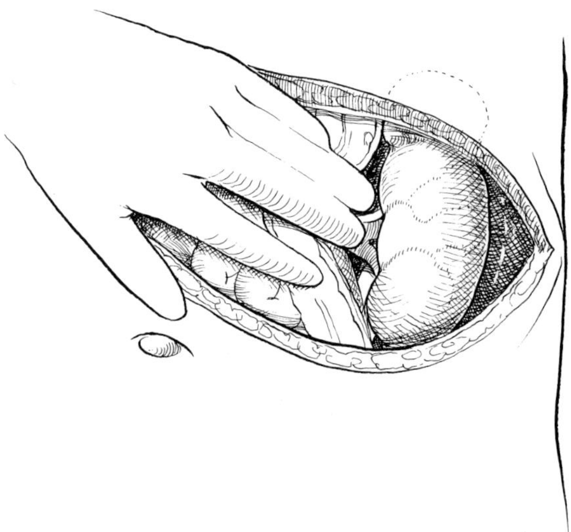

FIGURE 3. The posterior peritoneum can be cut just lateral to the ascending or descending colon, depending upon the side, and the colon reflected medially to expose the kidney and adrenal area.

kidney and the adrenal and pancreatic areas. If the kidney is dissected free in its lower portions and pulled downward, it tends to pull the adrenal and its tumor downward, and it can be more easily reached (Fig. 4). If the kidney is dislocated forward, the tumor and the adrenal tend to be dislocated forward as well. This brings them into still easier reach. Often the pancreas overlies tumors of the adrenal especially on the left side. The pancreas must first be recognized and then be carefully dissected away from the anterior surface of the tumor. The splenic vessels may run along the top edge of the tumor at this point, and must be carefully protected.

The adrenal tumor must be dissected out with great care, because a tear in the veins entering the renal vein can produce serious hemorrhage and obscure the field for long periods. If possible, the lateral and superior margins of the tumor should be freed first (Fig. 5) and the tumor then dissected away from its attachments to the kidney. This is usually done quite easily. The blood vessels supplying the adrenal tumor enter the tumor along a flat plane parallel with the great vessels, along the medial margin of the tumor. There is often a small vein leading upward to the diaphragmatic area, a small vein leading downward into the renal vein, and a larger set of vessels leading directly medially into the great vessels (Figs. 6 and 7).

When these largest vessels are clamped and tied, one must watch for a severe fall in blood pressure in cases of pheochromocytoma. A sustaining infusion into which norepinephrine or other pressor substances can be introduced must be kept running at this point and the blood pressure carefully monitored. Sudden shifts in the patient's position, such as follow the withdrawal of a sandbag, may precipitate sudden collapse and even cardiac arrest.

Some surgeons state that adrenal veins can be torn across with impunity and that there is little danger of hemorrhage from torn veins. It is more prudent, however, to try to clamp and ligate each vessel as it is encountered.

If the adrenalectomy is being done on a normal-sized adrenal gland, as in cancer of the prostate or cancer of the ovary or breast, or on a moderately enlarged gland, as in Cushing's disease, the gland can be dissected out with greater safety than when it is greatly enlarged, since the veins are often quite small. In patients

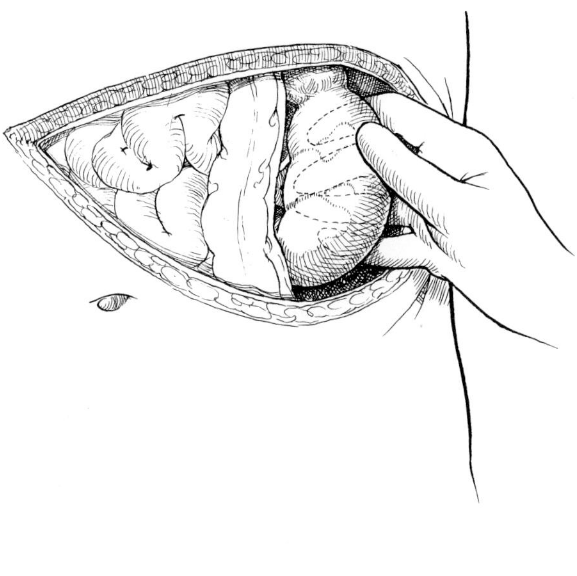

FIGURE 4. Adrenal tumors are often, but not always, attached to the kidney. It is therefore desirable to free up the kidney so that downward traction on it will draw both the kidney and the tumor into the wound, where it is more accessible. The tumor is frequently attached on the upper anterior surface of the kidney in the vicinity of the renal pedicle. The kidney vessels may appear to run under the tumor capsule, but usually can be easily dissected away from the tumor. Only rarely is it necessary to take the kidney out.

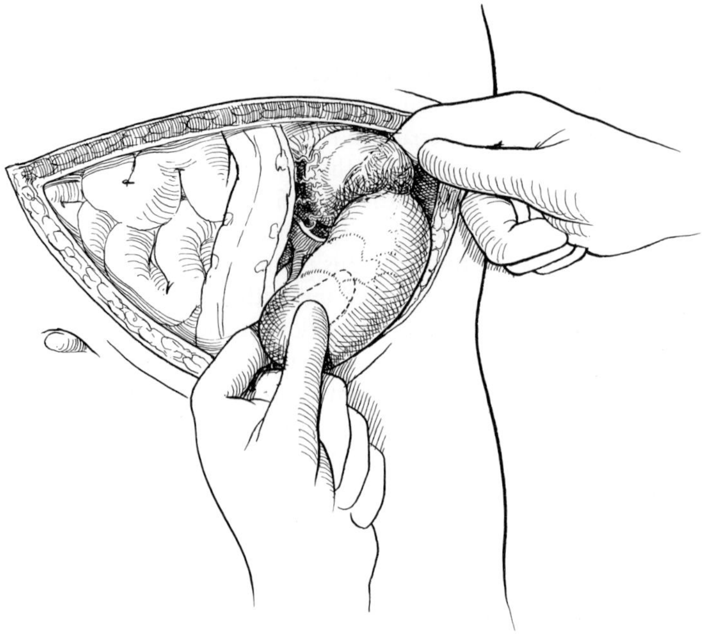

FIGURE 5. By scissor and finger dissection, the outer borders of the tumor are freed from their attachments until the many small vessels which supply the tumor can be isolated in a single plane running directly from the tumor into the aorta or vena cava. All the vessels tend to lie in this one flat plane. The tumor may also be dissected from its adhesions to the kidney with little risk of encountering blood vessels.

with Cushing's disease, care must be taken not to exert excessive pressure on the ribs or spine lest compression fractures result.

Only rarely is it advisable to attack an adrenal tumor through the flank. If this is done, the incision used for the removal of a kidney can be employed (see Chapter

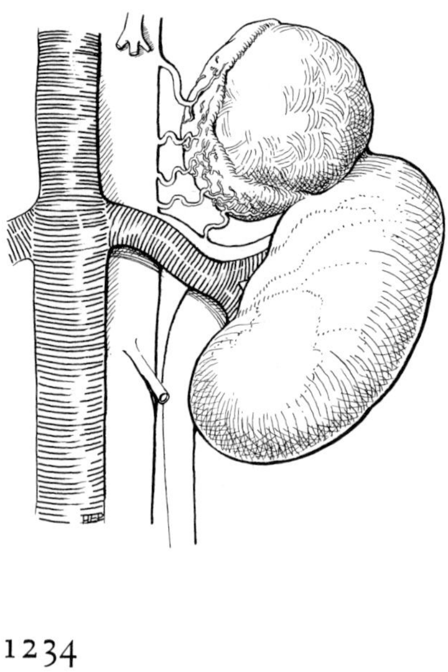

FIGURE 6. Usually the dissection reveals blood vessels running upward from the tumor toward the aorta and the region of the diaphragm, other vessels running directly from the tumor into the aorta and the vena cava, and still others running downward into the main renal vessels, near their origins at the great vessels.

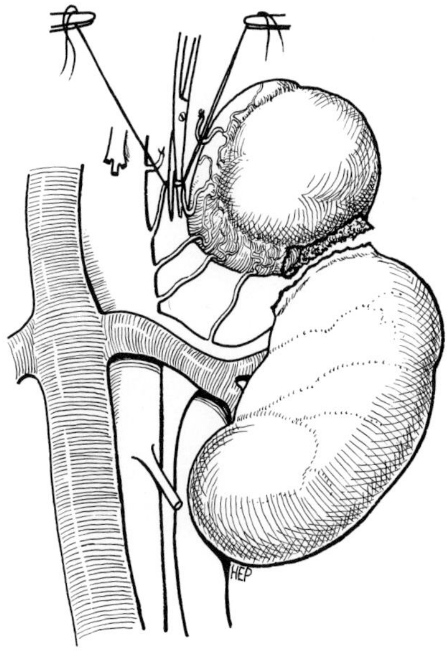

FIGURE 7. Each of the tiny vessels supplying the adrenal tumor is underrun with a small pointed clamp, such as an Adson clamp, and two black silk sutures are passed under each vessel. One of these is tied as near as possible to the great vessels; the other is then pulled laterally as far as possible toward the tumor and tied, and with the Adson clamp still remaining behind the vessel as a guide, the vessel is cut between the ties. The vessels can be cut successively, starting at the most available point. When the largest blood vessels are tied, the anesthesiologist must be notified, so that he may anticipate a possible blood pressure fall and increase the flow of pressor substances in an effort to counteract it.

114). It is our usual practice to remove at least half of the twelfth rib and extend the incision around parallel with the nerve fibers, to achieve whatever exposure is needed. It is well not to extend the incision too far posteriorly, lest the pleura be cut into and require repair. The incision can be extended anteriorly with great success and better exposure of the adrenal be thus obtained.

Bilateral simultaneous vertical incisions into the back of the prone patient have been advocated for simultaneous adrenalectomy. We do not believe that this procedure is wise, because the patient is placed under too much stress and the exposure is not as good as when the adrenals are removed one at a time. Serious complications such as cardiac arrest and death have been seen with this bilateral approach.

References

Cahill, G. F. Surgery involving the adrenals. *New York State J. Med.* 53:3, February 1953.

Cahill, G. F., and Melicow, M. M. Adrenal cortical tumors (the types of non-hormonal and hormonal tumors). *Surg., Gynec. and Obst.* 74:281, February 1942.

Cahill, G. F., and Melicow, M. M. Tumors of the adrenal gland. *J. Urol.* 64:1, July 1950.

Melicow, M. M. Tumors of the adrenal cortex and medulla in children. In Ariel, I. M., and Pack, G. T., *Cancer and Allied Diseases of Infancy and Childhood.* Boston: Little, Brown, 1960.

Melicow, M. M., and Cahill, G. F. The role of the adrenal cortex in somatosexual disturbances in infants and children: a clinico-pathologic analysis. *J. Clin. Endocrinol.* 10:24, January 1950.

XVIII. THE PELVIS

105. *Total Abdominal Hysterectomy*

LANGDON PARSONS

WHENEVER A REVIEW of the patient's symptoms and the physical findings calls for removal of the uterus for benign disease, a total hysterectomy should be performed. There is little excuse today for doing a supravaginal hysterectomy. On very rare occasions the surgeon may elect to amputate the cervix at the level of the internal os, but only (1) when the patient's condition deteriorates so rapidly that the surgeon is forced to complete the operation in a hurry, or (2) the surgeon encounters more technical difficulty than his experience can cope with when he finds that the bladder or rectum has become fixed to the uterus by pelvic inflammatory disease or endometriosis.

To make certain that the hysterectomy is being done for benign disease or is truly indicated, the patient should have a preliminary examination and a curettage, under anesthesia, before the abdomen is opened. If the surgeon will do this routinely, he will avoid performing a total hysterectomy for a benign polyp or placental remnant, or performing an inadequate operation for malignant disease which may be lurking in the endocervix or endometrial cavity.

The two most important factors which will insure the performance of a satisfactory total hysterectomy with minimum morbidity or mortality are (1) an adequate operative field unencumbered by clamps or adherent viscera, and (2) a thorough knowledge of the anatomy of the pelvic organs.

The following steps have proved helpful in meeting these requirements.

The Operation

Mobilizing the Uterus

PACKING BACK THE INTESTINE. In many instances the surgeon is far too anxious to get on with the removal of the uterus. Before proceeding with that, he should free up the small and large intestines so that they can be delivered out of the pelvis and kept free of the operative field with the minimum of packing with moist gauze. Forceful packing not only traumatizes the bowel, thereby increasing the likelihood of an uncomfortable convalescence through postoperative ileus or gas pains, but also increases the danger of postoperative atelectasis and pneumonia by interfering with the action of the diaphragm during the anesthesia. In addition, forceful packing may produce undue pressure on the large vessels that cross the brim of the pelvis. This may slow down the venous return from the veins of the leg and thereby lead to a thrombosis and fatal embolus.

The problem of packing back the intestine with the minimum of trauma can be made easier by employing a few simple expedients.

1. The patient should be properly placed on the operating table in an adequate degree of the Trendelenburg position. Hyperextension should be avoided.

2. At times the cecum, terminal ileum, and appendix are fixed low down over the pelvic brim and cannot be displaced easily with gauze packing. If the surgeon will incise the peritoneum along the lateral and inferior border of the cecum, the bowel can be displaced upward with ease. The defect in the peritoneum can readily be corrected at the time of reperitonealization.

In some instances the sigmoid with its redundant reflections obstructs the operative field. Again, incising peritoneal attachments will prove to be a useful maneuver, by permitting the sigmoid to be packed back without undue trauma.

3. When the symptoms and physical findings suggest that (1) small intestine may be attached to the pathological process in the pelvis, or (2) a tumor mass fills it, it is useful to pass a long Miller-Abbott tube into the small intestine prior to operation. The tube serves a double purpose. It allows the small bowel to thread itself on the bowel, with the result that there is much less of it to pack back and a larger operative field is created. It also provides a vent in case the bowel is damaged in removal, or resection of small intestine is called for.

FREEING OF THE ADNEXA. There is also a great temptation to proceed with the removal of the uterus before the uterus and adnexa have been thoroughly mobilized. This is particularly true when the basic pathology is pelvic inflammation. The first step is to free up the adnexa from their attachments to the back of the broad ligament and uterus. There is always a plane of cleavage in pelvic inflammatory disease despite the fact that the pelvic contents seem matted on first inspection. The separation should begin from below upward, employing the gloved hand rather than an instrument, after first gently determining the plane of cleavage. This can be done by gently rolling the tissue between the thumb and fingers. If the tissues do not separate with ease, the procedure should be abandoned and the structures brought under direct vision, for in all probability invasion of structures such as the rectum has occurred. Endometriosis, especially, has a propensity to invade. If the underlying pathology is endometriosis, the chocolate cyst cannot be separated from its attachment to the broad ligament without rupturing it. In this respect it differs from adnexal pathology of pelvic inflammatory origin.

APPLICATION OF TRACTION. One of the most important aids to a successful hysterectomy is the application of constant traction on the uterus in an upward direction. In most instances a tenaculum should be used to grasp the uterine fundus. If there is any reason to suspect malignant disease in the uterus, Kelly clamps should be placed across the tubal isthmus and ovarian ligament on both sides, rather than run the risk of dissemination of cancer by the trauma produced by a tenaculum.

The traction, once applied, should be maintained at all times until the uterus has been removed. By keeping the uterus on constant traction the anatomical relationships between the uterus and adjacent structures are maintained. If this is not done, the pelvic tissues tend to fall into accordion-like folds. The dissection becomes more difficult, the chances of maintaining a dry operative field are reduced, and the likelihood of producing damage to the ureter and bladder increases.

Mobilizing the Bladder

Development of the Peritoneal Flap. One of the practices that we have found of great value in carrying out a hysterectomy along anatomical lines is to develop a peritoneal flap off the bladder as the initial step in the operation. It should be done before the ovarian vessels are ligated or divided. If it is done later, the tissues are thrown into folds and the anatomical planes are lost. The bladder can be mobilized bloodlessly and with the minimum expenditure of time, effort, and risk. The anatomical relationship of the ureter to the uterine artery and cervix can easily be identified.

The uterus is drawn up and back, exposing the anterior leaf of the peritoneum of the broad ligament (Fig. 1). This is incised below the round ligament lateral to the midline. Kelly clamps are placed on the incised edge, and the index and middle fingers of both hands are inserted into the opening. With the fingers back to back, the areolar tissue can be gently separated in a bloodless plane. This creates a wide operative field and gives excellent exposure of the uterine vessels as they lie on the posterior surface of the broad ligament. The maneuver is repeated on the opposite side and the bladder is separated from the peritoneal reflection except in the mid-

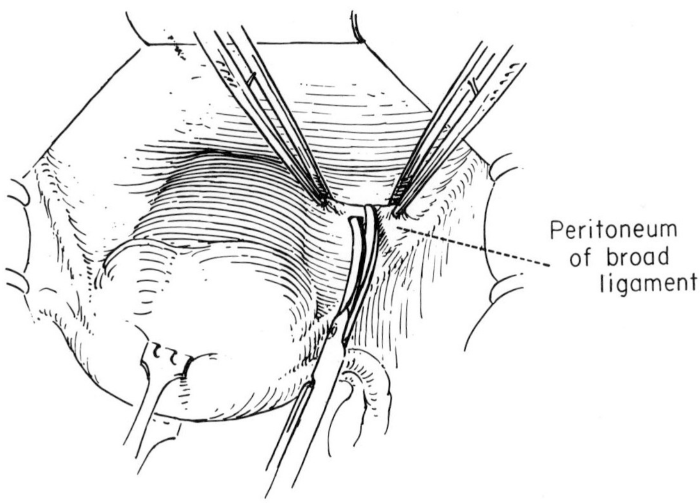

FIGURE 1. Traction is maintained with a tenaculum on the uterus. The surgeon and assistant pick up the anterior peritoneum lateral to the uterus. The peritoneal fold is then incised. (All figures in this chapter are reproduced from Parsons, L., and Ulfelder, H., *An Atlas of Pelvic Operations*, by permission of W. B. Saunders Company.)

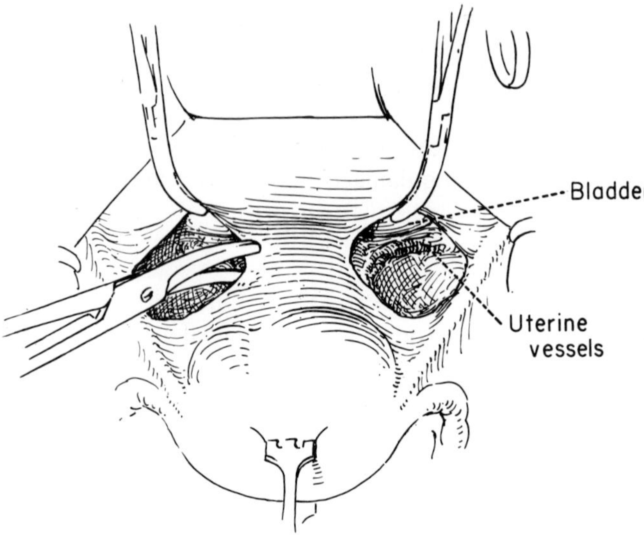

FIGURE 2. The maneuver of Figure 1 is repeated on the opposite side and the areolar space lateral to the bladder is developed bilaterally. The surgeon then divides the bridge of peritoneum between the two openings. Care must be taken to avoid damaging the bladder.

line (Fig. 2). The two incisions are then connected, care being taken that the dome of the bladder is not damaged. With the peritoneal edge held in traction the bladder edge is gently dissected from the peritoneal reflection (Fig. 3). This creates a peritoneal flap without attachments so that at the conclusion of the operation it can be drawn over the stump of the amputated vaginal canal as part of the peritonealization without drawing the bladder along with it. Postoperative urinary complications are thus reduced, because the position of the bladder is not disturbed.

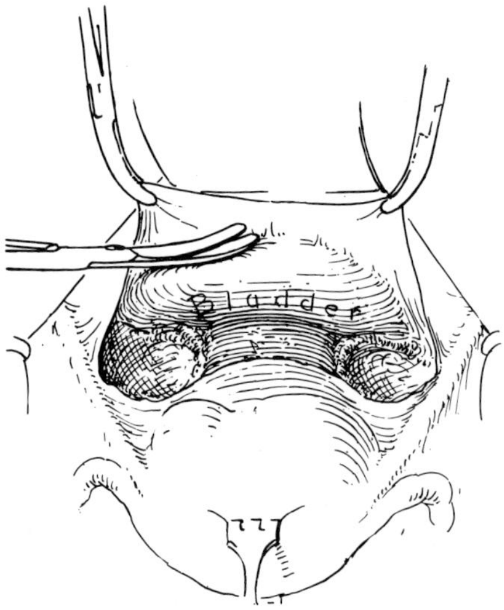

FIGURE 3. The bladder flap is held on tension while the surgeon divides the fine strands which hold the bladder to the peritoneum. The peritoneal flap, free of the bladder, is utilized in peritonealizing the pelvic floor after removal of the uterus.

Separation of the Bladder from the Cervix. The mobilization of the bladder from the cervix is essential if the entire cervix is to be removed. The majority of vesicovaginal fistulas encountered in gynecology today come, not from poor obstetrics, but from injury to the bladder in the course of total hysterectomy. After development of the bladder peritoneal flap, the bladder should be separated from the cervix by employing the same pill-rolling motion that is used in separating the adherent bowel from the uterus. The uterus is held on traction while the right hand grasps the cervix with the thumb on the anterior surface. Gentle downward pressure separates the bladder from the cervix bloodlessly. The bladder should also be freed from its attachments to the uterine vessels. It tends to be pulled upward on the vessels, leaving a crescent-like border of tissue. If the assistant and surgeon both grasp the bladder with forceps, in a transverse direction, this fold of tissue can be gently dissected off the vessels with minimal bleeding. When the bladder has been dissected away in this fashion, the chance of damaging the bladder wall by blind application of clamps to control bleeding is materially reduced.

Removal of the Uterus

Treatment of the Adnexa. The operator must now decide whether he wishes to remove the adnexa or not. Two main problems are encountered in the treatment of the adnexa:

1. If the adnexa are to be left in situ, the ovarian vessels and the round ligament should be ligated and divided separately. The round ligament should be sectioned closer to the uterus than the ovarian vessels. The ovary and its blood supply should lie easily, without tension, following reconstruction of the pelvic floor after the uterus has been removed. If the round ligament and ovarian vessels are intimately attached, the lumen of the vessels may be diminished by traction as the round ligament is pulled over and reapproximated to the vaginal cuff. This increases the chances that the retained ovary will later develop cysts.

Many surgeons feel that the major support of the vaginal apex comes from the cardinal ligaments, with the round ligaments playing only a subsidiary role. For this reason they approximate them to the angles of the transected vagina and do not attempt to attach the round ligaments at all. In this case the element of tension is no longer a problem.

2. If the tubes and ovaries are to be removed, it is of the utmost importance that the anatomical relationship of the ureter to the ovarian vessels be checked. They are in very close proximity at the point where they cross the common iliac artery. If bleeding occurs in the handling of the ovarian vessels, a hurried application of clamps or ligature can easily include the ureter. This is one of the commonest sites of injury to the ureter, largely because this anatomical relationship is not suspected. Injury can be avoided by simply tracing the course of the ureter as it runs up over the iliac vessels from the lateral pelvic wall. The peritoneum with the ovarian vessels should be elevated before clamps or stitch ligatures are applied.

Application of Clamps. One of the most important factors in simplifying the technique of hysterectomy is to plan the operation so that the operative field will not be cluttered with clamps. Following the application of each clamp, the

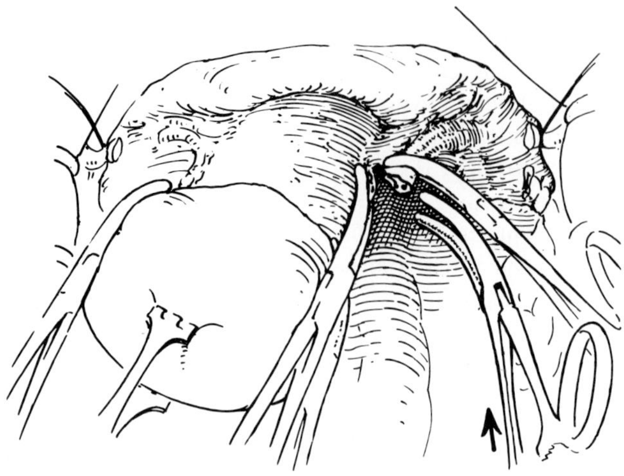

FIGURE 4. The uterine vessels are doubly clamped. This provides an element of safety should the tissue retract out of the clamp or the stitch ligature break while being tied.

tissue in it should be divided and a stitch ligature inserted and tied; the clamp is then removed. The only clamps in the operative field should be those used on the specimen side to control back bleeding. With the field of operation clear of clamps, the surgeon has free access to the structures in the pelvis and is in a good position to deal with any troublesome bleeding he may encounter.

The surgeon should pay strict attention to the manner in which he applies clamps to the uterine vessels. The vessels should be well delineated and their relation to the bladder established. The clamps are applied at right angles to the uterus, sufficiently far apart so that the tissue included can be divided, leaving a cuff. A second security clamp is placed on the cuff (Fig. 4). Stitch ligatures are then placed and tied as each clamp, beginning with the most distal, is removed. If for any reason the initial suture breaks, the clamp on the cuff will control the bleeding. From then on, all clamps are applied parallel to the cervix, medially and at right angles to the initial ligatures (Fig. 5). The length of the cervical portion of the uterus varies. The number of clamps and ligatures to be applied will therefore vary. Each clamp

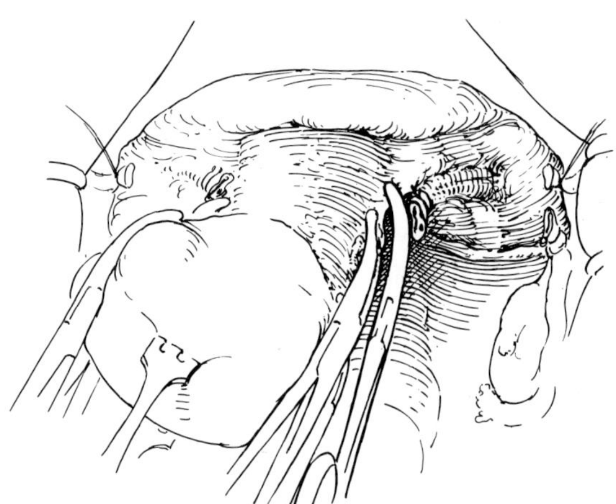

FIGURE 5. The bladder has been dissected off the cervix and anterior wall of the vagina. Thus the clamps, including a minimal amount of tissue, can be applied lateral to the cervix, under direct vision. When they are applied in this fashion there is little chance that the bladder or ureter will be damaged.

should include only the amount of tissue it can safely secure. For this reason we prefer to use Kelly rather than Kocher or other specially designed clamps. The operator will receive no prize for the smallest number of clamps used, and frequently will run into considerable blood loss if he tries to see how much tissue he can grasp with a clamp and include in his suture.

BLEEDING. The most likely site of bleeding is the so-called "bloody angle." This area lies distal to the point where the uterine vessels have been divided and ligated alongside the lower portions of the cervix and upper vagina. In this location the ureters are in close proximity to the operative field, and it is here that they are frequently damaged or included in a suture. There is a tendency to avoid this area because of the danger of encountering troublesome bleeding. The area must be dissected if the entire cervix is to be removed. Frequently, if these troublesome corners are neglected, examination of the specimen after its removal will show that enough vagina has been excised anteriorly and posteriorly, but some of the lateral portions of the cervix have been left behind.

This portion of the operation need not be bloody if the surgeon will adopt two simple routines:

1. After the uterine vessels have been secured with stitch ligatures and the cervical branches have been clamped, divided, and sutured, the operator should again direct his attention to the anatomical relationship of the bladder to the lower cervix and anterior vaginal wall. The position of the ureter can be detected by palpating the base of the dissection in the broad ligament with the thumb and the forefinger. A characteristic snapping sensation is noted when the ureter slips between the fingers. If the bladder has not been separated well down on the bladder wall anteriorly, that should be done now.

2. In most instances heavy bleeding in the area lateral to the cervix and upper vagina is due to inclusion of too much tissue in the clamp. If the tissue pulls out of the clamp after division, the bleeding points are hard to find and frantic clamping, done blindly, can readily result in damage to the ureter. Special hysterectomy clamps have been devised, but they are unnecessary, provided the operator takes the trouble to dissect the region adequately. This can be done by sectioning the uterosacral ligaments and securing them with stitch ligatures. The peritoneal bridge between the two is then divided and the tissue stripped downward off the cervix in a bloodless area until the posterior wall of the vagina is encountered (Fig. 6). When this is done very little tissue is left at the lateral angles and this can readily be contained in Kelly clamps (Fig. 7). They should be applied and the tissue divided, leaving a slight cuff of tissue beyond the clamp. This tissue is stitched serially, the number of sutures depending on the length of the cervix. The uterine specimen should show complete circumcision of the uterine cervix with a rim of vaginal tissue all around it.

ENDOMETRIOSIS. On rare occasions the rectovaginal septa may be infiltrated with endometriosis which adheres firmly to the posterior wall of the uterus. If this occurs, three recourses are open. (1) A plane of cleavage may be established by angulating the uterus sharply forward toward the symphysis. Frequently the tissue will separate, revealing the proper point of separation. (2) If this fails, it may be possible to enter the proper cleavage plane when the peritoneum, above the obvious

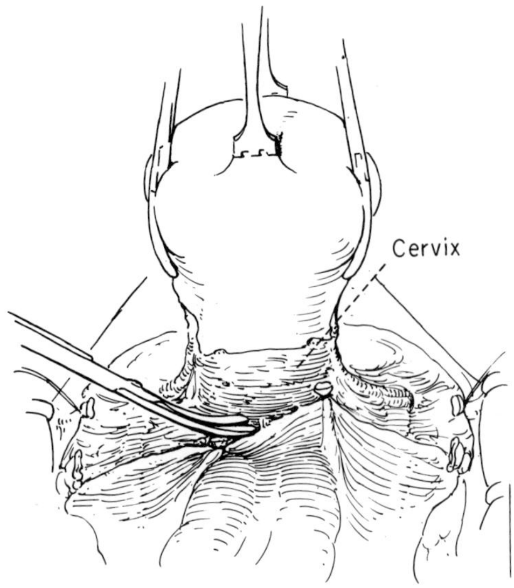

FIGURE 6. Further mobilization of the uterus is achieved by dividing and ligating the uterosacral ligaments. The peritoneum is then stripped off the back of the uterus. This step reduces the amount of tissue that must be included in the clamp placed on the cervical branches of the uterine vessels. The chance of troublesome bleeding and injury to the ureter is minimized.

point of attachment, is divided with a knife. (3) If the bladder is so closely adherent to the cervix that the operator is reluctant to proceed with the dissection, he may do so without danger by entering the fascial compartment through the oval-shaped aperture on the side of the cervix left when the uterine vessels have been divided. By introducing one blade of the Kelly clamp deep to the overlying fascia, the tissue enclosed may be divided without any danger of including the bladder. Or he may choose to incise this layer of fascia overlying the anterior wall of the cervix and proceed with the dissection. This is the so-called intrafascial hysterectomy. It is a very useful procedure in conditions in which the bladder is densely adherent to the cervix, but need not be done routinely. For pathological entities such as carcinoma in situ it would be contraindicated.

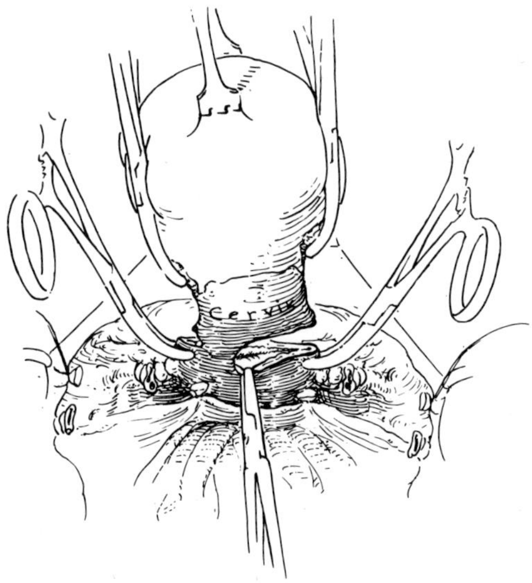

FIGURE 7. After the uterine vessels and their branches have been divided, clamps are placed on the lateral edge of the vagina. The vagina is then transected. The posterior vaginal wall is placed on traction with a Kocher clamp so that the surgeon sees the vaginal epithelium and its relation to the cervix.

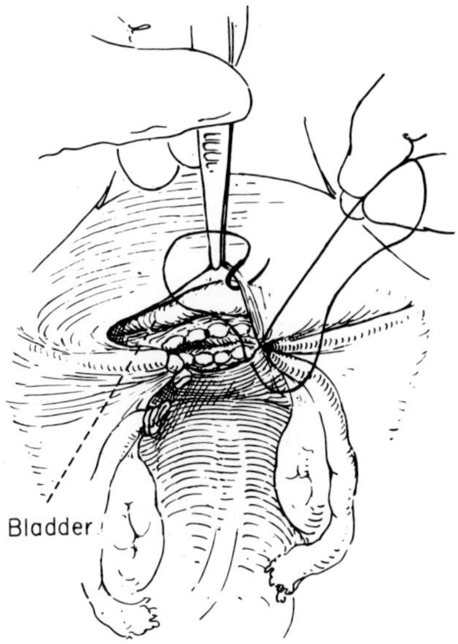

FIGURE 8. The vaginal cuff is sutured with a running lockstitch around its entire circumference. This maintains the vaginal canal as a tube and leaves the apex open. The anterior peritoneal fold is then utilized to peritonealize the raw areas of the pelvis and cover the open vagina.

Treatment of the Transected Vaginal Canal. The final danger point comes in the treatment of the transected vaginal canal (Fig. 8). We prefer to control the bleeding from the incised edges of the vaginal wall with a running lockstitch around the entire circumference. Others elect to approximate the anterior to the posterior vaginal wall with interrupted sutures, and ligate the bleeding points separately. Whichever method is used, there is great danger of including the bladder wall in the stitch ligature if the area where the stitch is to be applied cannot be adequately visualized. Blind application of such sutures is one of the major reasons why vesicovaginal fistulas occur after total hysterectomy.

There are two advantages in leaving the vaginal canal open, with only a peritoneal cover to seal it off. (1) If the walls of the vagina are approximated to each other and the upper part of the vagina is closed, the upper part becomes cone-shaped, and the vagina is foreshortened. When no attempt is made to bring them together, the vaginal canal remains as a tube and no loss in depth occurs. (2) With the canal open the ovarian and uterine vessels which are approximated to the angles of the vagina in the process of reconstruction of the pelvic floor occupy an extraperitoneal position. Any postoperative bleeding that may occur will immediately manifest itself.

Summary

Observance of the following recommendations has helped to make performance of an abdominal hysterectomy easier and safer in our experience.

1. An adequate operative field must be created and maintained.

2. To this end the tissue in each clamp should be secured with a stitch ligature immediately after it is divided. The operative area should be free of clamps.

3. The uterus should be held in constant traction by the operator, or his assistant, throughout the operation.

4. The uterus and adnexa should be mobilized and the anatomical landmarks established before any attempt is made to remove the uterus.

5. The bladder should be mobilized and its relation to the cervix and vaginal wall constantly kept in full view. No clamp should be applied without the operator's knowing exactly what is included in it.

6. To minimize the bleeding frequently encountered in the dissection around the lower portion of the cervix and vagina, only the amount of tissue that can safely be controlled should be included in the clamp. The number of clamps employed depends on the length of the cervix. The problem is simplified if the uterosacral ligaments are stripped down from the back of the uterus and ligated separately.

7. Bleeding from the incised edges of the vaginal canal should be controlled with a running lockstitch around the circumference.

8. Support to the vagina is maintained by suturing the cardinal ligaments to the corners of the amputated vaginal wall. After peritonealization, any bleeding from the vaginal cuff or from the ovarian or uterine vessels will manifest itself vaginally rather than intraabdominally.

References

ALDRIDGE, A. H. The choice and technique of operation for hysterectomy. *S. Clin. North America* 37:291, April 1957.

BURCH, J. C., and LAVELY, H. T. *Hysterectomy*. Springfield (Ill.): Charles C Thomas, 1954.

MEIGS, J. V., and PARSONS, L. Technique of total hysterectomy. In Cole, W. (Ed.), *Operative Technique in Surgical Specialties*. New York: Appleton-Century-Crofts, 1955.

PARSONS, L., and ULFELDER, H. *An Atlas of Pelvic Operations*. Philadelphia: W. B. Saunders, 1953.

TELINDE, R. W. Hysterectomy for carcinoma in situ. In Meigs, J. V. (Ed.), *Surgical Treatment of Cancer of the Cervix*. New York: Grune & Stratton, 1954.

106. *Radical Operation for Cancer of the Cervix: Wertheim Hysterectomy and Pelvic Lymphadenectomy*

LANGDON PARSONS

THE TERM "Wertheim hysterectomy and pelvic lymphadenectomy" is chosen deliberately in preference to "radical hysterectomy and node dissection." The basic objective in surgery for cancer of the cervix, the principal condition for which this operation is indicated, is the adequate removal of the local tumor and the immediate extensions from it. The removal of the nodes, though necessary, is a secondary consideration. It will profit the patient little if the node dissection is thorough and the removal of the primary tumor and the adjacent lymphatics is inadequate. Cancer of the cervix has a growth pattern that tends to keep it confined to the original site. Extension occurs into lymphatic channels or spread takes place along the line of least resistance, in tissue spaces. In stages I and IIa the nodes are involved in only about 20 per cent of the cases. Approximately 50 per cent of these patients will live five years or more, so the nodes should be dissected. Their lives will not be salvaged if the cancer at the primary site is not eradicated.

Any operation for cancer of the cervix must be radical in the sense of being adequate for the removal of the malignant disease—not radical in terms of the experience of the operator. Operations for malignant disease in the pelvis begin at the most lateral point of potential spread and move in the direction of the primary cancer, in contrast to operations for benign lesions, which are extended laterally only occasionally, to permit excision of the local growth. Too often the radical hysterectomy is only slightly more extensive than the procedure the surgeon is accustomed to employ for a benign fibroid. To repeat, because the point deserves constant emphasis: *the therapy should stress the adequate removal of the local disease and be less concerned with how well the lymph node metastases are managed.*

Preliminary Preparation

In the discussion of total hysterectomy, we emphasized the need for providing an adequate operative field and detailed several routines that make for greater ease and safety in the performance of hysterectomy. The same factors are magnified in importance when the extent of the surgery is increased. In the Wertheim hysterectomy it is also very helpful to pass a long suction tube through the nose into the small intestine. When this is done 24 to 36 hours prior to the operation, the small intestine tends to thread itself on the tube, thereby reducing appreciably the amount of packing necessary and the trauma incident to it. As a result, the problems of the anesthetist are lessened, the operative field is made more accessible, and the risk of both postoperative atelectasis and ileus is minimized.

The Operation

Mobilization of the Primary Tumor and the Adjacent Lymphatics

Exposure. It will help the operator appreciably if he will employ self-retaining retractors for the lateral margins of the wound but hand retractors for the angles. Fixed retractors at either end force the surgeon to operate through a rigid hole. It is very difficult to keep the dissection in tissue planes. We use chest instruments entirely; the added length permits better vision.

Early Mobilization of the Ureters. The operator stands to the patient's left side. After the operative field has been prepared as described in Chapter 105, the ureters are identified at the point where they cross the common iliac artery. By holding the uterus on upward traction, the parietal peritoneum is placed on stretch, which facilitates the placing of incisions lateral to the ureter. Stay sutures of silk are then placed on the medial edge of the incised peritoneum and clamped to hang outside the operative field. This leaves the ureter on the medial leaf of the peritoneum in constant view.

Development of the Peritoneal Flap. The surgeon then directs his attention to the vesicouterine field. The space of Retzius is entered lateral to the bladder by incising the anterior leaf of peritoneum as traction on the uterus holds it on tension. By gently manipulating the index and middle fingers of the two hands in opposite directions, while the assistant holds the uterus, this avascular space can be rapidly expanded, pushing the bladder gently in a medial direction. The obliterated hypogastric vessels, the external iliac artery and vein, and the obturator nerve come into view immediately. Stitch ligatures are then placed well out laterally on the round ligament before it is divided. The two peritoneal incisions are then connected. This exposes the external and common iliac vessels and demonstrates the intimate anatomical relationship of the ureter and ovarian artery and vein. With the ureter in full view, these vessels are secured with stitch ligatures and divided well up beneath the mobilized cecum.

Plan of Procedure. In the past I made it a practice to carry out the iliac lymphadenectomy as the first step in the dissection. In recent years the procedure has been modified because it is impossible to do an en bloc dissection of node and primary tumor such as is done in the breast. I now proceed with the removal of the primary tumor and adjacent lymphatic channels, leaving the dissection of the regional nodes until the end of the operation, when it can be carried out more expeditiously and with less danger, since there is more room in which to maneuver.

Development of the "Web." The key to an anatomical dissection deep in the pelvis is the development of the so-called "web" which contains all the lateral lymphatics as well as all the blood supply to the medially placed structures. This is made much easier by using the following technique. (1) Identify the internal iliac artery with its anteriorly placed superior vesical and uterine artery on the lateral pelvic wall. (2) Retract the medial leaf of the peritoneum, on which the ureter lies. (3) Gently insert the index finger alongside the rectum behind the terminal branches of the internal iliac artery—this space is always free and can easily be developed even when intensive radiation has been given previously. (4) Place the index and middle fingers astride the web, gently move the tips of the fingers anteriorly along its top, lateral to the bladder, and deep into the pelvis, and separate the areolar attachments. The block of tissue which is left contains the entire blood supply and lymphatic channels, and can easily be controlled with large Moynihan clamps (Fig. 1). The operator has the entire blood supply to the pelvis between his fingers much as he has it in the gallbladder area when he places his fingers in the foramen of Winslow.

Application of Clamps. Before clamping this tissue, however, it is necessary to separate the superior vesical artery, at its point of origin on the internal iliac,

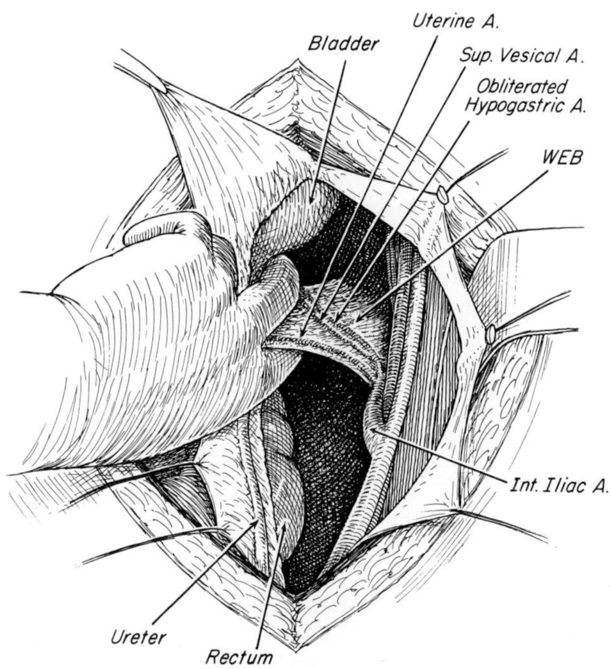

FIGURE 1. This is the web that contains the major blood supply to the uterus, bladder, and vagina as well as the middle hemorrhoidal artery. The avascular space lies posteriorly and just lateral to the rectum. By placing the pelvic organs on tension with the index finger below and the middle finger of the left hand (operator on left of patient) above the web and in the prevesical space, the superior surface is exposed with the vessels lying on it.

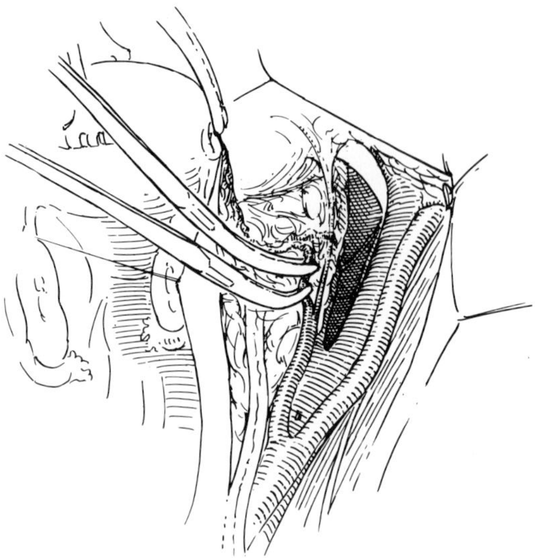

FIGURE 2. Cleaning of the external iliac artery and vein, and the internal iliac artery as well, provides a clear view of the uterine vessel and its relationship to the superior vesical artery. The latter must be preserved. The uterine vessel is being doubly clamped. The ureter lies on the undersurface of the peritoneal flap. (Figures 2 and 4–10 are reproduced from Parsons, L., and Ulfelder, H., *An Atlas of Pelvic Operations,* by permission of W. B. Saunders Company.)

from the uterine artery. The superior vesical artery must be preserved to maintain the integrity of the bladder. The uterine vessels are then clamped, divided, and secured with a double stitch ligature (Fig. 2). The vesical artery and its attachment to the bladder are now gently elevated so that a Moynihan clamp can be placed on the tissues beneath them as far laterally as possible, care being taken not to damage the internal iliac vein. A second clamp is placed on the medial side and the tissue between divided (Fig. 3).

To keep clamps out of the operative field, the tissue held in each clamp is secured with a stitch ligature immediately after it has been sectioned. The tissue in the medial clamp is secured first. This ligature can be tied by the assistant. With the clamp removed, the surgeon has greater freedom of access to the main clamp, which controls the major blood supply. The ligature securing the tissue in the main clamp must be tied by the surgeon because the angle is such that the tissue will retract out of the tie if the assistant should try to do the tying.

The process is repeated in progressive steps until finally the uterus, rectum, vagina, and bladder are completely free of all lateral attachments, except for the

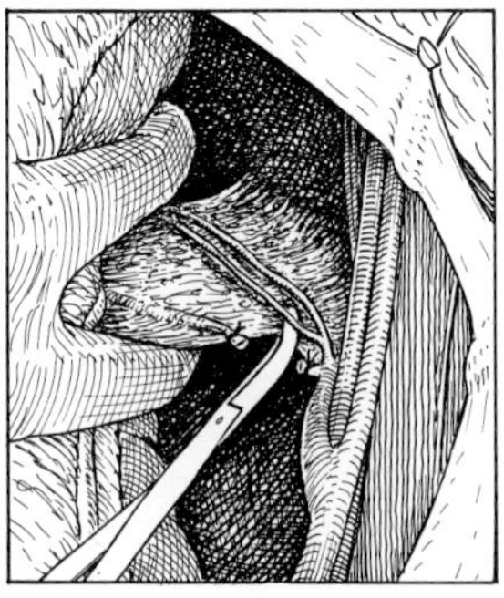

FIGURE 3. The superior vesical and the obliterated hypogastric are elevated so that they can be preserved, and a clamp is placed on the most lateral extension of the web. Care must be taken in placing this clamp to avoid sideswiping the internal iliac vein. A second clamp is applied medially and the tissue between divided; a stitch ligature is placed and tied on each individual clamp. Successive steps are taken in this manner until the tissues are entirely separated from the lateral wall.

superior vesical and obliterated hypogastric arteries. The surgeon then crosses to the patient's right side and completes the same steps on the left.

FURTHUR MOBILIZATION OF THE URETERS. It will be immediately apparent to the surgeon that the entire specimen has moved up toward him, where it is easier to get at as soon as the lateral attachments have been divided and secured. Easy access is important, because one of the tricky parts of the dissection is to mobilize the ureter so gently that its blood supply is not jeopardized any more than the dissection requires. This can be a bloody area. Since the lower arcades of the blood supply to the lower end of the ureter must be sacrificed, the only vessel left intact is the longitudinal vessel coursing on its surface. There is less chance of damage if the dissection can be made with the structures accessible, as they are when the lateral attachments are first freed.

The assistant holds the uterus on firm upward traction with one hand while he grasps the bladder transversely with long round-end forceps with the other. The surgeon also elevates the bladder wall in the same fashion as he gently dissects the wall of the bladder off the cervix and lower vagina. The objective is twofold: (1) to advance the bladder, and (2) to identify the lower end of the ureter as it runs alongside the lateral wall of the vagina to enter the bladder at its base. It is amazing how medially placed the ureter is at this point.

With the lower end of the ureter identified and the portion above the point where the uterine vessel crosses it held on tension by traction on the stay sutures, the surgeon gently inserts Moynihan clamps beneath the vessels over the superior surface of the ureter and divides the tissue between (Fig. 4). They are then secured with stitch ligatures. This maneuver unroofs the so-called canal in which the ureter runs. The ureter cannot be mobilized unless this unroofing is done. This is a very important area in the dissection also because any potentially malignant tissue must be removed from it. The ureter is then teased out

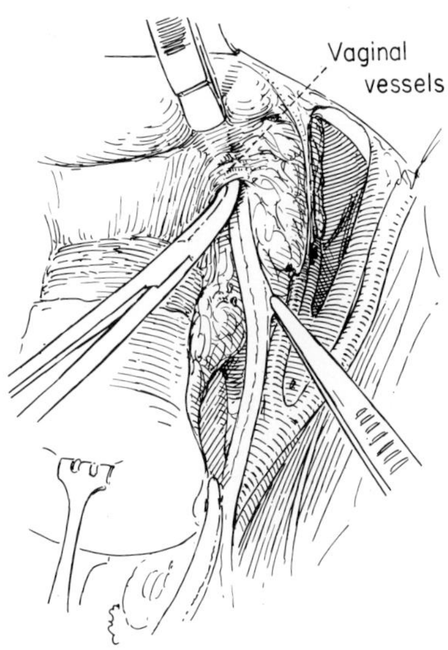

FIGURE 4. The ureter enters a tunnel of tissue (along the lateral wall of the vagina below the level of the cervix) containing a complex of vessels both above and below it. With the ureter held on traction and the bladder retracted with the forceps handle, a clamp is introduced into the canal, gently separating the ureter before the tissue is clamped and the canal unroofed.

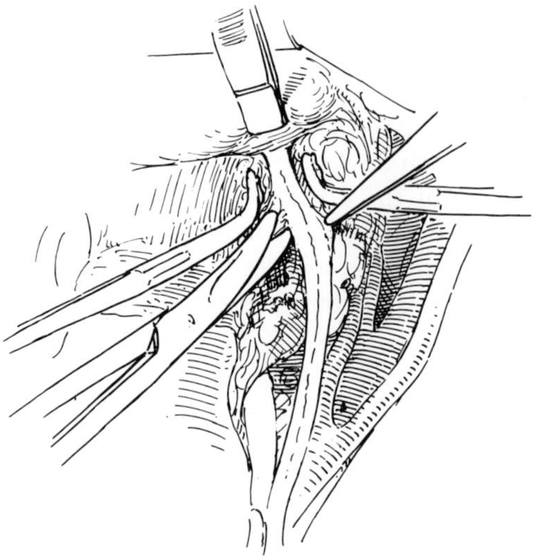

FIGURE 5. Under direct vision the ureter is gently dissected free from its bed throughout its length to the point where the ureter enters the bladder. The ureter must lie free so that the important paravaginal and paracervical tissue can be removed.

of its bed and the bladder advanced further downward until, with ureter and blood supply intact, it is free of the uterus and vagina (Fig. 5).

FREEING OF THE RECTUM FROM THE VAGINA. The surgeon now gives attention to separating the rectum from the posterior wall of the vagina. More of the cancer of the cervix spreads in a fore and aft direction than we formerly believed. The ureter is freed from its peritoneal attachment below the level where a small nutrient vessel comes to join it from the internal iliac artery. The uterosacral ligaments are divided as far posteriorly as possible and secured and stitch ligatures (Fig. 6). With large blunt-end scissors (rectal) the rectum is then separated from the posterior vaginal wall.

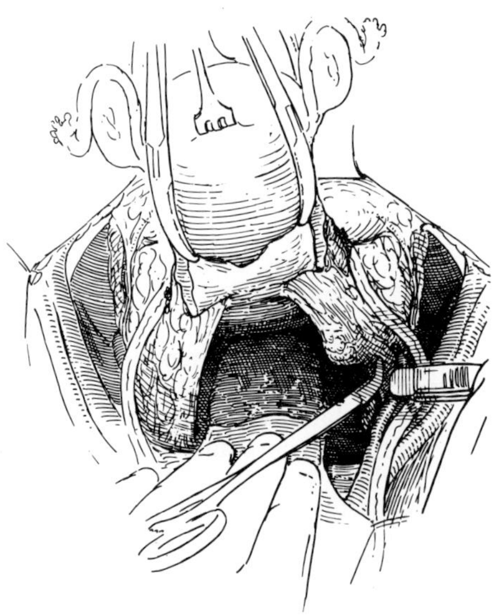

FIGURE 6. The ureters have been dissected free and the lateral margins of the web have been divided and secured with ligatures on the side wall of the pelvis. The rectum is retracted to expose the posterior attachment of the web, which is then clamped and divided.

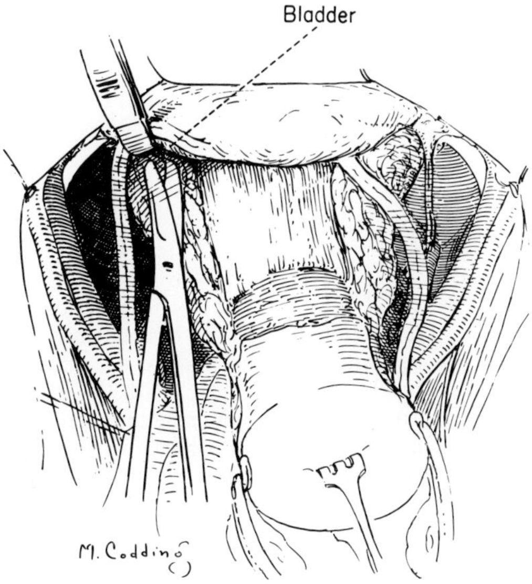

FIGURE 7. With the uterus and vaginal wall on tension, the undersurface of the bladder wall is dissected from the paravaginal tissue and the anterior vaginal wall.

Division of the Vagina. With the bladder and ureters mobilized anteriorly and the rectum posteriorly, the uterus with its lateral tissue, which contains the lymphatic channels (the so-called Franz Joseph's whiskers), stands out clearly. The dissection is completed by gently freeing the lateral tissue from the bladder anteriorly and the side wall of the rectum posteriorly and laterally (Figs. 7 and 8).

The vagina is then divided well down its length, and the bleeding from the cut edges controlled by stitch ligatures and by a running lockstitch which also serves to keep the canal open (Fig. 9). The most important part of the operation for cervical cancer has now been completed.

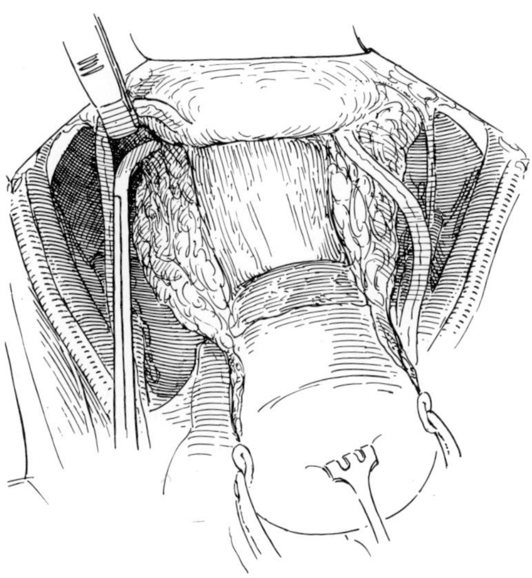

FIGURE 8. With the vaginal wall held in traction, the bladder wall and the ureter are retracted to permit the application of a clamp across the most distal portion of the paravaginal tissue.

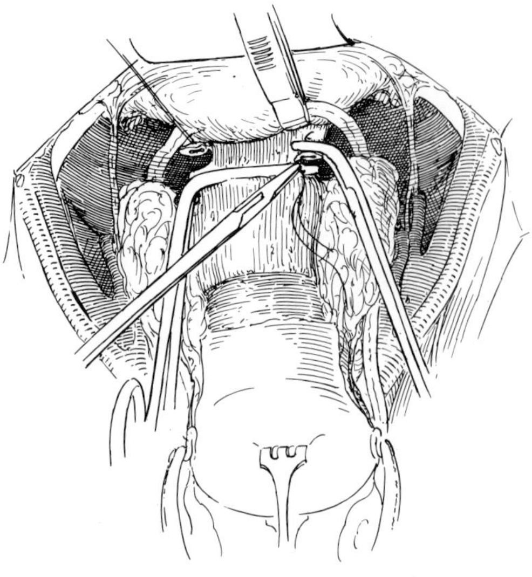

FIGURE 9. The lower limits of the dissection have been defined and the amount of vaginal wall to be removed has been determined. With the uterus on tension, a Wertheim clamp is placed across the vaginal wall to prevent spillage as the wall below it is clamped, divided, and secured with stitch ligatures.

Pelvic Lymphadenectomy

The surgeon now directs his attention to the lateral pelvic wall, where the regional nodes will be dissected. The dissection can be done more easily and the dangers minimized if the lymphadenectomy is begun lateral to the external iliac vessels along the medial border of the psoas muscle (Fig. 10). Only one, very small vessel, situated at about the level of the junction of the internal and external iliac arteries, holds these vessels laterally. By gently developing the area lateral to the vessels the surgeon enters the upper portion of the obturator space. In this space, troublesome venous bleeding can be encountered if the gluteal, pudendal, and internal

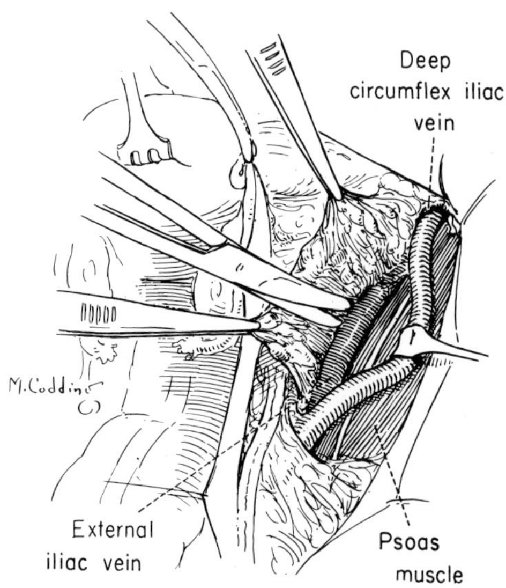

FIGURE 10. The nodal dissection begins on the lateral side of the external iliac artery. This provides access to the upper portion of the obturator fossa. The artery and vein are cleared of all tissue with scissor dissection as the assistant holds the fatty fibrous tissue on traction.

iliac veins are inadvertently damaged. By developing a lateral approach they may be dealt with from both the lateral and the under side of the external iliac veins.

The actual removal of the node-bearing tissue begins at Poupart's ligament and extends upward from that point on the anterior and posterior surface of the external iliac artery and vein. It is made easier by inserting one blade of the scissors in the adventitia of the artery. The fat and lymphatic tissue can be stripped away easily in this fashion. Rarely does metastatic disease from the cervix ever involve the wall of the artery. It may implicate the vein. If it does, the operator can either divide the vein above and below the point of attachment or mark the area with dura clips and leave it alone. The clips provide a target for the radiologist in directing therapy. In either case, only palliation can be expected, not cure.

After clearing the external iliac vessels as well as the internal iliac artery, the surgeon removes all tissue above the level of the obturator nerve out to the side wall of the pelvis. Beware of the internal iliac and gluteal vein. With the exposure that has been provided, they can be seen and avoided. The dissection then proceeds up along the side of the common iliac artery and inferior vena cava to the level of the bifurcation of the aorta.

Drainage

The operation is completed by placing drains through the vagina. The surgeon may elect to place catheters for suction drainage. The entire area is then peritonealized. Recently we have been translocating the ureters into the abdominal cavity, allowing them to lie free from the level of the internal iliac vessels to the point where they enter the bladder. This tends to keep the lower end of the ureter, with its damaged blood supply, free of a potentially contaminated area which lies retroperitoneally. The aim is to reduce the incidence of fistula. The bladder is placed on catheter drainage.

Wertheim Operation and Pelvic Node Dissection for Other Conditions than Cancer of the Cervix

The principal use of this operation has been for cancer of the cervix. Recently the operation has been applied to selected cases of cancer of the endometrium without muscle invasion and with only minor nodal involvement. When muscle is implicated, nodal involvement is more extensive and is found in approximately 15 per cent of cases. There is a suggestion that such patients may survive for long periods of time, even though positive nodes are present and the disease is extensive enough to warrant a pelvic exenteration. The Wertheim operation should be employed only in selected cases, for many patients with cancer of the endometrium are obese, hypertensive, and diabetic.

The exposure of the anatomical details of the deep pelvic structures which is employed in the Wertheim technique is most useful when the surgeon confronts such entities as a deeply placed sarcoma below the pelvic floor or a carcinoma of the rectum with lateral spread. It is my firm belief that this procedure should be used for most carcinomas of the rectum.

Summary

The basic requirements are (1) knowledge of the anatomy of the pelvic structures, (2) adequate exposure, (3) constant traction to provide the surgeon with a better chance to dissect in tissue planes, (4) suture of tissue included in each clamp directly following its section, to keep the pelvis free of obstructing clamps, (5) gentle handling of the bladder and ureter, and (6) adequate drainage.

References

Meigs, J. V. Radical hysterectomy with bilateral dissection of the pelvic lymph nodes. In Meigs, J. V. (Ed.), *Surgical Treatment of Cancer of the Cervix*. New York: Grune & Stratton, 1954.

Parsons, L., and Ulfelder, H. *An Atlas of Pelvic Operations*. Philadelphia: W. B. Saunders, 1953.

Yagi, H. Abdominal radical operation for carcinoma of the cervix (the Okabayashi operation). In Meigs, J. V., and Sturgis, S. H., *Progress in Gynecology*, Vol. 3. New York: Grune & Stratton, 1957. P. 535.

107. *Vaginal Hysterectomy and Vaginal Plastic Operations*

ABRAHAM F. LASH

Vaginal Hysterectomy

The technique of vaginal hysterectomy varies, depending on the size and position of the uterus and on associated pathology in the cervix, the endometrium, and the adnexa. The surgical maneuvers include an initial circular incision low enough on the portio to prevent shortening of the vagina; a posterior colpotomy for exploration of the pelvic cavity and exposure of the supportive ligaments; detachment of the uterosacral and cardinal ligaments from the cervix and utilization of these structures to support the vaginal vault; precise ligation of the uterine vessels; dissection of the bladder out of harm's way; removal of the corpus with or without the adnexa; and closure of the peritoneal opening and the vaginal vault.

Technique

The Normal-sized Uterus. To remove the normal-sized uterus vaginally, the vagina is separated from the cervix, after the circular incision has been made, by sharp and blunt dissection posteriorly exposing the peritoneum of the cul-de-sac (Fig. 1). The peritoneum is opened and fixed to the posterior vaginal edge with three interrupted fine catgut sutures which are left long and held by a forceps (Fig. 2). The anterior vaginal wall is then wiped off the cervix until the peritoneum is visible. The peritoneum is opened and fixed to the anterior vaginal edge by three interrupted fine sutures which are also left long and held by a forceps. A long retractor holds the bladder forward. The right uterosacral and cardinal ligaments are then dissected and developed, and clamped close to the cervix, cut, and ligated. They are fixed into the lateral vaginal edge (Fig. 3). This step is repeated on the left side. Next, the uterine vessels are clamped close to the cervix, cut, and ligated (Fig. 4). The corpus may now be brought anteriorly, exposing both cornua with the round ligaments, fallopian tubes, and utero-ovarian ligaments. These are clamped, cut, and ligated, with the sutures left long and held by a clamp.

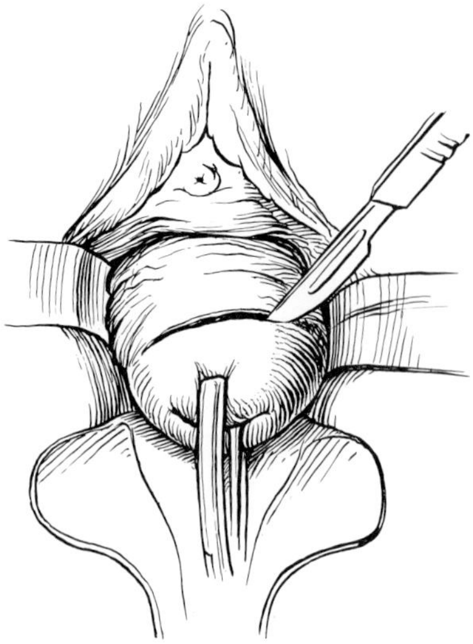

FIGURE 1. Vaginal hysterectomy. The incision around the portio is placed to avoid shortening of the vagina and injury to the bladder.

If the adnexa are to be excised, after one side of the components (round ligament, tube, and utero-ovarian ligament) of the upper broad ligament has been clamped and cut, the freed cornu is pulled down, exposing the whole corpus and opposite round ligament and adnexa. The fimbriated end of the tube is gently pulled down, exposing the infundibulopelvic ligament with the ovarian vessels. These are clamped, cut, and ligated. The whole uterus except the round ligament is thereby freed. Next, the round ligament is clamped, cut, and ligated; and again a long end of the ligature is left in a clamp. The opposite adnexa are dealt with in a similar manner. The anterior vaginal wall with its attached peritoneum is sutured to the posterior vaginal wall with the adjacent attached peritoneum, including the

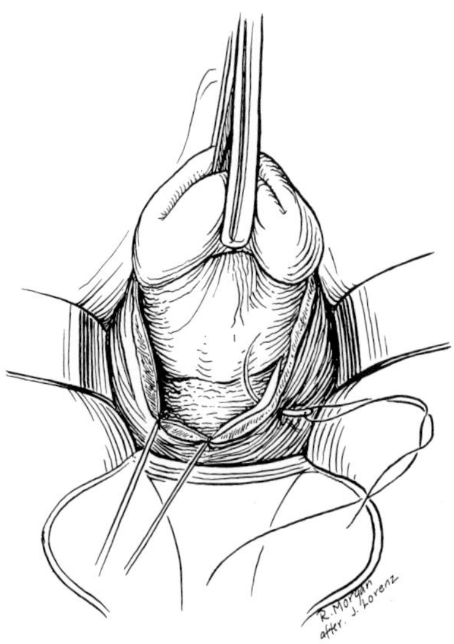

FIGURE 2. The posterior cul-de-sac has been opened. The peritoneum and posterior vaginal wall are held together by three long 00 chromic catgut sutures. The pelvic cavity may now be explored.

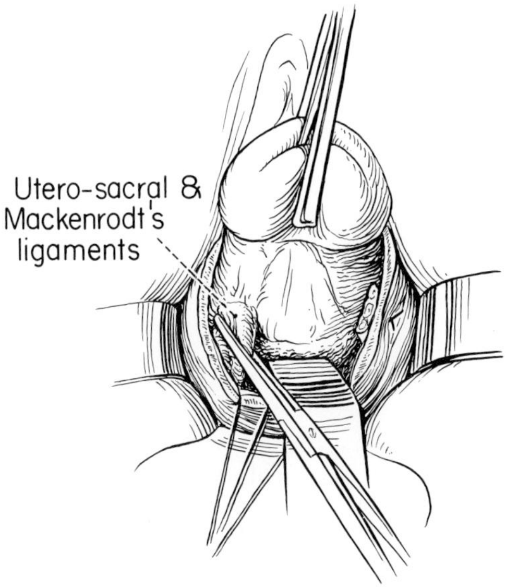

FIGURE 3. The supporting structures—the cardinal and utero-sacral ligaments—are fixed to the vaginal vault.

round ligament pedicles near the center of the vault (Fig. 5). A small opening is left in the center so that an iodoform gauze sponge can be inserted. The sponge is allowed to remain for 48 hours (Fig. 6).

THE LARGE UTERUS. A large uterus (size of a 16 to 20 week pregnancy), usually due to multiple fibroids, may be removed vaginally by the technique just described, with the following variation. After the procedure has been carried to

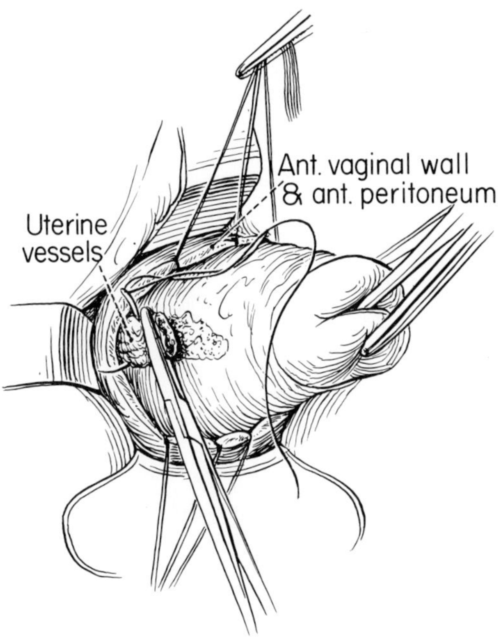

FIGURE 4. The anterior (vesico-uterine) peritoneum and the vaginal wall are held together. With the anterior retractor keeping the bladder out of harm's way, the vessel pedicles are clamped, cut, and ligated.

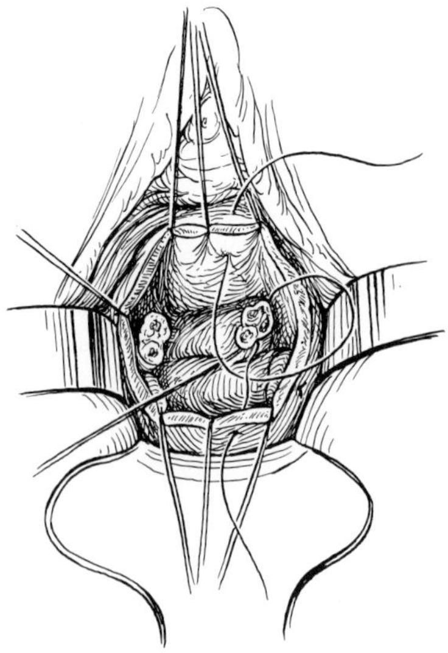

FIGURE 5. Ligament stumps are fixed in the midline of the vaginal vault, allowing a small space between them.

the point at which the uterine vessels have been ligated, an incision is started medial to the vessel stumps. It is advanced into the myometrium as high as one can reach with a long-handled scalpel. It is carried circumferentially in the corpus, and finally the greater part of the myometrium is peeled out of a thin shell of the fundus (Fig. 7). Single fibroids are shelled out and large ones are removed by piecemeal excision. With the size of the corpus decreased, the fundus can be brought anteriorly (Fig. 8). The rest of the procedure is the same as that described for the normal-sized uterus, either leaving or removing the adnexa.

An endometrial carcinoma and an in situ carcinoma of the cervix require the removal of the upper third or half of the vagina in addition to the hysterectomy.

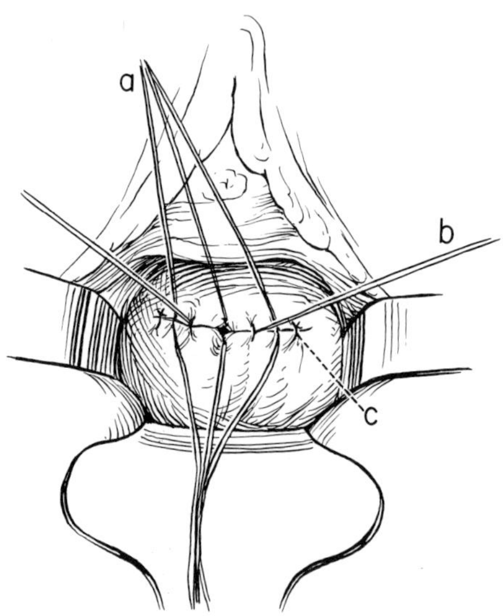

FIGURE 6. Vault closed with a central opening to allow insertion of iodoform gauze in the peritoneal cavity. All pedicles are extraperitoneal and are under the vaginal vault.

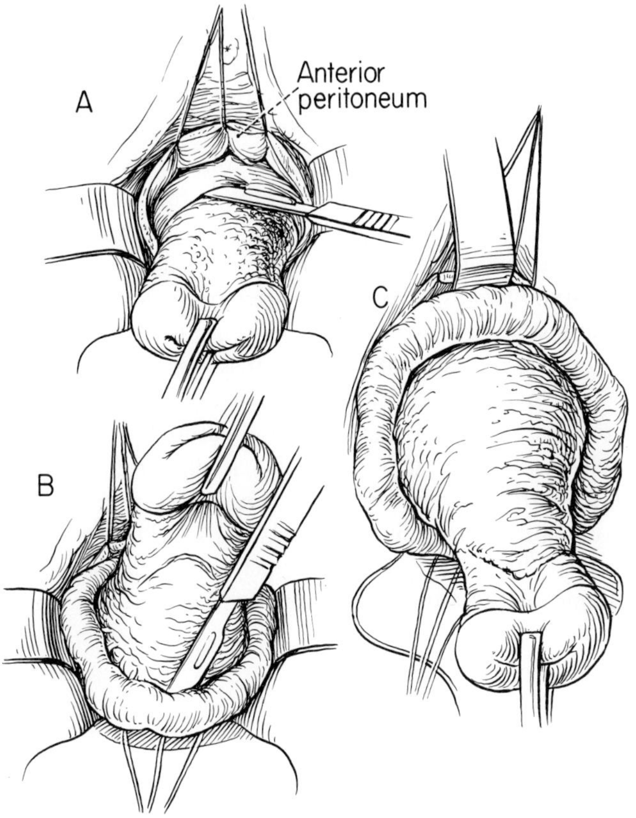

FIGURE 7. (*A*) The incision is started medial to the point where the vessels have been ligated and encircles the cervix. (*B*) The cervix is pulled firmly downward and then upward as the major portion of the myometrium is shelled out, leaving a capsule. (*C*) The major portion of the myometrium with its unopened endometrial cavity is delivered.

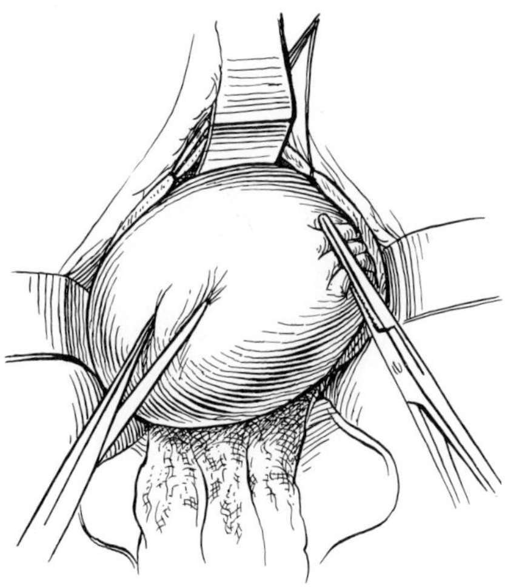

FIGURE 8. Remaining capsule of myometrium is brought forward, exposing the tube and the round and utero-ovarian ligaments. These are clamped on each side, the fundal capsule is removed, and the tubes and ovaries are inspected.

RADICAL VAGINAL HYSTERECTOMY. In the extensive or radical vaginal hysterectomy for early carcinoma of the cervix (stage I), the upper third of the vagina is brought down as a hood over the portio and suture closed. The bladder is dissected off the cervix, and the pillars are carefully followed to expose the ureters, which are traced under the uterine vessels. The vessels are followed to their origin and ligated near the internal iliac arteries. The parametrium is followed laterally to its pelvic wall origin, clamped, cut, and sutured. Thus, the extended operation includes more vagina and parametrium than the simple vaginal hysterectomy.

THE PROLAPSING UTERUS. Prolapsing uteri are removed in the usual manner, but the important step is to develop good supportive structures for the vaginal vault. Since enterocele is commonly present, it is essential to correct it. After the uterosacral and cardinal ligaments have been developed by sharp and blunt dissection they are separated from the uterus and sutured into the posterior vaginal wall. The cul-de-sac hernial sac (enterocele) is dissected from the vagina and followed up to its narrowest point. A purse-string suture is inserted at this point to close it, the redundant peritoneum is excised, and another closing suture is placed below the first one. This lowest point of the pelvic peritoneum may be fixed to the anterior periosteum of the sacrum. The remainder of the operation is then completed.

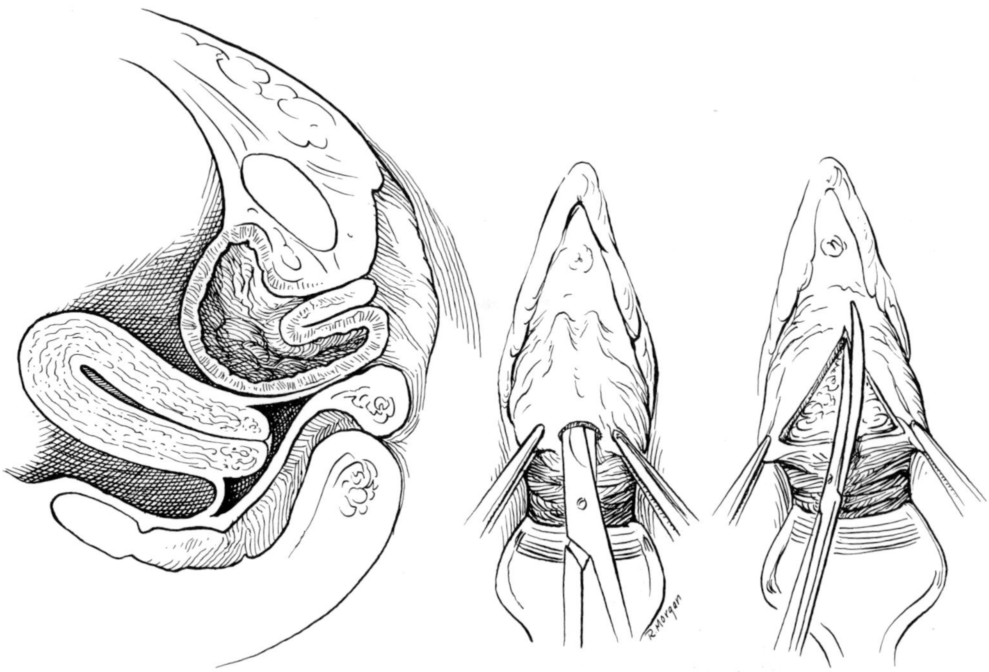

A B C

FIGURE 9. (A) Cystocele with uterus in situ. (*B and C*) Vaginal incision and dissection.

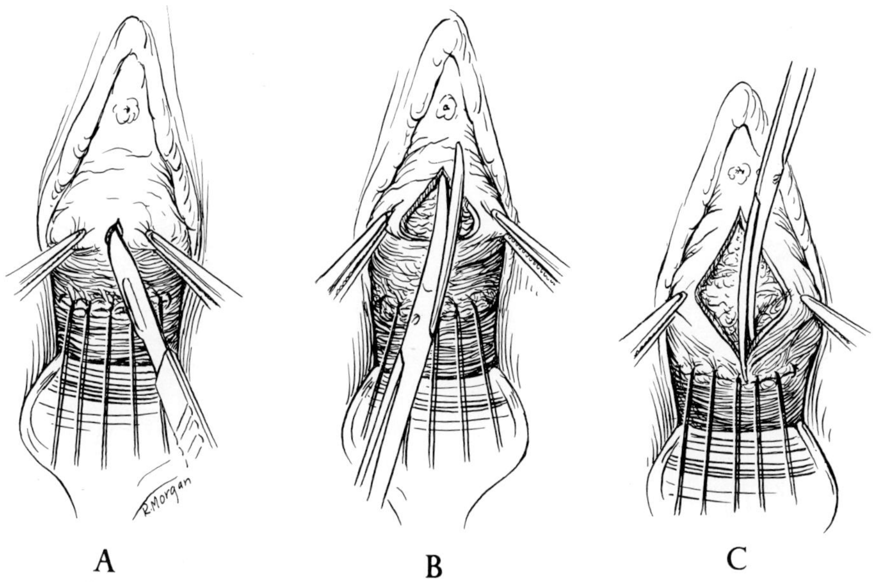

FIGURE 10. Cystocele repair after hysterectomy. (A) Vaginal incision. (*B and C*) Dissection of vaginal wall from fascia.

Vaginal Plastic Operations

The vaginal plastic operations commonly performed are occasioned by symptomatic urethrocele, cystocele, relaxed pelvic floor, and rectocele. The basic maneuvers are adequate dissection of the bladder and rectum, and correction of the hernia by proper use of the fascia for support (Figs. 9–11). Narrowing the urethra and bladder junction and elongating the urethra somewhat will overcome an incompetent sphincter and thereby correct stress incontinence.

The perineorrhaphy is accomplished by elevation of the posterior vaginal wall after the mucocutaneous junction has been excised, from the region of the orifices of Bartholin's ducts (junction of the middle and lower thirds of the vagina at the carunculae myrtiformes) (Figs. 12–14). The rectum is carefully dissected from the vagina. The prerectal fascia is utilized to overcome the hernial bulge due to the rectocele. The perineorrhaphy uses the pubococcygeus muscles and their fascia for establishing an adequate floor support, so that the vagina will be oblique and the anterior vaginal surface will lie on the posterior surface as in the normal state.

Vaginal vault hernias may be prevented by obliterating the cul-de-sac of Douglas when closing the vault after vaginal hysterectomy. If a deep posterior cul-de-sac is overlooked or ignored, after either a vaginal or an abdominal hysterectomy a vaginal vault hernia may result, as illustrated in Figure 15. The usual technique for repair for this hernia is exposure of the peritoneal sac, ligation of the neck of the sac, and closure after all hernial contents have been reduced into the pelvic cavity. The endopelvic fascia is utilized for repair below the ligated sac,

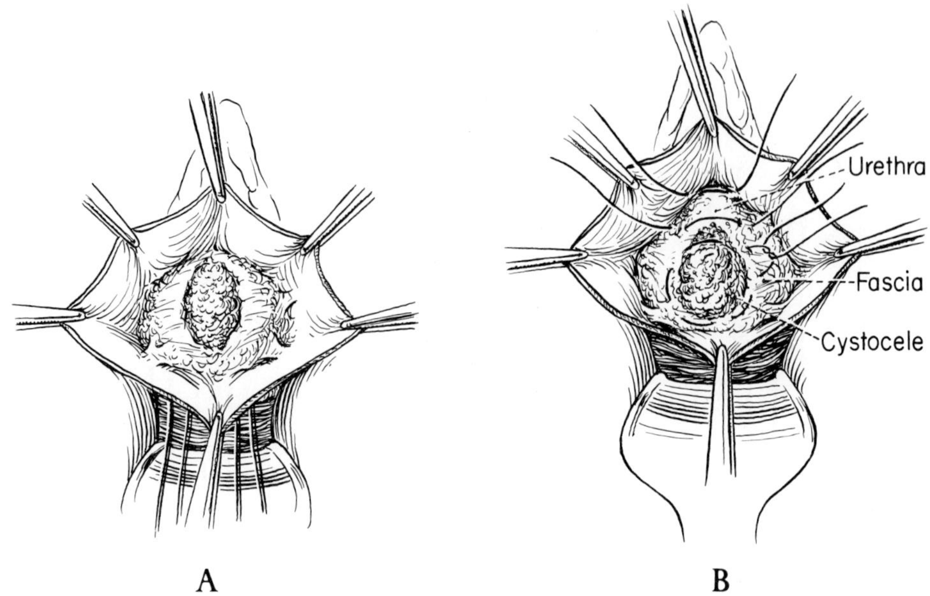

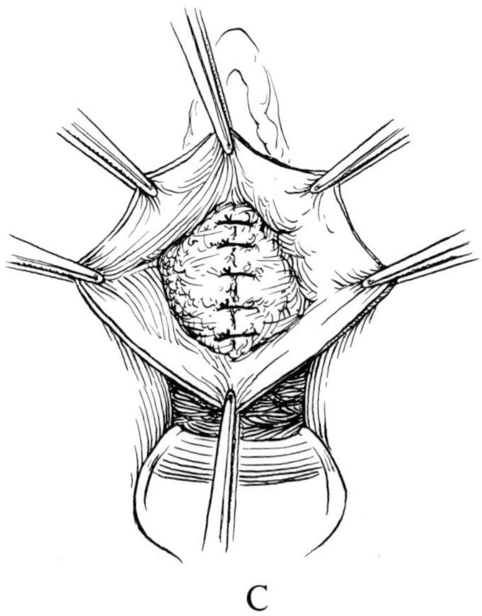

FIGURE 11. Cystocele repair and restoration of the urogenital diaphragm with narrowing of the urethrovesical junction and urethra. (*A*) Lateral fascia edges developed. (*B*) Purse-string suture in large, thinned-out fascia. (*C*) Fascial closure with restored urogenital diaphragm. The lower portion includes bladder pillars.

and then the vagina is closed without shortening. The restoration of the urogenital diaphragm and the pelvic floor follows, and helps to produce normal length of the vagina.

Special Comments

Troublesome conditions encountered in performing vaginal hysterectomy include an inadequate vaginal opening, associated pelvic pathology, intestinal adhesions, and bleeding during and after surgery.

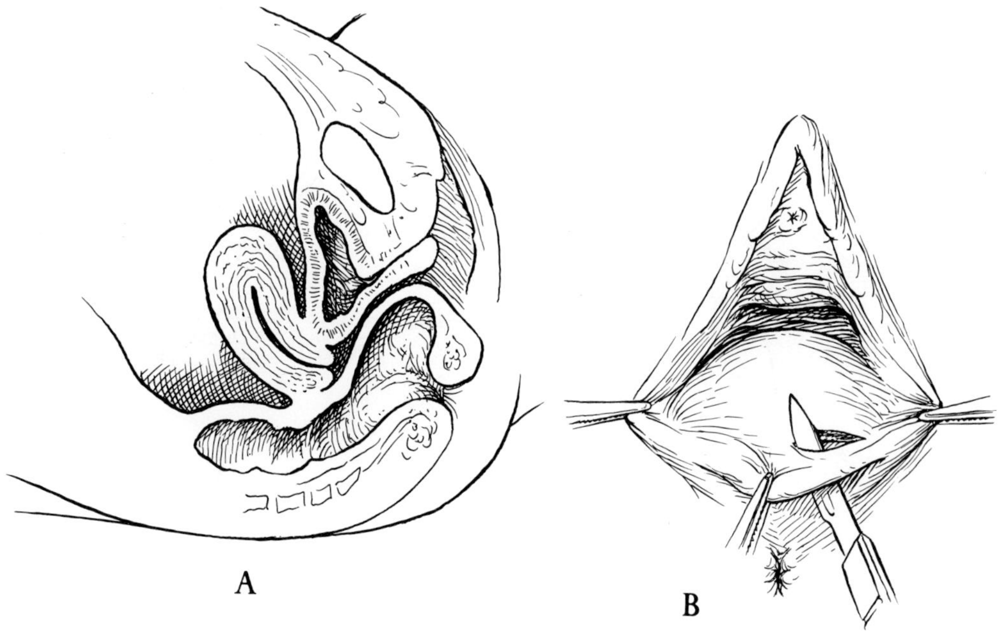

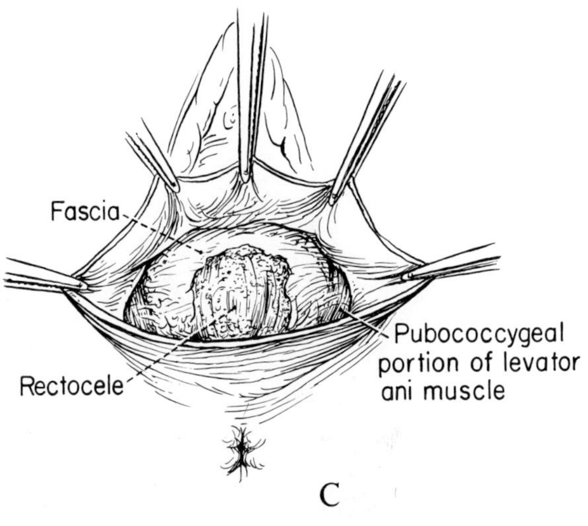

FIGURE 12. (*A*) Rectocele and relaxed pelvic floor. (*B*) Incision through the mucocutaneous edge of the vagina. (*C*) Dissection (sharp and dull) exposes the rectocele and the edges of the pubococcygeal portion of the levator ani muscle.

To enlarge the vaginal opening for easier access to the uterus, a median or posterior perineotomy or Schuchardt incision is very helpful. An enlarged vaginal approach is desirable in nulliparous and obese persons.

Infrequently, associated adnexal pathology (pelvic inflammatory disease or endometriosis) may make it impossible to enter the pelvic cavity. In the absence of any malignant growth, the major portion of the myometrium and the endometrial cavity may be removed, leaving a thin shell of myometrium which is obliterated by sutures, thereby accomplishing an extraperitoneal vaginal hysterectomy.

Previous abdominal operations are apt to leave adhesions or distorted anatomy. Under such circumstances the vaginal route may be preferable to the abdominal

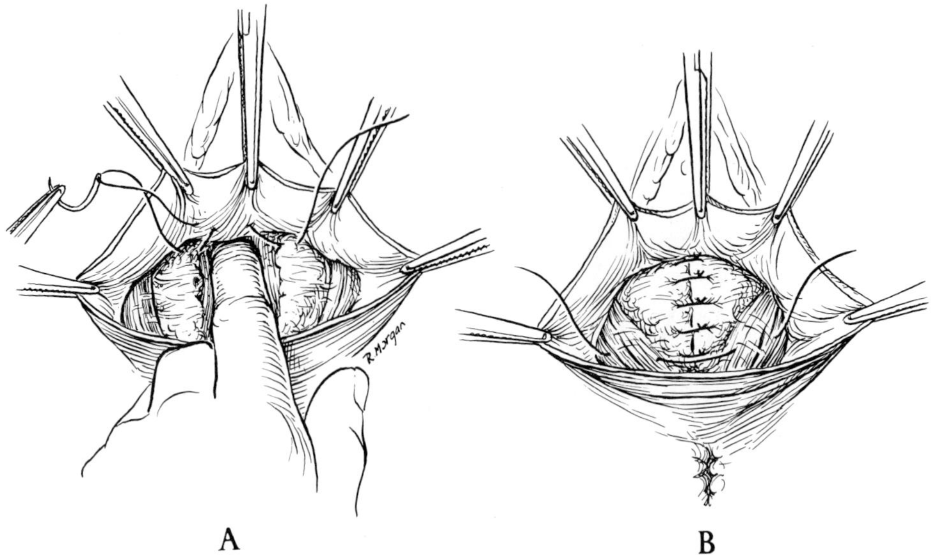

FIGURE 13. (*A*) Repair of the rectocele by depressing the rectum. The fascial edges become evident and serve for covering the bulging anterior rectal wall. (*B*) Completed fascial covering over the rectum.

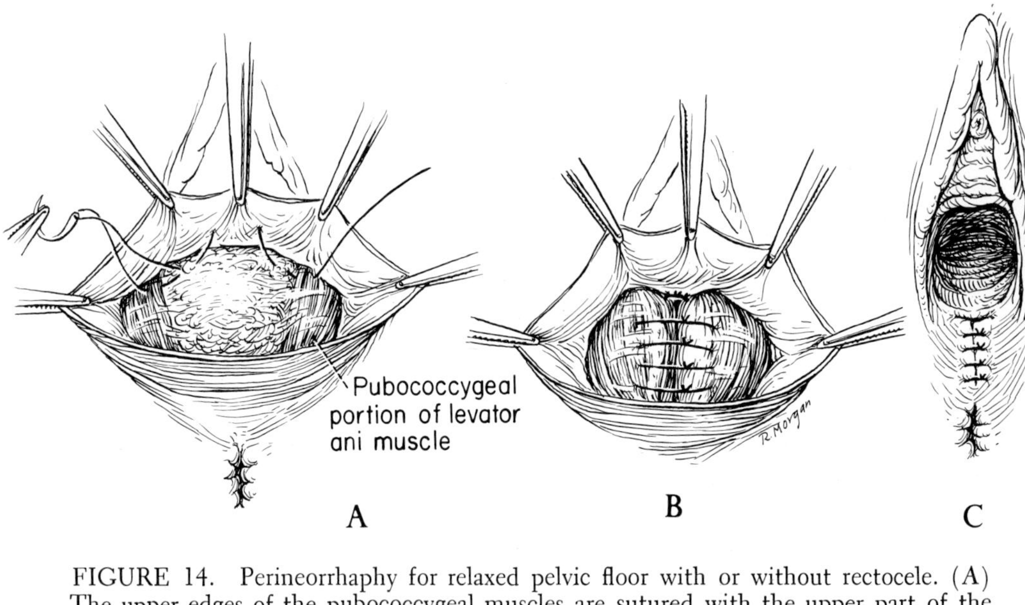

FIGURE 14. Perineorrhaphy for relaxed pelvic floor with or without rectocele. (*A*) The upper edges of the pubococcygeal muscles are sutured with the upper part of the posterior vaginal wall included in the first suture. (*B*) Pelvic floor restored by the musculofascial union of the two pubococcygeal muscles and fascia. (*C*) Closure of the perineal wound, illustrating the increased distance between the vaginal orifice and the anus (compare with Figure 12).

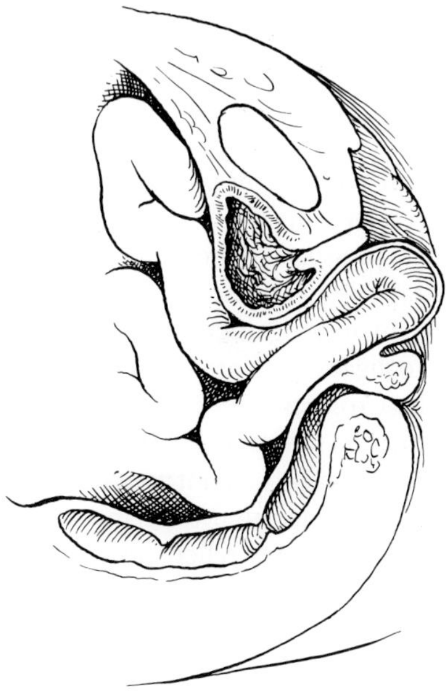

FIGURE 15. Vaginal vault hernia (enterocele). The repair follows the surgical principles of herniorrhaphy. The cystocele, rectocele, and pelvic floor plastic repair follow it.

approach for removal of the uterus. If pelvic surgery of unknown nature has been performed, the vaginal approach may be started, but if difficulties arise in the removal of the uterus and adnexa, that approach should be given up and the abdominal approach resorted to. This can be done with safety since the vagina has been properly prepared. Circumstances that may bring a shift from the vaginal to the abdominal approach are old fixation operations for suspension of the fundus, bowel adhesions resulting in intestinal lacerations when freed, extensive endometriosis, or unsuspected ovarian carcinoma.

To limit blood loss during vaginal hysterectomy, 0.5 ml. of surgical pituitrin intracervically is effective, but should not be used with cyclopropane anesthesia, for patients with cardiac disease, or for old people with myocardial damage. In the latter patients 3 to 5 drops of 1:1000 epinephrine solution in 100 ml. of normal saline solution injected around the cervix is a good local vascular constrictor. These procedures aid in separating the tissue layers, such as the vaginal wall from the cervix.

Opening the peritoneum of the posterior cul-de-sac *first* is desirable because pelvic structures are less likely to be injured; there is easy access to the pelvic cavity, allowing finger exploration and confirmation of an uncertain diagnosis. Strong traction downward on the cervix with tenacula and the retraction of the dissected vaginal wall upward prevent injury to the bladder and the ureters, and the retraction of the opened posterior cul-de-sac allows easy approach to the ligaments and the vessels of the uterus.

During surgery, adequate exposure is essential so that deep structures may be made superficial; rarely, with adequate exposure, is a vessel in the broad ligament not accessible and procurable if the ligature breaks or the pedicle slips through the forceps or ligature. Traction either on the cardinal ligament stump or on the round ligament and adnexal stump will always bring the vascular pedicle into view for reclamping and religating. Bringing the fimbriated end of the tube down exposes the infundibulopelvic ligament with the ovarian vessels for clamping and ligating. All pedicles are reinspected, insuring a dry field when closure is performed.

In the rare instance in which a ligature has been improperly placed or locked, and the vessel is not adequately secured, postoperative bleeding occurs, and is evidenced by a rising tachycardia and falling blood pressure. If no vaginal bleeding is seen, indicating that the hemorrhage is intraperitoneal, the abdomen must be opened and the bleeder controlled. If there is an intraligamentary hematoma and the bleeding vessel is not seen, it is simpler to ligate the internal iliac artery below its division from the common iliac artery than to seek the bleeding uterine vessel. With the control of the bleeding the clots may be removed. The ligation of the internal iliac vessels may be accomplished extraperitoneally or intraperitoneally and is an excellent method for control of pelvic hemorrhage due to many conditions. The ovarian vessels may also be reached by these routes when necessary.

When tissue is friable or a spurting vessel is seen on vaginal inspection, an 8-inch Kocher clamp may be applied and allowed to remain for 72 hours, opening it partially after 48 hours.

All these considerations suggest that it is well to know not only the technique of the operation but also to be prepared to cope with all intangible and unexpected complications.

XIX. THE SYMPATHETIC NERVOUS SYSTEM

108. *Splanchnicectomy*

REGINALD H. SMITHWICK

DENERVATION of the splanchnic bed is helpful in the management of essential and malignant hypertension. Most of these cases can be managed satisfactorily by antihypertensive drug therapy. For patients who do not respond satisfactorily, or who will not follow a medical regimen or are handicapped by the side effects of drugs, a conservative type of splanchnicectomy removing the sympathetic trunks bilaterally from the eighth to the twelfth thoracic ganglion inclusive and the great splanchnic nerves from the celiac ganglia to the midthoracic levels should be performed.

The splanchnic innervation is best exposed by an extrapleural transdiaphragmatic retroperitoneal approach. This also gives an excellent view of the kidneys, renal arteries, and adrenal glands; consequently, this same exposure may be employed in many cases of hypertension of renal origin and in virtually all cases of hypertension of adrenal origin, and for adrenal surgery in general.

A conservative type of splanchnicectomy is helpful in the management of pain problems involving the upper abdominal viscera. These may be divided into three groups: pain of biliary tract origin, pain of pancreatic origin, and upper abdominal pain of unknown origin. In general, a bilateral procedure should be performed. The afferent fibers carrying pain sensation from the viscera pass through the splanchnic nerves and sympathetic trunks. These may be effectively interrupted by resecting the sympathetic trunks bilaterally from the tenth to the twelfth thoracic ganglion inclusive, together with the great splanchnic nerves from the celiac ganglia to the midthoracic levels.

Technique

Intratracheal anesthesia should be employed. The patient is placed in the prone position, as for dorsal sympathectomy, with the chest and pelvis supported in such fashion that there is no pressure on the abdomen. The table is broken slightly to flatten the lumbar spine. Bilateral paravertebral incisions are made, centered over the eleventh rib and extending to above the tenth and below the twelfth rib

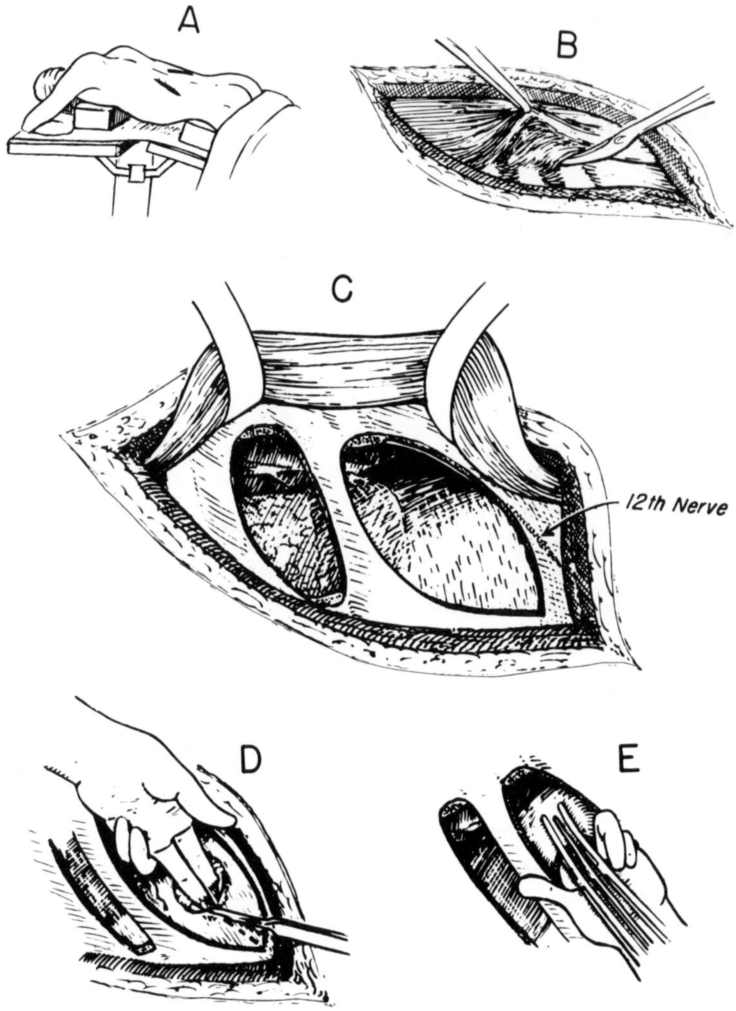

FIGURE 1. Exposure of the splanchnic innervation.

(Fig. 1A). The upper portions are placed 3 to 4 cm. from the midline over the lateral border of the sacrospinalis muscle group. They run downward and slightly outward to cross the twelfth rib at the lateral edge of the sacrospinalis muscle and then continue downward toward the iliac crest. The dissection is carried down through the deep fascia, through fibers of the latissimus dorsi muscle, opening the underlying sacrospinalis sheath from the top of the incision to below the twelfth rib. Below this point the deep dissection is carried downward and slightly laterally to the lumbodorsal fascia, incising the deep fascia and a few filaments of the oblique abdominal muscles. The lateral edge of the sacrospinalis muscle is elevated, exposing the underlying eleventh and twelfth ribs (Fig. 1B). A liberal portion of the former, about 7 cm., should be removed lateral to the transverse process. All of the twelfth rib is resected. The eleventh intercostal bundle is left intact. The twelfth intercostal vessels may be resected if in the way in the lower portion of the field, care being taken not to injure the twelfth nerve, which lies in a deeper plane under the lateral edge of the quadratus lumborum muscle (Fig. 1C). If one is concerned only with the adrenal glands or visceral pain problems, only the twelfth ribs need be removed.

The pleura is separated from the thoracic cage with gentle finger dissection. This dissection is best accomplished by working gently inward to the plane of the great splanchnic nerve, then upward to above the inner end of the eighth rib. The finger is then swept gently laterally and from above downward to the lateral end of the resected eleventh rib. An incision is then made through the renal fascia just lateral to the diaphragm. The perirenal fat protrudes through this opening (Fig. 1D).

The fascia is further divided laterally and downward, following which the dissection is carried medially and downward beneath this fascial layer and the diaphragm and over the psoas muscle to the lumbar spine. The diaphragm is then divided, together with the adherent underlying fascia, between clamps (Fig. 1E). There are always vessels of consequence in the diaphragm which require ligation. The ascending lumbar and at times the azygos or hemiazygos veins pass through the same hiatus as the trunk. Care must be taken to visualize these so that they will not be inadvertently injured, as serious bleeding may result.

After the diaphragm has been divided, the exposure is complete (Fig. 2A). The table is then tilted laterally about 30 degrees away from the operator. The kidney and its pedicle are inspected and the adrenal gland as well (Fig. 2B). It is wise to determine at this point whether or not an adrenal tumor is present. These are found in about 5 per cent of cases, although only an occasional tumor appears to play an active role in maintaining elevated blood pressure. If a tumor is present, it is removed. Unless a dramatic fall in blood pressure ensues immediately, one may proceed with splanchnicectomy. Renal abnormalities can be detected and handled with facility.

The sympathetic trunk is then elevated just below the eleventh ganglion. This is done best with a long Crile nerve hook. The trunk between the twelfth thoracic and the first lumbar ganglion is always very flimsy. The twelfth thoracic ganglion and its rami may lie entirely beneath the diaphragm, particularly in patients having a short twelfth rib. There are numerous variations in the anatomy of this region. The standard procedure, in my opinion, should be the removal of the sympathetic trunk from the eighth to the twelfth thoracic ganglion inclusive. The thoracic chain is divided below the twelfth ganglion and is removed from below upward to include the eighth ganglion. All rami as well as the trunk proximally and distally are carefully secured with tantalum clips. The portion of the dissection which lies above the ninth ganglion adds nothing to the completeness of the splanchnic denervation but may be an additional safeguard against regeneration. In removing the sympathetic trunk, all the lesser and least splanchnic nerves which have their origin in the excised main trunk are necessarily included.

The great splanchnic nerve is then identified, elevated upon a hook, crushed, doubly clipped, and divided just above the celiac ganglion. It is freed upward by

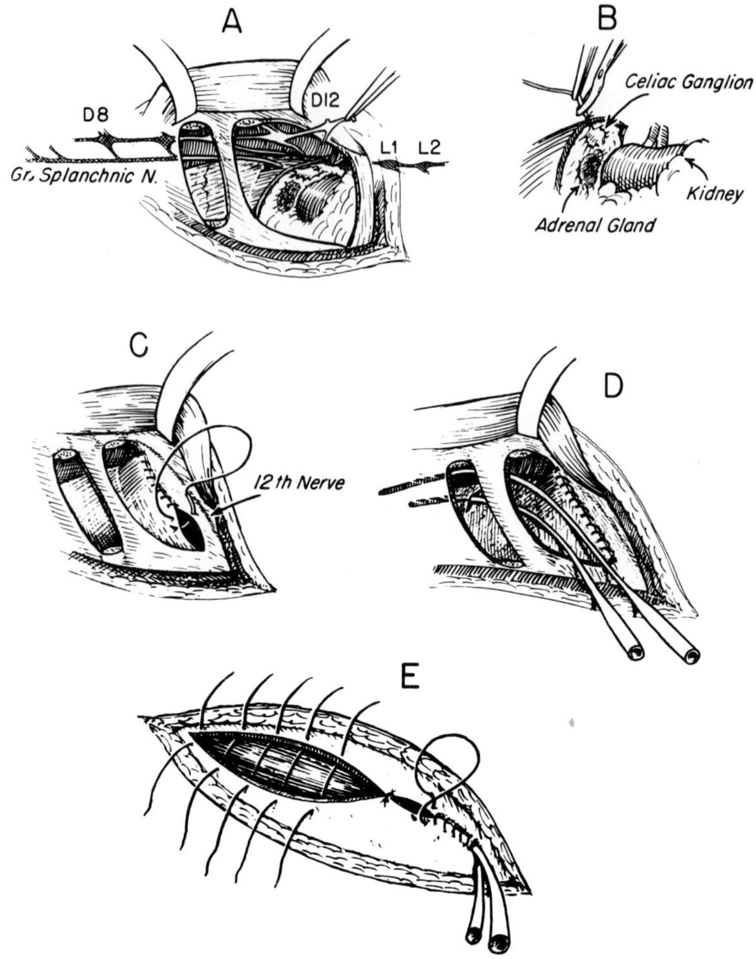

FIGURE 2. Removal of the sympathetic trunk from the eighth to the twelfth thoracic ganglion inclusive, and of the great splanchnic nerve from the celiac ganglion to the midthoracic levels. Closure of the incision.

manual dissection in order to avoid injuring the azygos or hemiazygos vein or the thoracic duct with which it is intimately associated. If it terminates in the sympathetic trunk at the seventh ganglion, as it occasionally does, it is removed up to this point. More commonly, a fine strand runs upward, and this is best avulsed with a long right-angle clamp.

The diaphragm is resutured and the renal fascia is then closed with a continuous catgut suture (Fig. 2C). A No. 24 French catheter is placed in the extrapleural space to aspirate any residual air which may remain after the wound has been closed. If there is an opening in the pleura, a second catheter is inserted within the pleural cavity (Fig. 2D). The lung is expanded with positive pressure and the catheters are removed after the incision has been closed in layers with interrupted sutures (Fig. 2E).

109. Lumbar Sympathectomy

REGINALD H. SMITHWICK

LUMBAR SYMPATHECTOMY is very helpful in the management of a variety of disorders including the more severe forms of Raynaud's disease, acrocyanosis, causalgia, posttraumatic painful neurovascular disorders, posttraumatic ulcerations, and edema and hyperhidrosis. It also is very helpful in the management of obliterative vascular disorders, especially peripheral arteriosclerosis with varying degrees of obliterative vascular disease, providing one selects the patients for operation with care.

The important sympathetic efferent fibers to the blood vessels and sweat glands of the legs pass through the first, second, and third lumbar ganglia. For vasospastic and other disorders without obliterative vascular disease, and for the latter when the popliteal pulse is present, removal of the second and third lumbar ganglia will suffice. For more extensive obliterative disease the first lumbar ganglion should also be included. Incomplete denervation due to accessory ganglia (Skoog) is not a problem as in the case of the upper extremity. Regeneration, while it does occur to some extent with the passage of time, does not detract significantly from the clinical results, as it may in the upper extremity.

Technique

The lumbar sympathetic trunk may be exposed transperitoneally, by a posterolateral retroperitoneal incision or by the anterolateral retroperitoneal approach. The latter is by and large the best and will be described. General intratracheal anesthesia may be used. In obese or muscular individuals, spinal anesthesia is the best. In most cases, a bilateral sympathectomy is indicated and both sides can be done at the same operation. With the patient in the supine position, transverse incisions are made opposite the umbilicus from the lateral border of the rectus sheath to the flank (Fig. 1). After skin towels have been carefully applied the dissection is carried down through the fat to the fascia. The fascia of the external oblique muscle is divided in the line of the skin incision from the lateral border of the rectus muscle to the flank. Several centimeters of external oblique muscle is di-

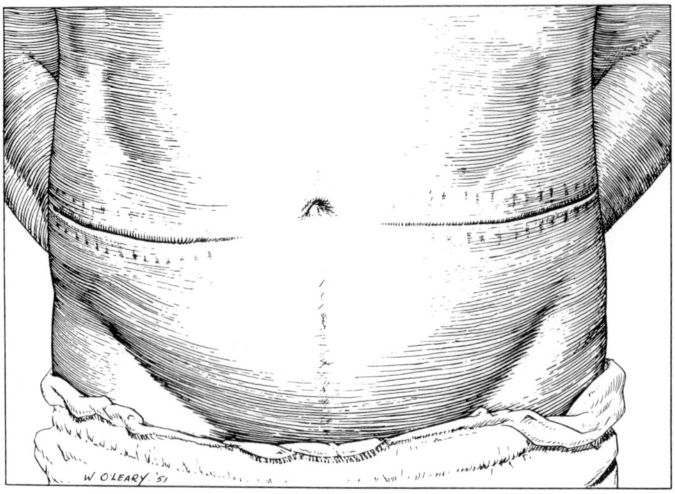

FIGURE 1. Incisions for the anterolateral retroperitoneal approach in lumbar sympathectomy. (Reproduced by permission of The Macmillan Company from White, Smithwick, and Simeone, *Autonomic Nervous System.*)

vided in the lateral aspect of the incision. This fascia and muscle is then separated quite widely by blunt finger dissection from the underlying internal oblique muscle. The fibers of the latter are then split in the line of their direction over a distance of about 4 inches. This muscle in turn is separated from the underlying transversus abdominis muscle. The fibers of the latter are then split in the line of their direction, which is transverse. Care should be taken to split this muscle, which is usually thin, in the most lateral part of the incision and continue the splitting process in a medial direction for about 3 inches. As the muscle becomes tendinous, it joins the peritoneum. If the foregoing directions are followed, inadvertent opening of the peritoneum will be avoided.

One then passes a forefinger posteriorly and slightly upward and inward along the course of the twelfth rib if palpable, or in the same direction if the rib cannot be palpated, until the finger passes over the psoas muscle to the vertebral column. If one dissects medially at a lower level, one will be in the wrong plane of cleavage, posterior to the psoas muscle.

One then separates the peritoneum from the psoas muscle and posterior abdominal wall by finger dissection from above downward to where the common iliac artery is felt and medially along the vertebral column. One should be able to palpate the second lumbar ganglion, as it is usually large and fusiform in shape. The back of the dissecting forefinger should always be toward the peritoneum to avoid opening it.

One then inserts a wide Deaver retractor in the center of the incision, retracting the peritoneum gently medially and upward. Usually three large wet sponges are needed for good exposure. These are tucked in beneath the retractor one at a time, shifting the retractor each time so that the sponge is between it and the peritoneum. This allows gentle retraction of the peritoneum and its contents without damage to either and gives excellent exposure of the central portion of the lumbar sympathetic trunk. An additional moist gauze sponge is then placed in the uppermost portion of the field. A narrow Deaver retractor is placed over this. Slight upward retraction on this, combined with gentle medial and upward traction on the other rectractor, gives an excellent view of the lumbar sympathetic chain. The secret of good exposure without trauma to the peritoneum or its contents is the amount of gauze packing beneath the retractors. The gauze packs also give indirect traction on the vena cava, lifting it away from the vertebral column and the region of the sympathetic chains and obviating any need of dissecting to obtain this exposure. The lumbar veins arising from the vena cava are also brought into view. This is important because, on the right side, the lumbar veins which normally pass posterior to the trunk may cross it anteriorly, especially one which arises at a level just above the third lumbar ganglion. Failure to detect this may result in damaging this vein. Bleeding from this source can be severe and difficult to control.

This exposure having been obtained, removal of the desired ganglia and intervening trunk is usually a very simple matter and takes but a few minutes. The trunk is best elevated with a long right-angle nerve hook just below the large second lumbar ganglion, and the dissection is carried upward to include it and also the first lumbar ganglion if desired. Dissection of the trunk is best carried out with Hartmann forceps. It is my custom to place dura clips on the trunk and the various rami before dividing them. As a rule, exposure of the third lumbar ganglion is facilitated by removing the narrow retractor in the upper portion of the field and replacing it over a gauze strip in the lower portion. This ganglion will usually be found close to the level of the common iliac artery.

Closure of the wound is a very simple matter and requires only two or three interrupted catgut sutures in the transversus abdominis and internal oblique muscles. One intercostal nerve normally crosses the middle of the field between the internal oblique and transversus abdominis muscles and need not be damaged. Care must be taken not to include it in the sutures when one is closing the defect in the transversus abdominis muscle. The external oblique muscle and fascia is then approximated with interrupted catgut sutures and the skin edges with interrupted silk sutures. The operation is repeated on the opposite side if indicated. With experience, it should take less than 30 minutes to do each side.

Reference

SMITHWICK, R. H. Lumbar sympathectomy in the treatment of obliterative vascular disease of the lower extremities. I. *Surgery* 42:415, August, 1957; II. *Surgery* 42: 567, September, 1957.

110. Dorsal Sympathectomy

REGINALD H. SMITHWICK

INTERRUPTION of the vasomotor and sudomotor nerve supply to the upper extremity is helpful in the management of Raynaud's disease, acrocyanosis, causalgia, posttraumatic painful neurovascular syndromes, hyperhidrosis, and various other circulatory disturbances.

Anatomical Considerations

A brief summary of the anatomical pathways of the sympathetic nerve supply to the upper extremity is advisable since it will clarify certain points in surgical technique. So far as is known, there is no important difference in the course of vasomotor and sudomotor fibers. The vast majority of these fibers emerge from the cord by way of the anterior roots of the second to the tenth intercostal nerves, inclusive. In some cases, there also may be an outflow along the anterior root of the first thoracic nerve. In about 90 per cent of cases, this is not significant. The usual course of a sympathetic fiber as it passes from the anterior root by way of a white communicating ramus to enter a sympathetic ganglion to form a synapse in the ganglion is shown in Figure 1G. That portion of the pathway before the synapse is preganglionic; after the synapse, it becomes postganglionic. The postganglionic fiber then returns to the intercostal nerve by way of a gray communicating ramus to be distributed to the periphery in the same fashion as are somatic sensory nerves. The synapse may occur in the same segment of emergence from the cord. It is believed, however, that most of the synapses having to do with the upper extremity occur in the third and second thoracic ganglia, the stellate ganglion (a combination of the inferior cervical and first thoracic ganglion), and the middle cervical ganglion. Gray rami pass from these ganglia to the cords of the brachial plexus and eventually reach blood vessels and sweat glands as do somatic sensory fibers.

The unusual course which sympathetic fibers may follow because of the presence of intermediate ganglia (Skoog, 1957), which are situated close to if not within the intercostal nerves, is illustrated by Figure 1H. Under these circumstances, sympathetic fibers may reach the periphery without passing through the sympathetic trunk at all. These accessory ganglia occur in man most frequently in the upper thoracic region. There is no way to predict which patients have them. The importance of this anomaly is that it makes it impossible to completely denervate the upper extremity by ganglionectomy alone. This circumstance will influence clinical results in perhaps 15 per cent of cases.

When there is an outflow from the first thoracic segment via Skoog's ganglia, nothing can be done about it. If there is an outflow from the second or third thoracic segment, it can be eliminated by resecting the corresponding intercostal nerves, including an intraspinal portion of both the anterior and the posterior root as depicted in Figure 1F. The second intercostal nerve commonly supplies a branch to the first thoracic nerve and thus contributes to the formation of the lower cord of the brachial plexus. The third intercostal nerve occasionally sends a branch to the second. Thus, in addition to fibers which normally reach the brachial plexus by way of gray rami arising from the second and third ganglia, sympathetic fibers from the second and third anterior roots can reach the upper extremity, if Skoog's ganglia are present, by way of these branches. Having studied a number of patients in whom, by error, the second thoracic ganglion was not removed in denervating the upper extremity, and having found evidence of substantial residual sympathetic control of blood vessels and sweat glands in such cases, I feel that complete and permanent abolition of the outflow from the second thoracic segment is of vital importance. Both because the third intercostal nerve may supply a branch to the second and because the third ganglion also sends gray rami to the plexus, it is essential that its outflow likewise be completely interrupted. This is best accomplished by intraspinal root sections of the second and third intercostal nerves. The second and third ganglia are also removed (Fig. 1B, C, D). Since ganglia below the third do not send gray rami to the plexus, they need not be removed. These are the reasons why intraspinal root section of the second and third intercostal nerves is an essential part of an operation designed to interrupt the vasoconstrictor nerve supply to the upper extremity. In dealing with sudomotor fibers, it is not necessary to use the same precautions against incomplete denervation or regeneration which one must employ when dealing with vasomotor fibers. To denervate sweat glands, all that is necessary is to remove the second and third thoracic ganglia. Any residual sudomotor activity after this operation is of no clinical importance and, for reasons unknown, there is little tendency for sudomotor fibers to regenerate, at least to the point where the clinical result in the case of the upper extremity is compromised.

Technique

Intratracheal anesthesia is used. Following induction, the patient is placed in the prone position. A firm hair mattress of appropriate size supports the chest and a second supports the pelvis in such fashion that the abdomen is free of pressure. The arm on the side to be operated upon, or both arms in a bilateral procedure, should be at the patient's side so that the medial border of the scapula will swing laterally away from the paravertebral area. Further to promote this, a small pillow is placed on top of the hair mattress directly beneath the upper two-thirds of the sternum. The head is in the midline with the neck slightly flexed. A side-tilting table should be used (Fig. 1A).

A vertical paravertebral incision or incisions 3 to 4 inches long are made, placed about 2 inches lateral to the midline. The incisions are centered opposite

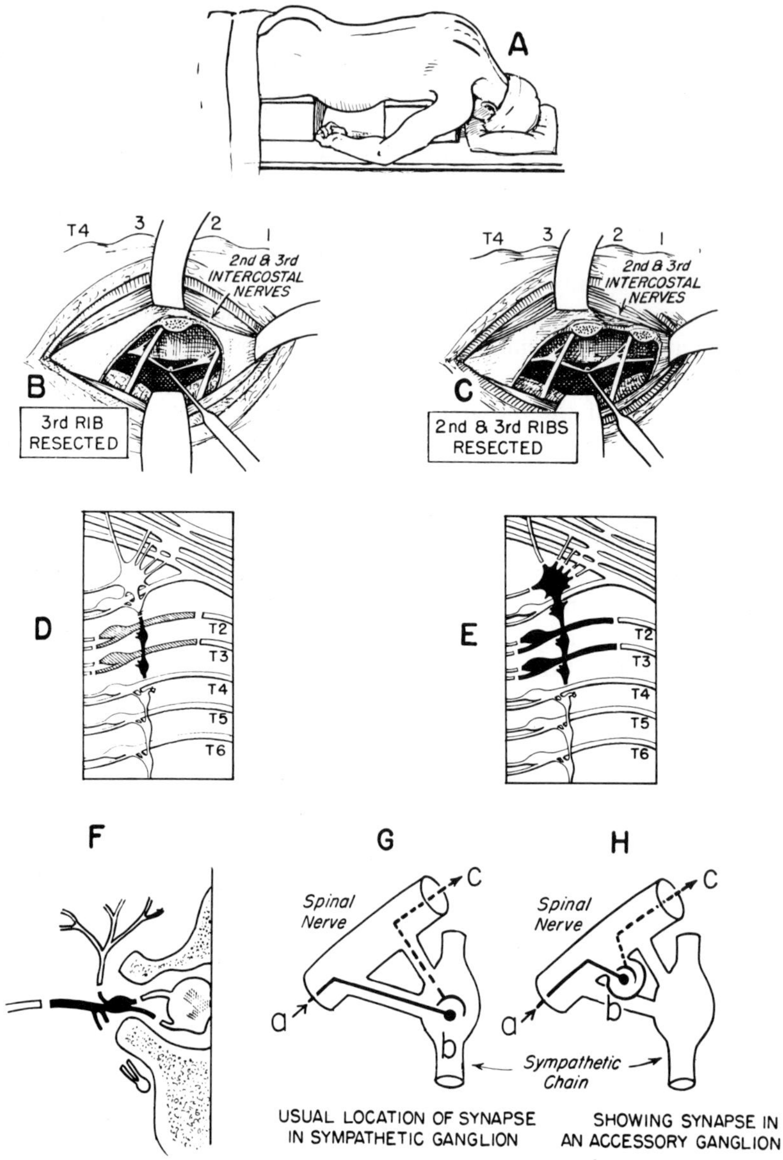

FIGURE 1. Anatomical and technical considerations in dorsal sympathectomy.

the interspace between the second and third thoracic spinous processes. After careful application of skin towels, the incision is carried down through the deep fascia to the trapezius muscle. The fibers of this muscle are incised vertically for a distance of 1 to 3 inches, depending on the subsequent details of surgical technique. This exposes the underlying rhomboid muscle, which is divided obliquely in the direction of its fibers. A finger can then be passed upward and downward beneath this muscle and the ribs palpated and counted accurately. If the incision is placed properly, the oblique split in the rhomboid will be directly over the third rib. The first rib is sometimes a little difficult to feel. The second is very prominent and beginners are apt to count it as the first. If one feels carefully over this prominent rib, the first rib will be identified with certainty. An x-ray is essential to exclude a cervical rib.

After identification of the third rib, the overlying longissimus cervicis muscle is split vertically, the intercostal muscles are separated by sharp (scissors) dissection from the upper and lower borders of the rib, and the inner 4 cm. is removed, including the periosteum. If one divides the external intercostal muscle and the fascia between it and the internal muscle layer close to the rib, one can then pass a finger around the rib, outside of the periosteum and between it and the pleura and the intercostal nerve, artery, and vein with minimal danger of injuring these structures. This technique is preferable to subperiosteal resections in this region. The tip of the transverse process is removed with rongeurs, and the underlying remnant of rib is removed for a centimeter or so. The pleura is then gently separated with a finger to the midline of the vertebral column, to a point above the second and below the third rib, and laterally to the resected rib end. One then has the exposure shown in Figure 1B. This exposure permits one to remove the second and third thoracic ganglia. Dura clips are applied to the communicating rami and to the trunk proximally and distally.

The operation just described is the procedure of choice when one is concerned with denervating the sweat glands, as in hyperhidrosis. If, however, the indication for operation is to interrupt the vasoconstrictor fibers to the upper extremity, the second and third intercostal nerves should be resected as well, dividing the roots intraspinally as shown in Figure 1D and 1F. The third intercostal nerve is picked up with a hook, care being taken that the intercostal artery and vein are not included. The nerve is divided at the lateral extent of the incision. It is followed to the intervertebral foramen, dividing the communicating rami running from the anterior aspect of the nerve to the corresponding thoracic ganglion. A dental spatula is then slipped about the dorsal branch of the intercostal nerve and the branch divided. This branch runs vertically and posteriorly between the transverse processes and is given off just lateral to the posterior root ganglion. The latter now comes into view and the spatula is inserted between the anterior and posterior roots at the proximal end of the ganglion. The posterior root is divided with a knife against the spatula blade, leaving the anterior root intact. The arachnoid is then pushed medially with the spatula and separated from the anterior root so that the latter, white and glistening, is free in the foramen. A small spinal fluid leak results. The root is then divided with scissors in such a way that the lateral centimeter is removed. The proximal end retracts within the canal and, after the meninges heal, theoretically it should not regenerate. The second intercostal nerve is treated in a similar fashion. The sympathetic trunk is then palpated. It lies on the anterolateral aspect of the vertebral column exactly where the head of the rib contacts the vertebral body. It is hooked between the second and third ganglia and is mobilized from below the third ganglion to above the second. The trunk is clipped and divided just distal to the third ganglion. Dissection is then carried upward to just above the second dorsal ganglion. The second and third ganglia are removed, clipping the upper divided end of the trunk below the first thoracic ganglion. Taking all factors into consideration, this is the preferred operation for vasomotor disorders. Certainly, if only one extremity is to be denervated, this operation should be performed, as it does not produce a Horner's sign. The latter, while not objectionable if bilateral, is unsightly if unilateral. This operation gives maximal protection against regeneration.

An alternate technique, preferred by some surgeons, is shown by Figure 1B, C, and E. In this, the stellate ganglion (a combination of the first thoracic and the inferior cervical) is removed in addition to the second and third ganglia, with resection of the second and third intercostal nerves. This produces a Horner's sign and should be employed only if both upper extremities are to be sympathectomized. The only advantage of this technique is that it interrupts any outflow which may be coming from the first dorsal segment via gray communicating rami from the first thoracic ganglion. It does not interrupt fibers which may reach the brachial plexus through the first intercostal nerve when intermediate (Skoog's) ganglia are present. Thus, the only advantage is a more complete original denervation in an occasional case. Experience has shown that this more extensive operation does not give additional protection against regeneration. To obtain adequate exposure, the inner portion of the second rib must also be removed. Judging from my experience, extending the operation as described in this paragraph for routine use is not worthwhile. I prefer the technique discussed in the previous paragraph and supplement it by removing the stellate ganglion at a second stage by the anterior cervical approach in that rare case in which residual vasoconstrictor activity of central origin, either because of incomplete denervation or because of subsequent regeneration, compromises the clinical result.

The incision is closed with catgut in the deeper layers and silk in the skin, bringing a No. 26 catheter out through the incision so that the extrapleural space can be aspirated with an Asepto syringe during positive intratracheal pressure after closure is complete. The catheter is then removed. If the pleura has been opened, a second catheter is placed within the pleural cavity and utilized in a similar fashion.

XX. THE EXTREMITIES

111. The Hand

J. WILLIAM LITTLER

THERE ARE FEW SURGICAL REGIONS wherein gentleness, technical precision, and imagination pay greater dividends than in the hand. This vulnerable structure, capable of willfully complex movements and endowed with strength, a sensibility akin to that of the eye, and aesthetic significance, is sometimes injured and further disabled, instead of salvaged, by another hand in the surgical attempt to restore its structural continuity and thus to set the stage for the healing process. A knowledge of the possible outcome of this intrinsic biological process determines what initially the surgeon can or should do. A misplaced incision, fixation of repaired tendons at sites inimical to free movement, cut nerve ends obturated by scar, counterrotated, mismated, are recurrent mistakes not always capable of correction later by even the most experienced surgeon. Indispensable is a keen knowledge of functional anatomy; and fortunately, with the tourniquet, a bloodless field enables an accurate identification of pertinent structures. Anoxia, however, is a critical factor and not infrequently determines the nature and extent of the operation. A rational surgical procedure, carefully executed on basic principles and at all times with an awareness of the immediate and later postoperative consequences, should reduce to a minimum those complications which negate a potentially successful anatomical and functional result. One may even say that it is the surgeon's conscientious, knowledgeable attention to detail which provides the greatest potential dividend to a cooperative patient.

This chapter will stress some of the more basic factors of hand surgery. Of necessity, many special procedures will be excluded. The incision, which is only a means to an end, but so important, can destroy the end result unless it is made in accord with subjacent structures. Faulty incisions have probably caused more secondary deformity in the hand than in any other part of the body. The design and use of free and pedicle skin grafts to complete the closure of wounds and to release contracture are of prime importance. Some techniques for tendon juncture will be considered. Dupuytren's contracture, the plague of surgical dissection, will be given special consideration.

Incisions and Skin Closure

The surgical exploration is in a sense somewhat akin to precise, three-dimensional navigation on surface and in depth, but the final result rests with time and the inherent biological response of specific tissues. Whereas simple but extensive skin incisions for exposure are the rule in extirpative work, complex and extremely accurate ones are required for many of the reconstructive problems in hand surgery. The structures with which we deal have been defined many times in numerous atlases, but only through a concentration on them in certain areas, and on their functional significance, can the problems of exposure and reconstruction be solved. It is distressing that so many hands are needlessly crippled through inappropriate incisions made electively or to enlarge an existing wound. The principles governing incisions in the hand, which literally can be cut to pieces without disability, demand that they be made through midaxial points and that they parallel flexion creases wherever possible (Fig. 1). Existing scars and recent lacerations should be excised or extended when necessary for adequate exposure to conform with this basic plan.

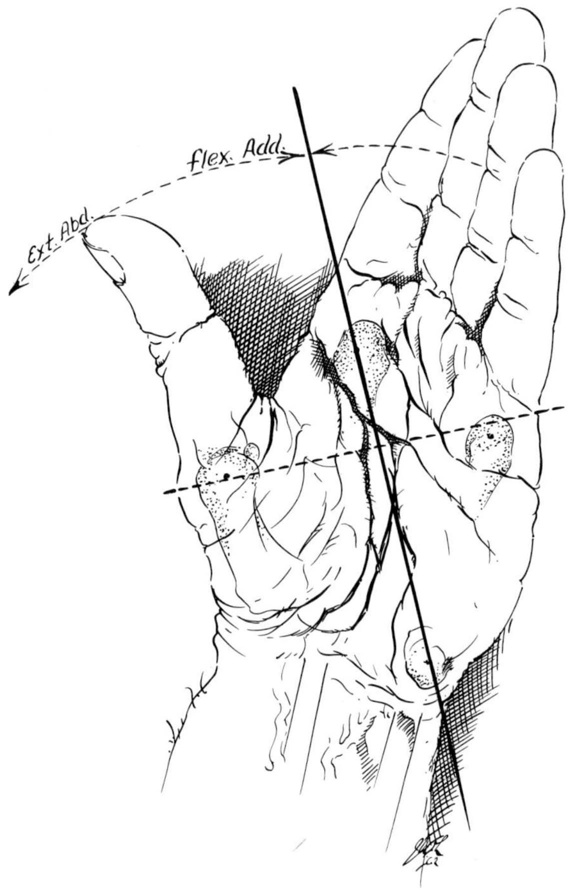

FIGURE 1. Oblique palmar line of the hand (line drawn through pisiform and second metacarpal head) dividing apposable units of the thumb (anticheir) and fingers. The lateral metacarpals adduct and abduct to and from this line. Central palmar incisions paralleling it are nondeforming; those at right angles to it will cause hypertrophy and contract the palm.

Many drawings of the allegedly correct placement of hand and forearm incisions are misleading, indicating about where they should be made, instead of demonstrating an exact relationship to the underlying structures. In the digit, the midaxial line is just dorsal to the midlateral, as indicated by the abrupt change between volar (papillary ridges) and dorsal skin. It is better to err a little to the dorsal rather than to the volar aspect in opening the digit, especially in the child.

As with incisional design, when certain areas of the hand are resurfaced the borders must be designed so that no restraint will be imposed on the essential mobility of the functional unit (Fig. 2). The elective incision, often necessarily modified by a laceration or scar, is the initial consideration in the surgical plan. Incisions are especially complex when a shift of tissue is a part of the procedure, for here a structural rearrangement requires a design which both permits exposure and anticipates transposition and closure, sometimes with the aid of free or distant pedicle skin. Exposure must be sufficient to reach all involved structures but leave no secondary deformity through scar contracture and joint restraint. Dissection in extent and depth must preserve important intact structures yet permit resection or repair of those damaged (Fig. 3). The cicatricial wake of injury and added surgery often leaves nerves and tendons fixed in a conglomerate mass, making their identification and isolation through dissection difficult and hazardous. By isolating the various important structures proximal and distal to the damaged areas, their continuity can be determined. This cautious liberation from scar is especially desirable in the case of nerves.

Prior to making the incision, a careful layout with methylene blue is very

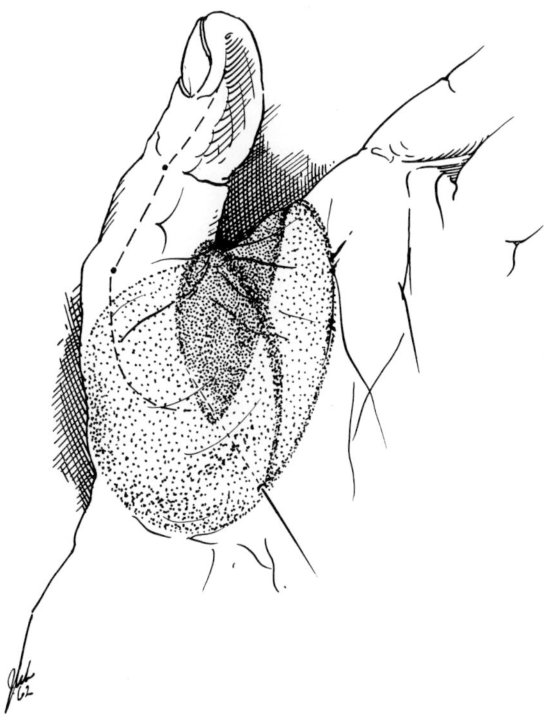

FIGURE 2. Functional cutaneous unit of the thumb. A pedicle flap of skin designed as shown to cover the thenar eminence with a triangular volar and dorsal extension fulfills the normal demand and permits unrestricted radiopalmar abduction on the axis shown. A midaxial incision on the radial aspect is the incision of choice for exposure of the flexor pollicis longus tendon and digital nerves.

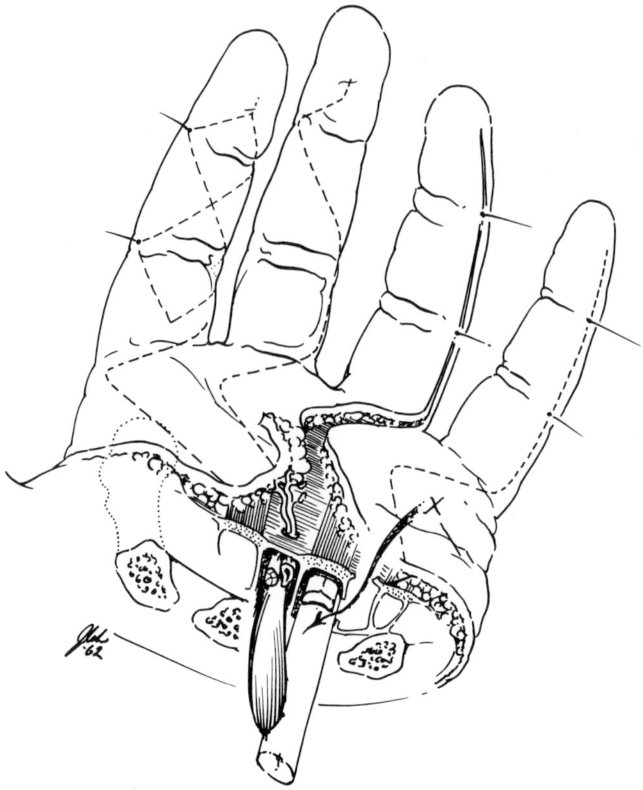

FIGURE 3. Schematic midpalmar transection approach to flexor tendons by opening first the ulnar adjacent lumbrical and neurovascular fascial tunnel. Easy access is then afforded to the tendons by dividing the septum from the deep fascia. A vertical neurovascular bundle to the palmar skin is shown perforating the aponeurosis between the heavier pretendinous fibers. The ulnar incisions shown will give exposure to any one digital flexor without secondary scar contracture (see Figure 7b). Each of the incisions has a common termination proximally between the eminences. Note the oblique phalangeal incision illustrated in the middle finger. As a rule, longitudinal incisions should not be made within the diamond patterns created by the oblique lines between joint axes (see Figure 4).

important. This can be modified where indicated. Furthermore, with tourniquet hemostasis the blue line accentuates the otherwise pale incision. In the hand and forearm the critical structures lie ensheathed by fascia beneath the skin and its thin panniculus. A vertical incision is carefully made just to the dermis; then the dermis is completely divided with shallow strokes. The underlying fat herniates as this is done. Small veins lie at this level, and the larger ones should be ligated with 6–0 plain catgut or cauterized. The fascial barrier is then encountered. In dissecting the skin and its fat from the volar aspect of the hand it is necessary to divide the fasciodermal fibers. These fibers restrain the palmar skin, especially at the creases, and are responsible for the initial change noted in the malady of

Dupuytren, when their retraction causes umbilication of the skin. Special oblique fibers, described by Cleland (1873), fix the skin to the phalanges on either side of the digit and constitute important surgical landmarks as septa between dorsal and volar compartments (Fig. 4). Elevation of the relatively inelastic palmar skin from the aponeurosis permits eversion of the edges and a better closure. The use of end-to-end mattress sutures is especially important in closing palmar skin. The skin is closed with its cross-section in mind, perfectly coapted, and never imbricated. When one is repairing nerves and tendons in the palm and forearm, it is judicious to excise an overlying area of investing fascia, and in the digit all but the strategic annular components of the fibrous tendon sheath (Fig. 5). Gentleness with the forceps in grasping skin edges is essential, and 4–0 silk rather than hooks or rakes is preferred for skin retraction. Major vessels are easily seen despite the tourniquet, and when divided must be ligated (with 5–0 or 6–0 plain catgut).

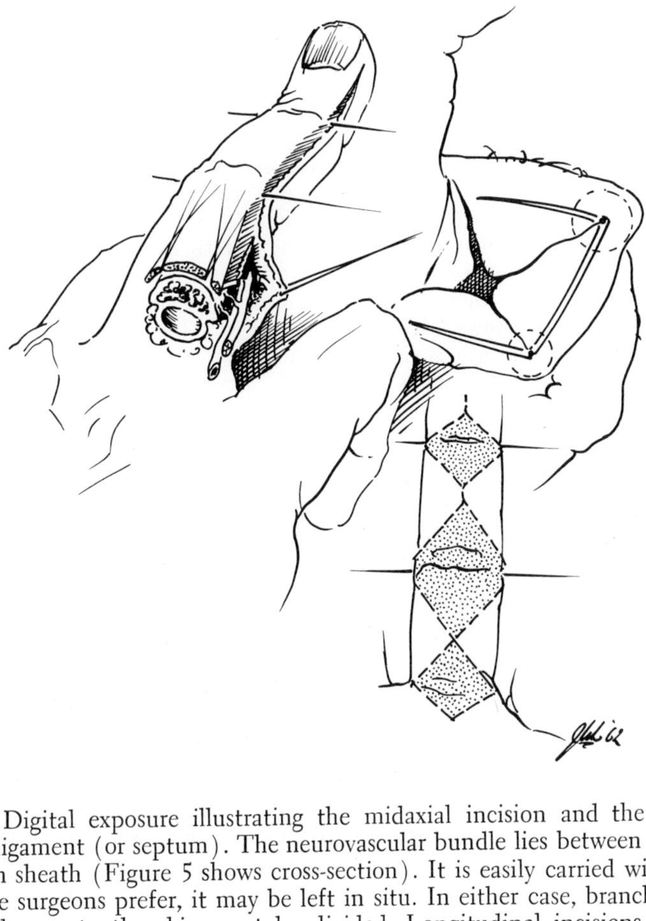

FIGURE 4. Digital exposure illustrating the midaxial incision and the division of Cleland's skin ligament (or septum). The neurovascular bundle lies between this septum and the tendon sheath (Figure 5 shows cross-section). It is easily carried with the volar flap or, as some surgeons prefer, it may be left in situ. In either case, branches to bone, joint, and tendon or to the skin must be divided. Longitudinal incisions should not enter the diamond patterns shown on the flexor aspect of the digit.

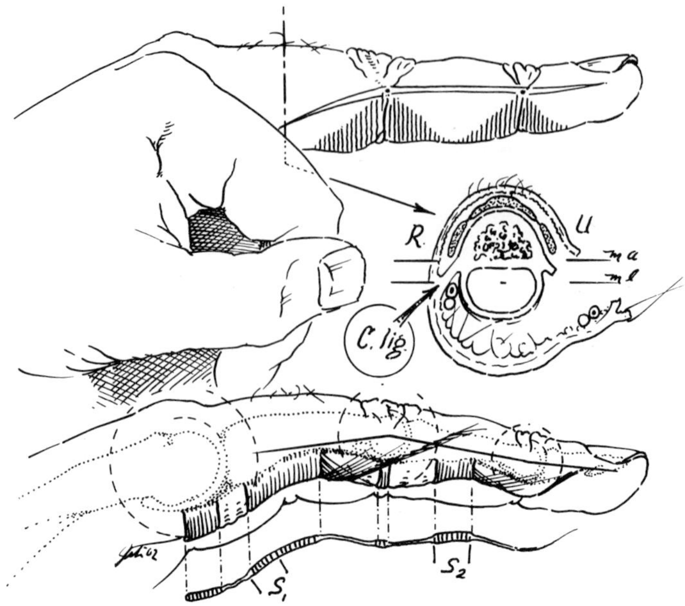

FIGURE 5. Relationship of midaxial incision to joints and fibrous tendon sheath. Note that the sheath is strategically thickened (annular ligaments) where stress is greatest, and thinned elsewhere to afford movement. S_1 and S_2 are the narrow segments to be preserved in resection of portions of the sheath in end-to-end tendon repair or grafting. Site of injury, however, determines optimum selection. The digital cross-section illustrates the slightly more dorsal position of the midaxial (m a) line over a midlateral (m 1) one and shows Cleland's ligament (C. lig.) or osseocutaneous septum. Entrance to the flexor sheath is made on the ulnar aspect (u) through the midaxial line, dividing Cleland's ligament (C. lig.) and carrying the neurovascular bundle with the volar flap.

The palmar aspect of the hand, unlike the dorsum and especially the forearm, has a tough corneal layer which disperses suture compression, preventing the cross-hatching which to some degree is inevitable in the forearm. The caliber and nature of the suture material, and the time it is in the tissues, determine reaction. Necrosis and local infection are the result of tension, inappropriate sutures, and poor immobilization. Interrupted 5–0 or 6–0 Dermalon on a cutting needle for skin closure is now my preference; however, No. 38 or No. 40 monofilament stainless steel wire, interrupted or continuous, is still preferred by many experienced operators. The appearance of the skin closure often indicates the quality of the deeper repair. Few or no deep sutures are required in hand surgery, and black silk sutures should never be buried in the shallow tissues over the dorsum of the digit—if anywhere!—for granulomas are formed all too frequently. Fine plain catgut (6–0 for skin closure) greatly simplifies postoperative care in youngsters, for whom immobilization of the hand in plaster for four weeks with an above the elbow cast is recommended following just about all procedures.

Excision of Benign Hand Tumors

The excision of benign hand tumors demands special attention to accomplish their complete removal without undue local destruction. The maintenance of structural integrity, especially of nerves, if at all possible during dissection, is incumbent on the surgeon. So important is this that a later section (Dupuytren's Contracture) is devoted to the resection of hypertrophied palmar and digital fascia. Large palmar lipomas, originating generally from the retrotendinous fat pad, and xanthomas of tendon sheath origin lie beneath the palmar fascia and the neurovascular system and infiltrate the potential palmar spaces, like a giant phlegmon. With expansion of the tumor the fascial space is distended and neurovascular bundles are attenuated over its surface, requiring caution and meticulous dissection for their preservation.

Tendon Repair

Figures 7 and 8 show some of the techniques I have used in tendon repair with good result.

Digital flexor tendons severed at any level from their muscular origins to their insertions into the terminal and middle phalanges constitute one of hand surgery's most frequent and difficult problems. The injury is often compounded by nerve division which is critically disabling through the loss of sensibility and intrinsic muscle function. The level determines the complexity of the nerve and tendon involvement. Unfortunately, the nature of surgical and biological repair often leaves the tendon ends bound by cicatrix to fixed structures at the site of injury, and little or no movement is transmitted to the interphalangeal joints beyond. The discouragement experienced by many surgeons in their attempt to restore nerve and tendon function is greatly reduced when certain principles are observed. Strict adherence to these principles, careful technique, and informed judgment concerning procedures will give good results in the majority of cases. A bloodless field, properly placed incisions for exposure, a knowledge of functional anatomy, and a repair only of pertinent divided structures with minimal overall tissue damage are essential to uncomplicated healing and restoration of useful function. It is far better, in most cases, to delay any primary nerve or tendon repair if surgical experience or operating conditions are unfavorable.

Primary repair of the ensheathed tendon at the metacarpophalangeal level is controversial, but most experienced surgeons prefer to close the skin, electing a secondary tendon graft procedure by which the junctures can be electively placed. However, if possible, digital nerves severed bilaterally should be meticulously coapted primarily with braided 7–0 eye silk on an atraumatic needle. The hand is then immobilized in an optimum position.

Following primary healing the interphalangeal joints are remobilized through a full functional range by diligent passive exercises performed by the patient. An early (within 14 days) secondary end-to-end tendon repair is possible at favorable sites, i.e. in the areolar areas proximal and just distal to the carpal ligament or near the terminal phalangeal insertion. A secondary tendon graft procedure can also be considered once induration has subsided and if the interphalangeal joints (particularly the proximal one) are mobile and sensibility is present through the integrity of one proper volar digital nerve. When both digital nerves have been divided, a primary or early secondary suture of these is mandatory, for a return of sensibility must precede tendon grafting. Pliable skin is also essential, since it is futile to attempt any reconstructive work through scar.

Source of the Graft

Selection of the tendon graft source is also controversial. It has been said that the caliber of the digital superficial flexor tendon is too great for a graft. This is obviously not true—certainly not in a child, and especially when superb results have been obtained in adults. With both flexors cut at the base of the finger, the ideal graft is the proximal segment of the superficial tendon. The next tendon of choice is the palmaris longus, which is generally easily obtained. A small incision is made at the wrist, isolating the tendon which is divided; with traction, its musculotendinous juncture is easily palpated in the midforearm, where through a small incision the tendon is exposed and withdrawn. It is unnecessary to make a longitudinal incision in the forearm to preserve paratenon. Paratenon is a proliferative tissue when injured, and is unimportant to gliding; furthermore, blood tracks between it and the tendon and a tube of scar develops, fixing the tendon in its bed. The plantaris may be used, but it is more difficult to obtain and unfortunately, like the palmaris longus, is absent in some 15 per cent of individuals. Toe extensors are always available but are the least desirable source.

Inlay of the Graft

With but one tendon to flex the two interphalangeal joints, a graft restoring profundus tendon continuity should move with greater ease through the proximal segment of the finger for coordinated flexion. The normal flexion arc of the finger is initiated by the intrinsic muscles at the metacarpophalangeal joint, followed by the middle and terminal phalanges. It is hard to gain smooth function without active proximal interphalangeal flexion (through the integrity of the flexor superficialis).

A tendon graft must be handled gently following removal, and only at its ends. It should be placed immediately in the prepared digital bed by passing it through two strategic pulleys, one at the base of the proximal phalanx and one at the midpoint of the middle phalanx (Fig. 6). The distal profundus tendon stump is split along its raphe, exposing a triangular area of bone bounded proximally by the volar plate. A core of bone is gouged from the cortex, and the graft is fixed with removable traction wire. This retention suture is passed through the phalanx and nail, and the two wires are tied over a button bringing the graft into the medullary cavity of the phalanx (Fig. 7). The profundus slips embrace the graft. To preserve

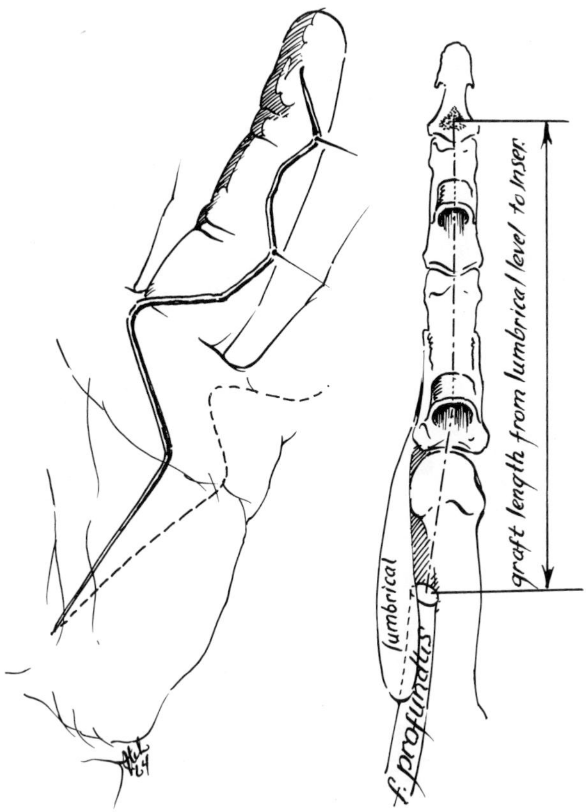

FIGURE 6. Combined digital and palmar incisions for graft restoration of ring finger flexor tendon. Strategic annular ligaments prevent tendon prolapse and provide efficiency for interphalangeal flexion.

the epiphysis in children, and when simpler union is desired, the graft can be joined to the profundus stump by a 5–0 braided steel mattress suture.

The length of the graft is adjusted so that the digits lie in progressively more flexion from the index to the little finger. The proximal profundus tendon graft juncture is made at the lumbrical level (Fig. 8). A special effort must be made to release the retracted proximal profundus tendon in the palm and to liberate the lumbrical muscle, which generally is found adherent about the tendon distal to its normal origin. If this tendon retraction is not corrected, the graft will be too long and profundus muscle power will be directed to the dorsal extensor apparatus through the lumbrical. The lumbrical embraces automatically the juncture. Silk is undesirable in suturing tendons, because a granuloma not infrequently develops.

Dressing and Aftercare

Skin is closed with 5–0 or 6–0 nylon or wire; the edges must be meticulously coapted. In infants and children the skin is closed with 6–0 plain catgut. With

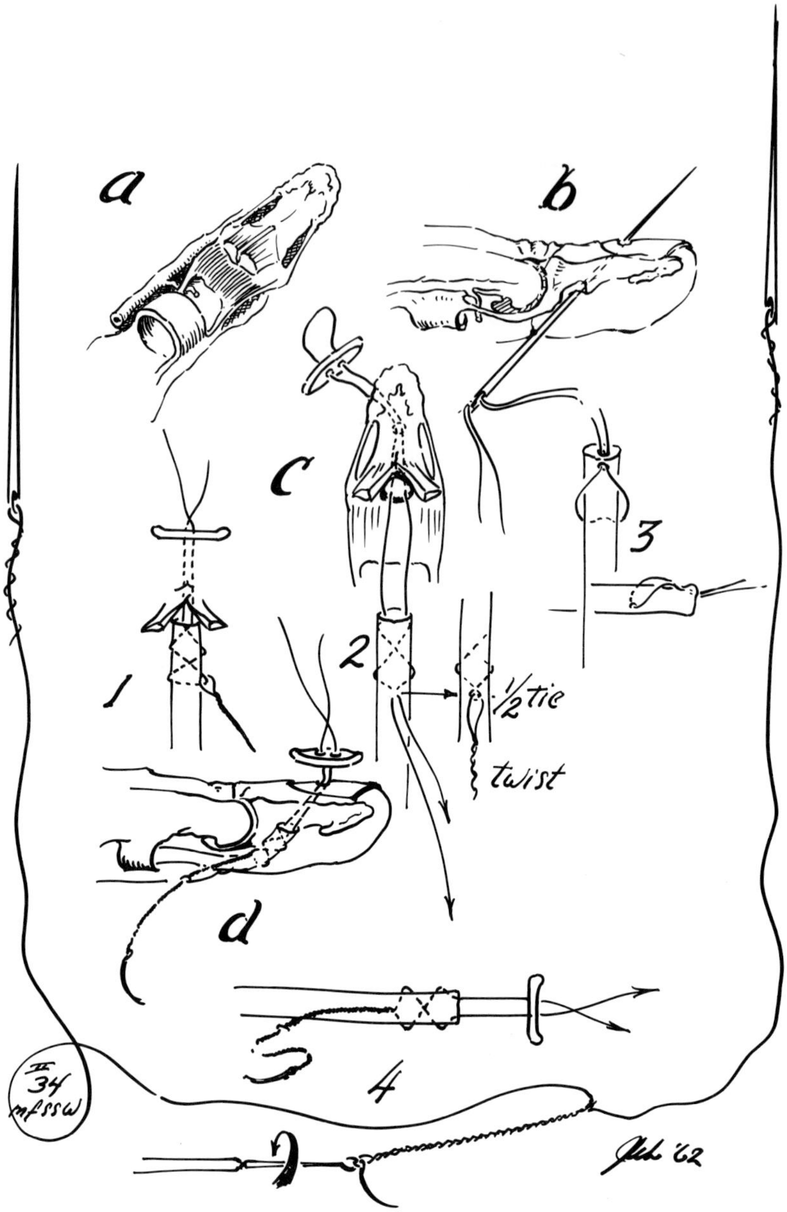

FIGURE 7. Preparation of terminal phalangeal tendon insertion and details of fixation through wire traction sutures. (*a*) Profundus stump, volar plate, and check ligaments. The vascular supply to the distal profundus vinculum brevis is shown entering beneath the check ligament; the profundus stump is split along its raphe, exposing the terminal phalanx and volar plate. (*b*) Dorsal cortex and nail perforated with Keith needle following step (*c*) wherein a triangular area of the volar cortex is exposed and opened with a gouge just distal to the plate. Bunnell "pullout" wire technique (*c*1) and modifications (*c*2, *d*4). Technique of Planas (*c*3): wire ends are tied over a button and removed by cutting one end with traction on the other.

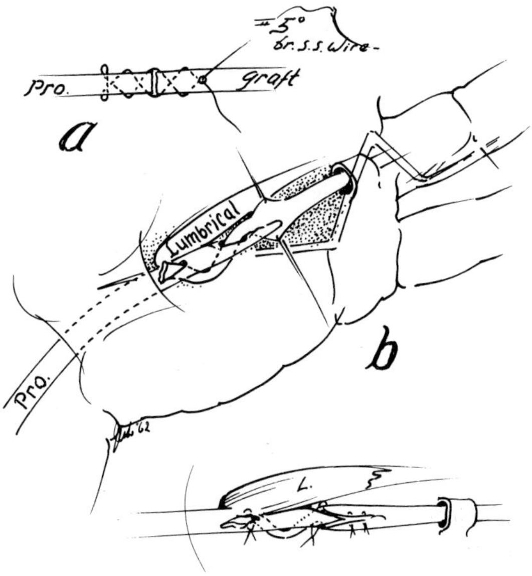

FIGURE 8. Tendon-to-tendon suturing with similar and dissimilar caliber ends. (*a*) Bunnell technique: end-to-end suture of cut tendon or one prolonged with graft of like caliber. Initially the juncture is accordioned somewhat when the suture is tied; an adjustment for some protraction must be made by insuring that the graft is not too long and that it holds the digit at operation with a little more tone than normal. (*b*) Brand-Pulvertaft technique: slender tendon graft united to a larger caliber tendon by interweave and embracement. Flat tendons, i.e. palmaris longus and plantaris, can be stretched laterally to enfold the profundus stump. Interrupted 5–0 braided stainless steel wire secures the juncture.

these sutures the young patients are left undisturbed for three and one-half weeks in a plaster encasing the dressing above the 90 degree flexed elbow. Excessive pressure and poor position can lead not only to a failure of the procedure, but to added disability. Moderate compression is applied through fluff gauze dressing, and maintenance of moderate wrist and finger flexion is insured by a dorsally reinforced plaster shell or gauntlet. A "functional relationship" is imperative between thumb and fingers; the wrist and proximal interphalangeal joints are never held for long periods in acute flexion. Immobilized coapted tendon ends will be sufficiently strong after four weeks to permit active but not too vigorous movement. The functional potential of repaired tendons should be reached within four months.

Notes on Aftercare

Constriction is a curse too often laid on the hand by improperly applied dressings or plaster, leading to pain, edema, and a disruption of the basic functional dynamics. The consequences of this error in management are severe, and most difficult to overcome, when the hand is not only tightly bound but also rigidly fixed in an exaggerated, nonfunctional position. The surgical effort is thereby negated and fresh injury is added which, with time, may be as devastating as gross tearing or crushing of tissues. It is illogical not to give the application of the dressing the same degree of attention as is demanded by the design and execution of the operation, for the outcome may depend as much upon one as the other.

The injured or operated hand is comforted by gentle, even anterior-posterior compression (not circumferential pressure) with the wrist supported in slight extension, the transverse and longitudinal arches upheld, the thumb in radiopalmar abduction, and the fingers progressively flexed ulnarward. Moderate departures are made from this basic position in order to afford relaxation of specific structures, but joints are never to be immobilized at the extremes of their ranges. An exception, unfortunately, is found when acute wrist flexion is necessary to allow coaptation of the ends of a nerve from which a segment has been lost. The wrist can be mobilized in full extension without undue discomfort or contracture. Moderate wrist and metacarpophalangeal flexion should be used to gain relaxation of flexor tendons. The proximal interphalangeal joints must never be held in full flexion. Extension here is preferable, as is some flexion at the metacarpophalangeal level. When immobilization reaches above the elbow, the forearm should be at 90 degrees flexion, and midway between pronation and supination. If dependent gravitational congestion is avoided, very little pain (practically none after the first day) is present in a hand that has been operated upon with delicate technique and dressed with due care. Excessive pain is a warning that must be heeded if the hand is to be rescued and skin necrosis, muscle ischemia, and altered joint mechanics are to be avoided.

Dupuytren's Contracture

No affliction of the hand has received more attention than the historically significant malady classically described by Dupuytren in 1831. The exhaustive etiological confusion concerning this palmar fascial contracture will not be expanded here; instead, the matter of surgical relief in certain disabling situations will be discussed.

The distressing operative morbidity for this condition probably parallels closely the morbidity in the nontreated cases. Realistically speaking, the functional and economic loss following surgical treatment has been so severe that most surgeons abhor the thought of any radical attack. The many stiffened joints, necrosed palms, severed digital nerves, lend poignant support to the thesis of nonintervention. Nevertheless, carefully performed on the selected patient, a resection of the involved palmar and digital fascia can afford great relief for serious disability. The foremost requirement is a rational selection of cases for a fascial resection or a subcutaneous palmar division. The lesion is not urgent, and it seems feasible to allow some progression rather than to recommend intervention the moment a nodule appears or the palmar skin is retracted at one point. The recent proposal that early excision of only the palmar nodule or plaque stems the development of a contracture may have merit, but it is well known that the disease can recur or develop elsewhere. This is especially true when it occurs first in the digit. Assurance of the benign nature of the process, progressive though it is, generally relieves the patient of undue anxiety.

When, however, hypertrophy and contracture of the fascia is established, with limitation of extension at the metacarpophalangeal and/or proximal interphalangeal levels, the operation is indicated before the skin is severely involved. The palm and digit pose two contrasting regions with respect to ease of fascial excision and prediction of the result. The palmar dissection is not so variable and intricate as is removal of contracted fascia from the fingers; and whereas metacarpophalangeal release is the rule, restoration of extension at the proximal interphalangeal joints often is not realized. The close relationship of the fascia to the dermis (Fig. 9) is such that surgical separation can be extremely difficult in advanced cases, and may occasionally necessitate excision of involved skin and the use of a free thick skin graft to complete coverage. Brachial plexus block analgesia (20 cc. of 2 per cent Xylocaine with epinephrine, or Carbocaine) is highly satisfactory for the procedure, and the pneumatic tourniquet is mandatory.

The dissection can be one of the most difficult known to the hand surgeon, and it is definitely not for the tyro. Certain fascial distributions demand special incisions for adequate exposure, yet these must be so designed that they will permit healing without secondary scar contracture or skin loss. In the more advanced cases, involving the proximal aspect of the digits, a Z-plasty (as recommended by MacIndoe) is of value for good exposure and a gain in skin length (Fig. 10). Exquisite care is required to separate the two thin skin flaps from the underlying fascia, and unfortunately their circulation is poor. When the proximal interphalangeal joint is restrained in flexion by contracted fascia and skin of the proximal segment, the limbs of the Z can be made at an angle of approximately 80 degrees (rather than the usual 60 degrees), for with the resection of the restraining fascia the joint release opens the proximal segment and allows the two flaps to alternate and fall vertically into position. Furthermore, the skin is tented abnormally by the bowstringing fascia, and the use of a Z incision takes advantage of this increase in vertical length. Unfortunately, the proximal interphalangeal joint, secondarily altered by an intrinsic contracture, is not always relieved by the fascial resection. This is especially true of the little finger. An interesting observation in a large series of fascial resections which I carried out was that a free skin graft was rarely needed, but the Z-plasty was often used at the base of the digit. Digital recurrences may require secondary excision of skin and fascia and the use of a full-thickness graft. A distant pedicle flap has been required only in a referred case in which, following an operation, the palmar skin necrosed and secondary healing led to a critical contracture. At all costs, hand function must not be jeopardized by the urge to excise the thickened fascia at the expense of crucial skin.

Palmar skin is nourished by vertical branches originating from the neurovascular bundles coursing deep between the longitudinal fibers of the pretendinous bands and roofed at the metacarpophalangeal levels by the transverse fibers. Diseased fascia in an advanced state unites with the overlying dermis through a contracture of the fasciodermal fibers, the normal intervening fat is lost, and skin and

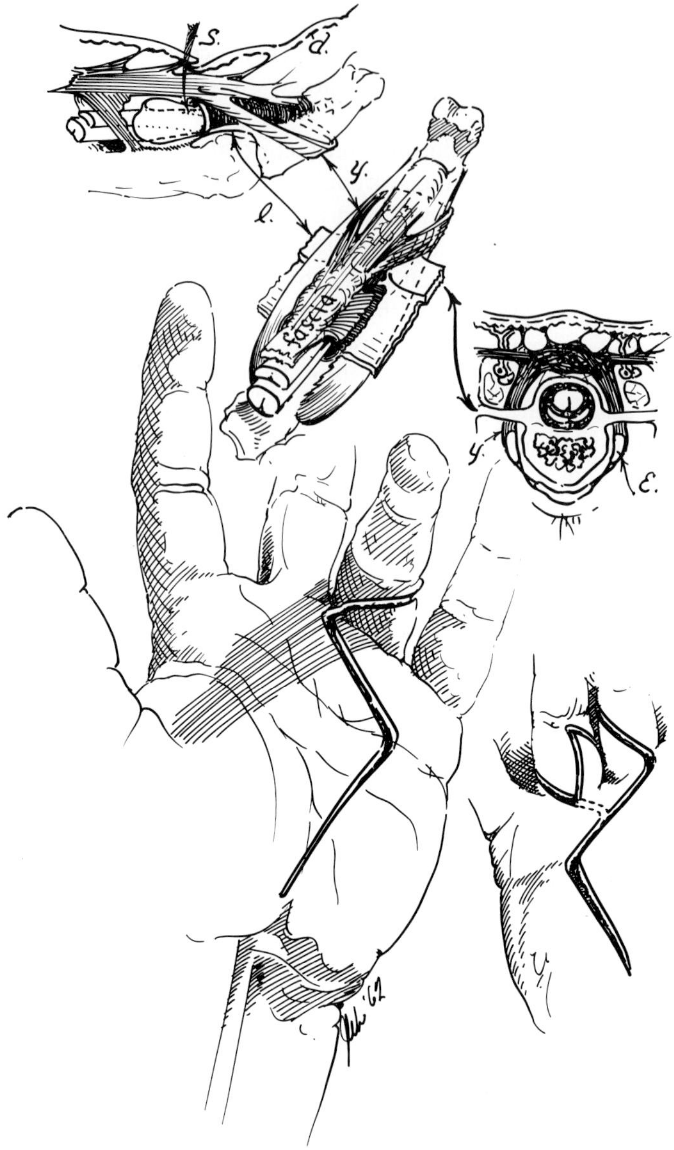

FIGURE 9. Fascial pattern and its relationship to the dermis (d), flexor sheath (s), intermetacarpal ligament (l), and extensor mechanism (e). Incision for exposure of the ulnar triangle of the palmar aponeurosis (pretendinous bands of the middle, ring, and little fingers) with a single oblique or Z incision extension into the digits. The many variations in the diseased fascal pattern require careful modification in design of the basic incisions for adequate exposure.

fascia become one, making separation difficult, at times impossible, and skin survival precarious. Fortunately, only limited areas are generally severely involved, and nourishment of the flap is assured, especially if one or more of the vertical

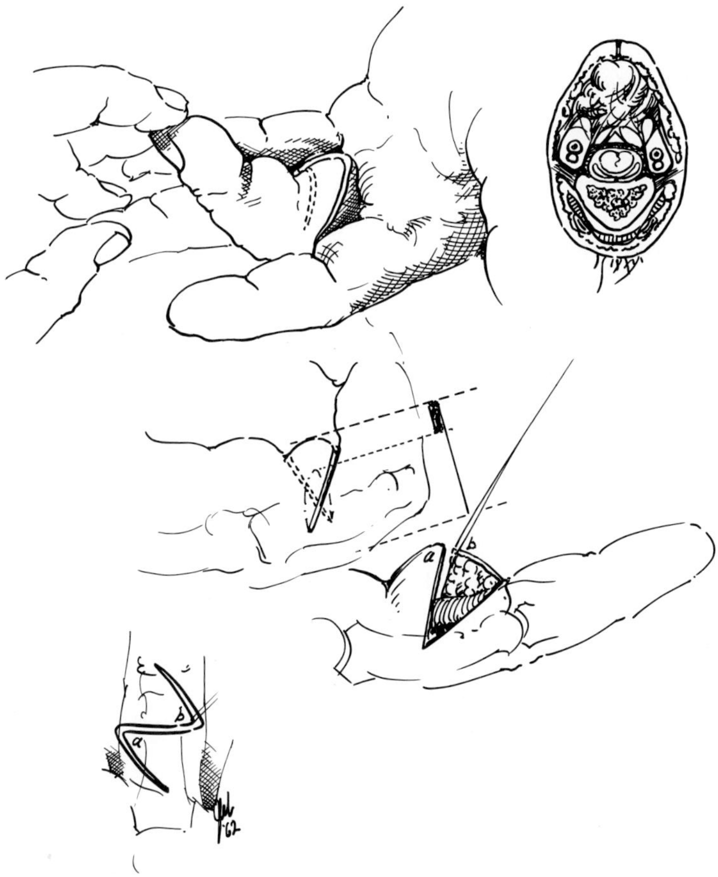

FIGURE 10. Z-plasty for exposure and resection of contracted fascia within the proximal digital segment. Transposition of the triangular flaps provides the desired skin length if the joint can be extended after removal of the fascia. With rotation of the two triangles, the gain in skin length is equal to the sum of the two altitudes minus one side; or more simply, the long diameter of the skin rhomboid has been rotated through 90 degrees into the longitudinal axis of the digit.

vessels can be preserved. The resection is made more difficult, but the result satisfies the effort.

Once the underlying abnormal fascia has been completely exposed, its vertical septa are isolated (with care for the lumbrical and neurovascular systems) and divided at the level of the deep fascia and intermetacarpal ligaments. Abnormally heavy septal extensions pass from the pretendinous bands bilaterally to the fibrous tendon sheath just distal to the intermetacarpal ligament, where they envelop the interosseous tendons and pass dorsally into the extensor hood. Traction on these yoke-like septa can flex the metacarpophalangeal joint. Preservation of the synovial cul-de-sac is precarious at this point where the heavy septa from the pretendinous bands encircle the proximal aspect of the fibrous tendon sheath. The relationship of the pretendinous band and its yoke to the tendon sheath is somewhat like that of the superficialis tendon to the profundus. An attempt must be made not to open the intact synovial sheaths, because blood within them produces discomfort, voluntary immobilization, and possibly a stiffened hand. The encircling fibers prevent metacarpophalangeal release when the pretendinous band alone is sectioned just distal to them at the metacarpophalangeal level in the operation known as subcutaneous fasciotomy. Prolongation of the pretendinous bands into the proximal phalanx is generally more to one side. In the fifth digit the fascia also arises as a prolongation from the common tendon of insertion of the intrinsic abductor and flexor muscles, or flexor sheath, bridges the proximal interphalangeal joint, and inserts into the fibrous tendon sheath and extensor mechanism.

The relationship of the neurovascular bundle to this fibrous extension is critical, for at the palmodigital level it often passes superficial and mesial to the band, and deep and lateral to it at the proximal interphalangeal level. (Variations are not exceptional.) Exquisite care must be exercised during the fascial resection not to damage this important vascular and tactile link. Whereas subcutaneous division of the pretendinous band can be made at the metacarpophalangeal level where it bowstrings the joint high above the deep laterally lying neurovascular bundles, such a division is fraught with disaster within the digit, where through encirclement the two are intimately combined (Fig. 11).

The fact that extension gained at the time of the fascial resection cannot be maintained when the contracted skin is closed is not of immediate concern. The

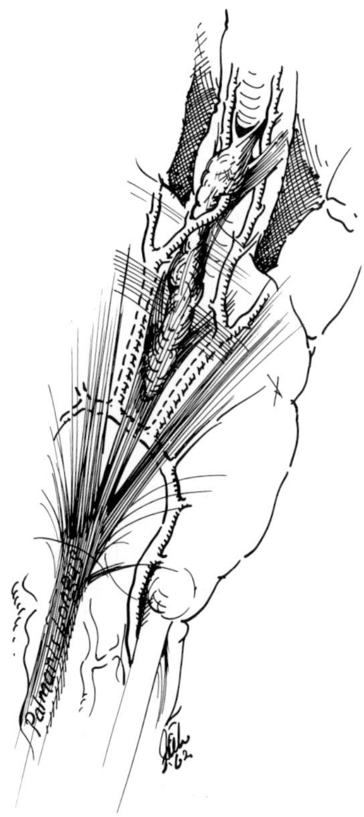

FIGURE 11. Relationship of hypertrophied palmar and digital fascia to neurovascular bundles. Resection of fascia demands exquisite care to prevent nerve damage. The finger with the cut nerve is far more disabled than the one moderately flexed by fascial contracture. The triangular component of the palmar aponeurosis shown is the area most frequently involved in the malady of Dupuytren.

chief factors are the resection of the involved fascia with preservation of viable skin and the gaining of primary healing with the hand in good functional position. Active metacarpophalangeal flexion and extension exercises can be started about four weeks postoperatively when all dressing support is removed. It is unnecessary for the early postoperative patient to practice vigorous hand activity, for if the synovial sheaths of the digit have not been entered they will be free of hemorrhagic irritation, and active interphalangeal movement will be possible and painless even early with the hand immobilized in a dressing supported by a plaster shell. Maintenance of the transverse and longitudinal arches of the hand with the wrist in extension and the metacarpophalangeal joints in some flexion, to ease the skin closure, is essential following the fascial excision.

Early unsupported activity causes swelling and induration of the unhealed palmar tissues. Dressing support for three to four weeks has been found eminently successful in preventing this complication. Immediate postoperative suction of the palm, for the control of any bleeding, has been advocated by Baron and others. I have not used this routinely, because hematoma is a rarity with good hemostasis, careful dissection and closure, and support of the palm by an anterior-posterior compression dressing and plaster shell. Furthermore, the necessary control of hemorrhage forces preoperative attention to the possibility of an altered clotting mechanism in the Dupuytren patient through a check of liver function and of bleeding and clotting time. At the end of a four-week period of immobilization the best treatment appears to be the use of silicone putty as an exercise medium for a progressive return of a normal supple hand.

Factors in Skin Grafting

The drum dermatome is unexcelled for taking a free graft for resurfacing the hand. With it a sheet of skin of the desired size and exact thickness can be obtained. Shim-stock is useful in determining the setting of the blade, since exact calibration is difficult even for the experienced. Whereas millimeters are important in the placement of hand incisions, fractions thereof are imperative in the taking of a split skin graft.

Skin donor areas vary in thickness in the young and old. The site of election is of extreme concern, especially in the younger female, and there is no excuse for the indiscriminate taking of even a small area of skin. Although today sites that can be concealed are limited and somewhat difficult to define, the favorable site is the gluteal region for a split free graft and the groin for a full-thickness graft. The donor area reaction can be violent in children, especially if the graft is thick and healing is delayed. Although the instrument is adjusted to cut from 0.008 inch to 0.010 inch, the resultant graft in the child will be near full thickness, that is, 0.015 inch to 0.018 inch, in some areas if the skin is excessively stretched over the drum as it is cut.

Either a primary or a secondary full-thickness (Wolfe) graft is desirable for the palmar aspect of the hand, since, with correct placement and a good take, contracture (unlike the situation with a split graft) is minimal. The dorsum of the hand accepts well the intermediate thick-split graft and does not provoke the contracture phenomenon that would result in the palm. The contracted thumb cleft is of special importance and the extent of involvement will determine whether a Z-plasty, free, local or distant pedicle graft is necessary for release of the adducted first metacarpal.

Near exact patterns of skin can be taken with a drum dermatome by outlining on both donor area and drum the pattern desired. To take a somewhat but not excessively larger area than is needed is obviously judicious. The glue on both areas is quickly and smoothly applied, care being taken not to overlap the drum edges, and allowed to set for approximately four to five minutes. The leading edge of the drum is then firmly applied to the skin and with a little stretch it is evenly rolled over the donor site. As the graft is cut its thickness is noted and, if necessary, a readjustment of the cam is made. A critical depth is obvious if the rete pegs of the corium are reached, as a pebbling of fat is visible through the dermal lattice. When sufficient skin is obtained the setting can be changed to zero, and with a final stroke of the blade (or with a scalpel) the graft is detached. The bleeding bed is nicely controlled by a surgical towel, moist with saline on one side, reapplied several times. In taking a full-width graft the skin must not adhere to the sides of the drum edge, for deep cutting will result. It is sometimes convenient to leave the skin attached to the drum and to cut (with a scalpel) the exact patterns of skin for smaller special defects to be covered. The design on the drum must obviously be the mirror image of that desired.

Free grafts should be sutured with interrupted or continuous 6–0 Dermalon or No. 40 wire, under a little stretch, for this restores the normal skin status and assures a better take. The recipient bed must be dry and the graft should transmit an even pinkness. Small clots are easily removed from beneath the graft by saline irrigation and/or a moist cotton swab stick. The blue of an underlying hematoma bodes partial or total loss of the graft, generally an unforgivable situation. If bleeding of the recipient bed is excessive after removal of the tourniquet, compression and ligation of vessels, it is often wise, when the area is great, to delay grafting for 36 to 48 hours. A careful inspection of the grafted area can be made 48 hours postoperatively, and if a collection of blood or serum is beneath the graft it can be expelled through small incisions. "Pie-crusting" need not be routine with free grafts on a clean site.

Wrinkling of a free graft and partial loss is not infrequent secondary to an irregular application of a compressive gauze dressing. Special relatively nonadherent porous elastic gauzes are of use as a prime cover, supplemented by gauze fluffs and Kling bandage compression. Whenever a free graft or pedicle flap is tented over a prominence, great care must be exercised to insure that ischemic compression necrosis does not occur. Once the hand has been carefully dressed well beyond the extent of the incision or grafted areas, it is held immobile in a favorable position by sheet wadding and a plaster shell. Immobilization, especially of the wrist, with the thumb and fingers in a functional relationship through a careful molding of longitudinal and transverse arches, is of the utmost importance for uncomplicated wound healing and preservation of useful function. Discomfort and edema are further minimized by moderate elevation. Bolus dressings (except for a free graft to an amputated finger tip) are not often needed in hand work. They are useful where circumferential compression is not possible.

A free graft should be protected (immobilized) four weeks or longer. At no time should the graft be rubbed when the hand is cleaned and redressed, for mechanical friction may cause a graft to corrugate and contract excessively. The donor site is dressed well beyond its borders with a medicated, not too fine mesh gauze, over which pure gauze dressings are secured. It should be kept dry during the first week by daily careful sterile application of fresh gauze down to the innermost pad. Early uncomplicated healing can be expected unless the depth of the graft was excessive or contaminated. Despite a good take of the free graft, the sutures should remain for at least 14 days, because there is some delay in border union, especially with a full-thickness graft.

Burns of the Hand

Serious burns are not often limited to the palm, because the inadvertent grasp of a hot object (or open electric conductor) is generally relinquished with reflex speed unless the hand is insensitive. The thick, corniferous skin of this area protects from third degree loss. More extensive and severe injuries are produced when the hand is caught between hot rollers, frequently used in laundries and other industries. Gross destruction involving tendons and other deep structures requires eventual pedicle coverage to support further reconstructive efforts. However, generally resurfacing in the palm should be accomplished with free full-thickness (rather than split) skin grafts with their margins properly oriented to lines of tension so as to avoid contracture.

The dorsal covering is much more vulnerable through its exposed position and thinner structure, especially when stretched tautly over the joints. As the hand is flexed, the dorsal skin area must expand, unlike the volar skin, which simply unfolds as the hand is opened.

Chemical and especially electric burns can be grossly destructive and their extent unpredictable. There may be deep soft tissue and bone involvement, and interruption of major nerves, tendons, and vessels. In the large majority of thermal burns, joints are not primarily involved, but necrosis and infection will expose them if meticulous primary care is not afforded. Injured tissue needs to be immobilized during the healing phase, for it either recovers or is further damaged and lost by exposure and infection. Immobilization of the hand in a functional position, with frequent dressings and debridement as necessary, will aid in the control of infection and help make apparent demarcation between healing second degree and definite third degree areas which must be excised and grafted. The aim of the surgeon is, without sacrificing sound tissue, to secure early healing of the wound so as to prevent devastating secondary joint stiffening and contracture.

The classical secondary dorsal burn deformity is manifested by a reversal of

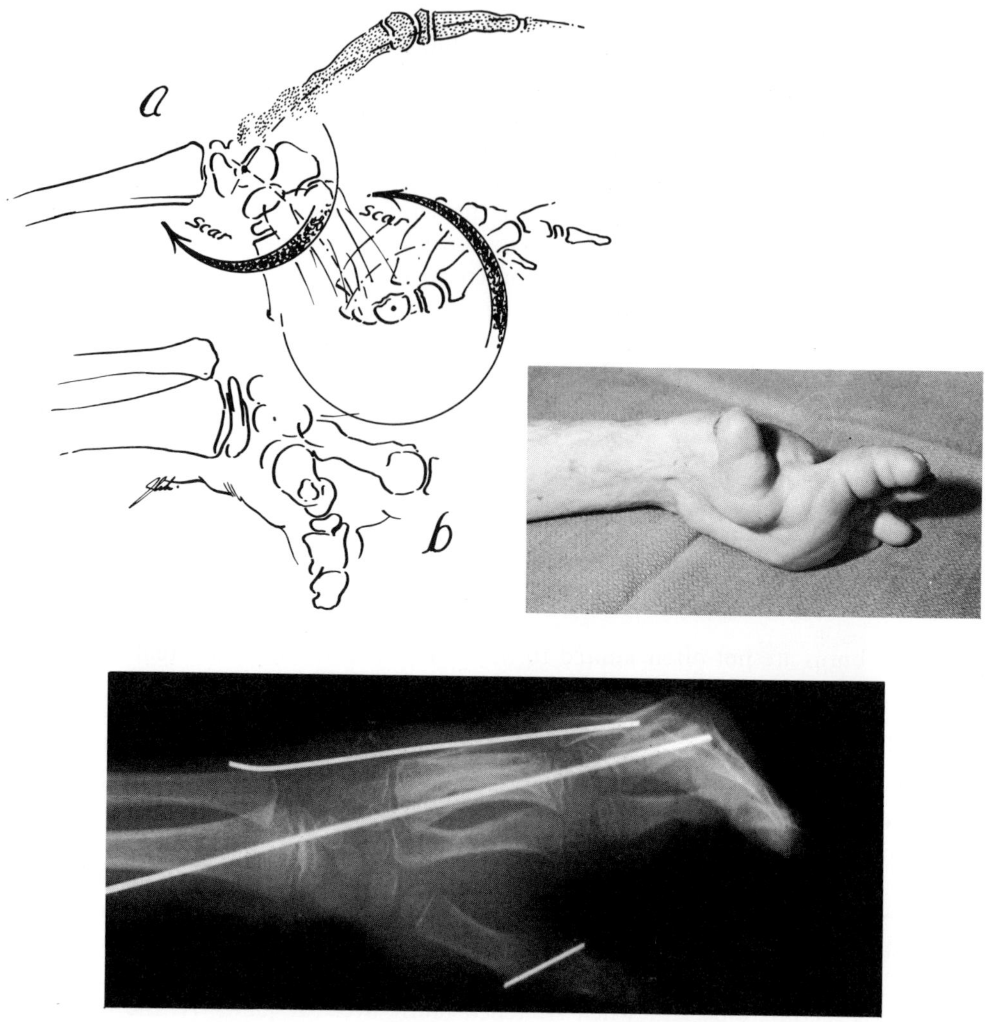

FIGURE 12. Deranged architecture secondary to thermal burn at age 1 year, nine years later. The longitudinal and transverse arches of the hand have been reversed by scar contracture and growth and the wrist is pulled into flexion. The arrows demonstrate the deforming forces. X-ray shows partial restoration through scar and extensor tendon resection, and joint fixation with Kirschner wires.

the longitudinal and transverse arches with an adduction contracture of the thumb imposed by the cicatrix (Fig. 12). The metacarpophalangeal joints are hyperextended and the proximal interphalangeal joints are often flexed, producing a claw hand not unlike that seen in a combined median and ulnar nerve motor paralysis. The nails may be grossly deformed and elevated from the matrix. With time the volar skin, though intact, contracts and becomes delicate from disuse, moist, and devoid of any significant corneal layer. The wrist may go into flexion through scar or atony of the extensors. Disuse atrophy is inevitable.

An understanding of the functional position and maintenance of the longitudinal and transverse arches of the hand is mandatory for the maintenance and restoration of function in a hand deprived of its dorsal coverage. If the functional position is relinquished to the inexorable cicatricial contracture of secondary healing or delayed skin grafting, the reversed arch deformity will result. Hyperextension of the metacarpophalangeal joints imposed by dorsal cicatrix is further complicated by secondary joint changes, specifically a contracture of the collateral ligaments, and eventually an alteration of the contour of metacarpophalangeal heads, and finally dorsal subluxation of the proximal phalanx.

In the average adult hand with full extension of the wrist and fingers, the distance from the radiocarpal joint to a point just beyond the proximal interphalangeal joint is approximately 5 inches. However, when a complete fist is made and the wrist is dropped, the distance is increased to nearly 7 inches. This 1½ or 2 inches of "excess" is necessary for full and unrestricted wrist and finger flexion. Loss of skin with cicatricial contracture will checkrein the fingers and permit secondary joint contractures. A similar checkrein is not infrequently seen following an injury or infection that produces marked edema over the dorsum of the hand and fingers, ballooning the skin and checkreining especially metacarpophalangeal joint function. The transverse skin from the radial to the ulnar border of the metacarpophalangeal joints of the thumb and little finger measures 5 inches with the hand flat and approximately 6 inches with a full fist. The necessary skin relaxation is essential for thumb abduction, and when dorsal skin has been lost the thumb and index web is involved and an adduction contracture is prone to develop, greatly limiting and checkreining the rotary palmar abduction movements of the thumb.

After excision of dorsal scar and mobilization of joints as far as possible, an attempt must be made to restore the transverse and longitudinal arches and to resurface the biconvex dorsal area with a thick-split graft. Elastic recoil from the restored position and a tendency for skin contracture demand rigid maintenance of the arches during the period of healing and graft maturation. This can only be adequately achieved over the required period of time by temporary buried Kirschner wire fixation (Fig. 12).

The interphalangeal joints are subject to great disability, especially the important proximal ones, where the subjacent extensor mechanism and joint are readily exposed with dorsal skin loss and where function is most difficult to restore. A boutonniere-like deformity is prone to develop with destruction of the central tendinous slip and volar displacement of the lateral bands. With time a secondary irreversible contracture of the joint occurs, involving all intrinsic structures. This is the reason primary or early excision of suspected devitalized skin and resurfacing is advocated for the protection of this most important area. In dissecting off the secondary burn scar, it is most essential to preserve the vascular coverage of the extensor tendinous mechanism. If paratenon is destroyed, a free graft will not survive over the exposed tendon and joint.

Not infrequently the dorsum of the distal interphalangeal joint is involved, with damage to the extensor tendon and the germinal layer of the nail. The extensor disrupts and the joint goes into full flexion. Though healed, the fragile scar epithelium easily breaks down under slight trauma, and recurrent infections develop. The joint should be fused at 20-degree flexion, eliminating the nail and its germinal cul-de-sac, but preserving the matrix just distal to the lunula. The proximal border of the matrix is sutured to the dorsal skin.

Use of Kirschner Wires

Kirschner wires are invaluable in the temporary support or realignment of bones and joints for skeletal traction and dynamic splinting, and for immobilization during the healing of free or pedicle skin grafts following scar excision. Such internal fixation, especially of joints, relieves soft tissue of undue pressure and the inevitable pressure when a mobile unit of the hand must be maintained in a favorable but difficult position for the prolonged periods required to gain bone union or skin healing. External support, however, is often possible after several weeks of Kirschner wire fixation. An intramedullary, transarticular Kirschner wire, deftly placed, will not damage a joint, nor will it impair an epiphysis. This latter factor is important in the management of the child's hand disabled by a congenital anomaly or injury, and especially in the management of severe secondary burn deformity, which often requires internal support for the correction of altered skeletal mechanics during the immobilization required for free skin grafts to heal and mature (Fig. 12).

When a Kirschner wire is left exposed, or when the skin overlying a buried wire breaks down under pressure, early removal is often necessary to prevent infection. Fortunately, complications are rare, but some difficulty besets the removal of wires if they have not been placed and cut with some foresight. The various structural problems and stresses require wires of appropriate caliber. Orthopedic screws and plates are seldom, if ever, required in contemporary hand surgery. The Kirschner wire, sometimes with a carefully fashioned bone graft, is highly effective in holding bones in alignment.

Ensheathment Syndromes

Compression or constriction of nerves or tendons occurs at specific sites in the forearm, hand, and wrist. The early symptoms of tendon incarceration are pain, restricted movement, and finally the "trigger" phenomenon of congenital or traumatic stenosing tenosynovitis. This is frequently encountered, both in infancy and in later life, as an involvement of the flexor pollicis longus at the metacarpophalangeal level. Here the intolerance or caliber discrepancy between the nodular tendon and the fibrous tunnel (annular ligament) is such that the terminal phalanx cannot be flexed or extended, depending upon whether the nodule is blocked distal or proximal to the pulley. A similar condition can restrict the fingers at the metacarpophalangeal level.

De Quervain's disorder, prevalent in women, is similar to the foregoing, but there is no triggering. It affects specifically the long abductor and short extensor of the thumb as they pass through their fibro-osseous tunnel just proximal to the styloid process of the radius. The classic carpal tunnel syndrome, also most frequently observed in women, is secondary to compression of the median nerve. The rigid confines of this fibro-osseous tunnel are such that any increase in content invariably affects the nerve, producing in varying degrees the signs and symptoms incident to median nerve blockage. Numbness, especially of the middle finger, night pain, and grasp insecurity are the general early symptoms. Synovial hypertrophy and villonodular tenosynovitis are the most frequent causes of compression. Division of the flexor retinaculum decompresses the compartment and affords relief. Recurrences are seen and other factors can affect the nerve at the carpal level and higher. A volar carpal ganglion or a displaced lunate will also provoke the symptoms, as will constriction of median nerve by fibrosed pronator teres and sublimi in Volkmann's deformity. The structure of the canal is such that the more radial the division of the ligament the less the tendency for tendon prolapse. However, this is of importance only when the wrist must be immobilized in flexion. Tendon prolapse is no problem following retinacular division for median nerve decompression, because the wrist is immobilized for three weeks in moderate extension, thus throwing the flexor tendon stress dorsally against the carpal floor.

Surgical Release

An incision 2 to 3 cm. in length is made in the distal palmar crease (Fig. 13). Here the skin is thin and attached to the fascia, which must be separated for the exposure and for an everted skin closure. The pretendinous fascial band can be split longitudinally, or better a segment resected together with its septa. It is at this level that fascia, synovia, and the proximal annular ligament conjoin to ensheath the two flexors (actually three, for here the superficial tendon splits and encircles the profundus and here the "trigger" phenomenon of the flexor tendons is encountered). With local analgesia and a tourniquet, which is tolerated easily by most patients for the limited procedure, the mechanics of the lesion are readily observed upon opening the synovial sheath. When the digit is extended and then actively flexed by the patient the caliber discrepancy between the tendon and fibrous sheath is obvious as the tendon snaps to and fro. In advanced cases the superficial tendon is shredded and degenerated. Some excess of synovial fluid may be present, but the granulomatous synovia of de Quervain's disease is rarely observed, except at the hiatus of the superficialis tendon. The mechanical aspect of the block is removed when the proximal fibrous ring is divided.

Increased disability can follow surgical release of (1) the flexor pollicis longus (metacarpophalangeal level), or (2) the long abductor and short extensor (distal radius). In both cases the proximity of a critical sensory nerve forces caution on the operator, who must be aware of the painful consequence of the nerve damage. The obliquity of the radiovolar nerve as it crosses the flexor pollicis longus at the metacarpophalangeal crease puts it directly in the field. There is a similar proximity

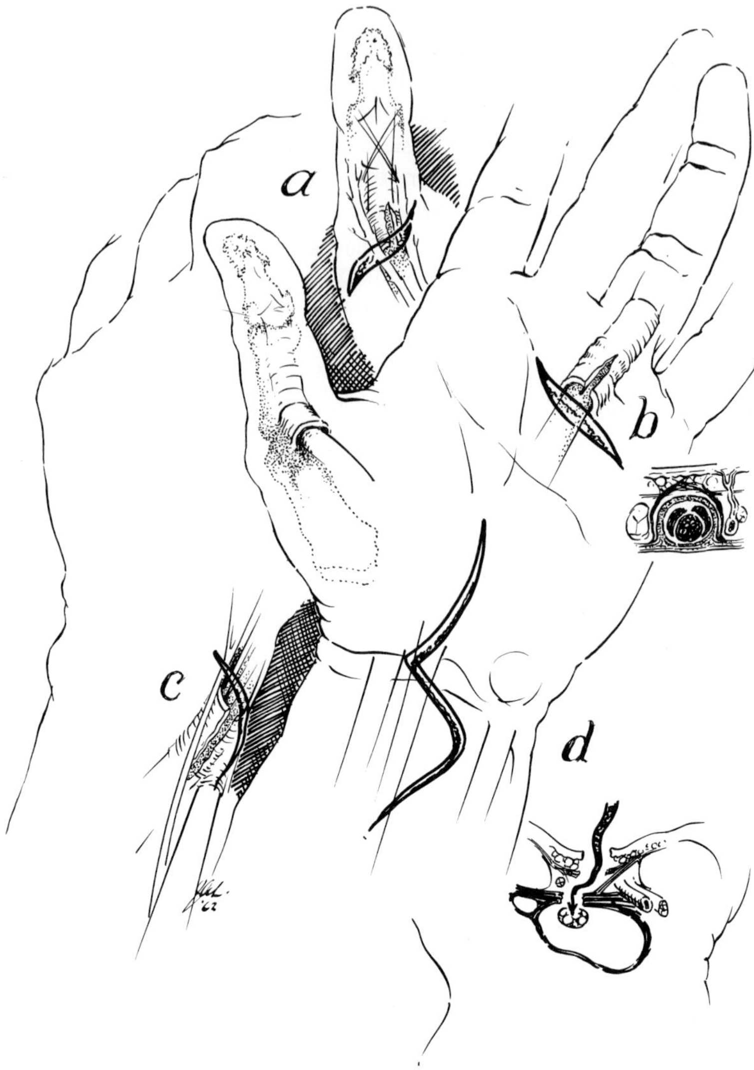

FIGURE 13. Incisions for exposure and release. (*a*) Long thumb flexor. Extreme care must be taken not to injure digital nerves. (*b*) Superficial and deep flexor tendons of the fingers as they enter the proximal annular ligament of the tendon sheath. The synovial cul-de-sac is not shown (see Figure 9). Insert shows the relationship of fascia to fibrous sheath. (*c*) Short extensor and long abductor of the thumb (de Quervain's disorder). Note the proximity of the superficial branch of the radial nerve coming from beneath the brachioradialis tendon to pass over the fibro-osseous tunnel. The extensor lies to the ulnar side of the compartment and is easily differentiated from the abductor (which may be multiple) by its greater amplitude. This can be noted directly when the operation is performed under local analgesia, or more simply by observing the effect of careful traction on the thumb. (*d*) The median nerve (carpal tunnel syndrome). Full exposure of the deep-lying volar carpal ligament is essential to insure complete decompression of the nerve. The palmaris longus (if present) is retracted radially and its fibrous extension over the carpal ligament is divided, exposing fat which overlies the carpal ligament. The nerve is exposed proximally just beneath the antibrachial fascia, and the ligament is completely divided in line with the nerve.

between the superficial branch of the radial nerve and the long abductor and the short extensor of the thumb over the radiodorsal aspect of the wrist.

The exquisitely sensitive neuromas developed in these operative sites following inadvertent surgical section are far more disturbing than the original lesion, and once established their transplantation to a less vulnerable site is often indicated.

Amputations

Finger Tip Amputations

Except for incised wounds, the most frequently encountered injuries of the hand are severed finger tips with loss of substance and length. If the tip or a portion thereof remains attached by a vascularized pedicle, it is worthy of replacement. If it is detached or contused, the cutaneous layer alone, trimmed of other tissue, may still be useful because of its unique qualities, as a free graft. Except in the thumb and index finger, where length is critical, primary closure by the simple and direct method of rongeuring exposed bone to allow approximation of soft tissue to form a well-padded stump is generally the preferred treatment. Bone shortening is seldom necessary in children, since even relatively large defects heal rapidly without primary closure as the shrinking wound draws intact soft tissue with good contour over the tip. Transverse losses through the nail and distal phalanx often are best covered with split-thickness skin grafts which preserve length, and with contracture result in good coverage as the remaining pulp is drawn centripetally distalward. When the injury is oblique, with a considerable loss of pulp, flap coverage is needed for replacement and for avoiding the excessive shortening necessary for primary closure. Cross finger or occasionally thenar pedicle flaps are preferred since they most closely simulate normal finger tip tissue and avoid the laboriousness of distant pedicle transfers. In elderly patients or those with arthritic tendency, one must be wary of joint stiffening in pedicle procedures.

The thumb and index finger should not be electively shortened. Amputation of the independent index at or near the proximal interphalangeal joint renders it essentially useless as an opponent for the thumb, so that the middle finger is used in its stead. The importance of tactile sense over the contact areas of the first two digits demands that substitution for tissue loss here be of the best quality possible. At times a transverse segment of the remaining finger pad can be advanced distally to the critical working area on bilateral neurovascular pedicles, and the less important proximal defect can then be covered with a properly shaped free full-thickness graft. Complete loss of the volar pulp tissue of these digits is best replaced, either primarily or secondarily, by a neurovascular sensory island transfer. A circumferential avulsion wound of a prime digit must be covered by a small glabrous tubed pedicle into which a sensory island can later be transferred. With extensive avulsion or degloving injuries, the terminal finger segments very likely will be beyond the circulatory limit, in which case coverage and reconstruction are best delayed until lines of demarcation become apparent. Avulsed skin relatively intact can be trimmed of subcutaneous tissue and used effectively for free graft coverage.

Major Digital Amputations

The only imperative indication for digital amputation is loss of blood supply. In general, injured digits should be preserved. Soft tissue filleted from a functionally impaired finger can be invaluable in primary closure of large wounds, and no viable parts should be discarded without evaluation of their possible use in immediate or delayed reconstruction as free grafts, or better as pedicle transfers. Amputation of digits without motion or sensation, rendered useless through disease or injury, allows fuller use of the intact hand. When total amputation is indicated, the index

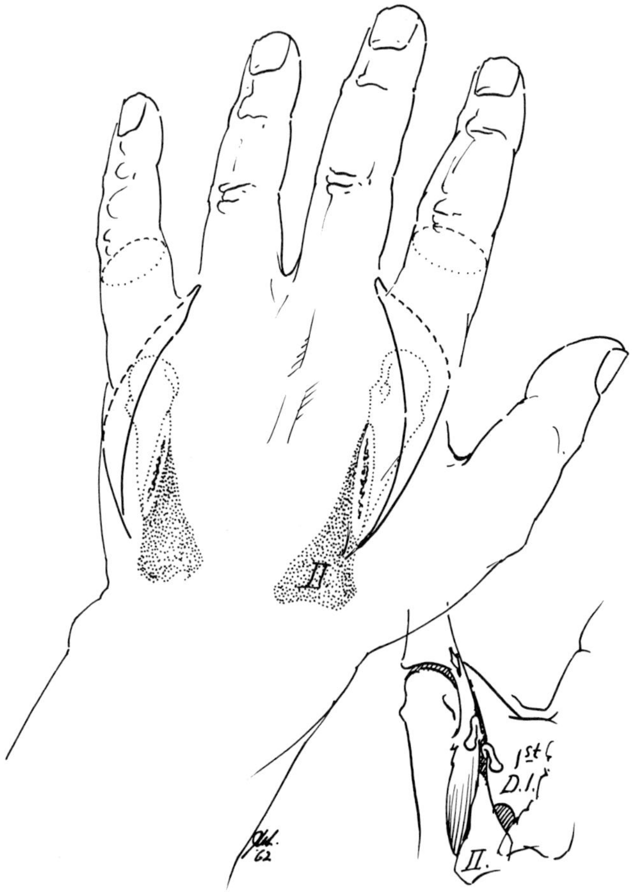

FIGURE 14. Partial resection of the second and fifth metacarpals generally improves the functional and aesthetic aspect of the hand when their respective digits have been amputated at the proximal interphalangeal levels. Insert shows transplantation of digital nerves to a less vulnerable site between the interosseous muscles, where they are anchored with fine plain catgut.

and fifth fingers should be removed with oblique section through the metacarpal bases so as to eliminate disturbing stumps and give a pleasing contour to the hand (Fig. 14). Digital nerves should be cleanly severed and the proximal ends placed in soft tissue away from areas of pressure and the grip of scar. Divided tendons should be allowed to retract—they are never to be sutured over an amputation stump.

Loss of the central fingers necessarily leaves a gap which may be troublesome to some patients. Transfer of an adjacent finger to the central metacarpal can give a better hand if the transverse arch is not broken and if some narrowing of the palm and loss of strength are acceptable.

Palmar Amputations

Oblique amputation of the ulnar portion of the hand reaching palmar level generally leaves the thumb intact together with enough of the more radial digits to form an effective holding and pinching mechanism. Major transverse amputations often require resection of central metacarpals in order to form a cleft between radial and ulnar units. Angulatory and rotational osteotomy of the lateral metacarpals can add greatly to the prehensile ability of such a hand by formation of a palmar cup. In more proximal, or total hand, amputations evaluation for the individual patient must be made of the benefits of a prosthesis versus those of the Krukenberg procedure with its advantage of preserving a sense of touch.

Radial oblique amputations of the hand involve disabling loss of the thumb. The type of reconstruction depends upon the extent of thumb damage as well as the concomitant finger injury. The index finger, because of its proximity and independence, is preferred for digital transfer to thumb position, and it can often be utilized even when damaged, since reduction in length is required in the transfer. When the thumb is lost distal to the metacarpophalangeal joint and intrinsic muscle control remains, a tubed abdominal pedicle incorporating a bone graft is useful to gain length. The neurovascular island transfer which supplies both discriminating sensation and arterial influx to the distal pedicle has given this method a new significance. For less extensive losses of the thumb, local flaps with a bone graft, perhaps augmented by an abdominal pedicle to help form the web, can be used to lengthen this prime digit. Excessive length is detractive—a pedicle-reconstructed thumb need not be as long as the normal.

112. *Amputations of the Lower Extremity*

FRANK C. WHEELOCK, JR.

Toe Amputations

The most commonly performed peripheral amputation is the amputation of a single toe (Fig. 1), a procedure which is done for peripherally located gangrene or neuropathic ulceration, for osteomyelitis of the distal phalanx, or for sepsis in an interphalangeal joint. Adequate circulation must be present, but palpable pedal pulses are not a necessity.

There are few absolute rules in surgery, but one is that *a toe should never be removed by disarticulation.* The large metatarsal head which one leaves by this method is covered with cartilage—a structure with poor blood supply and poor resistance to infection. Consequently, if the wound becomes infected, healing will be difficult, and even unlikely. The single toe amputation is always done through the proximal phalanx, leaving only a small segment of this bone behind. Except in special situations, medial and lateral flaps are utilized. In making these, the

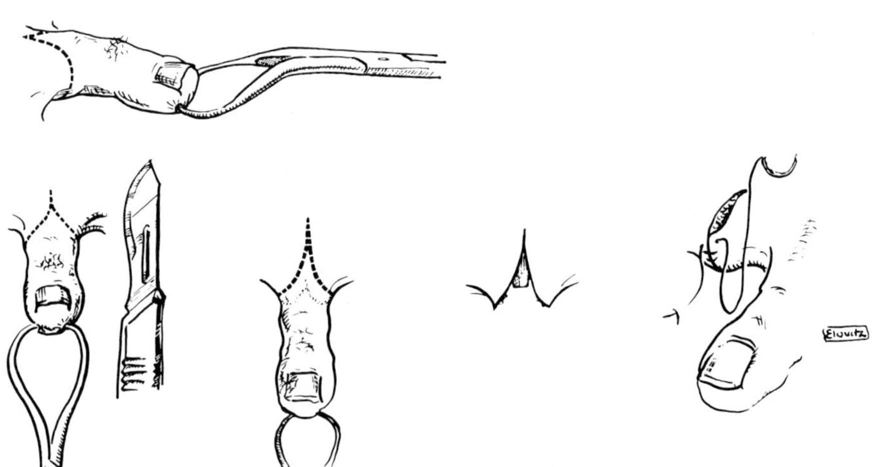

FIGURE 1. Amputation of a single toe.

adjacent toes are held apart with gauze and the scalpel is held at an absolute right angle to the skin to prevent beveling of the skin edges. The flaps must be long enough to avoid tension, which means that the most distal part of the incision is near the interphalangeal joint. The proximal point of the incision is a short distance up on the dorsum of the foot so that dependent drainage is assured if infection occurs and it becomes necessary to remove the sutures for drainage during the postoperative period.

During the amputation a towel clip holds the toe, and care is taken to avoid any contamination of the incision from the necrotic or infected area. The subcutaneous tissues and tendons are divided in line with the skin incision, and vessels are ligated with 4–0 plain catgut. The phalanx is cut with the bone cutter and rongeured back far enough to permit an easy one-layer closure with interrupted loosely tied No. 38 or No. 40 stainless steel wire sutures. Forceps or retractors are not used on the skin at any time lest they damage the relatively avascular tissues.

Occasionally when sepsis is present and the collateral circulation is fairly good, the skin may be left open and secondary healing allowed to occur.

Amputation of a Single Toe and Metatarsal Head

This procedure is less commonly utilized, as healing of the residual "dead space" may be quite difficult for two reasons. First, the remaining adjacent metatarsophalangeal joint capsules are relatively avascular, which hinders healing, obviously; and second, the adjacent metatarsals, being stiff, keep the area gaping until gradually fibrous tissue pulls them together. Closure of the space left by removal of the first or fifth metatarsals is obtained more easily than closure of the spaces left by removal of the others, which are held open by adjacent metatarsals on both sides of the defect. Whatever incision is used should be capable of being extended if necessary, in the direction the infection would normally take, and should also assure dependent drainage with the foot in normal resting position. In this procedure the danger of spread of infection to the next joint is a constant threat.

Removal of the first or fifth metatarsal is carried out through a racquet incision as shown in Figure 2. Care must be taken to leave enough skin distally to permit easy closure, whether by primary suture, delayed suture, or healing by secondary intention. The metatarsal is divided sufficiently far proximally to give a smooth contour to the foot, and the corner is beveled so that no sharp edge will push against the skin. Great care is taken not to enter an adjacent joint lest it become infected, and the infection lead to failure. Closure of the distal 80 per cent of the incision is usually carried out with fine wire interrupted skin sutures, and a cigarette-shaped gauze drain (no rubber) is placed in the proximal opening for dependent drainage. If all infected tissue is excised without contamination, the incision may be completely closed.

Amputation of the second, third, and fourth toes (Fig. 3) is similar except that the racquet handle extends down the sole of the foot. Again, one must have some skin in the web space to permit closure. The bone is divided fairly far

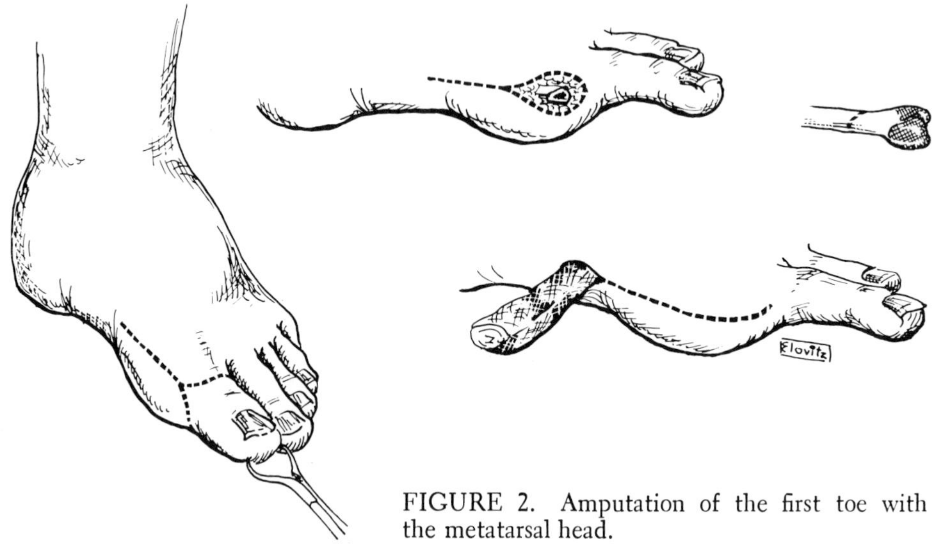

FIGURE 2. Amputation of the first toe with the metatarsal head.

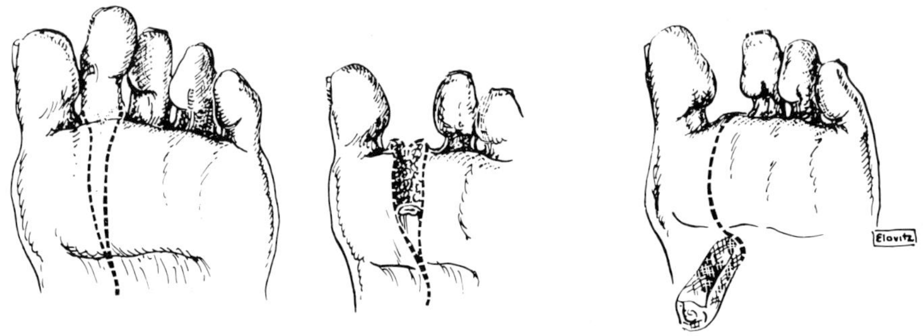

FIGURE 3. Amputation of the second toe with the metatarsal head.

proximally so that the adjacent metacarpals may eventually come together. All tissues are incised so that dependent drainage exists as the patient lies face up in bed; that is, the skin incision extends more proximally than does the incision in the fat and fascia, and in turn the bone is divided a little further out. These incisions are such that if saline were used for irrigation, it would run out, leaving no residual.

Again, distal closure with proximal drainage is usually performed, though healing without suture will eventually occur if the blood supply is adequate. Rarely, complete closure is possible.

Transmetatarsal Amputation

The transmetatarsal amputation is of great value in salvaging limbs when the location of the gangrene or the poor state of the circulation precludes successful toe amputations. Our experience at the New England Deaconess Hospital now encompasses more than 500 such amputations, and our enthusiasm for this procedure continues.

Being more proximally located than the procedures just described, this operation is carried out where the blood supply may be a little better. An added advantage is that no "dead space" remains. The plantar flap is used for closure because it is thicker and wider and has better circulation than the dorsal skin. A transmetatarsal amputation is done for stabilized necrotic process of the toe or toes or web spaces, or for small areas of gangrene of the skin over the first or fifth metatarsal head.

Technically the procedure is simple and straightforward (Fig. 4). The toes are covered with gauze and firmly held until they have been removed. This seems the only effective way of avoiding contamination from the areas of gangrene or ulceration. The incisions are carefully made without bevel and with firm pressure on the scalpel, frequently reaching the bone with the first stroke. The tendons are divided in line with the skin incision. The dorsal skin incision is gently curved, is just proximal to the metatarsal heads, and is not undermined at all. The plantar incision creates a flap which is used to cover the end of the foot and extends from points proximal to the first and fifth metatarsal heads to cross the foot just proximal to the web spaces. The flap is kept as thick as possible, but the sesamoid bones are not included. The metatarsals are divided proximal to their heads with a bone cutter and the ends are rongeured smooth; then they are carefully palpated to be certain that no loose fragments are left. The dorsum of each bone, the medial edge of the first metatarsal, and the lateral edge of the fifth metatarsal are beveled slightly to give a smooth contour to the shortened foot.

Hemostasis is checked and vessels are ligated with 4–0 plain catgut. The incision is closed without tension, using one layer of interrupted No. 38 stainless steel wire sutures, tied carefully to avoid crushing the tissues. Forceps are not used on

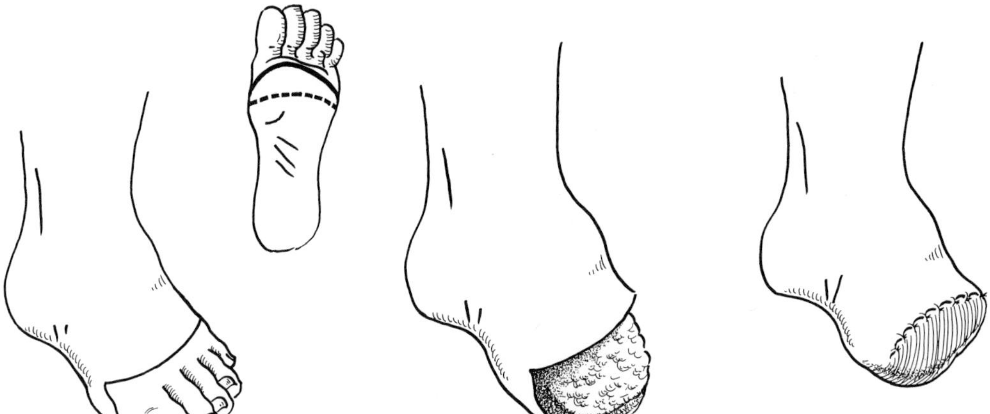

FIGURE 4. Transmetatarsal amputation. (Reproduced by permission of Year Book Publishers, Inc.)

the skin, and the needle is introduced in a dorsal to plantar direction to avoid ever lifting the dorsal flap. Retractors are never used on the dorsal flap during the operation, in an effort to avoid even the slightest trauma to this precarious skin area. All these seemingly trivial precautions are important, as failures are almost always due to necrosis of the dorsal skin.

A simple gauze dressing is applied, avoiding the use of elastic bandages, and occasionally a light posterior plaster splint is used if the situation seems precarious. Prolonged bed rest, frequently with the head of the bed elevated, is indicated, with inspection of the incision at suitable intervals.

Lower Leg Amputation

The lower leg amputation is being used with increasing frequency in preference to a supracondylar amputation. A palpable popliteal pulse is not necessary to accomplish this procedure, and on occasion we have succeeded when even the femoral pulse was absent; but there must be no gangrene and no line of temperature demarcation above the ankle. The operation can be done with the patient either supine or prone. A tourniquet is never used. The skin incisions, located about two-thirds of the way from the knee to the ankle, are so made that short anterior and posterior flaps of equal size are created (Fig. 5). The muscles are divided in line

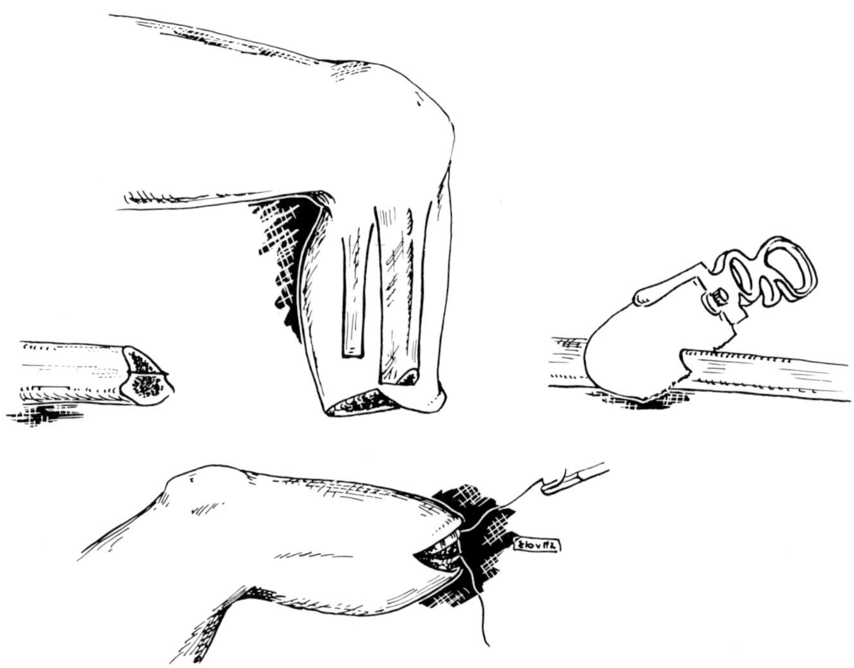

FIGURE 5. Lower leg amputation.

with the skin incision and allowed to retract, and then the vessels and nerves are divided. Great care is taken in elevating the anterior flap lest its precarious blood supply be damaged—it is of course very thin. The fibula is next dissected out and divided with heavy bone cutters or a Gigli saw an inch or more above the anticipated level of division of the tibia. The tibia is then divided with a saw—first making an anterior bevel, then cutting across the bone at right angles. The bone edges are smoothed with a file, and bone wax is used to stop bleeding from the marrow cavity if necessary.

After an extremely careful check of hemostasis, closure is obtained with interrupted 3–0 chromic catgut fascial sutures and interrupted skin stitches. Muscle is not brought over the bone ends. It is important that no "dead space" remain and that there be no tension on the suture line. No drain is used. The dressing is of gauze (elastic bandages are contraindicated), and a posterior splint is used to prevent a flexion contracture of the knee. In applying the dressing and the splint, pressure over the end of the tibia anteriorly must be avoided lest necrosis of the skin in this area result.

The Supracondylar Amputation

The supracondylar amputation is reserved for patients requiring a major amputation who are too debilitated to use an artificial limb or whose arterial insufficiency precludes a below the knee amputation. At this level healing should be no problem and the operation itself is simpler and quicker than the previous two described (Fig. 6).

The incision is circular and located exactly at the top of the patella. There should be no need to go higher; indeed, at higher levels the thigh is larger and therefore the operation much more difficult and the stump length most unsatisfactory. The "midthigh" amputation should be a great rarity.

After the incision has been made through the skin, fascia, and quadriceps tendon, if the extremity is held at nearly a right angle to the table, the hamstring muscles are put under tension and can be easily divided medially and laterally. Their ends retract and the sciatic nerve and the major vessels then stand out and are easily and quickly identified. The nerve is clamped before being cut, to facilitate identification for later treatment. The femoral vessels are ligated individually, and if clot is present in the femoral vein an interruption at the groin is indicated. The sciatic nerve is dissected out as high as possible, ligated with catgut, divided with the cautery, and allowed to retract far up among the muscles, where its end will not be caught in scar. With this simple method we have had very little trouble with neuroma formation or stump pain.

After a careful check for bleeding, the incision is closed with fascial sutures of 3–0 chromic catgut and interrupted fine skin sutures. The closure is transverse, and at the two corners there are slight protrusions or "dog-ears." These eventually

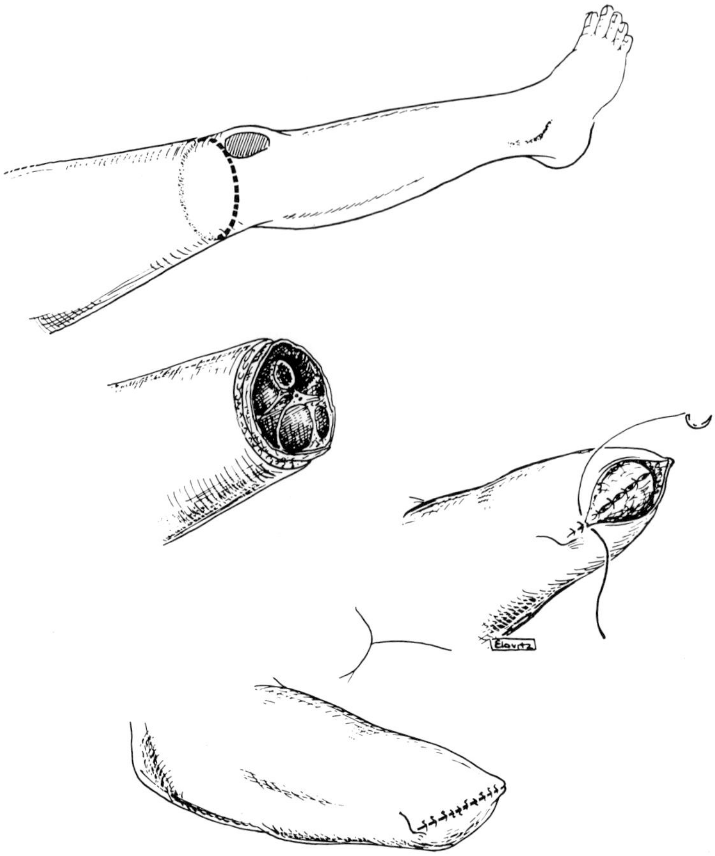

FIGURE 6. Supracondylar amputation.

smooth out and are not a problem. Again, the rule of no tourniquet, no tension, and no drain applies.

In a fat thigh the medial and lateral fascial sutures may be left out for an inch or so to permit inversion of the subcutaneous fat when the skin sutures are placed; otherwise the skin may be under too much tension.

A simple gauze dressing is applied with no splint. Postoperatively, appropriate exercises are used to avoid a flexion contracture of the hip.

113. *Radical Groin Dissection*

GEORGE T. PACK AND
PAUL E. REKERS

THE SUCCESSFUL TREATMENT of malignant tumors that arise in or metastasize to the groin depends on the complete removal of the primary neoplasm and associated lymph nodes. The procedure of groin dissection has varied in the degree of enthusiasm it has evoked and in its radicality. The radical operation of Stoeckel and Kehrer received little attention because of the associated high morbidity and mortality. Basset, in 1912, described a technique of groin dissection in which the inguinal ligament was split to enable a conjoined surgical removal of iliac and inguinal nodes. Taussig modified the Basset procedure by excluding the hypogastric nodes. Since that time the radical groin dissection with extirpation of the inguinal, iliac, obturator, and hypogastric lymph nodes has become standardized.

Indications for Groin Dissection

Groin dissections are performed for metastatic carcinoma and melanoma occurring in the skin of the lower extremity, the male and female genitals, the perineum, perianal zone, gluteal region, and the infraumbilical segment of the abdominal wall; for some lymphoblastomas; and for certain primary sarcomas which occur by chance in the groin or metastasize there. Cancers of the umbilicus, the infraumbilical or midabdominal skin, the skin of the anus and scrotum, the perianal zone, and the female genitals all are capable of metastasizing either to the right or the left group of groin nodes or to both groups. The dissemination toward both groins indicates the necessity for bilateral groin dissections. The entire procedure of excision of the primary and metastatic cancers in both groins may be performed in one, two, or three stages, but in our opinion the preferable plan is to excise the primary cancer and the lymph nodes in both groins en bloc, without interrupting the lymphatic connecting pathways, whenever it is technically possible and the condition of the patient permits such an undertaking.

The basic postulates for successful groin dissection are: (1) The primary cancer should be controlled or controllable. (2) There should be no clinical evidences of blood stream metastases. (3) The lymph stream must be centralward, with no evidence of blockage and retrograde extension. (4) It should be technically possible to excise all of the lymph nodes involved, or suspected of becoming involved, in the immediate neighborhood. (5) There must be some possibility of interruption of the lymphatic spread of the cancer by an excision of these nodes. (6) There should be evidence that the cancer has metastasized only to the regional group of nodes to be attacked in the groin dissection.

If the metastatic cancer in the inguinal nodes is intimately adherent to the femoral or external iliac vessels, it may be necessary to resect the vessels and perform subsequent anastomoses, transplantation, or ligation of vessels. When the neoplasm is inseparably adherent to the parietes, a hemipelvectomy may be necessary.

Groin dissection is not indicated in the face of numerous secondary nodules in the skin of the lower extremity, intervening between the site of the primary tumor and the groin, because such a radical procedure as groin dissection associated with hip joint disarticulation will not afford an opportunity for cure. This is particularly true in the case of malignant melanoma since this tumor, at the time of such widespread local extension, has usually invaded blood vessels, with resultant distant metastases.

Surgical Anatomy of Lymph Nodes and Related Lymphatics

Inguinal Lymph Nodes

The term inguinal nodes, as employed here, refers to all lymph nodes in the inguinofemoral region. The superficial inguinal lymph nodes, which average eight to twelve in number, are arranged in four main groups: the superolateral, superomedial, infralateral, and inframedial series (Rouviere-Tobias). These superficial inguinal lymph nodes drain in the major number of superficial lymph vessels from the skin of the lower extremity, the labia majora and minora, the praeputium clitoridis, the scrotum, the penis, the buttocks, the perineum, the lumbar, umbilical, and infraumbilical regions, and the cutaneous zone of the anus. Some (but not all) of these lymph nodes intercommunicate with each other by means of short lymph pathways (Fig. 1).

The number and size of the nodes seem to be influenced by the patient's age. For example, patients with malignant melanoma are usually in the younger age groups, and the lymph nodes appear to the surgeon and pathologist to be more numerous than in the elderly; whereas epidermoid carcinoma of the extremities and genitals occurs more often in elderly subjects, in whom the lymph nodes seem to have regressed or atrophied with age. An explanation is in order here. Although the lymph nodes in older people appear to have vanished, they really undergo involution and diminish in size; they do not actually disappear. For this reason, a dissection of the groin, and particularly the tissues along the femoral and external

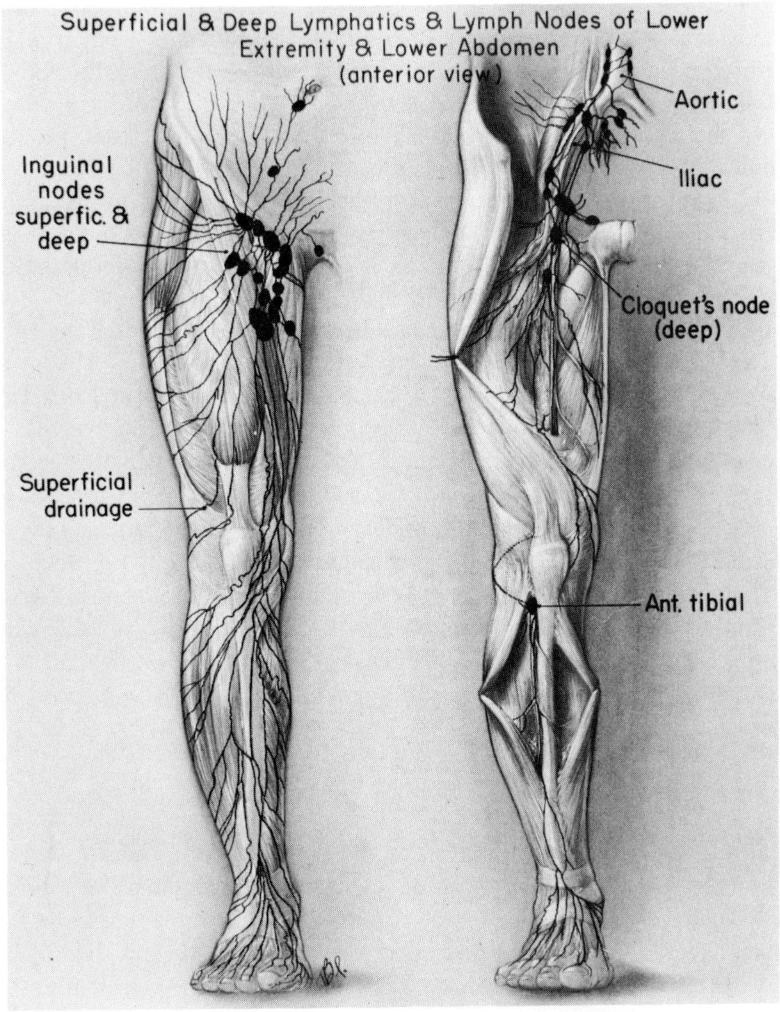

FIGURE 1. Lymphatics of lower extremity and lower abdomen (anterior view).

iliac vessels, must be meticulous in order to remove each and every one of these small intercalated nodes. If a groin dissection has been performed for metastatic cancer and a local recurrence develops which proves on study to be metastasis in a lymph node, it may be deduced that the dissection was not complete. Lymphatic vessels, after severance, may re-establish connection across the wound, but lymph nodes per se never regenerate.

Lymphatic Vessels of the Lower Extremity

The lymphatic vessels of the lower extremity may be divided into two sets, superficial and deep.

Superficial Lymphatic Vessels. The superficial lymphatic vessels are placed beneath the integument in the superficial fascia and are divisible into three sets: trunks which follow the course of the internal saphenous vein, trunks which accompany the external saphenous vein, and trunks from the gluteal region. Trunks which follow the course of the internal saphenous vein arise from a plexus on the dorsum of the foot. This plexus obtains lymphatics from all the toes, the sole, and both borders of the foot. The internal trunks, three or four in number, pass to the superficial inguinal nodes. The external trunks run upward and inward and end in the internal trunks. The trunks which follow the external saphenous vein number two or three. They take origin from the heel and from the posterior half of the outer edge of the foot and empty into the superficial inguinal nodes. The lymph trunks from the gluteal region join vessels from the anus and enter the superficial inguinal nodes.

Deep Lymphatic Vessels. The deep lymphatic vessels of the lower extremity are few in number and accompany the deep blood vessels. In the leg they consist of three sets, the anterior tibial, peroneal, and posterior tibial, which accompany the corresponding blood vessels, two or three to each artery. They ascend with the blood vessels and enter the lymph nodes in the popliteal space. The efferent vessels from these nodes accompany the femoral vein and join the deep inguinal nodes. From these nodes, vessels pass beneath Poupart's ligament and communicate with the chain of nodes surrounding the external iliac vessels. The deep lymphatic vessels of the gluteal and ischiatic regions follow the course of the blood vessels and join the gluteal and ischiatic nodes at the great sacrosciatic foramen.

Popliteal Lymph Nodes

The popliteal nodes are deeply placed in the popliteal fossa and are therefore all subfascial (Fig. 2). These three to six nodes are distributed along the course of the popliteal blood vessels. Although they receive afferent lymphatics from the knee joint, their practical importance in cancer diagnosis and therapy lies in the fact that they are intercalated in the paths of the lymph collecting vessels from the skin on the lateral aspect of the heel and the posterior half of the lateral border of the foot. It is only in this location that the lymph vessels are superficial, as they progress more deeply and finally become subfascial as they ascend the leg. There may be two or three small intercalated nodes intervening between the heel and the popliteal space; these nodes have been variously labeled as anterior tibial, posterior tibial, and tibiofibular lymph nodes.

These facts afford two valuable indications for the surgeon in planning treatment. Melanomas primary in the skin of the heel or lateral aspect of the foot should be treated not only by surgical dissection of the heel and groin dissection but by excision of the popliteal lymph nodes as well. Furthermore, it is possible for a melanoma or anaplastic carcinoma primary in this location to metastasize through the second relay if the popliteal nodes are involved without lodgment in the superficial inguinal nodes. Reliance on palpation of these nodes to determine the presence or absence of metastases in the groin would give a false assurance of

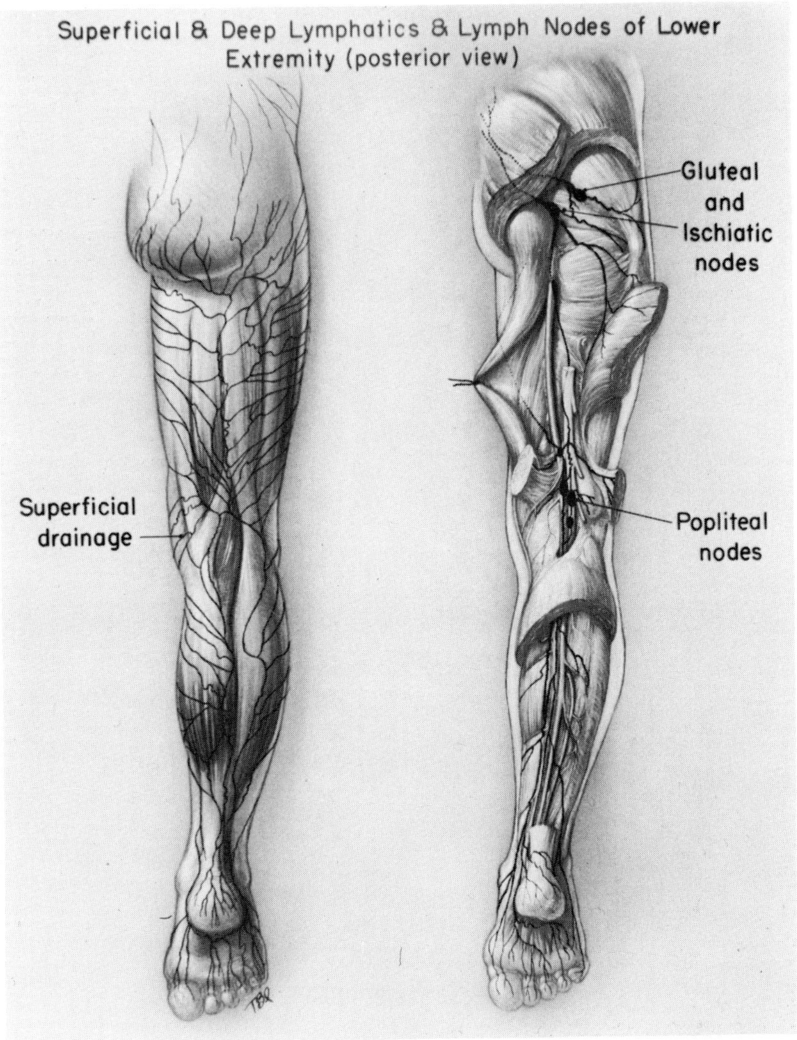

FIGURE 2. Lymphatics of lower extremity (posterior view).

safety. Only if the deep nodes were of sufficient size to be palpable could the surgeon be aware of their participation in the extension of the tumor. For this reason, it becomes imperative to perform a deep, radical groin dissection as an essential part of the treatment of all melanomas of the heel, particularly those which metastasize to the popliteal lymph nodes.

Lymphatics of the Pelvis and Abdomen

The lymphatics of the pelvis and abdomen constitute a continuous chain and it is customary to divide them into groups which are called the iliopelvic nodes and

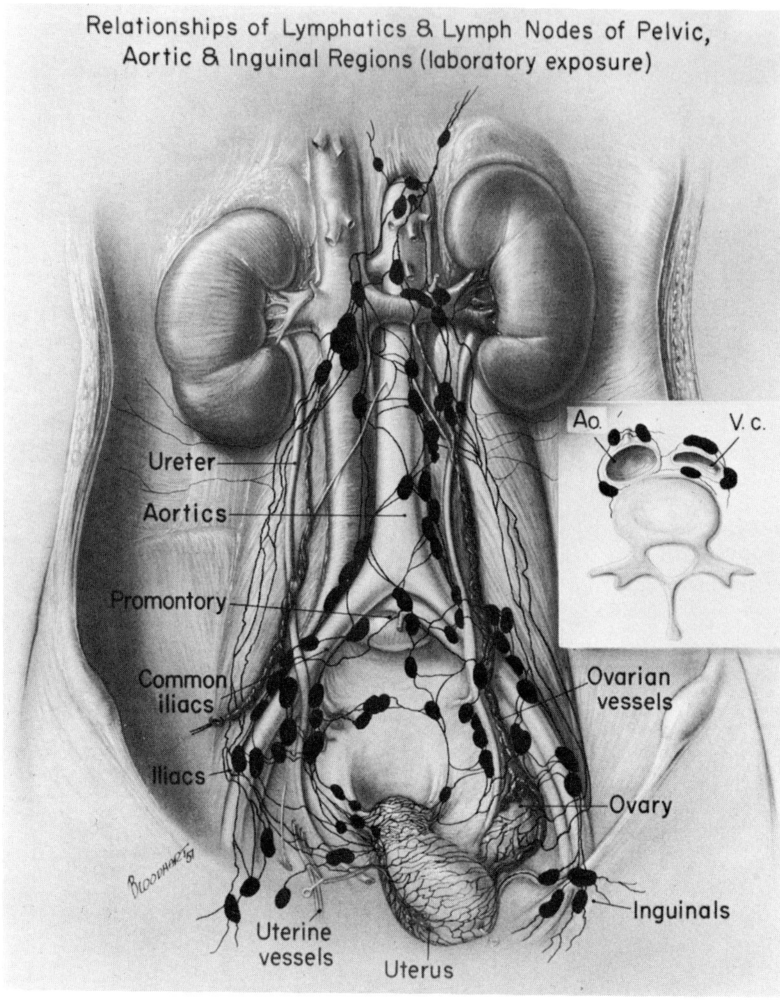

FIGURE 3. Lymphatics of pelvic, aortic, and inguinal regions.

the abdominoaortic nodes; the first group being below and the second above the level of the bifurcation of the aorta into the two common iliac arteries (Fig. 3).

Iliac or Iliopelvic Nodes. The iliopelvic nodes are at the level of the inlet of the pelvis or in the pelvic cavity. They follow the course of the blood vessels and are divisible into the external iliac, the internal iliac, and the common iliac chains and the pelvic nodes.

External Iliac Nodes. The external iliac nodes form chains around the external iliac vessels (Fig. 4). There are three chains of these nodes. An external chain of three or four nodes lies between the artery and the psoas muscle. The lowest node of the external chain is called the external retrocrural node. A middle chain of three nodes lies upon the front surface of the external iliac vein. The lowest node of this group is called the middle retrocrural node. An internal chain of three or four nodes is placed to the inner side of the external iliac vein. The

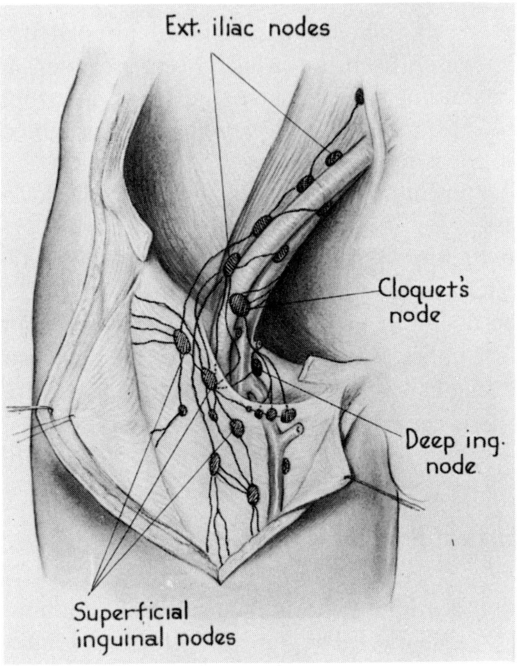

FIGURE 4. Superficial inguinal and external iliac nodes.

lowest node of this chain is called the internal retrocrural node, and is close to the upper node of the deep inguinal chain, the node of Cloquet. The obturator node belongs to the inner chain of the external iliac nodes. The external iliac nodes receive vessels from the superficial and deep iliac nodes, the glans penis or glans clitoridis, deep lymphatics from the umbilicus and lower part of the belly wall, the superior portion of the vagina, the uterine neck, the prostate gland, the bladder, the membranous portion of the urethra, and the internal iliac nodes. The obturator node receives deep lymph vessels from along the course of the obturator vessels. The external iliac nodes send vessels direct to the common iliac nodes and also lymphatics to join vessels from the internal iliac nodes on their way to the common iliac group. The nodes along the deep epigastric artery and those along the deep circumflex iliac artery are accessory chains to the main group of the external iliac nodes.

Internal Iliac or Hypogastric Nodes. The internal iliac nodes are placed along the internal iliac artery and its branches. The node on the middle hemorrhoidal artery is called the middle hemorrhoidal node. The lateral sacral node is on the lateral sacral artery. The internal iliac nodes receive lymph from the pelvic viscera, perineum, penile portion of the urethra, deep tissues of the posterior portion of the thigh, and from the buttocks. They send vessels to the common iliac nodes and also to the external iliac nodes.

Common Iliac Nodes. The common iliac nodes are found about the common iliac artery and are divided into an external group which lies upon the inner edge of the psoas muscle; a middle group, behind the artery; and an internal group, which lies upon the front of the body of the fifth lumbar vertebra or upon the sacrovertebral junction. They receive vessels from the external and internal iliac nodes and from the pelvic viscera, the vessels from the pelvic viscera ascending to the promontory of the sacrum and containing perhaps, here and there, interrupting nodes, known as sacral nodes. They also receive lymph vessels from the lumbosacral region. They send vessels to the aortic nodes.

The *epigastric nodes,* three or four in number, are placed alongside the lower portion of the inferior epigastric vessels.

The *iliac circumflex nodes,* two to four in number, are situated along the course of the deep iliac circumflex vessels; they are sometimes absent.

The common iliac nodes and the nodes about the lower portion of the aorta and vena cava may be called the lumbar nodes. The lymph nodes of the iliac chain are in intimate relationship with the inguinal and the abdominoaortic nodes and those within the pelvis by means of their corresponding lymphatic vessels.

Spread of Cancers of the Abdominal Wall and Gluteal Region

The lymphatics of the supraumbilical and infraumbilical regions do not communicate except by very small lymphatic capillaries. The integument of the infraumbilical region and the umbilicus proper drains through lymphatics terminating in the superficial inguinal lymph nodes. Carcinomas of the umbilicus, therefore, would generally metastasize to the lymph nodes of the groin rather than to the axillary lymph nodes. It is also possible for carcinomas of the umbilicus to perforate the deep fascia and spread by metastasis through the falciform ligament to lymph nodes in the hilum of the liver. Because there are numerous lymph nodules intercalated along the course of these anterior abdominal lymphatics superior to the inguinal ligament, radical groin dissection for carcinomas of the abdominal wall and umbilicus should include wide dissection of the subcutaneous fat and superficial fascia.

One possibility which should be borne in mind by the examining physician is the occasional metastatic involvement of a lymph node in the eleventh intercostal space posteriorly, where one of the posterior lymphatic vessels terminates. This node may reach a relatively large size and cause pain before it is detectable.

Although the skin of the gluteal region is drained by lymphatics which empty into the superficial inguinal lymph nodes, the possibility of occasional metastasis to the common iliac nodes by means of lymph vessels accompanying the sciatic nerve must be remembered. These lymphatics may perforate the fascia at the level of the gluteal fold in the upper posterior thigh and accompany the sheath of the sciatic nerve. These nodes are beyond the scope of excisional surgery and for this reason certain melanomas and anaplastic carcinomas of the gluteal skin may metastasize directly to the common iliac nodes without any intervening regional node involvement. This accounts for certain failures to cure these cancers by a wide excision of gluteal skin, fat, and fascia associated with homolateral groin dissection even when the primary and secondary tumors are thus removed en bloc.

Spread of Cancers of the Perianal and Perineal Regions

Cancers of the perianal and perineal regions also metastasize into the medial superficial inguinal lymph nodes, more commonly those of the inferomedial group. The cutaneous lymphatics on both sides of the perineum intercommunicate with each other extensively along the entire median raphe and for that reason there is every likelihood that the metastases, if they do occur, will be bilateral. The dissection should always be bilateral. The clinically involved side may require a radical groin dissection; the clinically uninvolved side may be treated simultaneously or at a second operation.

Spread of Cancers of the External Female Genitals

Clitoris. The lymphatics of the clitoris have the same distribution as those of the penis, and the same procedure should be followed in their treatment. (See the following section.)

Vagina. Although it has been stated in many texts on gynecology that cancers in the lower third of the vagina behave as do those of the vulva, this assertion is not entirely accurate. It is the hymen which is the definite boundary line. The mucous membrane of the vagina internal to this structure drains through its lymphatic network into the deep pelvic lymph nodes, and therefore is not concerned in this discussion. The hymen, vestibule, and fourchette all drain into the inguinal lymph nodes, and the metastases thereto are treated by the methods previously described.

Vulva. The lymphatic network of the vulva is extraordinarily copious and there is such intimate anastomosis with the opposite side that metastases may readily occur bilaterally or even contralaterally. All cancers of the vulva should be treated by a bilateral groin dissection. All of these lymphatics terminate in the superomedial group of superficial lymph nodes. If a radical vulvectomy is done in one or two stages, in the absence of clinical evidence of metastases to the nodes the dissection may, with reservations, be limited to the superficial, deep inguinal, and retrofemoral groups without removing the external iliac nodes above the inguinal ligament.

Spread of Cancers of the Penis

The character of the groin dissection is based on the portion of the penis involved by the cancer. For example, if the cutaneous envelope of the body of the penis together with the prepuce is involved, the first focus of metastatic deposit is in the superficial inguinal lymph nodes (superomedial group) and the groin dissection in some instances might be of superficial character without extension above the inguinal ligaments. If metastases do occur, even though they are palpable only unilaterally, a bilateral dissection should nevertheless be done because the collecting trunks at the root of the organ may separate and run to either the right or the left side.

If the glans is involved, the situation is infinitely more serious, because the lymphatics in this region may not terminate in the superficial lymph nodes but may penetrate directly into the deep inguinal nodes as well and sometimes into the external iliac or hypogastric nodes without intervening stops. Therefore, in the case of malignant melanomas and epitheliomas of the glans penis or glans clitoridis, one must suspect the possible presence of metastases to these deeper lymph nodes even in the pelvis, without the intervention of superficial lymph node involvement, and must guide one's surgical procedure accordingly.

The second anatomical fact which influences the choice of procedure is the existence of a small group of two or three prepubic lymph nodes which are situated in the midst of the presymphyseal lymphatic plexus which drains the lymphatics of the glans and in turn empties into the external iliac lymph nodes without a relay into the superficial inguinal nodes. Bearing these facts in mind, the surgeon has good theoretical reasons, at least, for extending the groin dissection above the inguinal ligament if the primary cancer involves the glans penis or glans clitoridis.

Spread of Cancers of the Scrotum

This site is one of the most dangerous locations in which cancer may occur. Successful end results in the treatment for epitheliomas of even low-grade malignancy are notoriously rare; and if conservative excision only is employed, practically no cures of malignant melanoma are ever obtained. The explanation of this tragic picture is the remarkable abundance of the lymphatic network throughout the scrotal skin. The collecting lymph vessels originate along the median raphe and anastomose freely with those of the opposite side. For this reason the metastases are nearly always bilateral. Accordingly, bilateral groin dissections are indicated. The local treatment of cancer of the scrotal skin necessitates an almost complete removal of this skin *en bloc* with the inguinal lymph nodes in order to effect a complete ablation of the disease. Again we emphasize that the lymphatics of the scrotal skin anastomose freely with those of the penis anteriorly and those of the perineum posteriorly. Therefore, a wide surgical removal of the skin should be done.

Problem of Retrograde Lymphatic Spread

Lymph flow is usually sluggish and contingent on muscular movements, adequately functioning valves, and absence of central obstruction. The direction of flow is usually proximal or central. The direction may be reversed by occlusion of the lymph vessels due to lodgment of tumor emboli or to the blockage of lymph nodes by cancer tissue. Subsequent emboli in the series may become piled up in this distended lymphatic, the valves of which become incompetent through distention. The resultant stagnation of lymph permits retrograde lymphatic permeation. As seen in the groin, particularly in the case of melanomas, this complication results in edema of the extremity and the rapid appearance of myriads of melanotic nodules in the subdermal lymphatics. This process may occur long after the primary tumor has been completely excised and in the absence of evidence of local recurrence.

This mechanism is of extreme practical importance and its operation must be avoided by the exercise of considerable judgment in the management of metastatic cancer in the groin. If a groin dissection is performed before the primary cancer has been removed or cured, or if a local recurrence develops at the site of the primary excision after a later groin dissection, this retrograde lymphatic embolism and permeation become speedily evident. The initial secondary nodules make their appearance usually in the neighborhood of the inguinal and femoral scar, where the emboli lodge in the blocked lymphatics. From this time on, one may readily see the successive, more or less orderly progression in the development of these nodules subcutaneously and intracutaneously down the thigh and leg. From these facts it is apparent that the timing of a groin dissection in relation to the date of excision or treatment of the primary tumor is of major importance. If metastases in the lymph nodes of the groin are clinically evident at the time the primary tumor is excised, a mistake may be made in the decision as to the proper time for groin dissection. For example, if a toe is amputated for subungual melanoma which has metastasized to nodes in the groin and the patient refuses hip joint disarticulation, the performance of a groin dissection at the same operative session rarely produces a successful result. If there should be tumor cells in transit, they may lodge in the groin wound and produce a diffuse uninhibited growth which cannot be controlled. If, on the other hand, the large lymph nodes are not removed shortly, there is the hazard of lymphatic blockage and retrograde extension down the thigh or toward the genitals. In either situation, the cancer progresses beyond the scope of curative surgery.

Elective Groin Dissection

"Elective" is a misnomer that is used here for the want of a better term. The operation called by this name refers to the elective removal of lymph nodes in the groin even though they are not palpable and there is no clinical evidence of metastases. If the primary cancer can be excised in continuity with the nodes of the groin, this dissection should be done routinely for all melanomas of the extremity and genitals. In a study made more than a decade ago, of seven dissections of this type for melanomas of the lower extremity, two of the patients had microscopically identifiable melanoma in the inguinal lymph nodes even though the surgeon at the time of operation found no gross evidence of involvement. In another group of ten similar axillary dissections for melanoma of the upper extremities, five patients, or 50 per cent of the series, showed microscopic evidence of metastases to the lymph nodes even though there was no gross evidence determinable preoperatively or during the course of the operation. It was our original contention that this early operation, although needlessly done in some instances, afforded the patient with metastatic melanoma in the groin a better and earlier opportunity of cure because it seemed reasonable that the fewer the lymph nodes involved and the earlier the involvement, the better would be the prognosis. In cases of epidermoid carcinoma occurring in the lower extremities, this routine dissection was not performed without evidence of nodal involvement, because this type of cancer seemed not to metastasize so frequently to inguinal nodes and there was a natural wish to avoid unnecessary operations of this major character. For epitheliomas of the scrotum and vulva, however, the bilateral inguinal dissection has been constantly employed even in the absence of palpably enlarged lymph nodes.

We have shown that an average period of 15 months elapses, from the time the primary melanoma is recognized, before the metastases in inguinal nodes are apparent. In earlier years, six weeks were permitted to elapse after the primary melanoma had been surgically excised before the second stage or elective groin dissection was done.

Unfortunately, when years passed and the results of analyses of those cases in which discontinuous operations in multiple stages were done became known, it was realized that the cure rate was unacceptably low. These tragedies were most apparent when the primary cancer (melanoma or epithelioma) was on the leg below the knee and had metastasized to the groin. Although there are some patients living and well for the definitive cure period or longer, who have had the primary cancer on the foot, for example, treated by excision and skin grafting, or amputation of a digit with groin dissection and preservation of the leg, the percentage of survivors is unhappily low. Our present inclination is to reserve the elective groin dissection for patients with the cancer in such close proximity to the groin as to make feasible the monobloc procedure of excision and groin dissection in continuity.

It is not an indifferent matter to decide whether to remove the primary cancer or to perform a block dissection of the regional lymph nodes as the first step in a two-stage procedure. The plan of treatment in which groin dissection is performed first, delaying the excision of the original cancer to a later date, is fraught with great dangers. The original cancer does not remain quiescent and metastases continue to occur. Either these malignant cells pour out directly into the fresh wound of the groin, where there is always abundant exudation of lymph, and in so doing may produce widespread, locally infiltrating, incurable recurrence; or, if the wound is healed to the point that the severed lymphatics are obstructed by the developing scar, the lymph stasis affords the proper setting for lodgment of emboli and retrograde lymphatic permeation, so that by the time the primary cancer is attacked the disease will have extended superiorly beyond the scope of excisional surgery. The ideal procedure, which can be achieved in some instances of malignant tumors of the genitals and upper thigh, is removal of the primary cancer and a metastatic cancer *en bloc*.

The proper way of handling, for example, melanoma of the foot metastatic to the groin is still an enigma. Our present scheme of management is presented here. In the absence of clinical evidence of suspicious lymph nodes in the groin, the primary cancer of the distal extremity is excised with skin grafting, or a digit is amputated, depending on the location of the neoplasm. Groin dissection is not done electively when it cannot be done in continuity. The patient is kept under close and frequent observation. If an enlarging node in the groin is discovered, it is removed for microscopic study; if metastases are found, the leg is removed by hip joint disarticulation with deep iliac nodal dissection. It has been our belief, substantiated by personal experience, that the lymph nodes in the groin should remain to exercise their function as catchment basins or filters for malignant cells which may be metastasizing at the time the primary cancer is removed.

The interval between the first appearance of the primary lesion and the confirmation of metastasis in lymph nodes of the groin is not the same for all malignant tumors. In our series, the average interval for epidermoid carcinoma is 30 months and for malignant melanoma only 15 months, which is in agreement with the usual greater degree of malignancy and the more rapid growth of melanoma. At one extreme, there is a case in which metastases in the inguinal nodes appeared 12 years after an epithelioma of the foot had been treated, and at the other extreme, an instance of simultaneous discovery of a primary melanoma of the vulva and enlarged inguinal nodes.

In patients who concurrently have active skin cancers of the feet or lower legs and proved metastases in femoral and inguinal lymph nodes, the hip joint disarticulation with deep iliac nodal dissection is done as the primary operation. It is most unlikely for any cancer as highly malignant as a melanoma to spread all the way from the foot to the groin, through the myriad lymphatics and their sluggish circulation, without some of the cancer cells becoming lodged en route in the tiny nodes intercalated along these pathways. A few long-term cures, however, in patients with the extremity preserved, attest to this possibility; but the chances are so few that we have no compunctions in advising and practicing the sacrifice of the extremity.

Do Sarcomas of the Soft Somatic Tissues Metastasize to Regional Lymph Nodes?

Although it is generally true that metastases of malignant tumors of mesenchymal derivation are blood-borne, an appreciable number of these sarcomas traverse the pathways of lymphatic drainage to lodge in regional lymph nodes. The three varieties of malignant mesenchymal tumors which more commonly metastasize to regional lymph nodes (seldom higher than 20 per cent) are rhabdomyosarcoma, malignant synovioma, and spindle-cell sarcomas of undetermined histogenesis. The anticipation of this occurrence now exerts a definite influence in planning the scope and technique of surgical treatment of these neoplasms.

Principles of Excision and Groin Dissection in Continuity for Primary and Metastatic Cancers

If a cancer is closely adjacent to the groin nodes into which it may metastasize, the operation may be so planned as to enable the surgeon to remove the primary tumor and the regional lymph nodes in one encompassing excision of skin and deeper structures. The procedure entails a wide sacrifice of skin overlying the cancer and an extension of this skin excision to include the skin overlying the lymph nodes. The skin flaps are then dissected widely back, and in the process the subcutaneous tissues are stripped from the skin. The underlying fascia is then removed, together with the specimen and the enveloping muscles, and the dissection is carried to the lymph-bearing regions, where a meticulous and radical dissection is carried out. Various bizarre-shaped incisions result, depending on the exact location of the cancer. As a rule, the wide excision of the skin and removal of so much subcutaneous fat and fascia will enable the surgeon to approximate the skin margins without employing a skin graft. The excised surgical specimen includes in continuity the primary cancer, the skin overlying it, the subcutaneous tissue and fascia containing the lymphatics intervening between the cancer and the regional nodes, the muscles and deep tissues enveloping the tumor, and all of the fatty, lymphoid, and areolar tissues in the region of the first relay of metastases.

Technique of Radical Groin Dissection

The patient is placed on the table with the corresponding thigh slightly abducted and externally rotated, with the knee slightly flexed over a small sandbag. In the male, the scrotal skin is superficially sutured over the genitals to the opposite groin, in order to withdraw the genitals from the operative field.

The skin incision differs from those previously described by Basset and Taussig inasmuch as it entails the removal of a wide ellipse (Fig. 5). The motives for removal of the skin are that it lessens the possibilities of local skin recurrence, it avoids the almost inevitable death and sloughing of the skin that follow the wide fascial dissection which is to be described, and it hastens wound healing. The upper extremity of the incision is situated 2 inches above and 1 inch medial to the anterior superior iliac spine. From that point it sweeps downward in a wide ellipse and then in a medial direction over the inguinal region, then the femoral trigone, to terminate at its lower extremity in the midthigh overlying Hunter's canal. After the skin edges have been defined by the scalpel, sterile towels are applied to the lateral wound edges by means of numerous tenacula, which are very helpful in facilitating subsequent dissection of fat and fascia from the skin.

With the tenacula elevated, the subcutaneous fat is dissected widely in all directions until the entire upper third or two-fifths of the anterior thigh, the in-

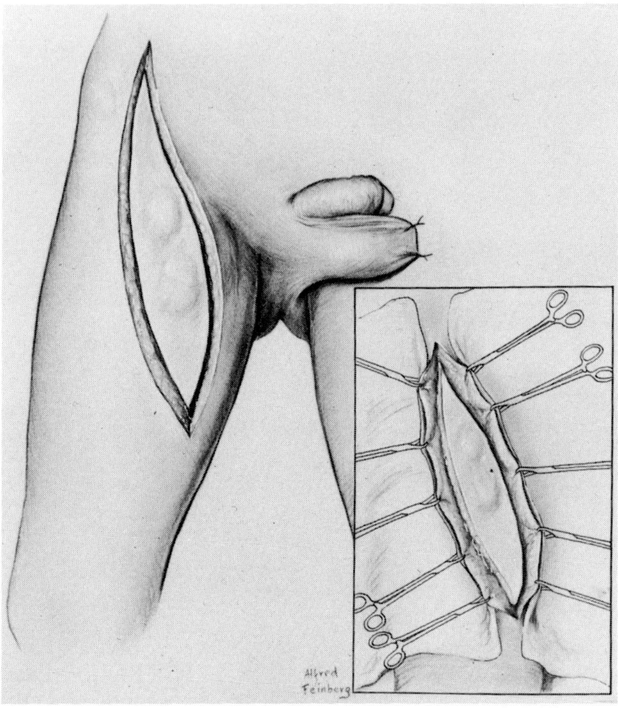

FIGURE 5. Ellipse incision for radical groin dissection. (Figures 5–8 are reproduced by permission from Pack, G. T., and Rekers, P., *Am. J. Surg.* 56:545, June 1942.)

guinal region, and the lower abdominal wall over the iliac quadrant have been denuded of skin. The dissection now continues deep to the underlying muscles, through the fascia, which is dissected with the fat and the lymphoid tissues en bloc in a medial direction. This dissection is started from above downward, exposing the inguinal canal and finally the femoral vessels. The adventitial layer of the artery and vein is stripped together with the fat and fascia intervening between these vessels. The internal saphenous vein is severed and ligated near its junction with femoral vein. The dissection proceeds from above downward, removing all the fascia from the muscles of the anterior thigh (sartorius, iliacus, pectineus, adductor brevis, rectus femoris) (Fig. 6). The sartorius muscle is retracted as the dissection proceeds down through Hunter's canal. The internal saphenous vein is again severed and ligated where it enters the operative field overlying the middle segment of the sartorius muscle. This bulk of tissue is then removed and the first stage of the groin dissection has been completed (Fig. 7).

The second step is now carried out. The inguinal canal is exposed, and incised from the external inguinal ring to the point where the round ligament or spermatic cord dips downward into the pelvic cavity. The canal is further exposed laterally by incising the external oblique fascia and the transversalis muscles down to the properitoneal fat. The occasional lymph node in the inguinal canal is sought for and removed if possible. The external oblique fascia and the inguinal ligament

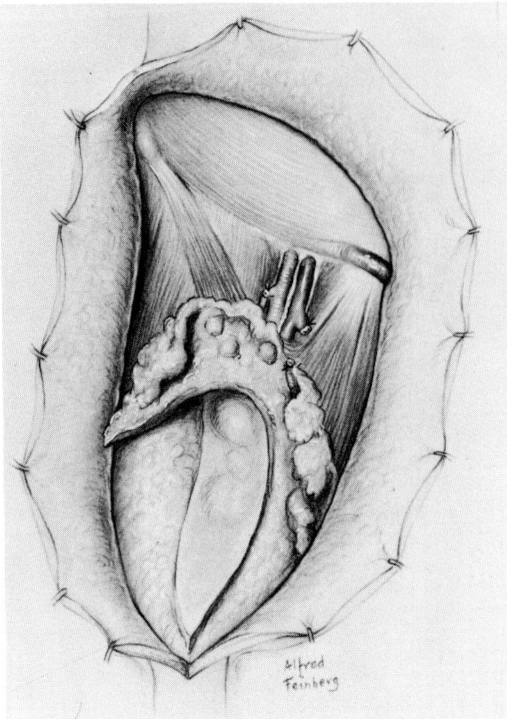

FIGURE 6. Excision of fascia from muscles of anterior thigh.

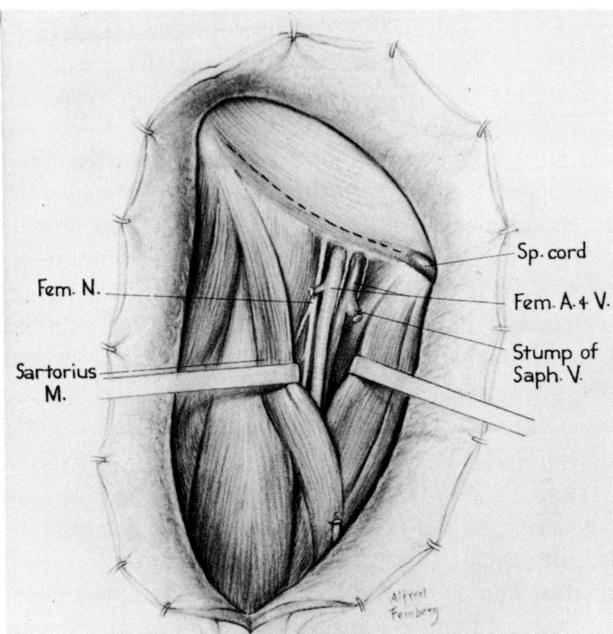

FIGURE 7. Exposure of muscles of anterior thigh and femoral vessels.

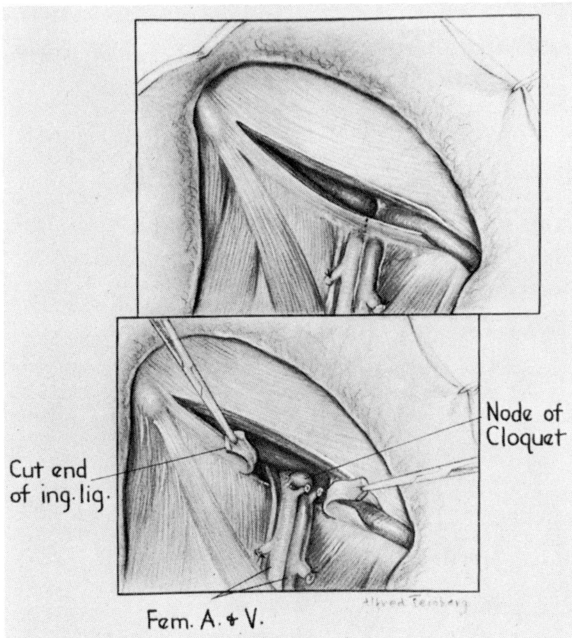

FIGURE 8. Incision of external oblique fascia and inguinal ligament.

are then severed about 2 inches from the anterior superior iliac spine, and the abdominal wall with the ligament is pulled medially after ligation of the deep epigastric vessels. This maneuver opens the femoral ring and improves the exposure of the vessels and lymphoid tissues situated retroperitoneally along the iliac vessels (Fig. 8). The lymph node of Cloquet is usually found resting anteriorly on the femoral vessels just within this ring. To secure even greater exposure, deep retractors are inserted to withdraw the peritoneum and abdominal viscera upward and medially out of the operative field. The peritoneal cavity is not entered during the dissection, which is carried out entirely retroperitoneally. The chain of lymph nodes and the fat and areolar tissue found along the external iliac vessels are dissected from above downward, including the nodes overlying the obturator foramen (Fig. 9). This exposure may be materially aided by preliminary ligation of the deep epigastric vessels where they come off at right angles from the external iliac artery and vein. The entire groin dissection is performed with the scalpel, and at the completion of the operation practically no fat or fascia should be left in the operative field except the normal structures necessary to reconstruct the inguinal ligament and canal.

Some surgeons have stressed a preference for performing the external iliac dissection first, continuing with the inguinal-femoral dissections later. The advantages of this sequence are more theoretical than practical. The completion of the preliminary superficial dissection affords a more adequate exposure, allowing the subsequent or continued deep iliac dissection to be radically performed.

The inguinal canal is then closed in the manner customary for herniorrhaphy.

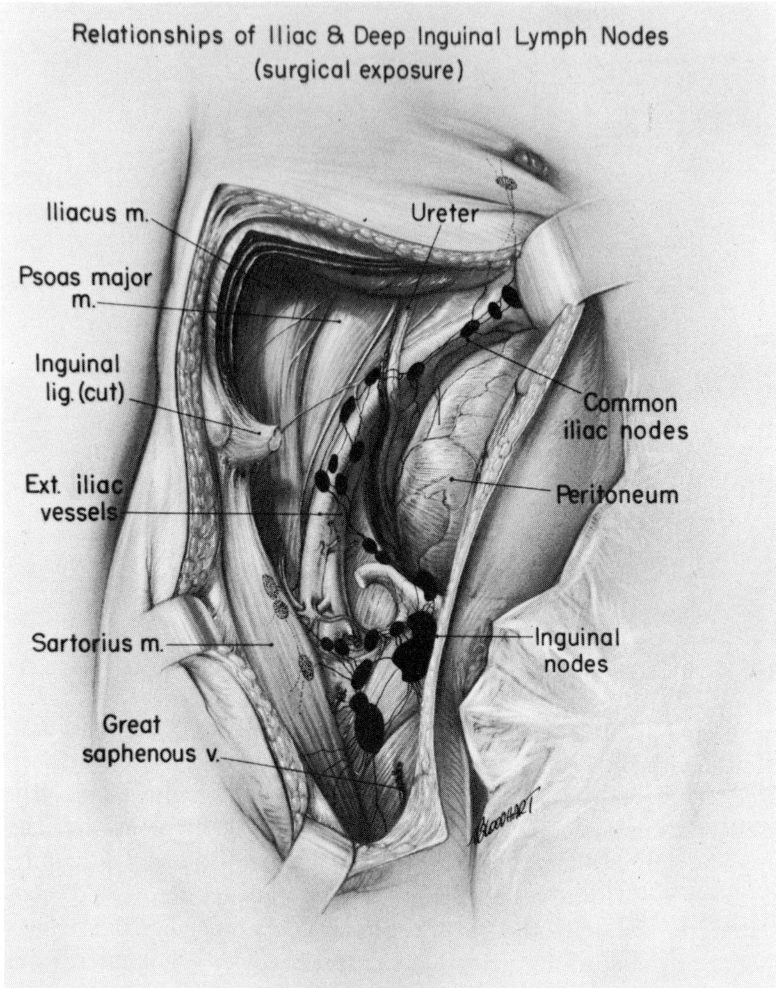

FIGURE 9. Exposure of retroperitoneal area revealing chain of lymph nodes.

The inguinal ligament is reconstructed and sutured around the femoral vessels without occluding them. The sartorius muscle is sometimes slightly sutured medially in an attempt to obliterate the so-called "dead space" of Scarpa's triangle and to protect the femoral vessels more adequately. All bleeding vessels are tied with silk ligatures, a practice which in our experience has greatly lessened the quantity of serous discharge. The serum which accumulates may be removed by aspiration. If the tumor is fungating through the skin or a radiation ulcer is present, catgut ligatures are employed and drainage is established through a standard incision placed in the most dependent portion of the wound on its medial aspect. The skin is usually closed by interrupted silk sutures. Continuous suction through a small sump drain during the immediate postoperative period prevents the accumulation of lymph and serum in the wound.

References

BASSET, A. Traitement chirurgical opératoire de l'épithélioma primitif du clitoris; indications, techniques, résultats. *Rev. chir.* 46:546, July 1912.

DASELER, E. H., ANSON, B. J., and REIMANN, A. F. Radical excision of the inguinal and iliac lymph glands. *Surg., Gynec. and Obst.* 87:679, December 1948.

LEE, E. S. Ilio-inguinal block dissection with primary healing. *Lancet* 2:520, September 10, 1955.

PACK, G. T., and REKERS, P. The management of malignant tumors in the groin. *Am. J. Surg.* 56:545, June 1942.

ROUVIERE, H. *Anatomy of the Human Lymphatic System.* Translated by Tobias. Ann Arbor: Edward Bros., 1938.

XXI. THE KIDNEY, URETER, AND BLADDER

114. Exploration of the Kidney and Nephrectomy

JOHN K. LATTIMER

EXPLORATION and most operations on the kidney, including nephrectomy, can usually be accomplished through a subcostal flank incision with division of the costovertebral ligament. However, still better exposure follows removal of the distal portion of the twelfth rib, with extension of the incision anteriorly. When the segment of rib is removed, the large twelfth intercostal nerve is not usually encountered. The incision can be extended medially, if necessary, with rapidity. Fibers of the eleventh intercostal nerve can be divided with less ill effect than those of the twelfth nerve. It is ordinarily not necessary to extend the incision more medially than the lateral margin of the rectus muscle.

Technique

A subperiosteal resection of the rib can be quickly and easily made. In using the rib-stripping instruments, it is very important not to penetrate too deeply beneath the rib, but to stay directly against its undersurface so that the pleura will not be damaged. It must be remembered that the lowest extension of the pleura reaches the twelfth rib and is almost always present under the posterior half of the rib. Hence the incision into the soft tissues, once the rib has been removed, must be carried caudally, watching carefully for the extension of the pleura and thus avoiding it. The anesthetist can help at this point by hyperventilating the lungs and making them move up and down with vigor. Once the pleura has been identified, the extrapleural space just above the diaphragm toward the back of the patient can be developed by finger dissection. The area directly below the diaphragm can be freed in a similar manner. The diaphragm can then be divided as deeply as is necessary to permit the lower half of the incision to drop away from the upper half, thus exposing the kidney and adrenal areas more thoroughly. Gerota's space should be opened widely and longitudinally, and the peritoneum freed from the undersurface of the abdominal wall and retracted anteriorly with a padded retractor. Efforts should be made not to cut into the pleura or peritoneum, unless it is necessary for greater exposure. Opening these sacs merely prolongs the operation, since they must be closed carefully.

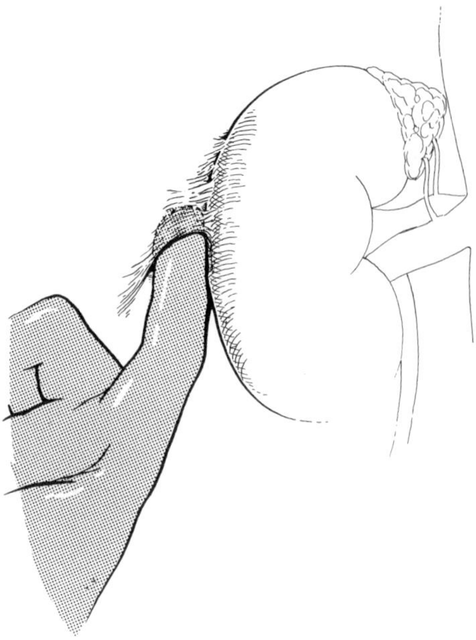

FIGURE 1. Rapid finger dissection can be used to free the kidney on its inferior and lateral surfaces.

If tumor is not suspected, the tissue plane closest to the kidney should be utilized for exposure of all parts of it. The parts most easily seen should be thoroughly freed first by finger dissection, to allow the kidney to drop down into the wound (Fig. 1). The lower pole of the kidney can then be pulled forward to expose the entire organ. The adrenal gland will usually adhere to the kidney, and should be dissected off, watching carefully for a branch from the renal vein into the adrenal gland (Fig. 2). As the kidney poles are freed, they can each be elevated by slings of Penrose drains.

Carcinoma

If a kidney mass is very large, it is wise to open the peritoneum and explore the peritoneal cavity to determine the extent of the mass and to ascertain whether there is any involvement of intraperitoneal structures. With the peritoneum open it is easier to dissect the peritoneal covering away from Gerota's space and its fascial layers.

If the kidney is being removed for tumor, it is advisable to carry the dissection into the region of the renal pedicle as quickly as possible, without disturbing the tumor. Once this is done, either a ligature can be passed around the vessels and tied, or a clamp can be applied and left in place until the dissection of the kidney and tumor mass is complete. Such a maneuver will greatly minimize blood loss during the dissection and prevent the dissemination of tumor cells into the blood stream. Care must be taken to detect any extension of the tumor tissue into the renal vein, which should extend medially and anterior to the aorta. Any thickened tongue of tissue extending into this area should be suspected of being a renal vein containing tumor.

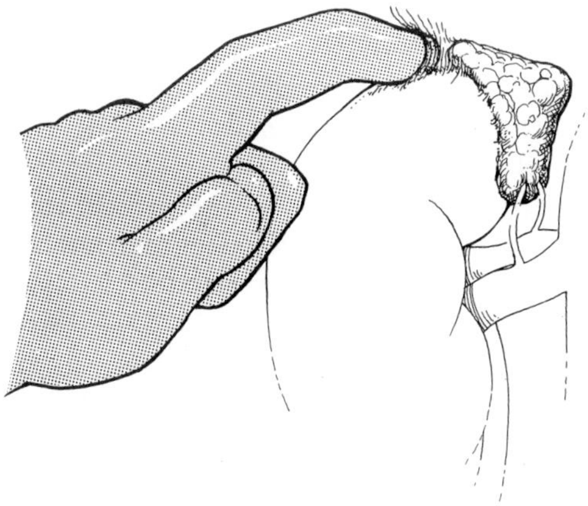

FIGURE 2. The upper pole of the kidney is freed completely from its attachments to the adrenal gland.

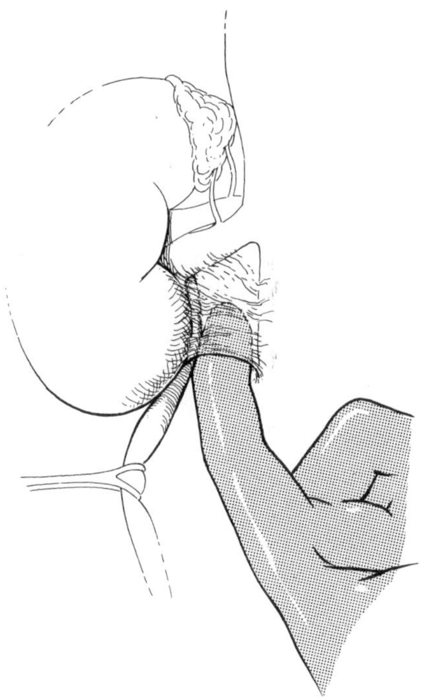

FIGURE 3. Dissection of the medial border of the ureter leads directly into the plane of the kidney pelvis and the renal vessels. Blunt dissection is combined with careful instrument dissection along the medial aspect of the kidney, to detect any aberrant vessels.

The dissection can then be carried around the tumor mass, removing as much of the fat in Gerota's space as possible but staying outside the perirenal fatty capsule. Since the upper part of the tumor mass will rest tightly against the diaphragm, there is little room for removal of a layer of fat in this area, but one should attempt to remove whatever fat is present.

It is wise not to cut the ureter until one is certain that the kidney can be removed. Then the ureter is cut and tied with a single tie of 3–0 chromic catgut and dropped back into the wound. The finger tips are then advanced upward along the upper half of the ureter, seeking a plane that will lead directly to the renal pedicle (Fig. 3). With finger dissection, this plane can usually be established and the layers of fat around the kidney can be removed with it.

Once the great vessels of the kidney have been fairly well isolated so that a pedicle about an inch in length has been developed, an additional "gathering" tie can be placed around the pedicle. When clamps are applied across the pedicle, one must be sure that the tips of the clamps are visible beyond the pedicle, and are not buried deeply in tissue where it will be impossible to get a tie under them (Fig. 4, insert). Three special kidney clamps with striations running longitudinally the full length of the jaws should be applied to the pedicle. If three clamps are applied, the pedicle can be cut between the two clamps closest to the kidney, after squeezing all clamp locks tightly to the last notch. It must be remembered that many of these pedicles will be under tension; hence, when the pedicle is cut, the stumps of the vessels will tend to spring medially and upward away from the operator, and may be lost to sight momentarily. Massive bleeding from the cut pedicle could be disastrous. Therefore, extra time is well spent developing the longest renal pedicle possible (Fig. 4). In general, it is not necessary to isolate and tie the artery and vein separately, since the incidence of arteriovenous fistulas in kidney pedicles which have been subjected to "mass" ligation is very low. The pedicle should be triply ligated with double sutures of No. 2 chromic catgut. This catgut is so heavy that there is little danger it will break and jerk the short pedicle out of the clamps, and it is so broad that it is unlikely to cut through the pedicle.

Massive hemorrhage, which might result if an arteriosclerotic renal artery or vein were to tear or be pulled away from the great vessels by some accident, may be checked initially with a large pad or towel, pressed into the wound with force and held there for about five minutes, in order to give the stumps of the vessels

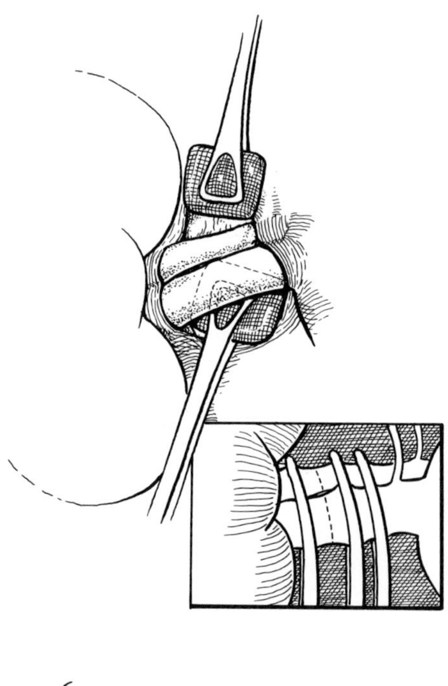

FIGURE 4. If nephrectomy is to be done, the vascular pedicle is freed to its maximum by dissecting and wiping away the covering tissues. *Insert:* When clamps are applied to the pedicle, the points must be seen to lie free of any soft tissue before the clamps are closed.

a chance to contract. If the rent is in the great vessels, pressure can be applied above and below the rent, and held for several minutes while transfusion and supportive measures are started. Then the margin of the pack may be moved away slowly until the bleeding point is located. It is dangerous to plunge into a bleeding pedicle area with clamps, because of the proximity of the duodenum, which may be caught in the points of such clamps. If the bleeding occurs after the renal artery has been cut, spasm of the end of the vessels and the drop in blood pressure will often check the bleeding. It is then easy to find the vessel and apply clamps.

If a renal tumor has adhered to any of the surrounding structures, the areas of the adhesion should also be removed, if possible. Even if the adherent areas look quite innocent, they should be removed, because of the possibility that tumor cells may be present.

It is our practice to drain all kidney incisions, because the escape of blood along the drain enables early detection of hemorrhage from the pedicle. If the urinary tract has been opened (even by the cutting of the ureter), the wound should be drained for several days. We close the abdominal wall in four anatomical layers, using continuous sutures of 0 chromic catgut, reinforced with two or three interrupted sutures, in each layer.

In particularly difficult cases, the "Nagamatsu approach" to the kidney may be utilized. The twelfth rib is removed and portions of the tenth and eleventh ribs are excised so that the chest wall can be rolled up like a venetian blind.

A thoracoabdominal approach is usually unnecessary for removing kidney masses, since a long abdominal incision, opening the peritoneum as well, is usually adequate. In closing any of these long incisions, it is well to place a row of interrupted sutures in the posterior angle of the incision before starting the remainder of the closure. This makes it easier to close the posterior angle portion of the wound without the risk of catching the pleura in the sutures.

Tuberculosis

When nephrectomy is done for tuberculosis, it is wise to divide the ureter last, after the vascular pedicle has been isolated and cut. The ureter can be followed upward to the lower portion of the vascular pedicle to find the proper plane of cleavage. The kidney should be brought out the anterior end of the abdominal incision with the ureter intact. The abdominal wound can then be closed around the ureter. After the abdominal incision has been completely closed and covered with protective padding, the ureter is transected between clamps, with a carbolized knife, leaving a stump one-half inch in length protruding through the skin. It must be remembered that the ureter may be under tension and will retract somewhat if it is released. A clamp can be left on the stump, which is attached to the skin by a few sutures of 3–0 plain catgut, for about five days and then removed. After removal of the clamp, the stump will drain for several days and will finally recede under the skin, which will heal completely. This maneuver prevents drainage of material from the end of the ureter into the depths of the wound and the formation of wound abscesses.

Papillary Tumor of the Renal Pelvis

If one is dealing with a papillary tumor of the renal pelvis, a complete nephroureterectomy should be done, including a cuff of the bladder, which should be opened to be sure the cuff is procured. If there is any doubt as to the diagnosis between papillary tumor and a radiolucent stone, and palpation of the unopened pelvis discloses no hard (stone) area, then nephrectomy may be elected, since papillary tumor cells implant into wounds readily.

Other Conditions

If the kidney has been explored for an equivocal mass, it may be cut into for biopsy and frozen section, and the pelvis or renal sinus may be opened to permit an exploring finger both inside and outside the kidney, simultaneously.

Very large hydronephrotic kidneys should be decompressed to uncover the pedicle more readily and to allow more precise evaluation of the amount of kidney tissue remaining, with a view to salvaging it.

Pyonephroses should be approached extraperitoneally and extrapleurally, when possible, to avoid contamination of the peritoneal and pleural cavities.

Calculous disease may require nephrectomy in the rare case in which long-standing obstruction or infection has brought about excessive destruction of a kidney; but nephrolithotomy is usually preferable if such conditions are not present.

References

NAGAMATSU, G. R. Dorso-lumbar approach to the kidney and adrenal with osteoplastic flap. *J. Urol.* 63:569, April 1950.

NAGAMATSU, G. R., LERMAN, P. H., and BERMAN, M. H. The dorso-lumbar flap incision in urologic surgery. *J. Urol.* 67:787, June 1952.

115. *Ileocystoplasty*

WILLARD E. GOODWIN

ENLARGEMENT OF THE BLADDER to increase its capacity, by attaching a segment of ileum, is a valuable and useful procedure in properly selected cases. It should be reserved for patients who have discomfort due to irreversibly small bladder capacity. It probably should not be done in the presence of malignant disease of the bladder. It is contraindicated in patients with obstructive lesions of the urethra, or neurological disease producing inability to empty the bladder. It is ideally suited to patients with contracted bladders due to tuberculosis, interstitial cystitis, or late results of irradiation or trauma.

Several different techniques for enlarging the bladder with segments of ileum have been described and employed by various authors (Fig. 1). We have had favorable experience with the use of the "cup-patch" technique described here, in which a segment of ileum is opened on its antimesenteric border and then sutured together in such a fashion as to form a "cup-like patch" which is attached to the dome of the bladder. This has the advantage of acting as a unified patch on the bladder and emptying normally without forming a diverticulum, or retaining urine.

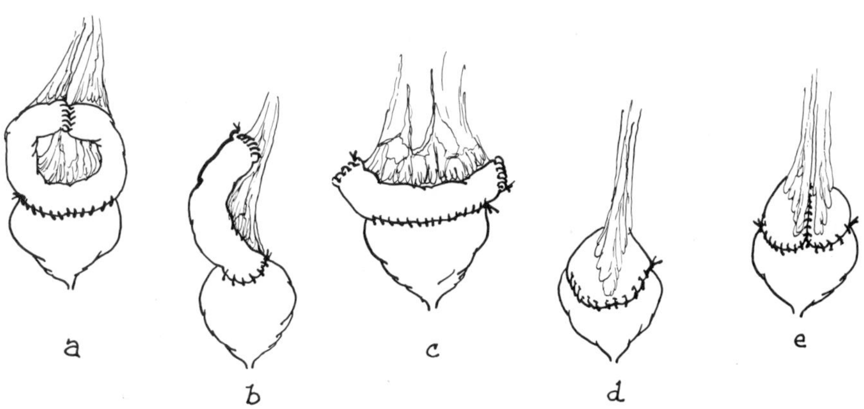

FIGURE 1. Types of ileocystoplasty. The type described in the text is type *e*.

As in other operations in which the ileum is employed to augment the urinary tract, it is desirable to prepare the bowel with a low residue diet and neomycin by mouth during the two days before the operation. Nasogastric suction is used before and after the operation to decompress the bowel.

Technique

The abdomen is opened through a generous lower midline incision. A transverse incision may be employed if desired, but the midline incision gives excellent exposure and allows more ease in handling the ileum.

Dissection of the Bladder

The prevesical space is developed and the bladder is dissected free on both sides in order to increase the ease of managing it. When possible, peritoneal flaps are stripped away from the back of the bladder so that the bladder is mobilized out of the pelvis. This is particularly important in cases in which there is long-standing fibrous change and the bladder is small and contracted, lying deep in the pelvis. The bladder is opened near the dome on its anterior surface and a generous biopsy specimen of the dome of the bladder is taken in order to get adequate information as to the nature of the fundamental disease. Both ureteral orifices are catheterized for identification. The posterior portion of the incision is carried down to a point about 2 cm. above the trigone. It is important not to go below this point, because of the danger of injuring the ureters or obstructing them. This dissection then leaves the bladder open along its dome from a point just above the trigone across the dome and downward on its anterior surface. The anterior portion of this incision is not carried to the vesical neck, because of difficulty in bringing the ileum down so far during closure. Bleeding points on the bladder are clamped and ligated, and the bladder is then packed off with a large dry sponge to await its use later in the operation. There is some advantage in doing the dissection of the bladder at the beginning of the procedure, as the surgeon thereby gains an idea of the size of the opening in the dome of the bladder with which he will later deal. Also it allows minor bleeding points to coagulate before the final closure is carried out.

Isolation of a Segment of Ileum

Following this dissection, a segment of terminal ileum is isolated in a routine fashion as is done for other operations in which the ileum is employed in urological surgery. A segment 25 to 30 cm. in length is used, with particular care to preserve the blood supply of the mesentery of the ileal segment (Fig. 2). This loop of ileum is usually taken from a point about 25 cm. proximal to the ileocecal valve. Normal continuity of the ileum is re-established by routine ileoileostomy.

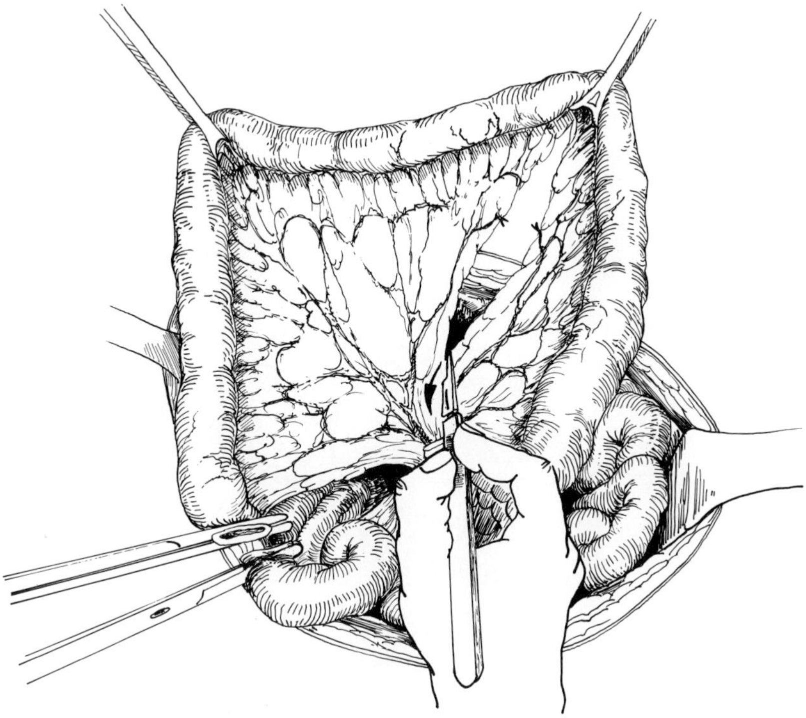

FIGURE 2. A suitable segment of terminal ileum is isolated with careful attention to preserving its blood supply.

The Ileocystoplasty

At this point the ileocystoplasty begins. The ileal segment is irrigated with saline and neomycin solution to cleanse it of any fecal material and mucus that may be present. Then it is boldly opened on its antimesenteric border along its whole length (Fig. 3a). This leaves a large, flat piece of opened ileum with its mesentery intact. There may be considerable bleeding from these cut edges, but no attention is paid to any but the largest bleeders, as the bleeding will be controlled by subsequent suturing.

Following this, the opened segment is fashioned in the shape of a U (Fig. 3b). The medial margins of the ileum are sewed together, using continuous 3–0 chromic catgut suture. This suture line may be placed either inside or outside of what is to be the lumen of the new bladder. It is usually easier to do it from inside. It is helpful to hold the ileum stretched out by using traction sutures at the bottom and on the two upper ends of the U-shaped segment of ileum. This allows more accurate suturing. The suturing is done in such a way as to produce hemostasis along the cut margin.

After this first suture line has been completed, the U-shaped piece of ileum makes a large, flat flap. This is again sutured on itself from top to bottom, in such a way as to make a cup-like structure which will form the dome of the new bladder

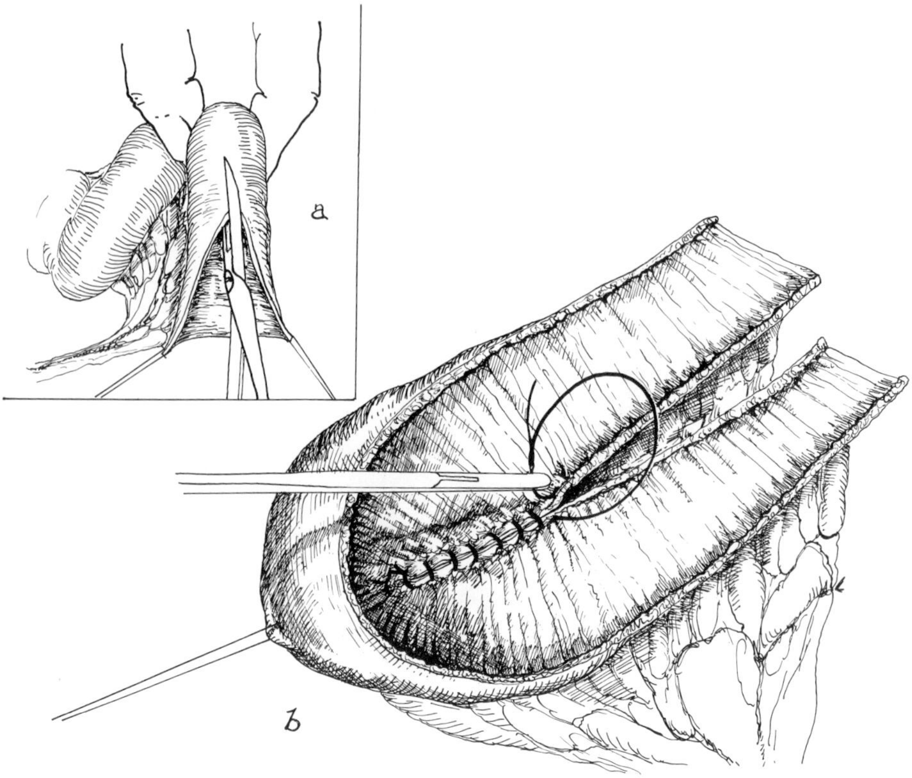

FIGURE 3. The ileum is opened boldly on its antimesenteric margin, creating a long, flat graft which is then formed into a U and sutured together along its medial margin.

(Fig. 4). The second suture line may again be started from the inside, but toward the end it is easier to complete the suturing from the outside. Chromic catgut (3–0) is used again as a continuous suture. After the suturing is complete, there is a cup-like structure with the mesentery of the ileum forming a kind of curved pedicle. When this closure is done properly, there is no further bleeding from the cut edges, the graft is completely viable, and the suture lines are watertight.

At this point, the dome-like new bladder is ready for anastomosis to the opened urinary bladder. It is gently mobilized downward until it can be brought into the pelvis. It is important in the beginning of the procedure to check the length of the mesentery to be certain that the loop of ileum that is used has a long enough mesentery to reach to the top of the urinary bladder without difficulty. The ileal segment lies posterior to the reanastomosis of the normal ileum, and its mesentery extends downward from the root of the mesentery of the normal ileum. The new cup-shaped ileal bladder lies just in front of the rectosigmoid. This cup-like structure is then pulled out of the peritoneal cavity into the pelvis until its cut margins lie extraperitoneally next to the bladder.

Anastomosis to the bladder is then begun (Fig. 5); 3–0 catgut is used. However, in this case a row of interrupted 2–0 chromic catgut sutures is placed along

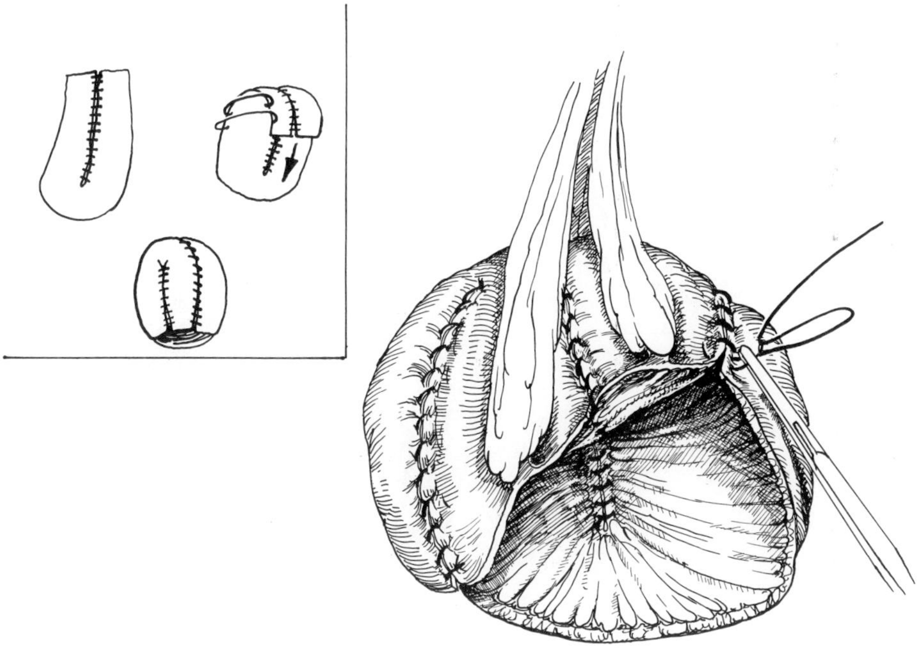

FIGURE 4. After the U has been fashioned to make a still larger flat graft, it is again sewed together from top to bottom, producing a cup-like patch which will be used as the dome of the new bladder.

the base of the bladder and the base of the new ileal cap to reinforce the suture line. After these have been placed, the anastomosis of ileal bladder to the urinary bladder is completed. It is easier to do this from inside the lumen of the bladder. Because it is important not to place the suture line too close to the ureteral orifices, the ureteral catheters should remain in place during the initial suturing in order not to compromise the ureters (Fig. 5).

The ileum is then sewed around the margins of the bladder, with careful approximation of mucosa to mucosa in the anastomosis. There may be some "dog-ears" of ileal tissue. If these are present, they may be excised and closed (Fig. 6). The posterior side of the anastomosis is completed first, leaving the anterior opening in the bladder to be attached to the ileum. All layers of bowel and bladder are brought together with this single suture line.

At this point it is important to place catheters for adequate drainage of the new bladder during the immediate postoperative period. There is often an unusual amount of mucus after such an operation, and it is advisable to have at least two catheters draining the bladder so that drainage will continue if either should become obstructed. A urethral catheter is introduced from inside out by passing a No. 20 red rubber catheter from inside the bladder outward through the urethra. Then the distal end of a Malecot catheter is led from inside outward through the urethra to follow the red rubber catheter and establish urethral catheter drainage. A second Malecot catheter is introduced through a stab wound in the anterior wall

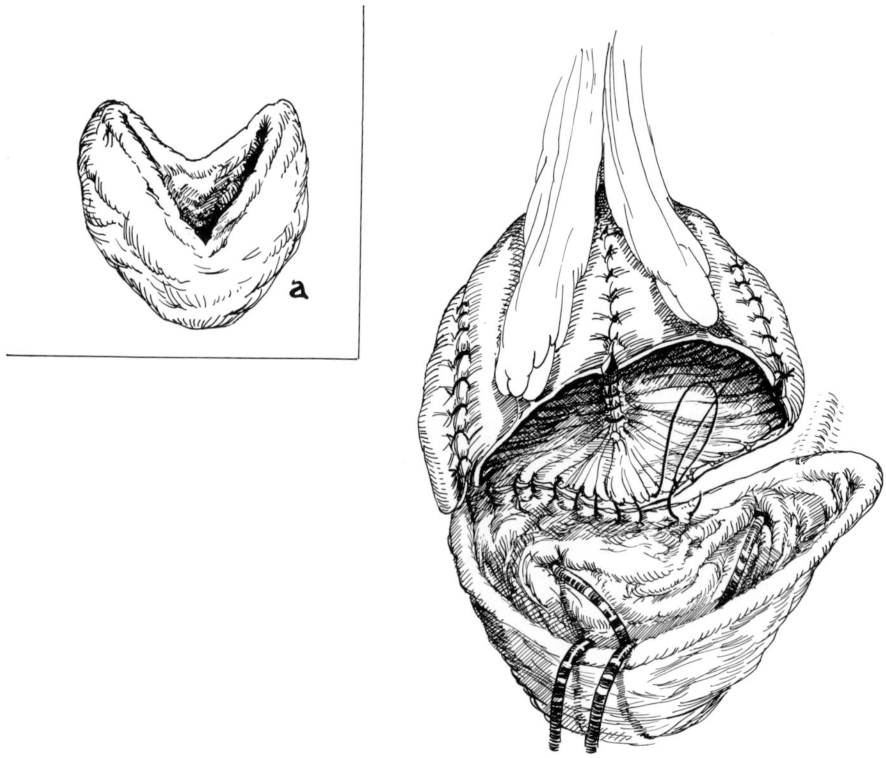

FIGURE 5. The cup-like ileal bladder is brought down to the opened dome of the urinary bladder and sutured to it. Ureteral orifices are identified by ureteral catheters.

of the bladder. This often has to be placed fairly low, toward the vesical neck. It is usually placed to the left or right of the midline and brought out through a stab wound in the lower quadrant.

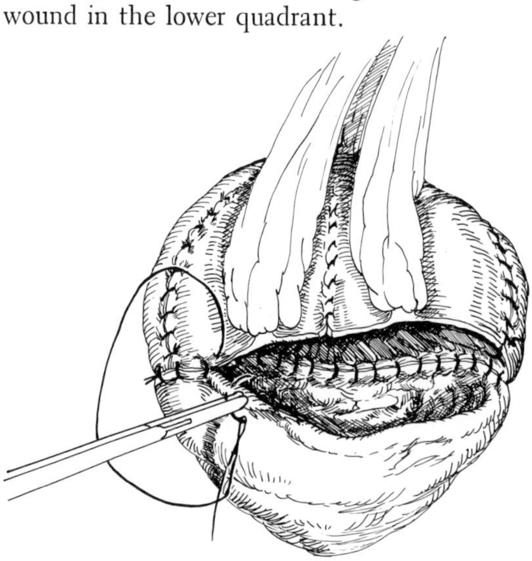

FIGURE 6. "Dog-ears" may be excised and closed, although this is not necessary.

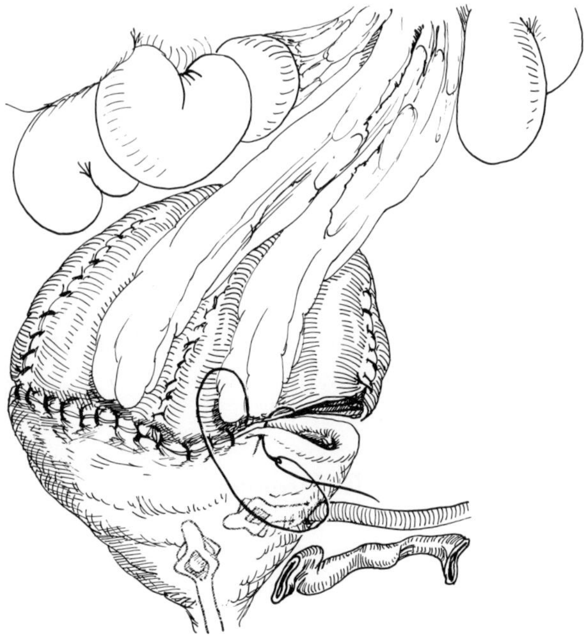

FIGURE 7. The "cup-patch" ileal bladder is mobilized further downward and sutured to the anterior opening in the dome of the bladder. Before closure is completed, urethral and suprapubic catheters are carefully placed.

The ureteral catheters are removed, and closure of the new bladder is completed from the outside (Fig. 7). If there is tension at the most distal portion anteriorly, it may be advisable to place additional stay sutures as a second layer. There is a difficult point at the most distal portion of this suture line where a kind of V develops. However, this is easily closed with careful attention.

General Comments

Postoperatively the key to the situation is to keep the bladder nearly empty of urine while healing takes place. It is assumed that the suture lines are probably not watertight, and catheter drainage is important.

In patients with interstitial cystitis and painful bladders, we have found it valuable to incorporate presacral neurectomy at the same time as ileocystoplasty. When this is done, it must be completed before the ileum is sewed to the bladder.

Once the new bladder is closed, the suture lines all lie extraperitoneally. The flaps of peritoneum may be brought upward loosely around the mesentery of the new ileal bladder. They are fixed with a few interrupted fine catgut sutures to the serosa of the ileum, insuring extraperitonealization of the suture lines of the new ileal bladder. Great care must be employed not to injure or distort the blood supply to the new ileal bladder.

In the beginning we were worried about the fact that there was a potential cavity behind the mesentery of the ileum which might act as a trap for loops of bowel. However, in this procedure it is impossible to obliterate this area, and nothing has been done about it. So far we have not seen complications from this source.

At the end of the procedure the omentum is mobilized as much as possible and pulled downward around the vascular pedicle of the new ileal bladder. It is then gently draped around the point where the bladder leaves the peritoneum, to add a further seal in the process of extraperitonealization of the new bladder.

The prevesical space is drained with Penrose drains on either side, usually brought out through stab wounds. The wound is closed in a routine fashion. Stay sutures are employed.

References

Goodwin, W. E., Winter, C. C., and Barker, W. F. "Cup-patch" technique of ileocystoplasty for bladder enlargement or partial substitution. *Surg., Gynec. and Obst.* 108:240, February 1959.

Goodwin, W. E., Turner, R. D., and Winter, C. C. Results of ileocystoplasty. *J. Urol.* 80:461, December 1958.

116. Replacement of the Ureter by Small Intestine

WILLARD E. GOODWIN

WHEN ONE OR BOTH URETERS have been damaged and it is impossible to restore the normal continuity of the urinary tract by using urinary tract tissues, it is technically possible and desirable to replace the ureter with an isolated segment of small intestine. This procedure, first performed in 1906 by Schumaker in an 18-year-old girl, was used rarely until about 1953 or 1954, when it was revived. Since then, it has been used successfully by a number of surgeons and has achieved general acceptance as a mode of restoring the irreparably damaged upper urinary tract in selected cases. The surgical technique is exacting and requires skill and imagination. Nonetheless, when it is properly and successfully performed, results are gratifying.

Technique

General Considerations

It is my preference to give a 24- or 48-hour bowel preparation with oral neomycin immediately preceding the operation. The small bowel should be decompressed by a nasogastric tube.

The isolated ileal segment is prepared in a routine manner. Several special precautions should be noted. (1) The segment of ileum should be slightly longer than is required. With a piece of suture material used as a measure, it is possible to calculate the exact distance that the segment is intended to fill. Toward the end of the procedure redundant portions of ileum may be excised and discarded. It is easy to make the ileal segment shorter, but very difficult to stretch a too short segment. (2) The segment must have a good blood supply, including a broad arcade in the mesentery. (3) The ultimate length of the segment should be the shortest possible to cover the required distance. Loops of bowel which are too long or redundant present the danger of absorption of urinary constituents and do not drain as well as segments that are exactly the right length. From 25 to 30 cm. is the optimum length for most total ureteral replacement operations. After the upper anastomoses are complete, it is often possible to remove excess ileum before completing the lower anastomosis. (4) The isolated segment should be obtained from a part of the ileum 25 cm. or more from the cecum.

When the segment has been isolated and the normal continuity of the ileum has been restored by reanastomosis, the loop, which now lies *below* the ileoileostomy, should be irrigated gently with saline and a warm solution of neomycin to wash out excess mucus and fecal material.

It is helpful to tag the distal end of the segment with a small suture for identification so that there is no confusion in establishing an *isoperistaltic* loop of bowel.

Exposure

In procedures of this type, in which a segment of intestine must be isolated and then later used to establish normal urinary tract continuity, it is often necessary to have perfect visualization and control of the kidney, the renal pelvis, the ureter, and the bladder, and in some cases to be able to see both sides. It is important to have maximum exposure. Our preference is a long midline incision from the xyphoid process to the symphysis pubis if both sides are involved. If only a single side is to be repaired, an elongated flank incision starting as a conventional kidney incision under the twelfth rib and extending medially to the lateral margin of the rectus abdominis muscle and then downward to the symphysis gives excellent exposure. The importance and value of perfect exposure for these long and sometimes complicated procedures cannot be overemphasized.

It is helpful to have a ureteral catheter in place to aid in identifying the ureter. This may be most simply placed by opening the bladder and passing it upward from the ureteral orifice under direct vision. This may be done early in the procedure, as it is an advantage to have the bladder open later at the time of the ileovesical anastomosis.

In patients with an established nephrostomy, it is sometimes helpful to pass a clamp through the nephrostomy opening into the renal pelvis in order to aid in identification of the pelvis from inside the abdomen.

The ileal segment may lie either intraperitoneally or extraperitoneally, depending on which seems easier and simpler. In general when the operation is for replacement of one ureter only, it is easier to make a "window" in the posterior peritoneum through the mesentery of the large bowel on either side and place the ileal segment in the retroperitoneal gutter. If it is necessary to replace both ureters, the ileum must lie intraperitoneally for part of this procedure.

Replacement of the Right Ureter

The cecum and ascending colon are mobilized medially and the ileum, with its mesentery, is passed laterally into the retroperitoneal space through a window in

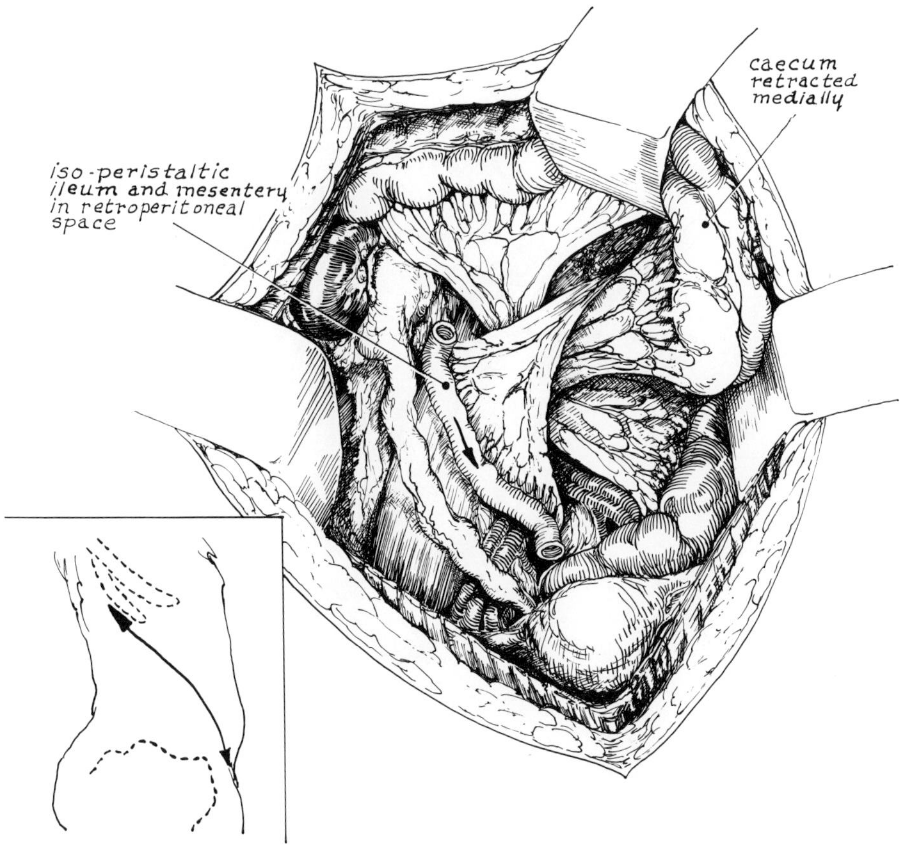

FIGURE 1. Technique of replacement of the right ureter.

the mesentery of the ascending colon. To achieve an isoperistaltic direction, it is necessary to perform a 90-degree rotation of the ileum on its mesentery (Fig. 1).

The lower end of the ileal segment crosses the iliac vessels at the same place that the ureter would cross them, and is led into the retroperitoneal area behind the back of the bladder (behind the round ligament in females).

Replacement of the Left Ureter

Replacement on the left side should probably always be done extraperitoneally so that the lower end of the ileum can pass into the back of the bladder without crossing over the sigmoid colon. The descending and sigmoid colon are mobilized medially by blunt dissection, and the space where the ureter lies in the left retroperitoneal gutter is developed. A window is made in the mesentery of the descending colon, and the isolated ileal segment is pulled through it so that it lies naturally in the retroperitoneal space. In this case it is not necessary to rotate the ileum, although there is a mild upward swing of the mesentery. It is important not to

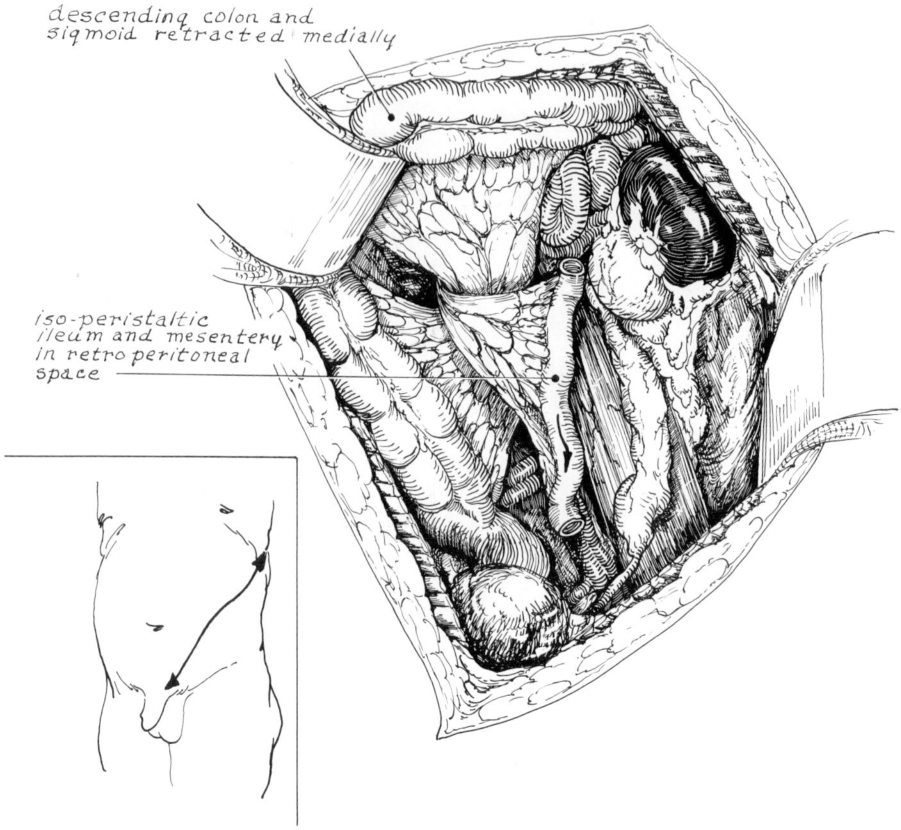

FIGURE 2. Technique of left ureteral replacement.

produce undue tension on the mesentery or to constrict it by having the window too small (Fig. 2).

Replacement of Both Ureters

In this situation it is usually simpler to have the urinary flow go from left to right to bladder (Fig. 3). Under some circumstances, we have established the flow in the opposite direction, from right to left to bladder. In either case, it must be isoperistaltic. The upper left ureter is identified in the retroperitoneal space, isolated, and brought through the mesentery of the descending colon, where it is anastomosed to the upper end of the ileum. The upper end of the ileum is first closed with continuous chromic catgut, placed as an inverting suture.

The ileal segment is then led across the midline to the region of the right ureter slightly below the point where it was anastomosed on the left side. Anastomosis of the ureter to the ileum is performed intraperitoneally after the right ureter has been led into the peritoneal cavity. It is then necessary to do a twisting type of rotation of the lower portion of the ileum in order to lead it as an iso-

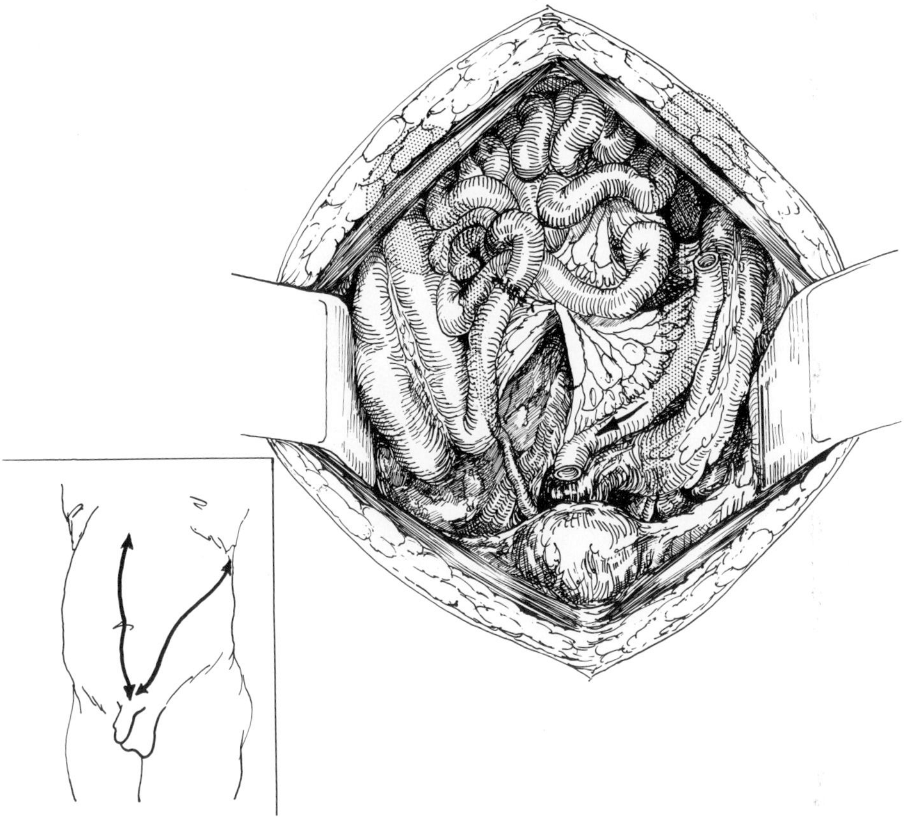

FIGURE 3. A long midline incision from the xyphoid process to the symphysis pubis is used for bilateral ureteral replacement. Left ureteral replacement started.

peristaltic segment downward to the back of the bladder, where it must then go extraperitoneally in order to be anastomosed to the back of the bladder.

In one case we led a loop from right to left to bladder after placing the whole ileal segment retroperitoneally by blunt dissection. This is technically possible in a patient in whom the retroperitoneal tissues have not been severely damaged by scar tissue and urinary extravasation. It would be difficult, if not impossible, in a patient who had previous retroperitoneal fibrotic changes from urinary extravasation. When the ileum is used from right to left to bladder, it is necessary to rotate it on its mesentery almost 180 degrees so that the most distal portion of the segment points downward to the bladder.

Anastomosis of the Ureter or Pelvis to an Isolated Loop of Ileum

The ureter is spatulated and attached to an opening on the antimesenteric border of the ileum as in Bricker's operation. Either interrupted or continuous sutures may be used. My preference is continuous sutures of 4–0 chromic catgut which are tied at each end in order to prevent a purse-string effect (Fig. 4). One or two

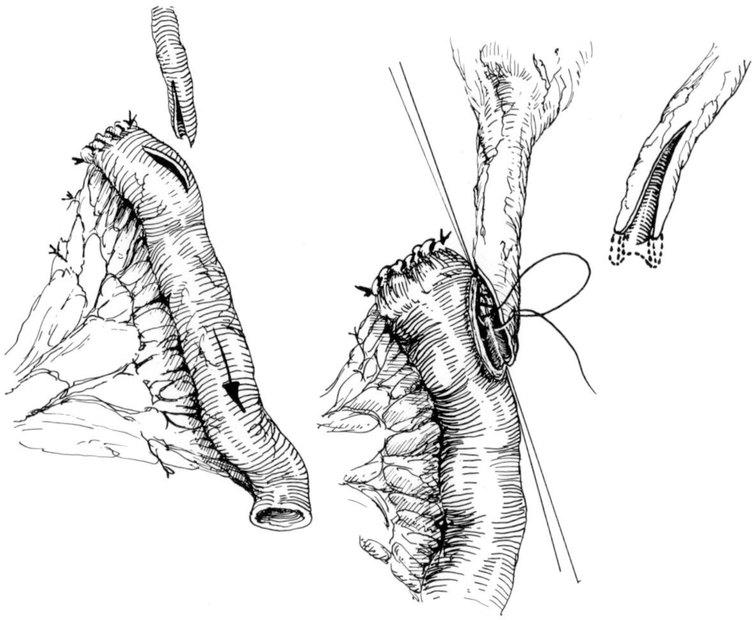

FIGURE 4. Technique of ureteroileal anastomosis. Atraumatic sutures of 4–0 chromic catgut are used.

stay sutures of heavier catgut may be employed to prevent tension on the suture line. Silk should not be used in the urinary tract because of the danger of calculus formation.

If the anastomosis is to be made from the pelvis to the upper end of the ileal loop, it is important to have the pelvis well mobilized before one attempts anastomosis. Great care must be exercised not to injure the renal vascular supply. The upper end of the ileal segment is left open and is cut along its antimesenteric border to make a long spatulated opening which will exactly fit the open renal pelvis. An attempt should be made to do the anastomosis in such a way that there is no pelvis lying redundant below the ileal segment. The stoma of the ileum extends downward to include the old area of the previous ureteropelvic junction. This anastomosis may be carried out with 3–0 or 4–0 chromic catgut, used either as continuous or interrupted sutures (Fig. 5).

In a few cases, we have opened the renal pelvis and lower calyces widely and anastomosed a long spatulated end of ileum to the opened lower half of the kidney along its medial surface (Fig. 6). When this is done, it is important to produce hemostasis in the cut surface of the kidney with interrupted catgut sutures. The anastomosis of the ileum to the widely opened pelvis is done with continuous chromic catgut sutures tied in several places to prevent a purse-string effect. All layers of ileum are anastomosed to the renal pelvis. Supporting sutures, from the outside of the ileum to the surrounding kidney, are placed to prevent tension and to try to establish a watertight closure.

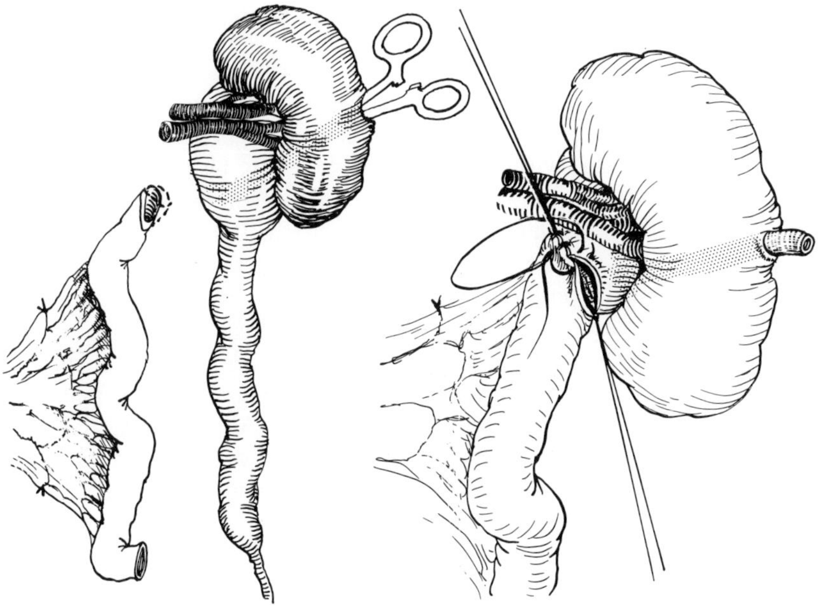

FIGURE 5. Technique of anastomosis of the renal pelvis to the upper end of an ileal segment.

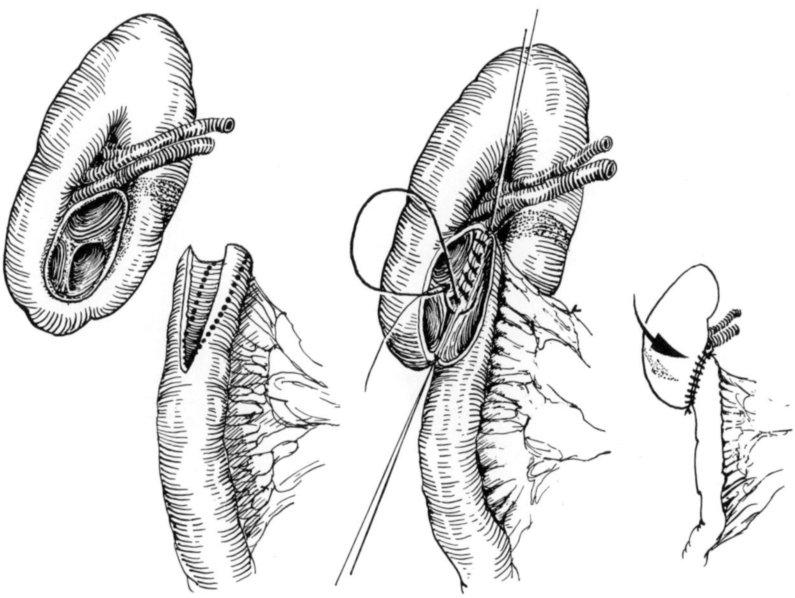

FIGURE 6. Technique of anastomosis of the lower half of the kidney and pelvis to a spatulated loop of ileum (operation devised for patients with recurrent staghorn calculi).

Anastomosis of the Lower End of the Ileum to the Bladder (Ileovesical Anastomosis)

The lower anastomosis is most conveniently done from inside the bladder. The extraperitoneal, retrovesical area should be developed by blunt dissection. It is usually possible to do this without too much difficulty, by using the index finger of either hand and working downward to the back of the bladder, with the other hand inside the bladder for identification of position. If there is extreme scarring from previous surgery, this may not be possible, and the anastomosis may have to be made higher on the posterior wall of the bladder. In any case, a space should be developed outside the peritoneum in order to do this.

After the lowest portion behind the bladder has been developed, the finger in the retrovesical position pushes upward to "tent up" the bladder in that area. The elevated bladder wall is grasped from within with an Allis forceps, and a circular window is cut out of all layers of the posterior bladder wall. It is very important to do this in order to prevent later stricture. After the window has been cut in the posterior bladder wall, it is possible to pass a finger from outside the bladder inside, marking the position where the ileum will lie.

Following this, a Babcock clamp is passed from inside the bladder outward, to grasp the lower end of the ileum, which is pulled into the bladder so that the distal end of the ileum now lies inside the bladder (Fig. 7).

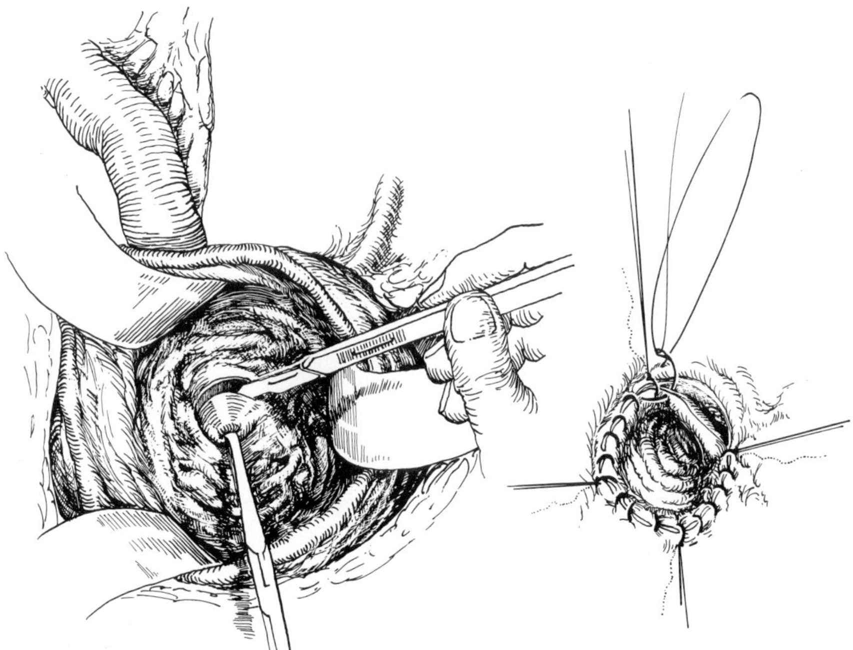

FIGURE 7. Technique of anastomosis of the lower end of the ileal ureter to the bladder. Note the cutting of the window in the base of the bladder, and that the anastomosis is placed as low as possible next to the trigone.

At this point, excess ileum is pulled into the bladder until the ileal segment lies in as straight a line as possible from the upper urinary tract to the bladder. It is important not to produce tension. Yet it is equally important not to leave redundant ileum. The ileum is then cut transversely, and the open end is sutured to the bladder with several interrupted chromic catgut sutures. This incision is carried around to the mesentery, and the redundant ileum is then resected. Bleeding points on the excess mesentery are ligated with fine silk sutures. The excess mesentery which lies inside the bladder is then pushed outward to lie in the extravesical space next to the ileum. Closure is completed by suturing the rest of the ileum to the bladder all the way around. Sutures include all layers of bowel and bladder.

General Comments

Ureteral splints and catheters may or may not be used. In any event, it is difficult to keep them in place. It is advisable in all ureteroileal anastomoses of this type to have urinary diversion above the point of the anastomosis. This can be established by a nephrostomy tube or ureterostomy.

The bladder is drained with a suprapubic or urethral catheter or both. It is my preference to use both, because during the immediate postoperative period there is often an excess accumulation of mucous material from the freshly handled ileum. This tends to plug catheters and causes urinary leakage. The use of two catheters in the bladder decreases this danger.

The mobilized colon is allowed to drop back into the normal position, covering the new ileal ureter. Closure is carried out in a routine fashion. If the ileum lies inside the peritoneal cavity, as in replacement of both ureters, it must be placed in as straight a line as possible. The mesentery of the ileal segment should be tacked down to the posterior peritoneum so that there will not be any pocket which might allow herniation of loops of bowel.

The bladder is closed in a routine fashion, using interrupted catgut sutures. The various sites of anastomosis are drained. A Penrose drain is usually placed near the region of the ileovesical anastomosis and brought out through a separate stab wound. The abdomen is closed in a routine fashion, with stay sutures used as an added precaution.

Postoperative Management

During the postoperative period, it is important to be certain that catheters remain open and do not become plugged with mucus. Nasogastric decompression should be continued for several days until bowel sounds are heard. Because of stretching of the isolated ileal segment in this type of procedure, there is often prolonged paralytic ileus. It is important not to feed the patient until this period is passed.

After healing is complete, usually in about 10 days, it is possible to clamp off the nephrostomy tube and allow the new urinary tract, partially composed of the ileal segment, to function. In some cases, edema persists, and there is no harm in leaving the nephrostomy drainage for a longer period. The suprapubic and/or urethral catheters may be removed after the tenth day.

When isolated segments of ileum are used as part of the urinary tract, it is important to be certain that the patient is in good condition, and does not have uremia, before embarking on the procedure. It is also important to follow serum electrolytes postoperatively to be certain that acidosis and hyperchloremia do not develop. Hyperkalemia has been reported as an added potential hazard, and serum potassium levels should therefore be obtained.

References

GOODWIN, W. E., WINTER, C. C., and TURNER, R. D. Replacement of the ureter by small intestine: clinical application and results of the "ileal ureter." *J. Urol.* 81:406, March 1959.

GOODWIN, W. E., and CROCKETT, A. T. K. Surgical treatment of multiple, recurrent, branched, renal (staghorn) calculi by pyelo-nephro-ileo-vesical anastomosis. *Tr. Am. A. Genito-Urin. Surgeons* 52:102, 1960.

GOODWIN, W. E. Replacement of the ureter by small intestine—the ileal ureter. In Riches, E., *Modern Trends in Urology* (Second Series). London: Butterworths, 1960.

117. Ureterosigmoidostomy (Open Transcolonic Ureterointestinal Anastomosis)

WILLARD E. GOODWIN

URETEROINTESTINAL ANASTOMOSIS to divert the urinary stream to the bowel has occupied the attention and imagination of many surgeons for a long time. Hinman and Weyrauch studied and categorized the principles of the various techniques employed up to 1936. Nearly all of them were carefully devised to prevent fecal contamination.

In 1953 we described a different approach to this problem, in which the anastomosis of the ureter to the intestine was done from inside the lumen of the bowel. We felt that with the use of modern antibiotics to sterilize the intestine before the operation, this procedure was safe and practical, and we have continued to use it almost exclusively for ureterosigmoidostomy. It has found favor in many quarters, and most surgeons who have employed it have continued to use it in preference to other techniques. It is particularly applicable when a diverting colostomy is done, leaving behind a rectosigmoid bladder. It can also be used for ureteroileal anastomosis in conjunction with ureteroileal cutaneous anastomosis to divert the urine to the skin (Bricker's operation). The procedure is not devoid of complications, but in our hands it has proved generally safe and satisfactory. The end results in patients of all ages have been as good as in similar operations done with other techniques, and sometimes better.

The advantages of this simple method of ureterointestinal anastomosis are appealing. The operation resembles reimplantation of the ureter into the bladder from inside, a procedure familiar to all urologists. (It is almost identical with the more recently described technique of ureteroneocystostomy as elaborated by Politano and Leadbetter.)

A careful mucosa-to-mucosa anastomosis is obtained under direct vision. An elliptical anastomosis, or anastomosis of a long open flap of the ureter, allows satisfactory anchoring of the ureter without occlusion of its lumen. The ureters enter the bowel posteriorly from behind the peritoneum, where they normally lie. There is minimal mobilization of ureters, and their blood supply is preserved.

The anastomosis is performed low in the bowel (below the sacral promontory) and allows pooling of the urine in the lower rectosigmoid in the recumbent position. The tunnel principle is employed in an attempt to produce a valve-like action.

The procedure is also simpler and quicker than many other types of uretero-intestinal anastomosis.

Preoperative Bowel Preparation

Since the bowel is open in this procedure, it is imperative that the patient have adequate preoperative preparation of the large bowel. Ideally this is done by beginning the preparation with a no residue, high protein diet 8 to 10 days before hospitalization. On the fifth preoperative day, the patient begins a soft diet, has a laxative, and takes Sulfathalidine, 2 grams every four hours. On the fourth preoperative day, the patient receives an enema. On the third preoperative day, the patient receives a laxative and is placed on a liquid diet which is maintained up to the time of surgery.

On the second day before the operation, oral neomycin is begun, 1 gram every six hours. Another enema is given. On the day before surgery, the patient receives a careful repeated flushing of the lower bowel until it is clear, and after that receives nothing by mouth except water, sweetened coffee or tea, and clear fruit juices, plus the medications. He continues on Sulfathalidine, 2 grams every four hours, and receives neomycin, 1 gram every four hours.

At 6 P.M. the night before surgery, the patient receives tincture of opium, 10 minims orally every three hours for four doses. No enema is given on the morning of surgery.

When this preparation is followed closely, the large intestine is clean and nearly sterile and is absolutely empty. Fecal contamination of the wound is at a minimum.

Technique

The abdomen is opened through a long lower midline incision or, if preferred, through a transverse incision. Adequate exposure is important.

If cystectomy is to be a part of the procedure, it is usually helpful to do it first, as the added space in the pelvis after the bladder is removed helps in the transplantation. However, cystectomy is not necessarily a part of this operation.

The patient is placed in Trendelenburg position and the small bowel and redundant sigmoid colon are packed off so that only the lower rectosigmoid occupies the lower part of the pelvis.

Mobilization of the Ureters

The ureters are identified at the point where they cross the iliac vessels, and an opening is made in the posterior peritoneum below this point. The lower portion of the ureters is dissected free by blunt dissection, and the ureters are transected low in the pelvis, approximately 3 to 5 cm. above the bladder.

By use of blunt finger dissection, the retroperitoneal plane of cleavage behind the rectosigmoid is developed, much as in colectomy. After this blunt dissection, it should be possible to pass the fingers of either hand through to the opposite side behind the colon. The free end of the ureter on each side is transfixed with a stay suture to aid in further management and handling of the ureter.

Ureterosigmoidostomy

After the preliminary dissection is complete, the anterior surface of the sigmoid is seized with Babcock clamps for stability, and the sigmoid colon is opened through a vertical midline incision on its anterior surface. The incision is usually about 10 cm. in length. It is advantageous to have ample room in which to work.

There may be some small bleeding vessels in the cut sigmoid colon. These may be lightly cauterized or may be ignored, as they will be caught up in the final closure of the bowel. If there are any fecal contents, it may be helpful to put a sponge in the lumen above and below the colotomy to wall off the area. It is important, if this is done, to remember that it *was* done and to remove the sponges before the end of the operation.

After the bowel has been opened, the fingers of the left hand are placed in the retroperitoneal space behind the bowel, and the posterior wall of the bowel is pushed upward and outward through the colotomy in order to make a smooth, firm surface on which to work. A long, superficial, vertical incision is made through the mucosa only. The incision is usually about 2.5 to 3 cm. in length and will ultimately be used for a trough in which to anastomose the opened end of the ureter. The right ureter is placed lower than the left. Both are placed fairly close to the midline.

After the superficial incision has been made, a small iris scissors with a blunt tip is introduced, and by blunt dissection a tunnel approximately 3 to 5 cm. in length is made submucosally and almost vertically along the posterior wall of the bowel. After this has been developed, a small curved clamp is introduced through the tunnel and then turned outward so that the curved tip points laterally toward the ureter. It is pushed by blunt dissection through the remaining fibers of the posterior wall of the bowel and between the vessels of the mesentery. Care must be taken not to use undue force and not to injure the mesenteric vessels. It is important to keep pointing this clamp posteriorly and to stay behind the peritoneum. An undesirable but common occurrence is for the operator to find this clamp coming into the peritoneum along the lateral margin of the intestine. The clamp is passed laterally toward the region of the ureter, and when its point is seen the stay suture on the end of the ureter is grasped and the ureter is pulled into the bowel (Fig. 1). This leads the ureter into the intestine along its posterior wall, through the long tunnel that has been developed.

After the right ureter has been introduced into the bowel, the same procedure is performed on the left side, bringing the left ureter in through a similar

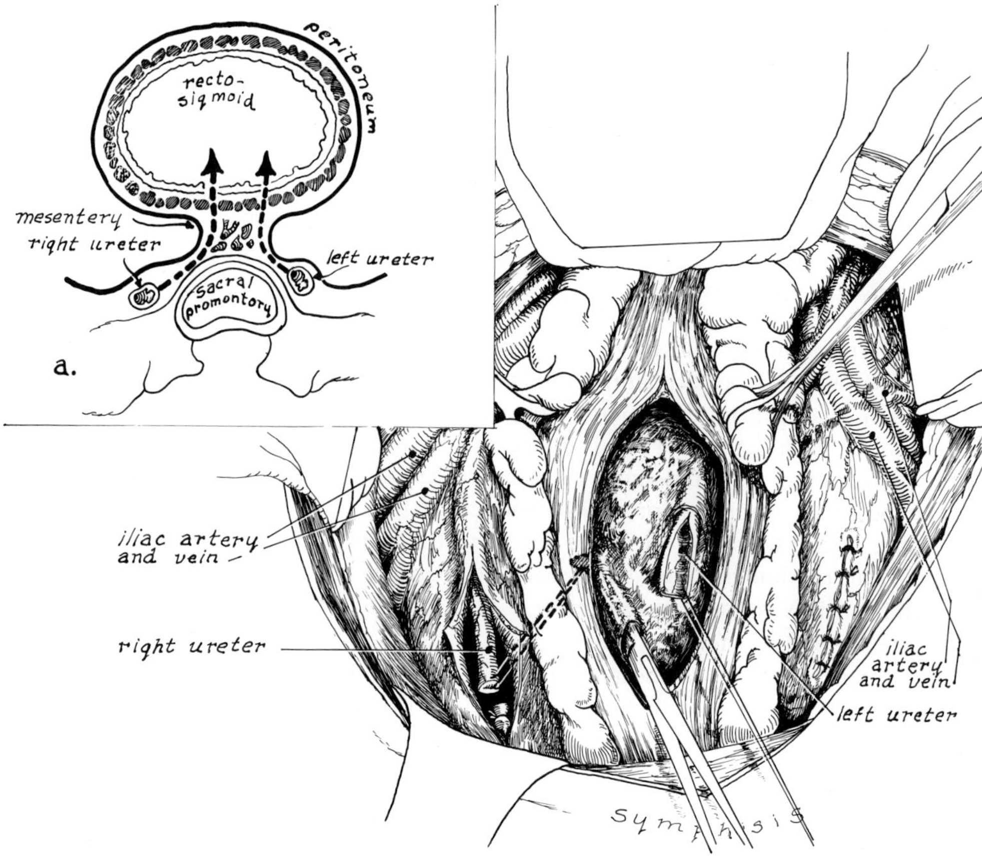

FIGURE 1. Operative field viewed from below; symphysis at the bottom of the field. The sigmoid colon is opened widely by vertical incision through a taenia coli to expose the posterior wall of the bowel. Insert *a* shows the path that the ureters will follow retroperitoneally, when brought into the bowel from behind.

incision higher up. It is helpful to lead both ureters into the bowel before one begins the anastomosis.

The redundant lower end of the ureter is to be discarded, but it is first opened vertically with a long incision which leaves the ureter lying open and flat in the mucosal slot which has been made for it. The stay suture is left in place for management during the beginning of the anastomosis. It is important that the ureter be allowed to lie freely, without any tension. Experience and judgment are required to know how far to open the ureter before beginning the anastomosis.

The first stitch of the anastomosis is placed at the upper portion of the ureteral stoma; it goes through all layers of the ureter and engages only the mucosa of the intestine. Chromic catgut (4–0) is used on an atraumatic needle.

After the apical suture has been placed, companion sutures are placed on each side of it through all layers of the ureter so that the ureter is attached to the mucosa of the intestine. This procedure fixes the point of the true stoma of the ureter.

After this fixing has been accomplished, the flayed open end of the ureter, which is longer than is necessary, is cut at the proper length so that it fits exactly into the mucosal slot which has been made for it. Then the distal end of the ureter is sutured to the bowel with a number of interrupted chromic catgut sutures which include all layers of both ureter and bowel. The remaining ureter, between the sutures, is anastomosed in a similar fashion. This produces a long, slot-like tongue of ureter which acts as a fixation to prevent retraction and which heals to form a kind of little trigone in the posterior wall of the bowel (Fig. 2). After this procedure has been completed on the right side, the same thing is done on the left side. Again the redundant distal end of the ureter is cut off and discarded, and the long slot-like tongue of open ureter is used for fixation.

This procedure may be done either with or without ureteral catheters. Probably ureteral catheters add a safety factor, although they have some disadvantages.

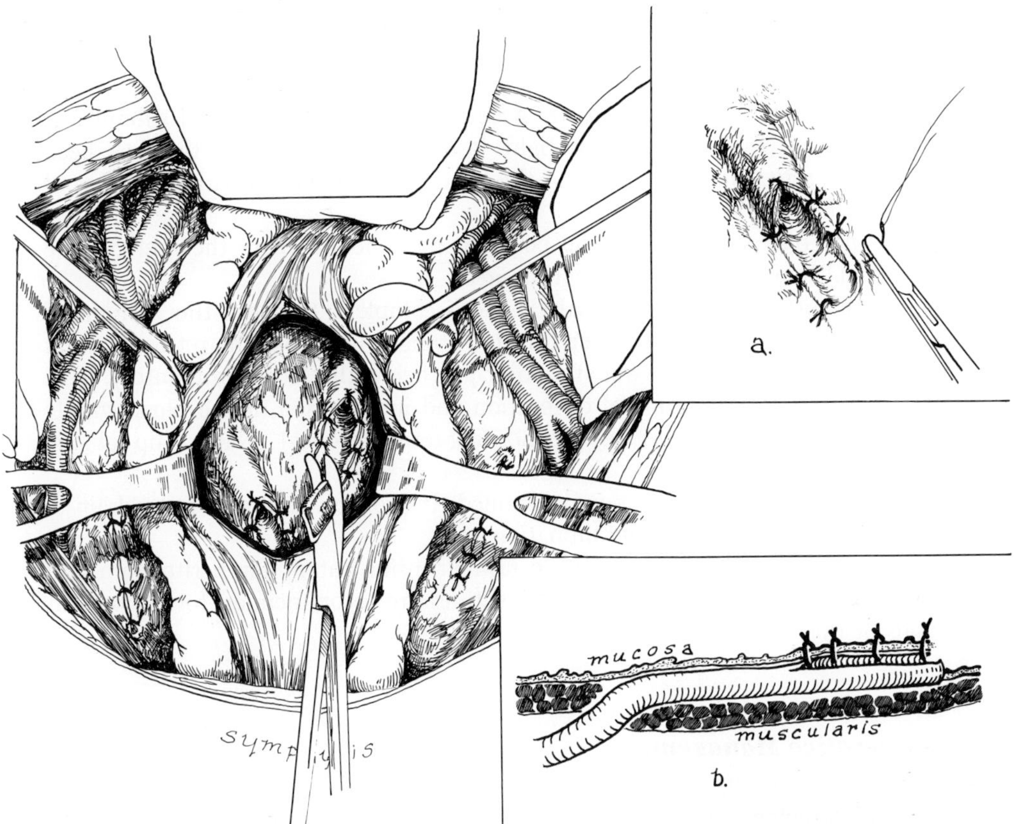

FIGURE 2. Operative field from below after incision of the bowel mucosa and development of the submucosal tunnel. The ureters are brought into the bowel through a short tunnel (insert *b*) made with the iris scissors and a small curved clamp. The redundant ureter is cut off and discarded, leaving a long slot-like tongue of open ureter for fixation in the bowel (insert *a*).

If ureteral catheters are employed, it is important to use the soft, red rubber, Bardam marked catheters. These are placed at approximately 20 cm. They must drain perfectly before they are fixed in place. A fine suture of 5–0 catgut (eye suture) is used for fixation of the catheter and is placed through the mucosa only, above the point of the anastomosis. It is then tied to the catheter to hold it in place.

The distal ends of the ureteral catheters are then led out through the anus. This is done by passing large rectal tubes down the bowel from inside out. After they have been secured outside the anus by an assistant, the ends of the ureteral catheters are introduced into the large rectal tubes. The rectal tubes are pulled out, and this allows the ureteral catheters to exit through the anus. It is important to hold the catheters with a clamp to be sure that they will not be dislodged during this maneuver.

The Closure

At this point the closure of the bowel is begun. A continuous inverting suture of 3–0 chromic catgut on an atraumatic needle is used for mucosa and submucosa, and the mucosa is closed in watertight fashion (Fig. 3). After this has been achieved, the serosa and muscularis of the large bowel are closed with a number of interrupted fine silk sutures.

It is not necessary to close the posterior peritoneum where the ureters were mobilized, although it may be done if desired.

It is important, before the final closure is complete, to check the position of the ureters and to be sure that they run in a straight line from the retroperitoneal space into the back of the bowel at a point just below the sacral promontory. This orientation insures only minimal dislocation and interruption of the blood supply of the ureters. It also preserves the normal retroperitoneal relationship of the ureters to the large intestine.

The wound may or may not be drained. It probably is desirable to drain it because of the likelihood of contamination.

The wound is closed in a routine fashion, using catgut for peritoneum and fascial layers, and silk for the skin. Stay sutures are recommended for support in wounds of this type.

Postoperative Management

If ureteral catheters are used, they are attached to straight drainage devices. In addition a mushroom catheter is placed just inside the anus to drain any additional accumulation of blood or urine. If ureteral catheters are not used, we often employ a mushroom catheter inside the anus and a rectal tube extending upward, approximately 4 inches inside the anus, to drain this area. These rectal catheters must be kept open. It is necessary that they be removed and reinserted if they are plugged.

If ureteral catheters are used, they are usually left in place for approximately

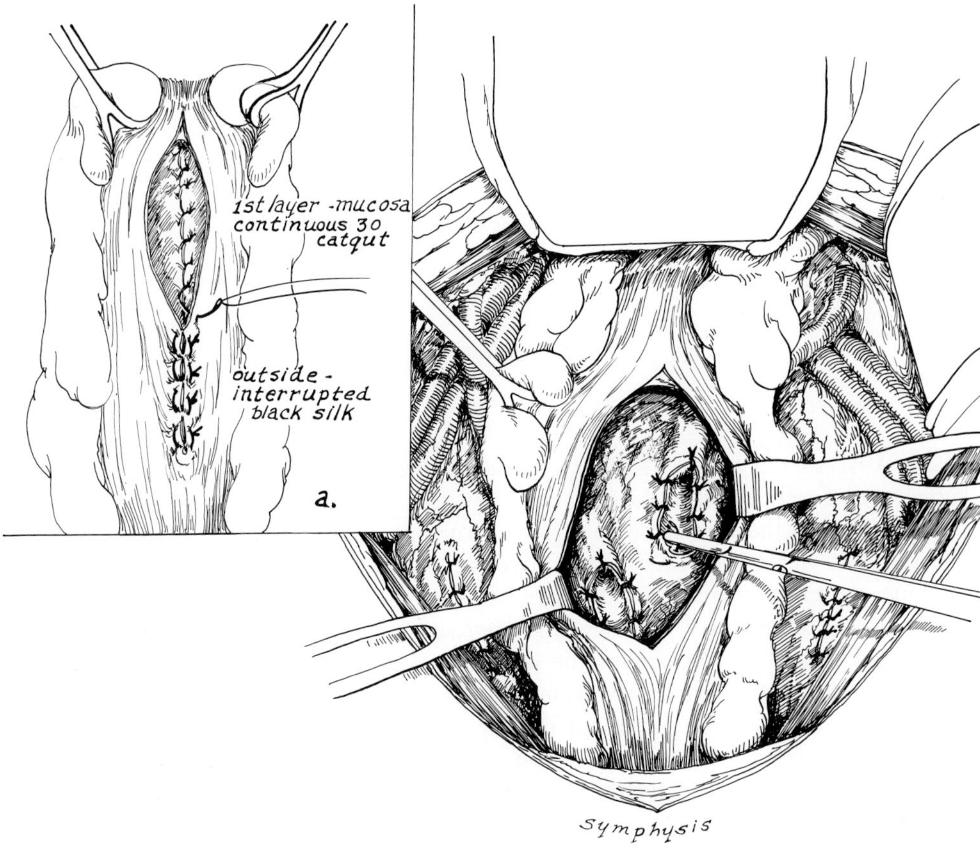

FIGURE 3. Operative field from below. Direct anastomosis of the ureter to bowel mucosa is performed with interrupted fine catgut sutures. The colotomy opening is closed in two layers with catgut for the mucosal layer and interrupted silk for the external layer (insert *a*).

seven days and then removed. The patient is usually allowed nothing by mouth after this type of procedure, and usually has nasogastric suction for three or four days. He may be permitted to resume oral nourishment after that time. Antibiotics are not used postoperatively unless there is some specific indication. Further management of the patient after the operation is the same as for any other type of ureterosigmoidostomy.

References

Goodwin, W. E., Harris, A. P., Kaufman, J. J., and Beal, J. M. Open, transcolonic ureterointestinal anastomosis. *Surg., Gynec. and Obst.* 97:295, September 1953.

Hinman, F., and Weyrauch, H. M., Jr. A critical study of the different principles of surgery which have been used in uretero-intestinal implantation. *Tr. Am. A. Genito-Urin. Surgeons* 29:15, 1936.

118. *Cystectomy*

WYLAND F. LEADBETTER

REMOVAL of the urinary bladder is always a formidable procedure. An intimate knowledge of pelvic and abdominal anatomy and a broad surgical experience are prerequisites for the surgeon who does this surgery. All the techniques for bowel resection and anastomosis may be utilized; ileostomy and colostomy will have to be done; ureterointestinal anastomosis of one or more types must be performed; major arterial injury may necessitate arterial suture, anastomosis, or replacement by graft. The ultimate success of the operation depends in large measure on the outcome of associated urinary diversion procedures. Serious early and late complications involving the bowel and upper urinary tract occur, and the surgeon must be prepared to cope with them. No surgeon can be considered a competent urologist until he has mastered the technical details of the various operations for urinary diversion and cystectomy.

Our present concept of cystectomy is not that it is a single operation, an easily described operative technique, but rather that it embraces a series of increasingly radical operations, each of which has application under certain circumstances.

Simple Cystectomy

Simple cystectomy implies that the bladder alone is removed, without the urethra in the female and without the prostate gland and seminal vesicles in the male. This limited operation is certainly not necessary or even desirable in the female, since removal of the urethra has no deleterious effect and in fact eliminates a source of possible continued infection and irritation. Simple cystectomy may be desirable in the male in an effort to preserve sexual function in younger persons, but it should not be done at the risk of leaving malignant disease behind. The best indications for this operation are nonmalignant conditions which may be listed as the exstrophic bladder after urinary diversion, the residually infected neurogenic bladder or persistently infected bladder of interstitial cystitis after urinary diversion, the rare case of severe pelvic trauma with irreparable bladder injury or destruction, the unusual nonmalignant lesion such as diffuse neurofibromatosis, radiation cystitis with uncontrollable bleeding, and persistent generalized papillomatosis without involvement of the prostatic urethra.

Total and Radical Cystectomy

The more radical operations, always performed for malignant disease, are total cystectomy, radical cystectomy, and pelvic exenteration. The primary indication for these operations is the presence of infiltrating malignant disease of the bladder base or bladder neck, or widespread tumor of the bladder which may not be treated in any other manner.

Total cystectomy implies removal of the bladder, prostate, and seminal vesicles in the male, the bladder and the urethra in the female.

Radical cystectomy is probably conceived and carried out somewhat differently by different surgeons. The technique I employ in the male consists of outlining by incision pelvic peritoneum to be removed with the bladder, en bloc dissection of the tissues from about the common and external iliac vessels, the hypogastric vessels, and the lateral pelvic walls, and in continuity reflection of the dissected tissue onto the bladder so that this tissue and the bladder and prostate are removed as a single mass of tissue. In the female, a similar gland dissection is done and then the broad ligaments, uterus, and cervix if present, together with most or all of the vagina, the bladder and urethra, are removed en masse. This operation in the female requires both abdominal and perineal stages.

The purpose of the radical operation is to remove as many lymph glands directly concerned with lymph drainage from the bladder as possible, together with all intervening tissues containing lymph channels from the bladder to the nodes. The initial hope that metastases from the bladder to lymph nodes occurred by tumor embolization rather than by lymphatic permeation has unfortunately not been substantiated, because cure of bladder cancer has been rare in the presence of involved lymph nodes. The problem, yet to be solved, is the removal of all lymph channels coursing from the bladder to the external and internal iliac lymph nodes. The reason this has not been possible, I believe, is that some lymph channels pass through the posterior bladder pedicles deep in the pelvis around the rectum onto the pelvic wall in relation to pelvic vein radicles. Their removal poses a very difficult surgical problem. In the female, removal of the uterus, cervix, vagina, and broad ligaments seems desirable to eliminate possible lymphatic extension from the bladder to these organs whose lymphatic channels are so closely related to those of the bladder base and urethra. Further technical improvement in radical cystectomy may be possible but depends on more accurate knowledge of the lymphatic pathways from the bladder to the external and common iliac nodes. One advantage of the radical procedure as contrasted with total cystectomy is the widest possible removal of paravesical tissues. If, in a given case, lymph gland metastasis has not occurred but the lesion has locally extended through the bladder wall, cure is possible and the patient is given the best chance for survival. Removal of all pelvic peritoneum is necessary to accomplish this.

Pelvic Exenteration

Pelvic exenteration has a very limited use in treating carcinoma of the bladder, because the rectum is rarely involved if the disease is still operable, but cases in which it is applicable are seen and they must be recognized so that potentially curable lesions are not missed. The main use for this operation has been for the eradication of coincidental primary lesions of the rectum and bladder, which have been encountered several times. It has also been used for carcinoma of the sigmoid widely involving the bladder. The operation involves the same general techniques described for radical cystectomy except that the rectum is removed with the other organs. It is somewhat simpler in that the hypogastric arteries may be divided distal to the superior gluteals, allowing a cleaner dissection of the pelvis. Removal of the levator ani muscles and the extreme lower end of the rectal canal may or may not be desirable.

Urinary Diversion Procedures

The more general use of cystectomy, regardless of specific indications and techniques, has been possible only since the development of safe urinary diversion procedures. I still utilize ureterosigmoidostomy without proximal colostomy on occasion if the upper urinary tract is functionally and anatomically normal, because results have often been entirely satisfactory, but more use has been made of the rectosigmoid bladder and the ileal conduit. One reason has been that many patients have had obvious pyelonephritis, or intravenous pyelograms have demonstrated hydroureter or hydronephrosis—sometimes a nonfunctioning kidney with hydronephrosis on the other side. Conventional ureterosigmoidostomy or the rectosigmoid bladder should not be considered under these circumstances. Undoubtedly the use of the ileal conduit has decreased both immediate and late complications, and many patients are now alive who would formerly have died from renal failure.

Cystectomy and urinary diversion should be done as a one-stage procedure whenever possible. Older patients seem to withstand one well-done major procedure better than two procedures which, to be effective, must usually be carried out as close together as possible. With experience, operating time and blood loss may both be considerably reduced. Cystectomy should not be done with the hope of palliation in the presence of gross involvement of retroperitoneal lymph nodes or other metastases. Urinary diversion followed by deep roentgen therapy may provide a period of control under these circumstances. Cystectomy may occasionally be necessary in the presence of pelvic lymph node or other metastases to control serious hemorrhage, but should be done with full knowledge that only temporary relief is possible.

Preoperative Management

The important preoperative consideration, aside from proper assessment of bladder pathology and search for distant metastases, is adequate visualization of the upper urinary tracts so that information as to function, presence or absence of hydroureter or hydronephrosis, calculi, or tumor of the upper urinary tract is obtained. Coincidental neoplasms of a ureter or the renal pelvis are occasionally found and should be searched for. A barium enema must be obtained if ureterosigmoid anastomosis is to be done in any form. This may be difficult or even impossible if a severe degree of sigmoid diverticulosis is present.

Preoperative preparation includes evaluation and treatment of cardiac or respiratory problems. If bleeding has been present or the patient is debilitated, blood volume must be restored. The bowel must be prepared by catharsis, enemas, the use of a low residue diet for several days, and sterilization with one of the mycin drugs. We prefer neomycin given for two days in doses of 250 mg. every six hours. The morning of operation a final enema is given, making sure that it is completely expelled. General anesthesia via intratracheal tube is preferred. After anesthesia has been established the bladder is thoroughly lavaged with normal saline until clear, and 2 ounces of 1 per cent neomycin solution are injected and the catheter removed. If the rectum is to be used for diversion, the rectum and sigmoid are similarly cleansed and a large rectal tube is sutured or taped in place.

Techniques

Incision

The first consideration is the incision. Regardless of the procedure planned, in the male it is done through an abdominal incision. Perineal dissection to free the prostate and seminal vesicles is a preliminary procedure I have advocated and done many times, but more experience has shown that it is not necessary. It does add to the length of the operation, and unless abdominal exploration has been done previously and the lesion been found operable, one may encounter a situation, when the abdomen is opened, that prevents cystectomy and has rendered the perineal dissection unnecessary and even undesirable. In the female, a preliminary dissection of the urethra and vagina is desirable if the bladder lesion is known to be operable (see Figure 7), but otherwise the perineal stage should be accomplished after abdominal exploration and dissection of the bladder and pelvic organs from above.

When urinary diversion is to be done by ileal conduit it is desirable to place the abdominal incision well away from the projected site of ileostomy so that it will not contribute to irregularity of the skin which may interfere with easy application of the urine-collecting device. I therefore have been in the habit of utilizing a left paramedian incision for ileal conduit diversion and cystectomy unless the right abdomen is so scarred from previous surgery that it seems wise to locate the ileal stoma on the left side. Under this circumstance a right paramedian incision is made. The incision should extend from the symphysis well up toward the xyphoid to provide adequate room for exploration and surgery. When urinary diversion has been previously done a low transverse incision placed just above the symphysis with each end curved upward toward the anterior superior spines of the ilia is very satisfactory for cystectomy.

Exploration

The second consideration is exploration for possible metastases in the liver or retroperitoneal and pelvic lymph nodes. This must be thorough and is sometimes difficult if the patient is obese. If the liver is negative and no nodes can be palpated there is no problem, but if enlarged nodes are palpated the highest one must be removed for frozen section. If this is found to be negative a lower node should be removed and sections made. If no positive nodes are encountered above the pelvic brim the local lesion in the bladder is observed and palpated in an effort to decide whether cystectomy will be worthwhile. Sometimes this is very difficult to determine if the lesion is in the bladder base and has extended somewhat. Involvement of peritoneum over the bladder surface is not necessarily a contraindication to cystectomy even if a loop of small bowel or the sigmoid is adherent and possibly involved, because this may be resected with the bladder and the bowel repaired. Although cure cannot be expected if positive pelvic lymph nodes are found or if the lesion has extended outside the bladder wall, it seems worthwhile to do cystectomy if a good margin can be assured about the local lesion. Differences of opinion exist in regard to this, but there is fundamentally no problem, because cystectomy should not generally be done for palliation.

Preparation of the Ureters

If cystectomy is decided upon and if urinary diversion is planned as part of the procedure, an appendectomy should next be done (if the opportunity is present) because the development of acute appendicitis after ileal conduit diversion presents unusual difficulties of diagnosis and treatment. The next step is the isolation and division of the ureters at the pelvic brim. Lymphatic involvement of the lower ureters is frequently encountered; hence, the lower ureters should never be used for diversion in the presence of malignant disease of the bladder or prostate. Both ureters are found in the retroperitoneum by making two short incisions in the posterior peritoneum. On the left the sigmoid colon usually must be sharply mobilized to allow this. The ureters are divided, their distal ends ligated, and the proximal ends intubated with appropriate catheters which are sutured in place and allowed to drain outside the operative field. Leakage of urine into the peritoneal cavity is undesirable since it may lead to infection and peritonitis. Division should be done early in the operation so that the bladder, emptied just prior to surgery, does not fill with urine to create a mass interfering with exposure and increasing the hazard of spillage from the bladder and the dissemination of tumor cells and bacteria into the wound if the organ is torn or urine leaks from the urethra immediately after it is cut. The intubated ureters must be carefully placed in the wound so that retractors will not injure them or interfere with circulation in their terminal portions.

Simple Cystectomy

MOBILIZATION OF THE BLADDER. Assuming, for purposes of discussion only, at this point, that cancer is not under consideration and that simple cystectomy is to be done for benign disease, the bladder is freed from the transversalis fascia either by blunt dissection with the fingers, or by sharp scissors dissection if the bladder is adherent as a result of previous surgery, until the bladder neck is exposed. The peritoneum is stripped from the vertex and posterior wall of the bladder to its base. In the course of this stripping, the urachus and umbilical arteries are divided. Lateral dissection of the bladder from the iliac vessels is usually accomplished by blunt dissection with the fingers, which exposes both vasa; these are divided and ligated. The pelvic stumps of both ureters are freed to the bladder wall. The hypogastric arteries are deliberately exposed and dissection is made downward along these vessels until the superior vesical arteries are encountered. In the male, these are the first anterior branches. In the female, sometimes the superior vesical branch comes off the uterine artery; consequently, enough dissection must be done to make sure that the artery ligated is in fact the superior vesical. These vessels are clamped and divided, and each end of the vessels is ligated to prevent back bleeding. The inferior vesical arteries may be found by further dissection along the hypogastric trunk; they are clamped, divided, and ligated. This effectively interrupts all major arterial blood flow to the bladder. The technique is easy and dispels worry relative to major arterial bleeding. Further dissection slightly below or distal to this level exposes the vesical veins which unite with veins from the prostatic plexus in the male and the vaginal plexus in the female to form the hypogastric veins. These may be clamped and divided at this time, but the usual practice has been to accomplish this in the course of subsequent isolation and division of the posterior bladder pedicles, since, if veins are torn before one pedicle is divided, troublesome bleeding may ensue which is difficult to stop.

REMOVAL OF THE BLADDER. Removal of the bladder may be accomplished in two ways. In the female, the easy method is to establish a line of cleavage by sharp scissor dissection in the midline at the bladder base between the vaginal and bladder wall. As the bladder base is dissected and pulled upward, the posterior pedicles on either side of the bladder base which bind the bladder to the vagina are encountered. These contain the nerves, lymphatics, and veins of the bladder. Finger dissection behind the lateral to the bladder base will help to delineate these more clearly so that they may be clamped from above downward and divided. This type of dissection and mobilization is continued until the bladder neck is reached.

At this point the bladder neck is clearly identified anteriorly and the urethra is skeletonized to some extent. By pulling upward and backward on the bladder a right-angle clamp can be placed across the urethra just distal to the bladder neck and the urethra divided distal to the clamp. This prevents any spillage from the bladder. After the bladder has been removed, bleeding points beneath the symphysis or on the surface of the vagina will usually require suture ligation. There is a rich venous network in this area which often is torn in the course of cystectomy. The tissue of the bladder pedicles held in clamps must be suture ligated since these contain the vesical veins. This method of cystectomy may be termed the antegrade method.

One may reverse the procedure, and approach the bladder neck and urethra first, divide the bladder neck, establish a plane of cleavage between it and the vaginal wall by sharp dissection, and follow this up to meet the dissection from above, clamping and dividing the posterior pedicles as one proceeds. There is no particular choice between the two procedures except that there is more chance of tearing the bladder and spilling its contents into the wound if the retrograde method is used.

In the male, the retrograde method is preferred because the purpose is to save the prostate gland and seminal vesicles without damaging or destroying the autonomic nerve supply on which ejaculation depends. The bladder neck is exposed anteriorly, opened, and aspirated of fluid, to prevent spillage of bladder contents so far as possible, and then the entire circumference of the bladder neck is divided just above the surface of the prostate. After this has been completed and the bladder base pulled upward, a plane of cleavage can be established between the bladder base and the fascia overlying the ejaculatory ducts and seminal vesicles. With the upward traction on the bladder base continued, this plane is followed upward until a finger insinuated under the bladder base meets the dissection of the posterior bladder wall from above. The posterior pedicles are then identified and developed by blunt dissection on either side of the bladder base until they may be clamped and divided from above downward, first freeing one side and then both sides of the bladder base. All bleeding points must be suture ligated, and special care must be taken to include tissue in the clamps which hold the pedicles. It is well to save a bit of bladder just above the base of the prostate for suture over the prostatic orifice to prevent the development of a suprapubic prostatic urethral fistula, which may start as an abscess deep in the wound.

Following simple cystectomy the pelvic peritoneum is preserved, being repaired if necessary. Urinary diversion is done and the wound closed in layers without drainage of the pelvic cavity unless gross contamination by infected urine has occurred.

Total Cystectomy

The only difference between simple and total cystectomy in the female is the removal of the entire urethra in the latter procedure. This can usually be accomplished by dissection from the abdominal side by putting traction on the bladder and following the urethra to its meatus by scissor dissection. If more careful dissection and the removal of more periurethral tissue is desired it should be done by perineal operation.

Mobilization of the Bladder and Prostate. In the male, the bladder is freed as described above. The prostate is dealt with by wiping away loose connective tissue from about its anterior and lateral surfaces. The endopelvic fascia on both sides of the gland is perforated with the scissors lateral to the periprostatic venous plexus, which can be easily seen on the surface of the gland. The index finger can then be inserted into this break in the fascia (Fig. 1) to separate the fascia anteriorly toward the puboprostatic ligament and posteriorly around the rectum. One then works a finger around the prostate to its apex on the surface of

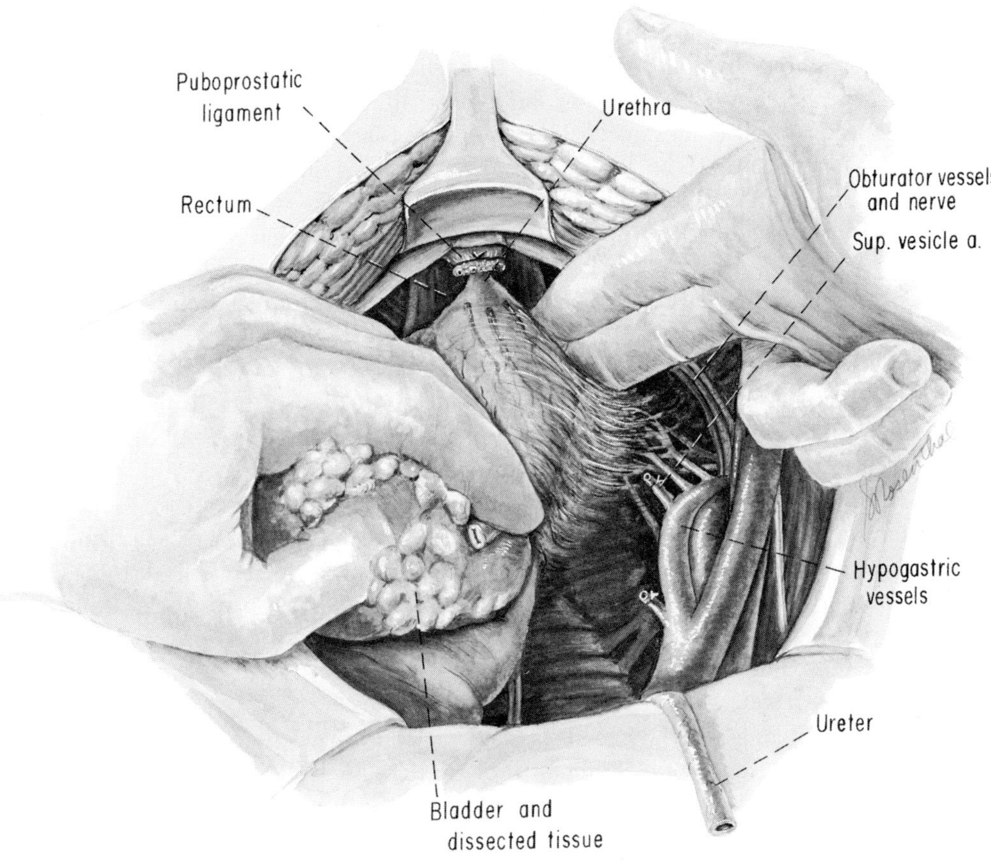

FIGURE 1. Bilateral gland dissection has been completed. The right pelvis is demonstrated. It will be noted that the arterial supply has been interrupted at the origin of vessels from the hypogastric artery. The puboprostatic ligament has been divided and ligated. The operator's fingers demonstrate blunt dissection of the lateral prostate to the apex of the gland to free the membranous urethra, which will be severed next. To the right of the bladder base is shown the deep pelvic attachment or pedicle of the bladder which must be separated from the rectum and divided before the bladder base can be mobilized. (The figures in this chapter show steps in a radical cystectomy. Figures 1–3 have been placed in the section on total cystectomy because they illustrate equally well certain phases of that procedure.)

the triangular ligament on both sides, thus freeing the lateral surfaces of the gland. By pushing down firmly on the prostate and pressing medially from each side on the anterior surface of the gland, the puboprostatic ligament is stretched and the tissue consolidated toward the midline, so that a curved clamp can be placed about the ligament from above downward. This maneuver is particularly important because on it depends ligation of the dorsal vein of the penis. If this vein is torn, serious bleeding results. The vein is difficult to suture secondarily, situated as it is on the undersurface of the symphysis. Care must be taken to place the tip of the clamp well down toward the surface of the triangular ligament to be certain of occluding the venous channels. Tissue on the undersurface of the clamp is then divided with a sharp knife close to the clamp. This division frees the prostate from the symphysis.

Considerable back bleeding from the surface of the prostate usually occurs. It may be ignored temporarily or be immediately controlled by deep sutures through the prostatic substance. The tissues in the clamp placed on the puboprostatic ligament must be carefully ligated. In doing this, the clamp must not be pulled or angulated, or it will tear the vein or pull off. Properly done, this ligation prevents bleeding from the dorsal vein of the penis, which is usually the chief source of bleeding in the performance of cystectomy. Considerable experience is necessary before the ligation can be routinely and satisfactorily accomplished.

After bleeding has been controlled, the apex of the prostate is inspected. A finger worked underneath and around the apex above the rectal wall is used to free the membranous urethra and apex of the gland from the rectum beneath. If the rectum cannot be separated easily, one should not attempt vigorous dissection, because rectal injury may result.

Removal of the Bladder, Prostate, and Seminal Vesicles. By upward traction on the prostate the membranous urethra just at the apex of the gland is visualized, and divided over a finger if one can be passed behind the urethra. If not, the urethra still must be divided, but one must take great pains to divide only the urethra. The apex of the gland and the urethra are grasped with a right-angle clamp or tenaculum (Fig. 2) and pulled upward, and a plane of cleavage is established on the rectal wall between the prostate and rectal wall. It is probably best to develop a plane on the rectal fascia just beneath Denonvilliers' fascia because this allows a more radical removal of tissue. This is not always possible and does increase the chance of rectal injury. When the prostate is sufficiently freed the urethra should be securely suture closed to prevent spillage of urine and tumor cells during subsequent forceful manipulations. As the prostate is pulled upward, continued dissection frees the prostate entirely from the rectal wall. Further dissection in this same plane carries one upward behind the ejaculatory ducts and the seminal vesicles, which must be freed beyond their tips. At this point a finger can be worked up between the rectum and bladder base to meet the dissection from above. Upward traction on the bladder and finger dissection of the rectal wall from the tissue binding the bladder posteriorly on either side of the bladder base (bladder pedicles) will delineate the pedicles and allow them to be clamped from

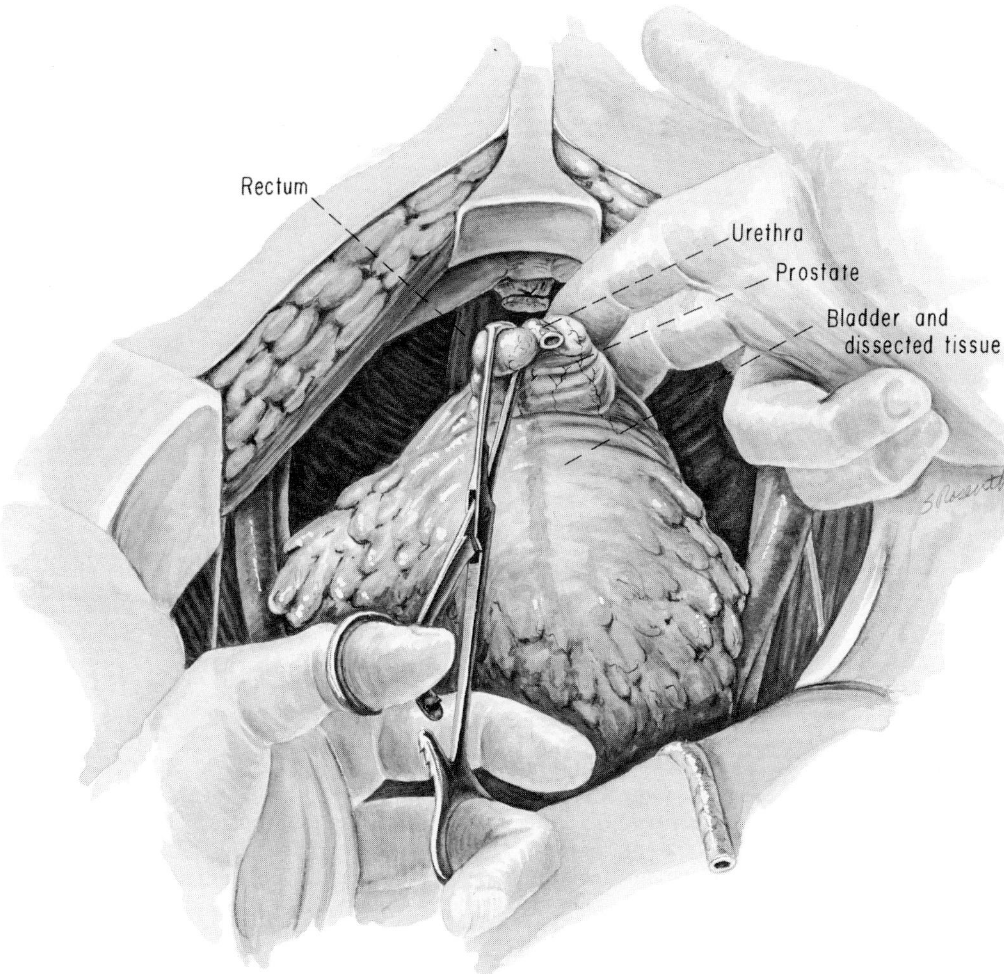

FIGURE 2. The gland dissection has been completed, the membranous urethra divided, and the prostatic apex separated from the rectum. As this dissection on the rectum is continued upward, the midline bladder base will be undermined with a finger to meet dissection from above, and the lateral attachments will be isolated for clamping and division.

above downward deep in the pelvis and lateral to the rectal wall (Fig. 3). This must always be done with a finger between the pedicle and the rectal wall so that the rectum will be pushed medially and not be included in a clamp. One pedicle at a time is clamped and divided, because until one pedicle has been divided, direct vision is difficult and the operator has to depend mostly on feel to place the clamps. It is best to suture ligate the tissue held in the clamps on one side before proceeding to clamp and divide the opposite pedicle. Too many clamps in the wound are cumbersome. Once the bladder has been removed, any actively bleeding points can be secured. Most troublesome bleeding is apt to come from the region of the

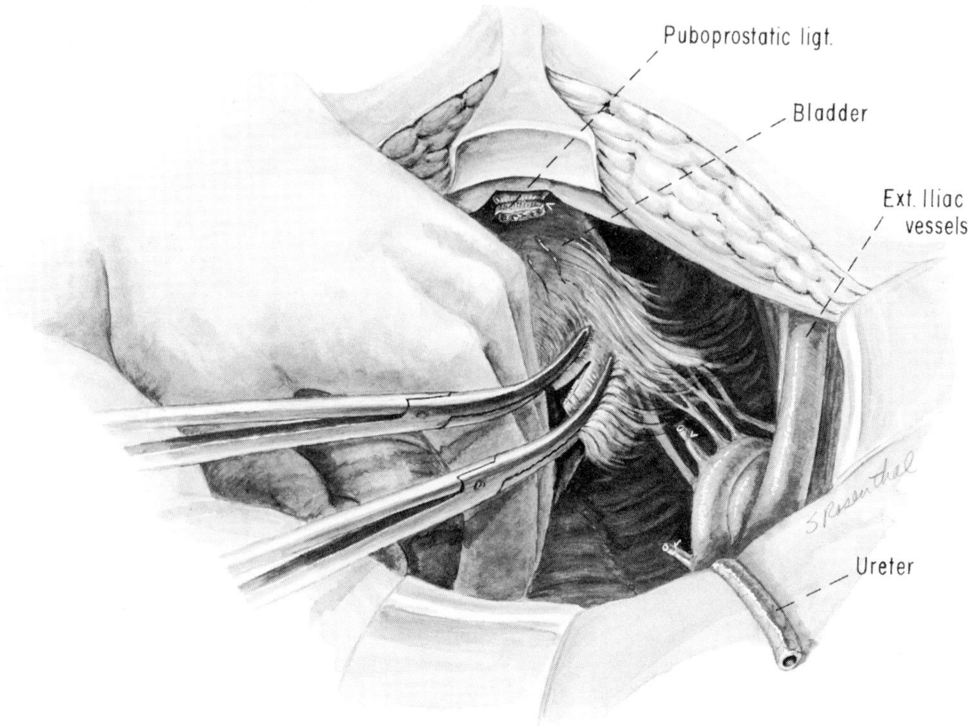

FIGURE 3. The bladder and prostate have been completely mobilized except for the pedicles attaching the bladder base on either side of the rectum to the deep pelvis. The right pedicle is being clamped and divided. This contains the connective tissue, lymph channels, nerves, and veins which deeply bind the bladder base about the rectum. Once this pedicle has been divided, the right side of the bladder base is free and cystectomy is completed by dividing the pedicle on the left side. The rectum must be retracted medially from the pedicle so that it is not injured when clamps are applied.

triangular ligament, which is always traumatized to some extent in the course of freeing the prostate and dividing the membranous urethra. Packs can be placed, but it is much better to obtain suture hemostasis at this point.

Urinary Diversion Procedures. After cystectomy has been accomplished by these methods, urinary diversion by whatever method is considered desirable is done and the wound closed. Since the pelvic peritoneum is saved and closed in this operation, a space is left in the pelvis. This is likely to become infected if a drain is left; thus it seems best not to drain unless gross contamination of the wound has occurred. The peritoneal cavity is never drained after a diversion procedure. If one does not drain and the pelvic cavity does become infected, it may be drained by passing a sound and then a catheter through the urethra into the pelvis. One advantage of closing the wound without drainage is that the large loss of plasma and electrolytes through wound drainage during the first few days is prevented. Accumulated fluid in the pelvic cavity is gradually absorbed.

Radical Cystectomy

Radical cystectomy rather than total cystectomy is my preference for the treatment of extensive or basilar infiltrating lesions of the bladder, not because many additional survivals or cures can be expected (we have two five-year survivals without evidence of disease in the presence of one or two positive lymph nodes), but because a much wider and more complete removal of perivesical tissue is accomplished, which undoubtedly gives a better chance of survival to patients without gland metastases.

Study of the nodes aids in establishing the prognosis. So far as is known, gland dissection does not lead to dissemination of the disease. We are using deep roentgen therapy more and more before cystectomy, and like to have evidence of lymph gland involvement if it is present.

Radical cystectomy is performed somewhat as follows after preliminary exploration, ureteral division and catheterization as described above.

Preparation for the Resection. The anterior bladder wall is separated from the transversalis fascia by blunt dissection. The peritoneum over and about the bladder is incised from the urachus to the rectovesical pouch in a wide circle to include most of the pelvic peritoneum (Fig. 4). In the female, both round ligaments and tubes are divided in the course of this circumscribing, and the peritoneal incisions are carried around the base of the uterus in front of the rectum. Preparation for pelvic gland dissection is made by stripping the lateral peritoneum from the iliac fossae and retracting it upward under Deaver retractors. In the male, the spermatic cords are identified during this stripping. The vasa are divided and ligated and the spermatic cords freed and retracted upward and laterally out of the immediate operative field (Fig. 5).

Gland Dissection. Gland dissection from about the external iliac vessels is begun at the femoral ring by first skeletonizing the deep epigastric vessels. The main lymphatic channels about the external iliac vessels at the femoral ring are easily identified and are either clipped or tied off with fine silk. This materially decreases the flow of lymph from the lower extremities into the wound, and the resulting unnecessary protein and electrolyte loss if the lymph is drained. The iliac vessels are stripped cleanly and the psoas muscles are cleanly exposed. In the course of this stripping, the obturator fossae and the side walls of the pelvis are cleaned of all loose areolar tissue. Obturator vessels may be divided without concern. Care must be exercised at this point not to injure the radicles of the hypogastric veins, which vary a great deal. Dissection is carried upward, exposing the hypogastric vessels and cleanly dissecting out all tissue about and behind the iliac and hypogastric vessels.

Attention is then transferred to the common iliac vessels just at or slightly below the bifurcation of the aorta. Incisions are made in the posterior peritoneum lateral and parallel to the rectum sufficient for good exposure. All tissue is dissected from the common iliac vessels, including that in the lumbosacral fossae, and from the brim of the pelvis. In the course of this dissection, both ureteral stumps are freed and incorporated with tissue from this area. Lymphatics at the upper limit of the dissection are tied or clipped. All tissue is reflected toward the

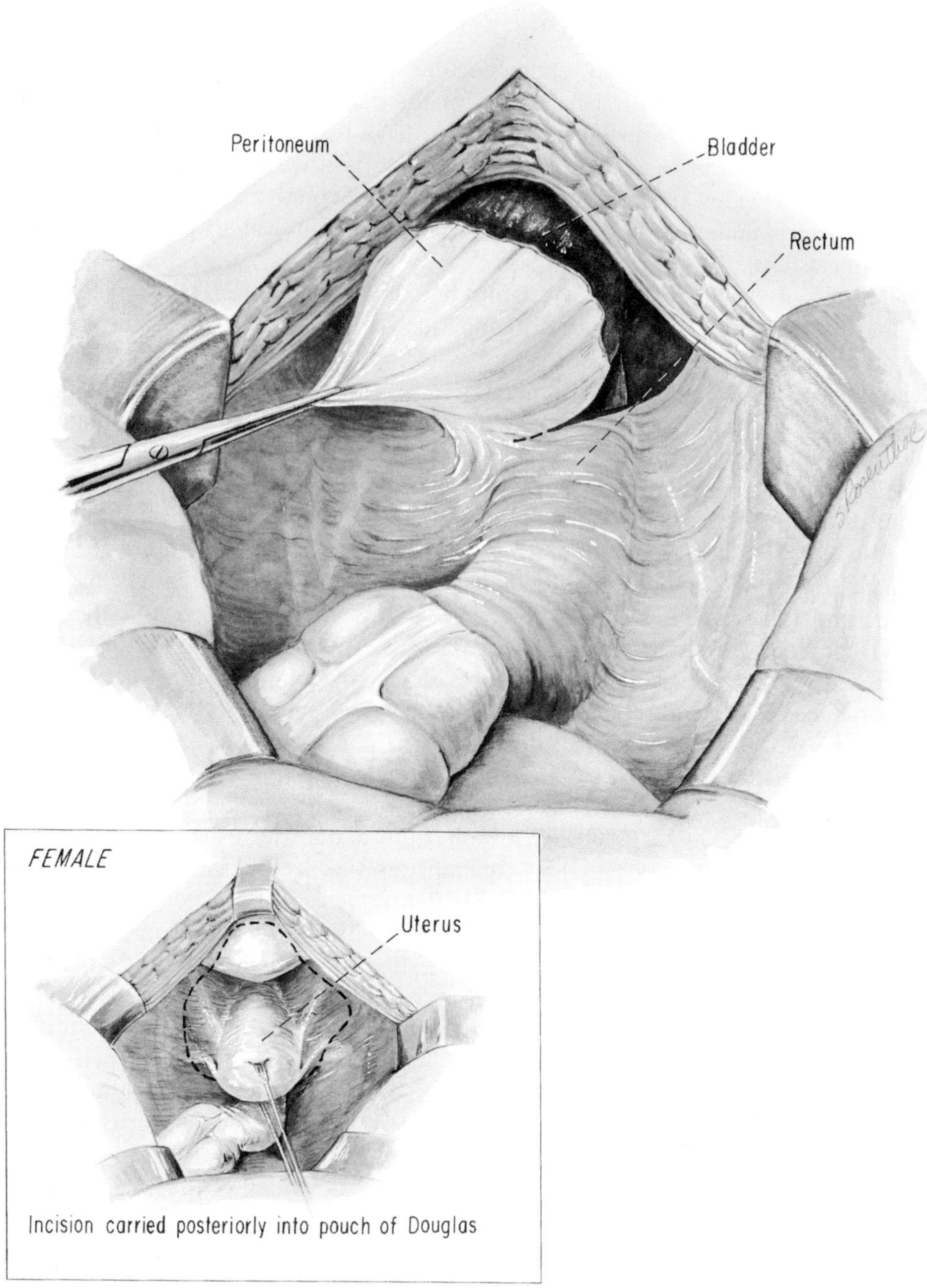

FIGURE 4. The exposure necessary for radical cystectomy is illustrated, and the initial peritoneal incisions about the bladder in the male and pelvic organs in the female are shown. Lateral extensions of the initial incisions upward on each side of the rectum to provide wide exposure of the retroperitoneum for gland dissection are necessary.

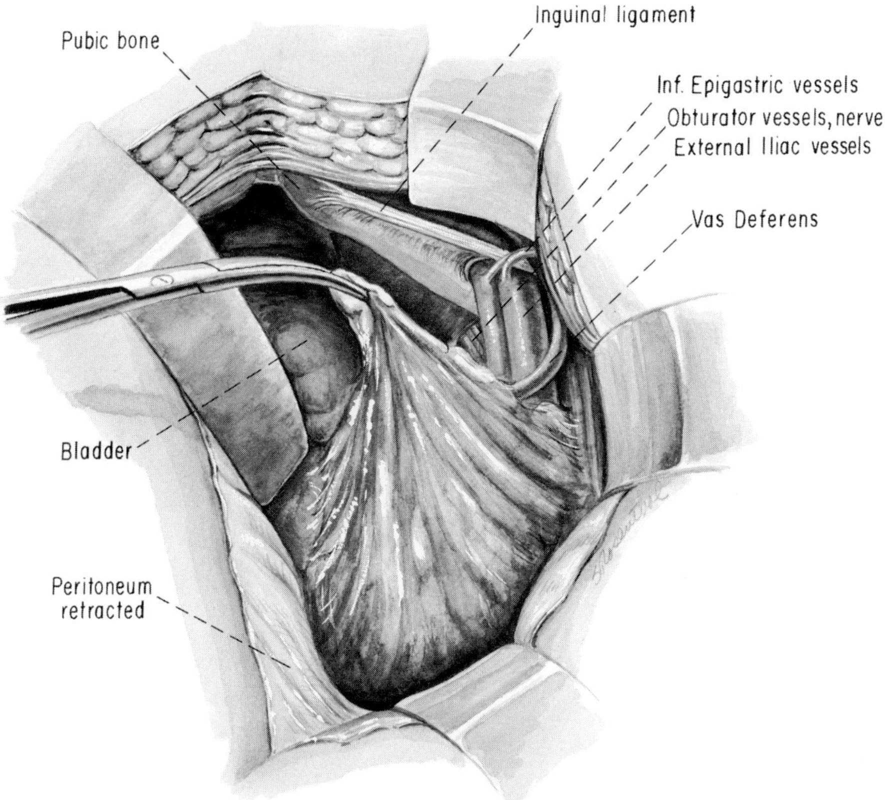

FIGURE 5. The right pelvis in the course of pelvic gland dissection is illustrated. The peritoneum has been stripped and retracted from the right side of the pelvis. The spermatic cord has been retracted upward out of the field. Gland dissection has been begun at the femoral canal, exposing the deep epigastric, external iliac, and obturator vessels. This dissection will be continued upward along the vessels until the hypogastric artery is exposed. Then dissection is transferred to the bifurcation of the aorta to free all tissues about the vessels, which will be pushed medially and incorporated and removed with the bladder. (See Figures 1–3.)

bladder, and dissection of the hypogastric vessels is completed, to the uterine or superior vesical artery. These vessels are clamped, divided, and ligated, and the dissection is continued with division of all arterial branches passing to the bladder, prostate, or vagina. The pelvic walls are further cleaned toward the bladder pedicles. This exposes the radicles of the hypogastric veins in the deep pelvis. These may be interrupted at this time or may be clamped and divided when the bladder is mobilized and its pedicles clamped and ligated.

Radical Cystectomy in the Male. Cystectomy in the male is then completed as outlined above by mobilizing the prostate, dividing and ligating the puboprostatic ligament, dividing the urethra, and stripping the prostate and seminal vesicles from the rectum. The posterior bladder pedicles are clamped and divided as deeply in the pelvis lateral to the rectum as possible. Additional dissec-

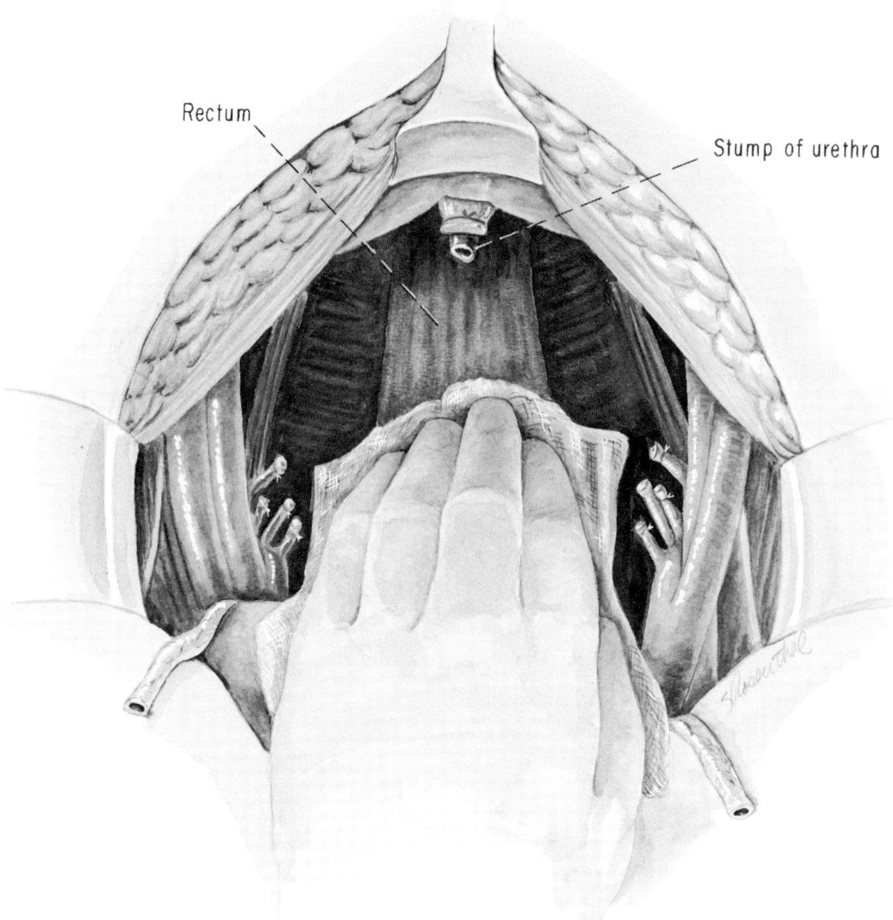

FIGURE 6. The pelvis after cystectomy.

tion of tissue from the pelvic walls about the venous radicles may be desirable after the bladder has been removed. A clean pelvis is left (Fig. 6).

Radical Cystectomy in the Female. Radical cystectomy is somewhat more difficult in the female. After the gland dissection and division of the arterial supply to the bladder, uterus, and vagina, the problem is to establish a plane of cleavage between the vagina and the rectal wall. The best method seems to be to place a tenaculum on the uterus, pull it up and forward to demonstrate the vaginal apex, and with scissors develop a plane close to the vaginal wall. The vagina and bladder are bound down around the rectum laterally by rather dense connective tissue which must be clamped and divided lateral to the rectum. This frees all tissue from the posterior pelvic wall and rectum, and dissection can be continued as far toward the pelvic outlet as practical. Much venous bleeding is apt to occur, and vessels must be secured as dissection progresses. At this point the patient is changed to lithotomy position if she has not been positioned for a combined approach, and

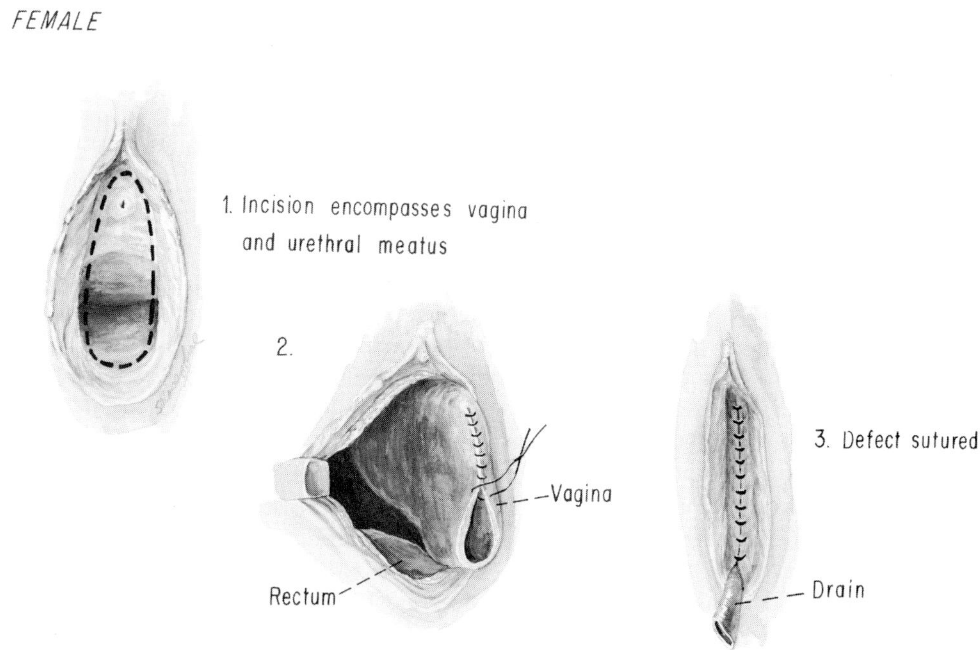

FIGURE 7. Radical cystectomy in the female requires removal of the vagina and urethra along with the bladder, uterus, and broad ligaments. These illustrations demonstrate the perineal phase of the operation: (1) the incision; (2) the incision deepened about the vaginal cuff and urethra and closure of the vagina to prevent leakage of urine and seeding of the wound by cells; (3) the closure, and placement of the drain.

dissection of the vagina and urethra completed from below (Fig. 7). An incision is made about the vaginal orifice and urethra inside the labia minora. This is deepened first just beneath the symphysis so that all tissue from beneath the symphysis is included in the specimen. Care must be exercised, as the incision is carried posteriorly around the vagina, not to injure the rectum. After the vagina and urethra have been freed sufficiently, the vagina is suture closed over the urethra so that spillage of bladder contents into the pelvis will not occur. Dissection is then carried upward until the dissection from above is met. The specimen is removed from above. The vaginal wound can usually be closed in two layers. If drainage is to be established, a vaginal drain is placed. The abdominal wound is closed without any effort to reperitonealize the pelvis. Usually the sigmoid is redundant and can be placed in the pelvis to cover much of the raw area.

General Comments

Radical cystectomy can usually be accomplished in two hours in the male but requires more time in the female. Cystectomy and urinary diversion requires at least five hours. Blood loss must be carefully estimated and replaced as the operation progresses. Serum loss is considerable, so that more blood or blood and plasma is necessary than blood loss suggests.

Pelvic exenteration presents no additional problems. We find that it can generally be accomplished as quickly as radical cystectomy, and more readily, because of the ease with which the rectum can be freed from the hollow of the sacrum and because ligation of the hypogastric trunks below the posterior gluteal vessels simplifies hemostasis. The hazard in this procedure is bleeding from pelvic veins, which may be difficult to control. This should not be attempted by clamping, but rather by the use of deep sutures.

Injury to the common or external iliac artery occasionally occurs with any of these operations when dissection is difficult. A simple laceration can be easily sutured, but division is more difficult to handle. Bulldog clamps should be available at all times; they provide a simple way of arresting bleeding. If division of an external iliac artery occurs, the ends may be reapproximated by mobilizing the distal artery into or below the femoral ring. Reanastomosis should be done carefully, with removal of clots and the local use of heparin. If a segment of artery has been removed which creates a defect that cannot be bridged by mobilization of the distal artery, a graft must be inserted. Blood flow to the limb must be assured before the arterial repair is considered satisfactory. Ligation and division of any veins can be done safely, but repair should be made if possible. Considerable prolonged swelling of the lower extremity is to be expected if the external iliac vein is tied, and the entire lower extremity should be wrapped in elastic bandage as soon as possible. Rectal injury calls for immediate temporary colostomy because leakage of fecal material into the open pelvis spells disaster, and primary healing in the presence of gas and feces will not occur.

Wound closure following radical cystectomy and urinary diversion must be done very meticulously and without drainage unless considerable soiling of the peritoneum and pelvis has occurred. Wound dehiscence is a very serious and often fatal complication in older persons. We have found that two operating teams, one to do cystectomy and the other to establish urinary diversion and to close the wound, are excellent for the performance of this long operation. Wound closure consists of placing nylon stay sutures through all layers of the abdominal wall three-quarters of an inch apart. The peritoneum cannot be closed in the lower portion of the wound, but it should be closed with continuous catgut as completely as possible. The rectus muscle should be reapproximated and the rectus sheath very carefully and solidly brought together.

Our mortality for total cystectomy and urinary diversion done for benign disease is approximately 5 per cent. That for radical cystectomy and urinary diversion approaches 15 per cent. This seems excessive, but it must be considered from the standpoint of age and associated degenerative diseases. Many patients were very poor risks. Most deaths have occurred as a result of respiratory complications or cardiac mishaps. Pulmonary emboli have been the cause of death in a few. We have come to think that gastrostomy done at the time of surgery is preferable to use of a Levin tube in patients with severe respiratory problems. Adynamic ileus, with the constant threat of intestinal obstruction, has been the most troublesome complication. Fortunately, most intestinal problems subside with patience and adequate intestinal decompression. Intestinal obstruction may be a fatal complication if secondary operation is required in the presence of peritonitis or localized sepsis. Fortunately, leaks from ureterointestinal anastomoses have not occurred. Late intestinal obstruction has been encountered. Each patient must have an intravenous pyelogram as early in convalescence as possible, to determine the status of the upper urinary tract. Poor functional results must be recognized early.

119. Ileal Segment Urinary Diversion

EUGENE M. BRICKER

DIVERSION of urinary excretion to the intestinal tract was done many years ago, at least as early as 1888 when Tizzoni experimentally transplanted the ureters into an isolated segment of ileum. Since that time, practically every imaginable way of using the intact intestinal tract or segments of intestine as substitutes for the urinary bladder has been attempted. In more modern times Blair, in 1916, transplanted the ureters to a segment of ileum which in turn was anastomosed to the sigmoid colon, and Seiffert, in 1934, described the use of an isolated segment of jejunum which acted as a conduit for the urine from the ureters to an external stoma. The development of rubber cements that provide a watertight attachment of an external appliance to skin has had a marked effect upon continued attempts to solve the problem of urinary diversion in the past fifteen years.

The use of pelvic exenteration as a means of controlling advanced pelvic cancer led to the need for a method of disposing of the urine from both ureters in the absence of the rectum. Several methods of solving this problem were attempted, but the resulting urinary complications were of such magnitude that it seemed doubtful such extended surgery was justifiable. Starting in 1950, we began the practice of transplanting the ureters to a short segment of terminal ileum in patients undergoing pelvic exenteration. The intestinal segment conveyed the urine to the external abdominal wall, where it drained into a glued-on appliance. Following the adoption of this procedure, we found early postoperative and late urinary complications to be so greatly diminished that the technique has been used essentially unchanged up to the present time.

The results of over 300 urinary diversion operations employing intestinal segments have been reported in *Annals of Surgery*, October 1962. The operative mortality attributable to urinary diversion was 3.4 per cent in 263 patients having pelvic exenteration, and 2.3 per cent in 44 patients having operations of lesser extent. Twenty-five per cent (65 of 260 adequately followed patients) had late renal or other complications attributable at least in part to urinary diversion, though in roughly half of these patients the complication was minor. However, in 3 of the 260 patients the complication was fatal. The overall incidence of clinically recognizable pyelonephritis in the last postoperative period was 14 per cent.

Hyperchloremia and acidosis were not observed as a complication in this group of patients. Similar results have been achieved by other observers, and have led to the rather widespread adoption of the technique.

Basic Principles

The basic principles contributing to the results produced by this method of urinary diversion appear to be the following:

1. The segment is isolated from the fecal stream.
2. The shortness of the bowel segment does not permit excessive absorption of urinary constituents into the blood stream.
3. The bowel segment, if functioning properly, does not act as a reservoir for the urine, but is essentially empty at all times.
4. The absence of any type of sphincter mechanism or external obstruction produces a minimum of back pressure and ureteral reflux.
5. The method of ureterointestinal anastomosis is simplified and allows primary healing with a minimum of scar tissue formation that may produce obstruction.

Preparation of the Patient

The patient is prepared as for any major surgery. Intravenous pyelograms are procured as a record of the preoperative renal status. Fluid and electrolyte balance is established, and the hemoglobin, blood, and extracellular fluid volume are brought to normal. A good urinary output is desirable, as is a normal blood urea nitrogen. However, the operation is not contraindicated by bilateral ureteral obstruction and an elevation of the blood urea. Intestinal preparation is accomplished in the usual manner, using one of the sulfonamide drugs for four or five days before operation. The patient is placed on a liquid diet the day before operation and given castor oil unless it is contraindicated by some degree of intestinal obstruction. Every effort is made to have the small intestine as well as the colon completely empty and deflated at the time the operation is done. Preoperative nasogastric suction is not used.

Technique

The Ileostomy Site

Before the abdomen is opened, the site for ileostomy is selected (Fig. 1). In selecting this site, consideration must be given to the size of the bag and the configuration of the abdomen. It is essential that the bag be worn over flat skin and that

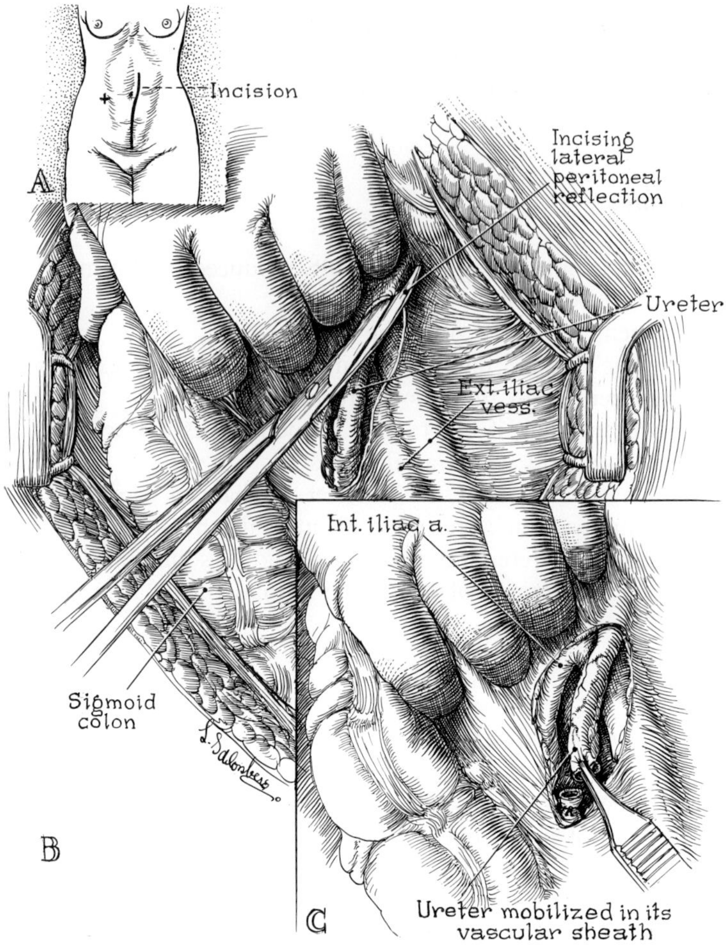

FIGURE 1. Before the abdomen is opened, the site for the ileostomy stoma is scratched on the skin. If the operation does not entail removal of the colon and rectum, the left ureter is exposed by an incision through the lateral peritoneum of the sigmoid mesocolon. After sectioning of the ureter, the proximal end is elevated with its vascular sheath intact.

the anterior superior iliac spine and the costal margin not impinge upon the edge of the bag flange regardless of the position of the patient. The stoma must be far enough from the umbilicus for the flange of the bag to stay glued to the skin throughout its entire width. With these considerations in mind, a site is usually chosen lateral to the umbilicus by the width of the bag flange. The individual variations in the length of the abdomen and in the bony protuberances make it impossible to have a fixed rule regarding the location of this stoma. The two most important landmarks are the anterior superior iliac spine and the umbilicus. If there are scars on the right side of the abdomen, it must be made certain that they will not interfere with adherence of the bag.

A midline incision is used. The umbilicus is not excised, since excision may remove just enough skin to produce distortion of the skin surface that may result in poor adherence of the bag.

Mobilization and Preparation of the Ureters

The ureters may be transected at any level, depending upon the need. In the standard case, the optimum level for transecting the ureters is about 2 cm. below the point at which they cross the iliac artery (Figs. 1, 2, and 3). In patients not having pelvic exenteration or resection of the colon, the ureters are exposed through longitudinal incisions through the peritoneum, and are transected at the selected level. The distal ureter may be ligated or removed, depending upon the operation that is being done. The proximal end is carefully elevated for 3 or 4 cm. with its vascular sheath intact. It is highly important that the adventitia of the ureter containing its blood supply not be stripped down to bare ureter. The proximal ureteral ends are not ligated, but are simply tucked out of the way until the primary operation has been completed. The small amount of urine that drains into the wound and peritoneal cavity is of no consequence unless there is definite pyelonephritis, in which case the ureter may be ligated and handled as aseptically as possible.

After completion of the primary operation, the ureters are prepared for transplantation to the ileal segment. The left ureter must be passed through the sigmoid mesocolon if the sigmoid has not been removed (Figs. 1 and 2). The most satisfactory path for this transfer is beneath the superior hemorrhoidal artery and vein,

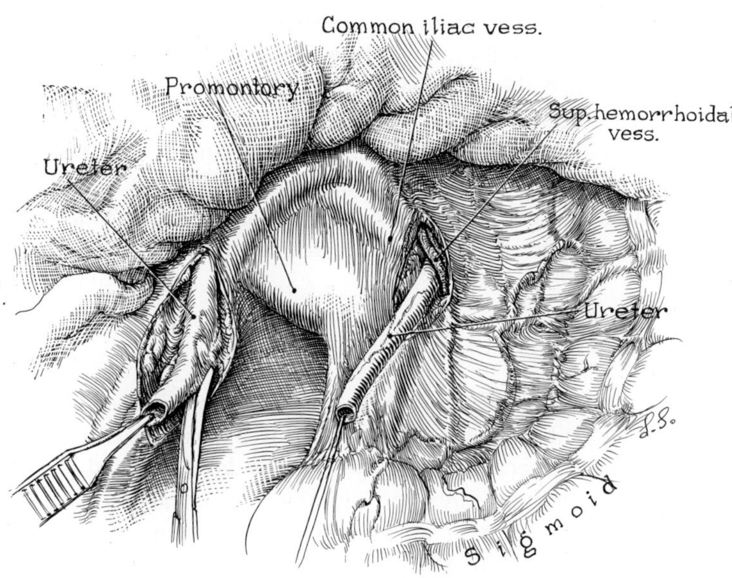

FIGURE 2. The right ureter is exposed through a longitudinal incision over the pelvic brim, and the proximal end is mobilized. The left ureter is drawn through an incision in the sigmoid mesocolon posterior to the superior hemorrhoidal vessels.

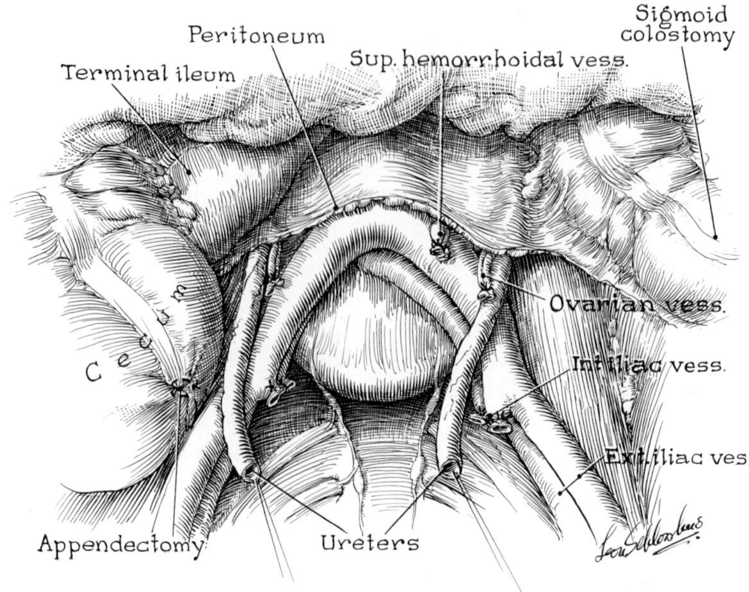

FIGURE 3. The appendix is removed. If a pelvic exenteration has been done, the anatomical relationships are essentially as illustrated in this figure.

and it can best be established by inserting the finger through the peritoneal incision on the left side and moving it onto the promontory of the sacrum, beneath the superior hemorrhoidal vessels, and across to the right side of the sigmoid mesocolon, at which point a peritoneal counterincision is made and the ureter drawn through (Fig. 2). We do not hesitate to use instruments on the end of the ureter at this stage, since the terminal centimeter or so will subsequently be discarded. The tunnel through the sigmoid mesocolon must be ample, and directed so that the ureter passes through it easily without angulation and without impinging on a peritoneal edge. Patients having pelvic exenteration present no problem in getting the left ureter over to the right side (Fig. 3). With both ureters now ready for anastomosis to the intestine, attention is turned to fashioning the ileal segment.

Isolation and Preparation of the Ileal Segment

Before the segment is isolated, the appendix is always removed. The best level for isolating the segment from the small intestine appears usually to be about 6 to 8 inches from the ileocecal valve. However, the level selected should be that which appears to be mechanically most suitable for the individual situation. So far as we are aware, the variation in physiological function of different levels of the small intestine is of no significance in determining the suitability of a segment as a urinary conduit. The important factors are purely mechanical and anatomical. In patients with obese abdominal walls we usually design the segment far enough away from the ileocecal valve for well-developed vascular arcades to make it pos-

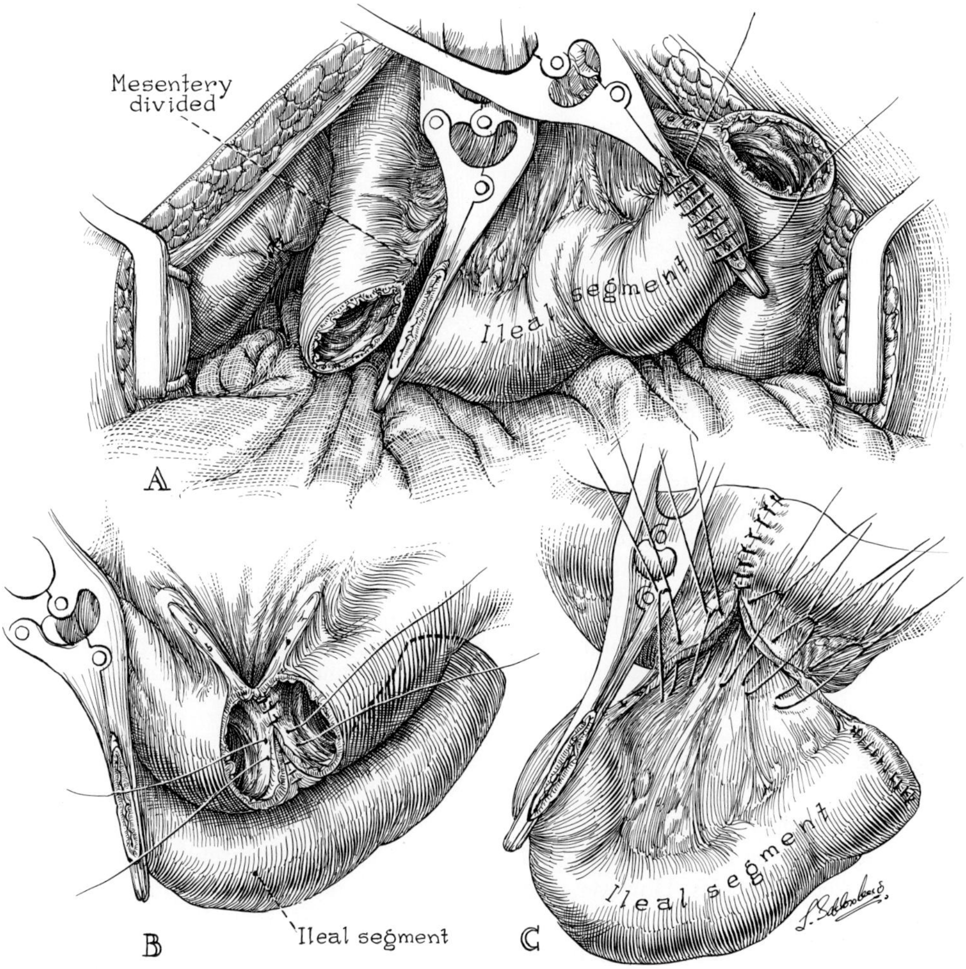

FIGURE 4. The ileal segment is isolated at the selected level. The mesenteric incisions are made no deeper than necessary to accomplish the isolation of the segment and to allow an end-to-end anastomosis of the remaining bowel to be done anterior to the vascular pedicle of the segment (A). The proximal end of the isolated segment is closed immediately with a running inverting catgut suture in two layers. Continuity of the bowel is then restored by end-to-end anastomosis with interrupted fine silk sutures in two layers, turning in a minimal amount of bowel edge (B). The mesenteric rent between the anastomosis and the vascular pedicle should always be closed. We usually do this as the final step after delivering the external stoma (C).

sible to undercut the mesentery for a short distance, to allow the distal end of the ileal segment to be brought through the thick abdominal wall without tension (see Figure 5). In the average or thin patient, bringing the distal end of the segment through the abdominal wall presents no problem.

The average segment is planned to be 6 or 7 inches in length. This length allows the external stoma to reach the skin level without tension. The patient with an obese abdominal wall may require a slightly longer segment. We never have

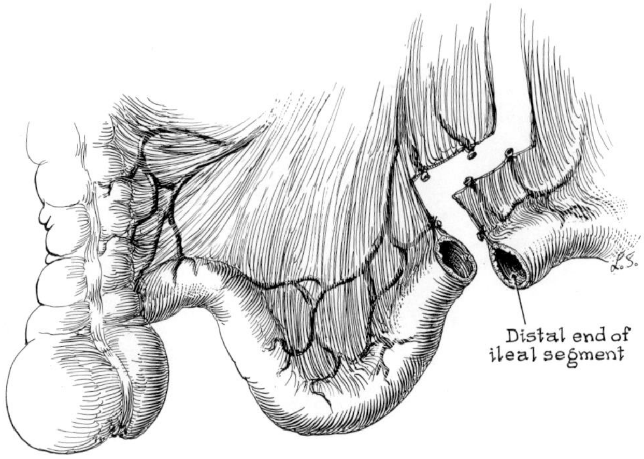

FIGURE 5. In patients with an obese and thick abdominal wall, it is necessary to plan the ileal segment so that the distal end can with certainty be withdrawn through the abdominal wall without tension. Accordingly, we select a higher site, where the vascular arcades are well demarcated, and undercut the mesenteric incision as indicated in this figure. This fashions a pedicle out of the distal end of the segment and facilitates its delivery through the abdominal wall. One must be certain that the blood supply of the segment end is adequate, and it must not be jeopardized, in passing through the abdominal wall, by tension, twisting, or too tight an opening through the musculofascial layers.

occasion to make a segment over 10 inches in length. The cuts into the mesentery are usually made only 2 or 3 cm. in depth (Fig. 4). It is of great importance that the blood supply of the four cut bowel ends be completely adequate. In the standard case this is no problem, and does not even require careful identification of the vascular arcades. However, the proper management of the patient with an obese abdominal wall requires the most careful attention, in fashioning the ileal segment, to both its level and its mesenteric pedicle (Fig. 5). Only two crushing intestinal clamps are used, one on each end of the segment to be isolated (Fig. 4). The proximal end is immediately closed with two rows of running inverting 3–0 chromic catgut sutures. The distal clamp is left in place until it is time to deliver the end of the segment to the external stoma. The bowel ends to be anastomosed are left open without clamps, and an immediate end-to-end anastomosis is done. It is our practice to do this anastomosis with two rows of fine silk. First a mucosal row of fine interrupted silk sutures is placed around the entire circumference of the bowel, and then the serosal layer of interrupted sutures is placed. It is quite easy to rotate the bowel 180 degrees to expose the entire circumference for the careful application of the second row of sutures. As little of the bowel as possible is incorporated in the sutures forming the anastomosis. The end-to-end anastomosis is done anterior to the vascular pedicle of the isolated segment.

The Ureteroileal Anastomoses

With the segment isolated and the end-to-end anastomosis completed, attention is turned to anastomosis of the ureters to the proximal end of the segment. The small intestine can be packed and retracted out of the way within the abdomen, or it can be lifted out of the abdomen and protected by moist laparotomy gauzes. The anastomoses can best be done with unrestricted exposure. The proximal end of the isolated segment is carried down to the region of the promontory of the sacrum in proximity to the left ureter.

It can be seen easily that anastomosis of the left ureter to the end of the segment in this position will leave a hiatus formed by the segment, the ureter, the posterior abdominal wall, and the inferior surface of the mesentery of the small intestine (Fig. 6). This is an appreciable hiatus through which the small intestine could easily herniate, and for this reason it should be closed. Closure is accomplished by suturing the end of the segment and its vascular pedicle to the peritoneum of the posterior abdominal wall and the inferior surface of the mesentery of the small intestine with fine interrupted silk sutures. Care must always be taken not to place these sutures deeply enough to get into the blood vessels supplying the segment. The exact method necessary for closing the hiatus is always apparent as the operation is being done, though it may vary in detail from case to case.

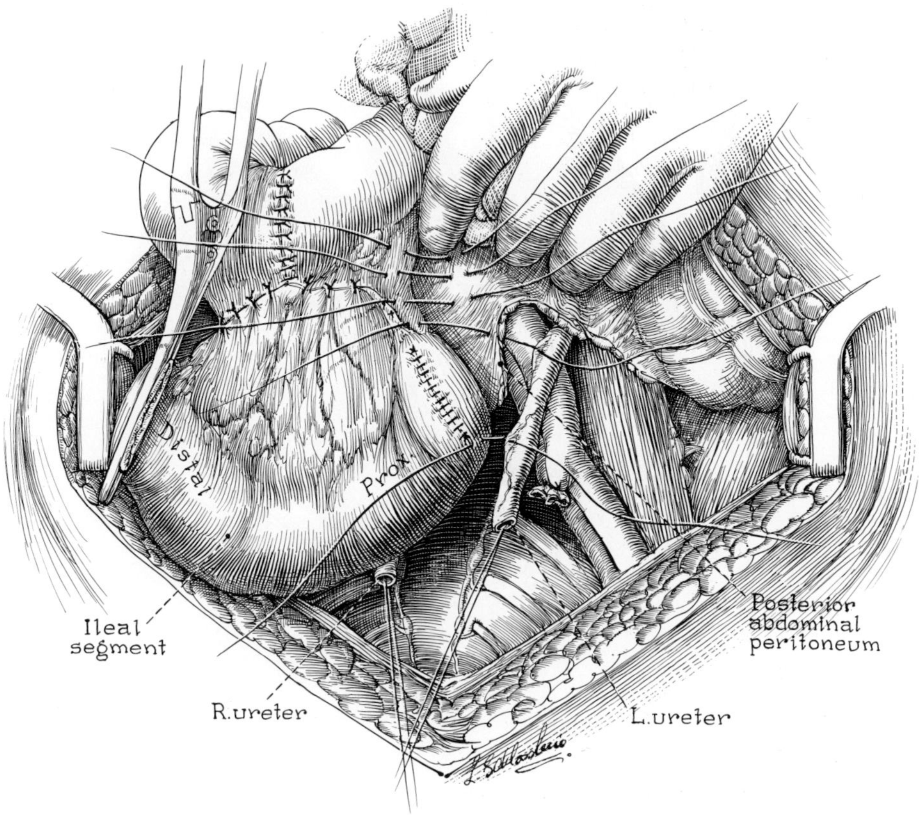

FIGURE 6. Before anastomosis of the ureters to the segment, the hiatus formed by the segment, the vascular pedicle, the posterior peritoneum, and the ureter must be closed.

After the hiatus has been closed, the left ureter is brought into proximity with the proximal end of the intestinal segment and the anastomosis is begun (Fig. 7). First, three fine silk sutures are placed between the vascular sheath or adventitia of the ureter and the serosa of the segment about 1 cm. from the blind end of the segment. The two lateral sutures are left long and hemostats are hung on them for stabilization. The middle suture is cut. Next, a pointed blade is used to make a small incision through the layers of the bowel, 4 or 5 mm. from the first row of sutures. If this incision is made by stroking the bowel wall so that the individual layers bulge through the small serosal incision, the mucosa will protrude and its edges will be visible when the incision is completed. It is quite difficult to identify the mucosal edge of this small opening if the incision is made as a stab with the pointed blade. The final opening through the bowel wall should be no larger than the diameter of the ureter (Fig. 8). As the bowel incision is being made it may be gently sponged or cleared with a low pressure sucker. It is unnecessary

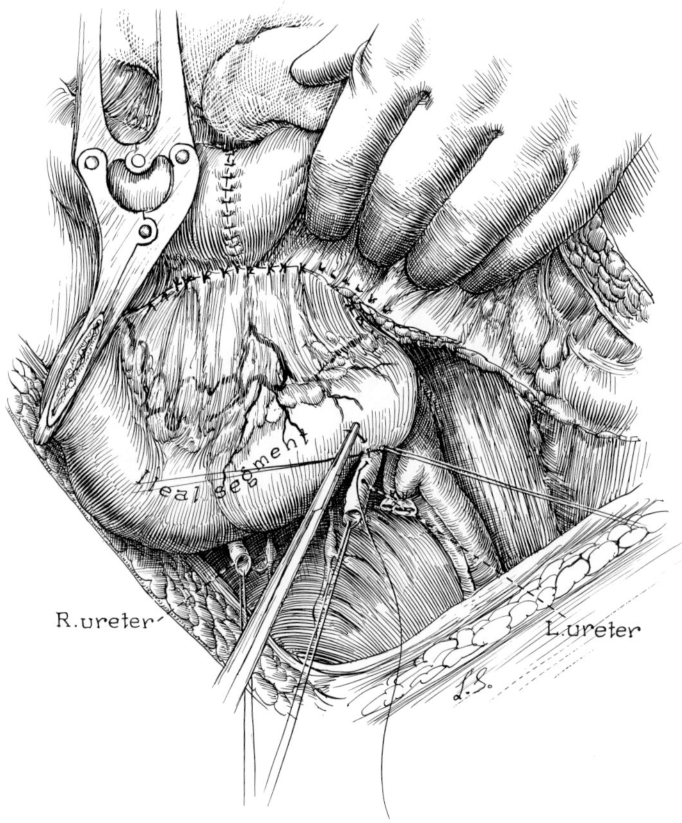

FIGURE 7. Both ureters are anastomosed to the segment near its proximal end, the left ureter first. The anastomosis is done in two layers, the first being a posterior row of three fine silk sutures placed between the serosa of the bowel and the adventitia and vascular sheath of the ureter. Excess ureter is trimmed away before the internal row of fine catgut sutures is placed.

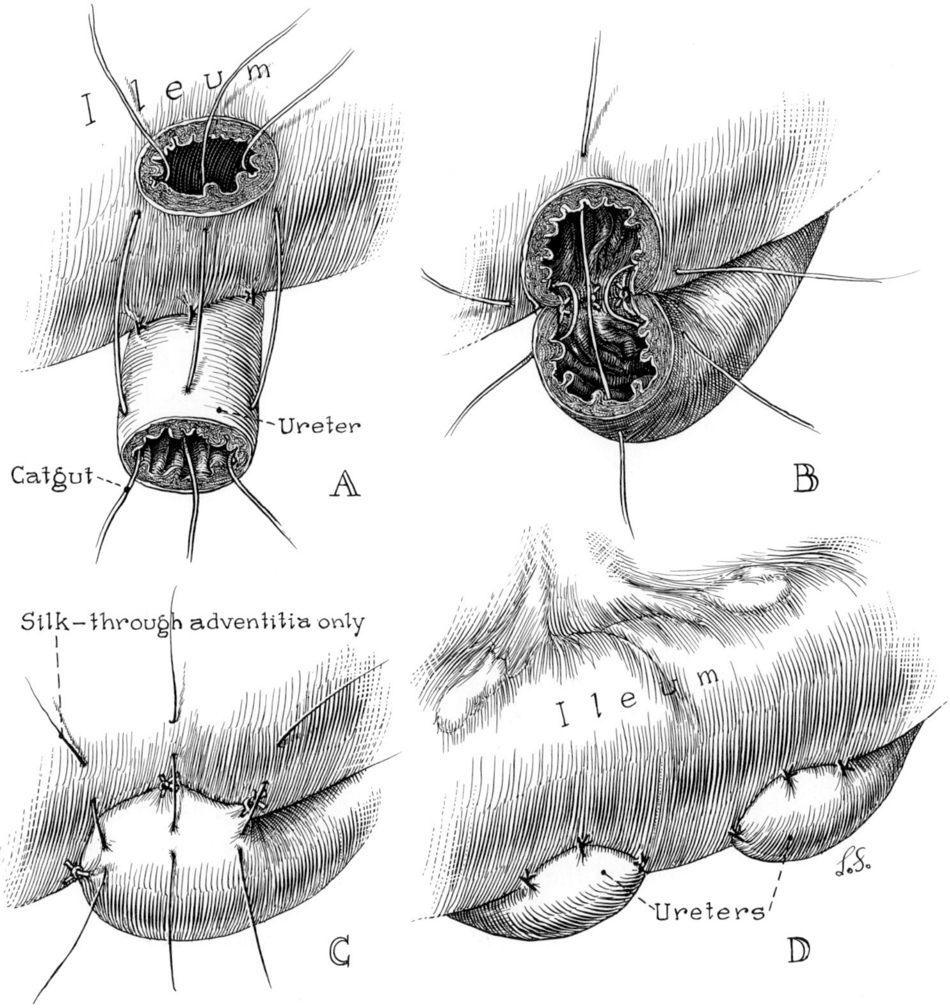

FIGURE 8. The opening into the bowel is made no larger than the diameter of the ureteral lumen. Although this is referred to as a mucosa-to-mucosa anastomosis, actually the fine catgut sutures of the inner row pass through the entire thickness of both the ureter and the small intestine. After the catgut sutures have been placed, three or four fine silk sutures are added to complete the external row, the sutures incorporating the serosa and the vascular sheath and adventitia of the ureter. The silk sutures must not perforate the lumen of the ureter.

and inadvisable to clamp and tie small bleeding vessels. This will only distort the bowel opening and complicate the anastomosis. Furthermore, the slight bleeding points encountered are eventually controlled as the anastomotic sutures are placed. A little digital pressure on the bowel segment while the incision is being made through its wall will help force the mucosa out through the serosal opening so that it can be seen easily.

During these early stages of the anastomosis the end of the ureter can be manipulated by a straight artery clamp applied to its tip. The ureter is thus easily moved about and positioned, and it is unnecessary to apply other instruments to it. After the first row of sutures has been placed, and after the opening has been made into the bowel segment, a knife or sharp dissection scissor is used to amputate the excess end of ureter to which the artery forceps has been applied. From this time on, the ureter is not grasped with an instrument. Chromic catgut (4–0) with an atraumatic needle is passed through the entire ureteral wall from inside out, taking about 1 mm. of the entire thickness of the ureter. The needle is then inserted through the serosa of the bowel opening and through the pouting mucosal edge. One end of this suture is then left long and hung with a small clamp for stabilization of the anastomosis as the other sutures are placed. Another similar suture is placed on the exact opposite side of the ureter. Although small pointed vascular thumb forceps are used, it is usually unnecessary to take hold of the ureteral edge with an instrument as the anastomosis is being done. The placement of a third catgut suture between the two previously placed will complete the posterior row of the anastomosis in a normal-sized ureter.

The anterior row of catgut sutures is then placed in a similar manner, but with the knots tied on the outside of the lumen (Fig. 8). It makes no difference whether these small knots are inside or outside the lumen. It is simply easier to tie the posterior row with the knots on the inside and the anterior row with the knots on the outside. Introduction of a pointed thumb forceps into the lumen of the ureter will facilitate passage of the needle through the ureteral wall without catching the other side. As the anterior sutures are being placed, it is important to reach a slight way down the external surface of the ureter and engage the point of the needle in the vascular sheath before passing the needle through the ureteral wall. If this is not done, the ureter may gradually extend itself out of the adventitia and vascular sheath and become so thin that it is difficult to work with. The needle is then passed through the mucosa of the bowel and out through the serosa. This must be done with great care, and the bowel mucosal edge must be carefully identified to make certain that the needle does not inadvertently catch the mucosa on the other side of the opening and thus partially occlude the lumen.

During all this manipulation it is of great importance not to tear the mucosa of the bowel and make the opening larger than the lumen of the ureter, since this will require more sutures for closure. The more sutures that have to be placed the greater is the chance for technical error. Five catgut sutures, or six at most, are enough for the circumference of the normal-sized ureter. Dilated ureters require proportionally more sutures but are much easier to manage because of the increased size. After completion of the circumferential row of catgut sutures, three or four anterior silk sutures are placed between the vascular sheath of the ureter and the serosa of the bowel, care being taken not to perforate the lumen of the ureter with the sutures. This completes the anastomosis. The temptation to place another suture here and there, to add security, should be avoided. A total of five or six catgut sutures for the internal row and six or seven silk sutures for the external row is enough.

Attention is then turned to the anastomosis of the right ureter, which is done in exactly the same manner as the anastomosis of the left. This anastomosis is made only a centimeter or so away from the first, both being near the end of the ileal segment. If the ureters are not placed near the end of the segment, a proximal pouch of the segment may result which may empty poorly. The uretero-intestinal anastomoses act as a point of fixation of the ileal segment, and it is desirable that this point of fixation be at the end of the segment rather than elsewhere. The right ureter is hidden beneath the mesentery of the small intestine and there is no potential hiatus or tunnel through which the bowel can herniate. It is therefore not necessary to obliterate a potential space as is essential when the left ureter is brought to the end of the segment. The operator should use good mechanical judgment in placing the segment and in doing the anastomoses, so that the ureters will drain freely into the segment. If the ureters have been cut a couple of centimeters below the pelvic brim, it will usually be found that there is more ureter than is necessary to accomplish the anastomisis. For this reason, we do not hesitate to manipulate the ureter by clamping its end, since a bit of the ureteral end will be discarded before the anastomosis is completed. After the ureter has been trimmed it should be manipulated as little as possible with instruments, since the resulting trauma may interfere with healing.

The Ileostomy

Following completion of the ureteroileal anastomoses, the distal end of the segment is made ready to be delivered through the external stoma. A circular opening, 1 inch in diameter, is made through the skin at the previously determined site. This can most expeditiously be done by tenting the skin up by traction with an Ochsner clamp applied at this spot and then slicing off the skin in such a manner as to leave an opening of the desired diameter. Before one makes the opening through the remaining layers of the abdominal wall, it is advisable to grasp the fascial layers of the abdominal incision on the right side and to place them on approximately the same tension that will exist after the wound is closed. An incision is then made through the fascial and muscular layers down to and through the peritoneum. If the layers are under proper tension, this can be done quite easily by cross-cutting the muscle and fascia with a knife through the skin opening and enlarging the opening to the desired amount with sharp scissors as the muscular and fascial layers are palpated with the fingers of the left hand passed into the opening from the peritoneal side. The pulse of the inferior epigastric artery can usually be palpated with the left hand, and an effort should be made to avoid the artery by carrying the opening lateral to it. The size of the opening through the layers of the abdominal wall depends upon the thickness of the abdominal wall and the amount of adipose tissue in the mesentery of the end of the ileal segment which is to be delivered through it. Ordinarily we make this opening no larger than two fingerbreadths in diameter, and in thin patients smaller. After the opening has been completed, a long Kelly clamp is inserted through it from outside in and the end of the ileal segment is gently grasped as the Payr clamp is removed. The end of the segment is then gently drawn through the opening in the abdominal wall without twisting its mesentery. Upon being delivered to the outside, the edges of the ileum are grasped with small pointed forceps and the circumference is sutured to the skin edge by interrupted 3–0 catgut sutures (Fig. 9). For double security and to bring the ileal mucosa to the skin edge without tension, the catgut sutures are passed through the skin edge, through the serosa of the ileum about 2 cm. from the edge, and then through full thickness of the bowel edge. All efforts are aimed at getting an ileal opening flush with the skin which will heal by first intention and which will not distort or retract the skin surface. A segment end that will not reach the skin surface without tension indicates poor planning of the segment.

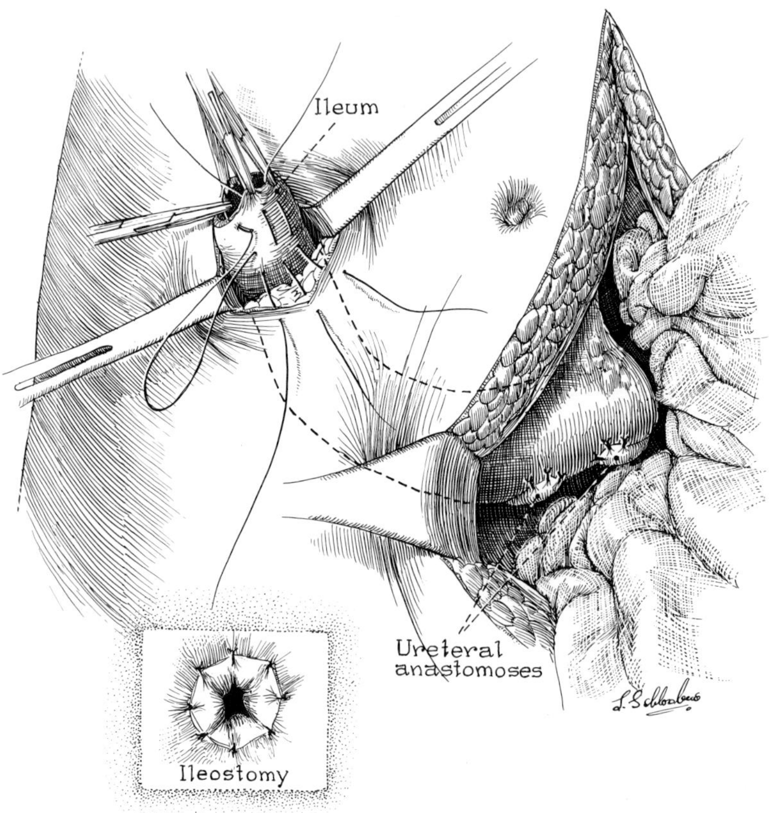

FIGURE 9. After completion of the ureteroileal anastomoses, the distal end of the segment is drawn through an opening prepared at the previously selected site in the right side of the abdominal wall. It may at times seem advisable to deliver the segment to the external stoma earlier in the course of the operation, in order to establish anatomical relationships before the ureters are anastomosed. Catgut (3–0) is used to suture the edges of the segment to the skin edges. A mild eversion can be accomplished by passing the suture through the skin edge, through the serosa of the bowel about 2 cm. proximal to its edge, and then through the edge of the bowel. Placing the sutures in this manner decreases the chance of retraction.

The hiatus formed by the end-to-end ileoileal anastomosis over the vascular pedicle of the ileal segment is next closed (Fig. 4C). We usually postpone this part of the procedure until the external stoma has been delivered, since we cannot be sure of the various relationships until this is done. The hiatus is closed by suturing the cut edges of the mesentery to the peritoneal surface of the vascular pedicle, taking care not to introduce the needle deeply enough to rupture a blood vessel and produce a hematoma in the vascular pedicle.

Before the abdomen is closed, the relationships of the small intestine, anastomosis, segment, and cecum are carefully checked. An occasional patient will have a redundant cecum that hangs loosely deep in the pelvis. This position of the cecum forces the terminal ileum to angulate itself over the ileal segment as the

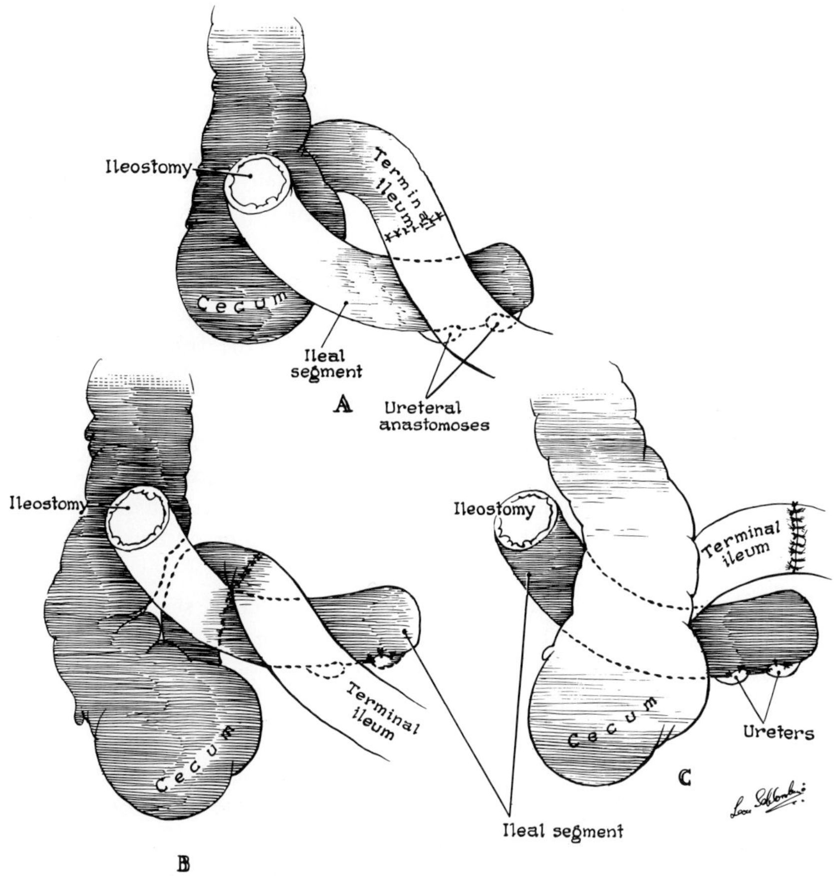

FIGURE 10. The relationship of the cecum and terminal ileum to the ileal segment when the cecum is attached high in the right iliac fossa is as illustrated in A. If the cecum is redundant and hangs low in the pelvis, the relationship, indicated in *B*, is undesirable and might lead to intestinal obstruction. This can be corrected easily by incising the lateral peritoneal reflection of the ascending colon and transferring the cecum medial to the ileal segment as indicated in *C*. (Reproduced by permission of W. B. Saunders Company from Bricker, E. M., *S. Clin. North America*, August 1956.)

segment traverses the abdominal cavity to the anterior abdominal wall (Fig. 10B). When this situation is exaggerated or appears to be mechanically unfavorable, it can be corrected easily by incising the lateral peritoneal reflection of the cecum and ascending colon, freeing them from the retroperitoneal attachments, and drawing the cecum and terminal ileum medial to the ileal segment rather than letting them remain in the lateral position (Fig. 10C). This is never necessary when the cecum is attached high in the lumbar gutter (Fig. 10A). No attempt is made to suture the ileal segment to the lateral abdominal peritoneum in order to close this large lateral hiatus. We have not found it necessary.

General Comments

Patients having ureteroileostomies in conjunction with pelvic exenteration do not require drains through the abdominal wall, since there is free drainage through the pelvic and perineal defect. However, if the operation is of more limited extent and does not provide free drainage through the pelvis, a rubber dam drain is inserted into the depths of the pelvis and brought out through the inferior angle of the wound. Its purpose is to take care of any leakage of urine from the anastomoses, an extremely rare occurrence.

It has long been my practice, before closing the abdomens of patients who have had pelvic extenteration or other extensive pelvic operations, to insert a long intestinal tube to the level of the ileocecal valve. This tube has perforations throughout its distal 3 or 4 feet and serves to splint the bowel in a favorable position to prevent kinks. At the same time, it keeps the bowel decompressed through suction. We cannot yet prove that this technique reduces the incidence of postoperative intestinal obstruction in patients having pelvic exenteration, but it is my distinct clinical impression that it not only reduces the danger of this complication but is of very great value in controlling ileus or obstructive symptoms when they do appear.

The abdomen is closed with interrupted figure-of-eight steel wire sutures by the method of Tom Jones. The superficial portion of the wound is frequently only partially closed, the remainder being left open for delayed primary closure with adhesive strips on the third or fourth postoperative day.

A transparent plastic bag is glued over the ileostomy stoma before the patient leaves the operating room. The bag allows accurate measurement of urinary excretion through the early postoperative period and at the same time does not obscure the ileostomy stoma from visual inspection. This temporary bag is used for three or four days, after which the standard urinary ileostomy bag is applied.

Postoperative Management

The postoperative management is the same as that for any other patient after major abdominal surgery with a resection of the small intestine. If the long jejunostomy tube has been used, it is kept on suction until the fifth or sixth postoperative day and until there is evidence that intestinal function has returned to normal and the patient is on an increasing diet. It is then simply clamped off until the twelfth or fourteenth postoperative day, at which time it is removed. If in the meantime the patient develops symptoms that warrant it, the tube is irrigated and put on suction.

The skin around the urinary ileostomy is carefully watched and the temporary bag is changed as necessary to protect the skin during the early postoperative period. Urinary excretion is usually evident an hour or so after completion of the operation. However, occasionally the total urinary excretion may be quite small in the first 12 to 24 hours. Assuming the patient is adequately hydrated, this is not alarming, since we have frequently seen the urinary excretion increase rapidly to normal as late as the second postoperative day. A possible explanation is that there is enough obstruction from edema at both ureterointestinal anastomoses to hold up excretion until sufficient pressure is built up to effect it, or until the inflammatory reaction begins to subside. If the anastomoses are carefully done, it appears that the chance of bilateral obstruction is very small; it has occurred only twice in our series of 307 operations. If the urinary output appears alarmingly low in the early postoperative period, a catheter can be inserted into the segment in order to be sure there is no obstruction at some level in the abdominal wall. We have found that leaving a catheter in the segment for drainage is not very satisfactory, since the catheter tends to plug up with mucus. A retrograde pyelogram with Hypaque solution can be of value in demonstrating whether or not a leak is present and whether or not the anastomoses are patent enough to allow reflux of the opaque medium.

As soon as it is apparent that urinary outflow is adequate and that the ileal stoma is viable and healing satisfactorily, a permanent ileostomy bag is applied. The flat, glue-on type of bag appears to be the most suitable. We prefer a bag with a valve in the dependent end for emptying the urine. The patient is taught as early as possible to apply this bag himself, the lesson usually starting on the tenth to twelfth postoperative day. The problems of using the bag are no different from those encountered when the bag is used for a terminal ileostomy, except that they are less severe because urine is less irritating to the skin than is the fecal stream from the terminal ileum. Nevertheless, it is good practice to fit the bags as precisely to the external stoma as possible. It is our practice to keep a supply of a standard-size bag with a standard aperture of 1 inch, and we fashion the external stoma to fit this aperture. Very seldom is it necessary to have a bag custom made.

Patients vary greatly in the frequency with which the bag is changed; from once every two days to once every seven or eight days. Associated odor is due to lack of cleanliness, to carelessness in the management of the bag, and especially to spillage of urine on the skin, bag, and clothing when the bag is emptied. I have been convinced by one or two very intelligent patients that odor can be prevented completely, the most important factor being the elimination of spillage.

Postoperative intravenous pyelograms are obtained before the patient is discharged from the hospital. Subsequently, intravenous pyelograms are obtained at six-month intervals for a year or 18 months, and thereafter at increasing intervals or as indicated.

A discussion of the complications resulting from this operation has been presented in *Annals of Surgery,* October 1962.

References

BUTCHER, H. R., JR., SUGG, W. L., MCAFEE, C. A., and BRICKER, E. M. Ileal conduit method of ureteral urinary diversion. *Ann. Surg.* 156:682, October 1962.

CORDONNIER, J. J., and NICOLAI, C. N. An evaluation of the use of an isolated segment of ileum as a means of urinary diversion. *J. Urol.* 83:834, June 1960.

120. Revision of the Vesical Outlet

VICTOR F. MARSHALL

REVISION of postsurgical contracture and congenital narrowing of the vesical neck, rather than the removal of gross obstructions such as benign prostatic hypertrophy, will be discussed in this chapter. When clearly defined obstructing tissue is present, transurethral resection is usually adequate; but when the obstructing element is ill-defined, transurethral excision often provides only an incomplete improvement and is not without the risk that incontinence may result. Furthermore, among the sequelae is additional fibrosis with recurrent obstruction. Two more reliable techniques are available for revision, and both may be employed in the same case if indicated.

Enlargement of the Anterior Vesical Outlet

The first of these procedures is the Y-V plastic enlargement of the anterior part of the vesical outlet (Fig. 1). After suprapubic exposure, the bladder is opened by an incision which constitutes a limb of an imaginary Y. The central point of this Y is in the midline at the junction of the bladder and the urethra. The two upper

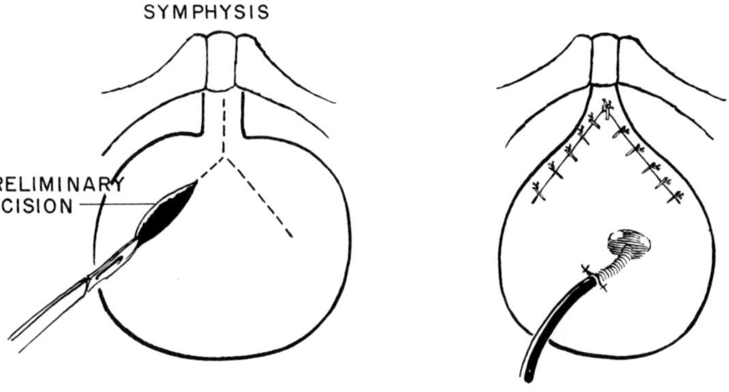

FIGURE 1. Anterior Y-V enlargement of the vesical neck.

limbs of the Y diverge from this point at about 90 degrees to each other. Each limb can be of liberal length: for example, 5 cm. is usually not excessive even in a child. The stem of the Y incision goes down the midline of the upper portion of the urethra to a point at least 1 cm. below the area where the obstruction of the neck is considered to be. In actual practice, this preliminary opening of only a limb of the Y permits inspection and palpation of the vesical outlet for evaluation. Assuming that a Y-V plasty is indicated after this evalution, the incisions for the other limbs are made and bleeding points controlled by ligation with fine plain catgut. If no more than the Y-V procedure is to be performed, the apex of the V portion is drawn down to the end of the longitudinal incision in the top of the urethra and secured there with several interrupted sutures of 00 plain catgut. A tapering wedge of flexible tissue is thus interposed in any ringlike constriction and the outlet becomes more funnel-shaped.

Although not always necessary, it has generally seemed safer to provide a small cystostomy site in the upper portion of the bladder for drainage during the healing period. Accordingly, a small stab wound is made in the dome of the bladder immediately below the peritoneal reflection, and a double Malecot catheter, 16 to 20 French size, inserted. A chromic catgut suture is passed through the bladder wall immediately above the cystostomy site, and the ends of this suture are passed through the rectus muscles on either side and tied, so that the cystostomy site will be suspended upward and away from the vesical outlet.

The closure of the plastic area does not then need to be completely watertight, but it is preferable that the fluid delivered through the cystostomy not flow out when the bladder is only mildly distended. In the usual case the ureteral orifices are readily visualized and are well away from the suture lines; but if there is any doubt as to their location, ureteral catheterization should be employed and the catheters removed only after it is clear that no sutures compromise the ureters. A small drain is left in the space of Retzius, and the abdominal wall is closed in routine fashion. A transurethral catheter is not left in place. The drain can usually be removed in three days. Since about twelve days are required for firm healing, the cystostomy is permitted to drain freely for that period and the tube is then removed if there are no indications to the contrary. A voiding cystourethrogram made by filling the bladder with a contrast medium through the cystostomy tube, just before the catheter is removed, provides useful information concerning function.

Wedge Excision of Obstruction on the Floor of the Vesical Outlet

When the constriction of the vesical outlet appears to be principally in the posterior half, the second procedure mentioned may be more valuable. The approach and inspection are the same as in the procedure just described. An adequate view of the interior of the bladder must be obtained. Identification of the ureteral orifices by catheterization is necessary so that these structures will be constantly visualized and not compromised. The incision is made as a small U, beginning at the posterior

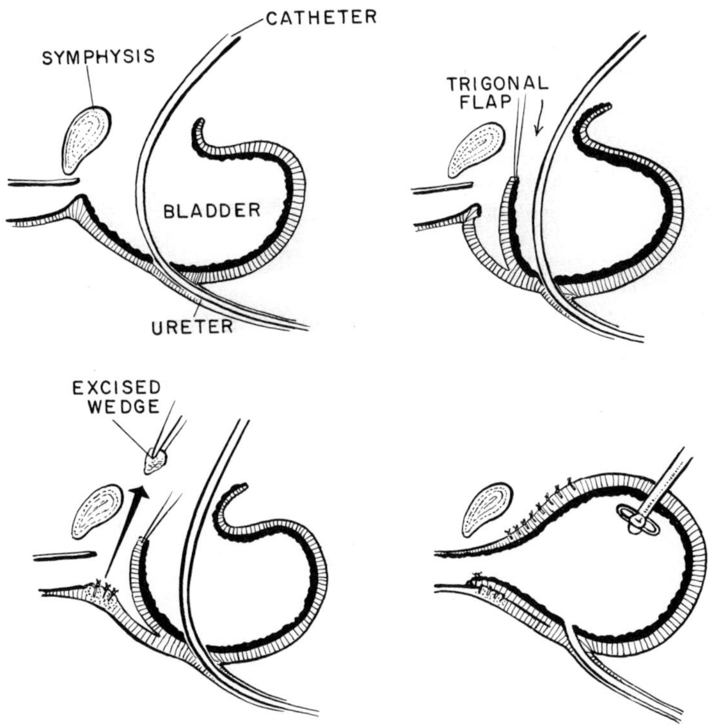

FIGURE 2. Plastic wedge excision of obstruction on the floor of the vesical outlet.

edge of the vesical outlet and passing downward into the urethra for a distance of about 1 cm. (Fig. 2). A traction suture is placed on the tip of this tissue, and by sharp dissection the mucosa with a thin layer of trigonal muscle is raised backward off the underlying structures to within a few millimeters of the ureteral orifices. The abnormal tissue on the floor of the vesical outlet is thus exposed. A traction suture is placed in the center of this offending tissue, and with scissors or scalpel a liberal wedge excision is made to remove it. To facilitate healing and in particular to interpose mucosa between the cut ends of the abnormal tissue, the flap of trigone is returned across the defect and sutured to the floor of the posterior urethra with two or three single plain catgut sutures. A suprapubic drain is inserted and a temporary cystostomy is formed, as previously described.

The Combined Procedure

In some instances it is profitable to carry out Y-V enlargement of the upper portion of the bladder as well. The combination of the two procedures has been especially successful in cases of acquired severe fibrosis. In such cases the long limb of the Y divides the anterior commissure of the prostate and care must be taken to stop short of the prostatic apex. Even in extreme cases such as complete closure of the vesical outlet following prostatectomy, the combined technique has nearly always resulted in an adequate and permanently open vesical outlet. In certain cases in which vesicoureteral reflux is present, it may be advisable to correct that dysfunction either at the same operation or subsequently.

References

Bonnin, H. Cited in Nesbit, R. M., and Crenshaw, W. B. Treatment of bladder neck contracture by plastic operation. *J. Urol.* 73:516, March 1955.

Young, B. W. A retropubic approach to vesical neck obstruction in children. *Surg., Gynec. and Obst.* 96:150, February, 1953.

121. *Immediate Repair of Intrapelvic Rupture of the Urethra by Synchronous Abdominal and Perineal Approach*

ALAN H. HUNT

MARION DESCRIBED the operation of primary anastomosis of the ruptured anterior urethra. Stricture formation was thereby reduced. Our object is to extend the use of this procedure to traumatic ruptures of the intrapelvic part of the urethra, which is made accessible for surgical suture by division of the triangular ligament.

The patient is prepared for operation as soon as he has recovered from shock. He is placed in the lithotomy-Trendelenburg position (Lloyd-Davis, 1939). The shaved abdomen and perineum are covered with Vi-DRAPE occlusive dressing. A urethral catheter is passed to establish the diagnosis.

The *abdominal surgeon* makes a midline suprapubic incision, opens into the cave of Retzius, and evacuates the hematoma. A temporary pack is placed in the cavity. He then opens and empties the bladder and demonstrates the upper part of the torn membranous urethra by passing a metal sound from within the bladder.

Meanwhile the *perineal surgeon* has passed a catheter up from below and exposed the upper end of the separated distal part of the urethra by the following approach. A transverse incision, arched forward, is made across the middle of the perineum. Dissection is carried inward, posterior to the urethral bulb and the triangular ligament, into the hematoma.

The attachment of the triangular ligament to the pubic arch is then defined by palpation. (It is often found that one side is already separated as a result of the fracture, in which case the following maneuver is needed only on the other side.) The posterior edge of the triangular ligament is divided with scissors, the cut being started near the ischiopubic ramus and then extended from behind forward and inward between the ischiocavernosus and bulbocavernosus muscles (Fig. 1). This enables the central part of the triangular ligament to be hinged anteriorly. The cuts are carried forward only as far as is necessary to bring the tip of the urethral catheter and distal torn end of the urethra into view (Fig. 2).

The abdominal surgeon then removes the pack and, with fingers in the bladder, gently presses the trigone and the prostate downward and forward into

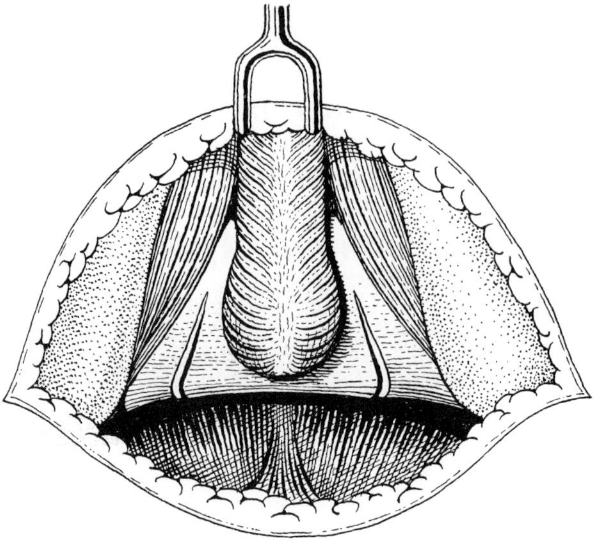

FIGURE 1. Method of dividing the triangular ligament.

the perineal wound. The sound above and the catheter below are then partially withdrawn and manipulated so that the ventral edges of the divided ends of the urethra are brought into apposition. The end-to-end anastomosis is then done, using fine plain catgut sutures on atraumatic needles, the knots being tied outside the lumen. The stitching is begun at the deepest (ventral) part of the urethra with a central stitch and then one on each side of it, the triangular ligament being

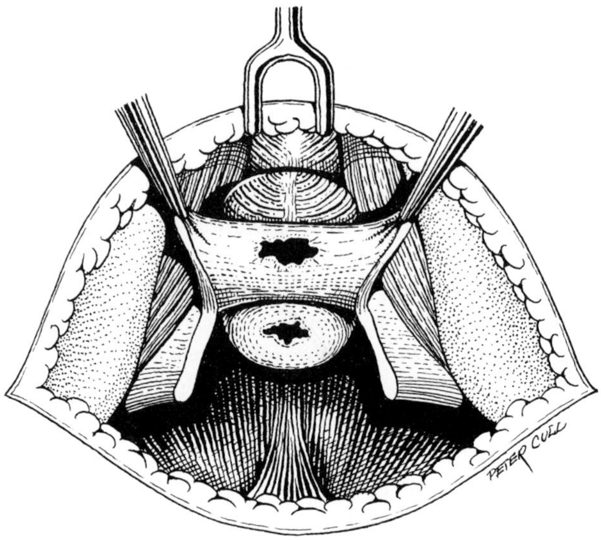

FIGURE 2. Triangular ligament hinged forward to give access to the ruptured membranous urethra for end-to-end anastomosis.

hinged fully forward. The other stitches are inserted in pairs, left and right, from deep to superficial, the triangular ligament being returned to its normal position as they are put in. The abdominal surgeon continues to press the prostate down, so as to present the rupture to the perineal surgeon, until the anastomosis is complete.

Hemostasis is secured at each stage of the operation. It is not necessary to suture the triangular ligament back into place. A penile catheter can be passed up into the bladder and retained there if the surgeon prefers, or the urethra may be left unsplinted if the tear is clean and the anastomosis precise. A suprapubic catheter (de Pezzer or Malecot) is inserted into the bladder, the cave of Retzius is drained, and the abdominal wound is closed in the usual manner. The perineal wound is closed except for a small drain of corrugated rubber.

Postoperatively, the wound drains are removed on about the third day and the suprapubic catheter on the fifteenth. Free drainage through the urethral catheter will allow the suprapubic wound to heal. The penile catheter can be removed by the twenty-first day. Subsequent instrumentation should be done gently and infrequently.

References

Hunt, A. H., and Morgan, C. N. Complete rupture of membranous urethra. Treated by anastomosis without indwelling urethral catheter. *Lancet* 2:330, September 19, 1942.

Lloyd-Davis, O. V. Lithotomy-Trendelenburg position for resection of rectum and lower pelvic colon. *Lancet* 2:74, July 8, 1939.

Marion, G. *Traité d'Urologie*. Vol. 2. Paris: Masson et Cie, 1940. P. 1224.

XXII. THE SCROTUM AND PENIS

122. *Exploration and Biopsy of the Testis; Epididymectomy*

JOHN K. LATTIMER

Exploration of the Testis

Any enlargement of the testis should be explored if it does not transilluminate and is not obviously infected or edematous (as from torsion of the cord). If a tumor is suspected, the testis itself should not be exposed first. Instead the spermatic cord should be isolated low in the inguinal region well above the testicular mass, and the spermatic cord and mass freed in all directions possible, without disturbing the tumor or exerting any pressure upon it. If the cord is long, it may be exposed immediately below the external ring; if it is short, the inguinal canal is opened and the cord isolated in the canal. A soft, rubber-shod intestinal clamp should be applied to the cord well above the mass, and the mass quickly delivered into the wound for exploration (Fig. 1A).

If there are strong indications of tumor, some surgeons recommend removing the testis without further exploration. If there is doubt about the diagnosis, the entire scrotal wound is covered with an impervious sheet of plastic or rubber, which is drawn tightly about the cord, well above the testis (Fig. 1B). This impervious sheet is covered with thick layers of gauze to absorb any liquid or cells which might be spilled when the tunica vaginalis is opened. The tunica vaginalis should then be opened quickly. If a tumor diagnosis is obvious, the testis is removed immediately. If the testis is enlarged but the diagnosis is still uncertain, an incision should be made directly into the testis, over the firmest area and deeply enough to make sure that a deep-seated nodule does not lie far down within the normal testicular tissue. Adequate exploration may demand an incision halfway through the testis at one or more points. A frozen section of doubtful tissue can be done, but the diagnosis is usually obvious upon section of the testis, with compressed tumor tissue pouting above the cut margins of the tumorous nodule. If no tumor is found, the testis can be repaired, particular attention being given to the tiny vessels immediately below the tunica albuginea, which bleed freely as soon as the clamp on the cord is released, if they have not been

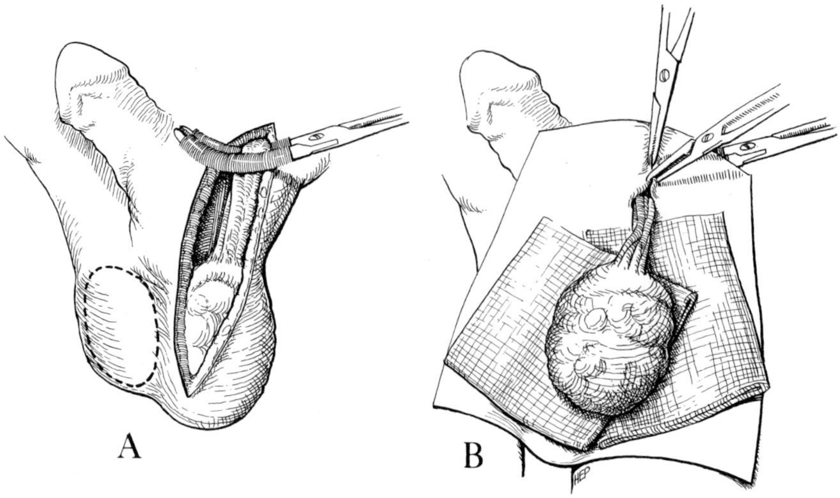

FIGURE 1. (*A*) The spermatic cord is isolated above the testicular mass and the cord and mass freed in all directions without disturbing the tumor. A rubber-shod intestinal clamp is then applied to the spermatic cord, and the mass extruded from the scrotum. (*B*) An impervious sheet of plastic or rubber is placed beneath the testis and its mass, and secured tightly around the cord. Dry laparotomy pads are placed under the mass.

secured. If a tumor is encountered, the testis should be removed at once, with an uncontaminated assistant doing the removal above the impervious drape and outside the field of biopsy. The surgeon should then change gloves and gown, and all instruments used in the biopsy should be discarded, because of the danger that they may have been contaminated by cells of the testis tumor.

If a seminoma is reported on frozen section, the wound is closed after section of the cord high in the inguinal region pending further sections of the excised testis to determine whether radiotherapy will be sufficient or whether further node dissection is advisable. If a more malignant form of testis tumor is reported, a node dissection should be done immediately, extending to the level of the renal vessels, through a midline incision, or through two flank incisions, if the patient's permission has been granted in advance. Otherwise, the wound is closed and the patient apprised of the necessity for a node dissection, which can be done at a later time.

Nontumorous enlargements of the testis include spermatocele, which is a cyst of the head of the epididymis entirely within the tunica vaginalis. Such cysts are filled with sperm-laden fluid and can be dissected out intact. Care must be taken to remove all small cysts of the area, lest they grow into large spermatoceles at a later date.

The hydatid of Morgagni may be present anywhere along the epididymis or as an an appendix to the testis. This structure may twist if on a long stalk, causing edema suggestive of torsion of the testis, but the process is usually more localized and of shorter duration.

Torsion of the testis is usually easily recognizable as a large swollen mass, retracted high into the upper portion of the scrotum and becoming very painful when downward pressure is applied to it. A suspected torsion usually becomes edematous, and must be explored immediately or atrophy of the testis will result. Testes should not be removed if there is the slightest evidence of viability, since they have surprising ability to recover even after torsion for prolonged periods. It is essential that the other testis be explored at a later date and be fixed in place, lest the second side twist as did the first. Torsion is usually due to an unusually long spermatic cord which permits the testis and epididymis to revolve within the tunica albuginea like the clapper in a bell.

Biopsy of the Testis

Biopsy for purposes other than establishing a tissue diagnosis is usually performed to determine the capacity of the testis for spermatogenesis. It is done with either local or general anesthesia. The testis should be compressed against the skin of the scrotum by the application of a rubber tourniquet around the spermatic cord in such a way as to stretch the skin of the scrotum over the testis. A 1 cm. incision in the skin is made directly over the front of the testis and carried down quickly through the tunica vaginalis to the tunica albuginea. A small incision is made in the tunica albuginea, approximately 7 mm. in length. The sides of this incision should immediately be grasped with mosquito forceps to prevent the incision from shifting out of the field. A small cluster of tubules is then teased or squeezed from the testis and amputated with tiny scissors. Bleeding is usually confined to the margins of the wound in the tunica albuginea, since most of the blood vessels of the testis are immediately under this layer. Ligatures of the bleeding points along the margins or suture ligatures of these areas will usually control any bleeding. A single suture in the tunica albuginea, of plain catgut, is used if there is gaping of the edges, but no sutures are necessary if there is not excessive separation or gaping of the wound. The incision in the skin is closed with one or two sutures of plain 3–0 catgut and the tourniquet released. Earlier release of the tourniquet may help to stop the bleeding, but makes the location of the incision more difficult.

Epididymectomy

In performing epididymectomy for tuberculous or other abscesses, it is preferable to make a vertical rather than a transverse incision in the scrotum so that the other half of the scrotum will not be entered if the incision has to be extended. All scrotal incisions heal well and unobtrusively. Furthermore, if it is desirable to exteriorize the cephalad end of the ductus deferens, as in operating for a tuberculous lesion, this can be done through the upper end of a vertical incision quite easily. The tunica vaginalis is incised on its anterior border, where it overlies the testis, to approach the epididymis (Fig. 2A).

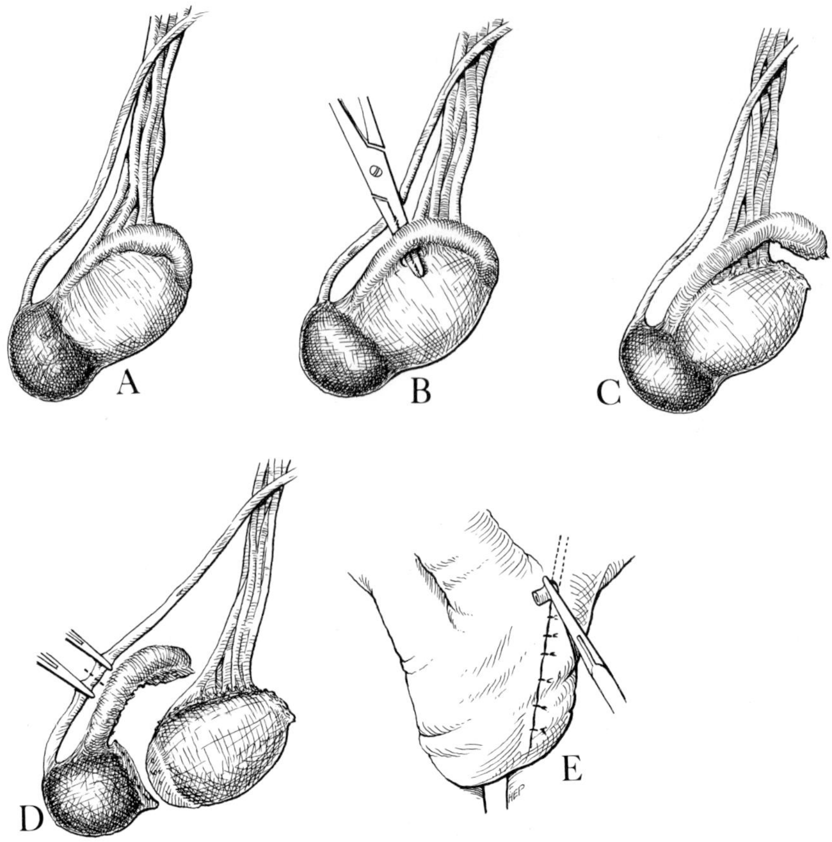

FIGURE 2. (*A*) The testis and its accompanying structures are delivered into the wound. (*B*) A clamp is thrust through the thin membrane which holds the middle of the epididymis to the testis, just above the blood vessels. (*C*) The opening is extended upward to divide the efferent tubules at the junction of epididymis and testis. (*D*) The dissection is then carried downward and the abscess, which is usually in the tail of the epididymis, is shelled away from the testis. The ductus deferens is then divided with a carbolized knife if an infection such as tuberculosis is under consideration. (*E*) The cephalad stump of the ductus deferens is brought out through the skin and a clamp placed across it. A few plain catgut sutures are inserted to hold it to the skin. The scrotum is closed in two layers with plain catgut.

If the epididymis is not greatly distorted, the dissection is best commenced by underrunning the epididymis in its middle portion, where it is attached to the testis by a very thin membrane. This membrane is perforated with a clamp, thus isolating the attachments of the epididymis at the head and tail (Fig. 2B). It is easiest to attack the efferent tubules at the head of the epididymis, dividing them by sharp dissection, where they enter the upper end of the epididymis (Fig. 2C). The small blood vessels encountered are secured with very small mosquito forceps and tied with 3–0 plain catgut ligatures. The dissection is then carried downward to separate the tail of the epididymis from the lower end of the testis (Fig. 2D).

In cases of tuberculous abscess, this area of the epididymis may be thickened, or occupied by cold abscess cavities surrounded by nodules of fibrous tissue. Sharp dissection is often necessary, following the plane of the tunica albuginea and leaving the tunica intact if possible. The ductus deferens can then be followed to the level of the upper end of the scrotal incision and amputated with a carbolized knife. The proximal stump of the ductus deferens is brought through the upper end of the incision so that approximately one-fourth inch of stump protrudes through the skin (Fig. 2E). This is sutured to the skin with 3–0 plain catgut. The scrotum is then closed in two layers with plain catgut. A clamp is left on the stump for five days. With the passage of time this stump will drain a modest amount and then recede below the skin, and the skin will grow over it. Thus, if an abscess should form at this point in the future, it would be located immediately under the skin and could be drained easily.

Any such operation for tuberculosis is covered by chemotherapy.

The dissection described avoids tearing the blood vessels which enter the testis from the medial side of the middle portion of the epididymis. Rarely, tuberculosis may invade the upper end of the testis, which then becomes involved in the caseous tuberculous process. After the diseased portion has been excised, the remainder of the tunica albuginea can be sutured loosely over the end of the testis and the wound irrigated with streptomycin and neomycin solutions.

Reference

Girgis, A. S., and Lattimer, J. K. The chemotherapy of genitourinary tuberculosis with regimens using cycloserine. *J. Urol.* 87:9, January 1962.

123. *Orchidopexy*

JOHN K. LATTIMER

Technique

The Incision

The incision for orchidopexy can ordinarily be made transversely, following the crease of the abdominal wall over the middle or upper portion of the inguinal canal. Even when it is necessary to extend the incision on the abdominal wall upward an unusual distance, this can be accomplished by lengthening the transverse skin incision medially and laterally, still following the line of the natural crease in the abdominal wall. One must watch for the hernial sac, which often turns cephalad after coming out through the external ring. The scalpel may cut into such a sac, or into the testis if the testis lies unusually high in the subcutaneous fat. The hernial sac can be dissected out from the point where it comes through the external ring. The fibers of the external ring can be divided directly with the knife, or first a small incision can be made in the aponeurosis of the external oblique muscle, just above the external ring, and a grooved director passed through this incision under the aponeurosis and out through the external ring. The scalpel can then cut down on the grooved director, insuring that no damage will be done to the underlying spermatic cord. One must watch for the ilioinguinal nerve, which comes out through the external ring along with the spermatic cord. The incision in the fascia of the external oblique muscle is then carried upward to a point approximately 1 inch above the internal inguinal ring. At this time it is well to dissect out the ilioinguinal nerve throughout the length of the incision, freeing it from the testis and spermatic cord and far up into the muscle of the conjoined tendon, so that it can be kept out of harm's way. Next, with traction on the hernial sac and testis, the sac and cord can be dissected by blunt and sharp dissection, upward to the internal inguinal ring. With the cord still intact, it is easy to open up the retroperitoneal space lateral to the cord and above the internal inguinal ring.

Dissection of the Spermatic Cord into Its Three Components

The first lengthy step in orchidopexy is to dissect out the testis and the spermatic cord, far up beyond its trifurcation into hernial sac, spermatic vessels, and ductus deferens. The ductus deferens is ordinarily easily dissected out and is quite elastic. The hernial sac, also, can usually be dissected readily from the vessels and tied, toward the end of the dissection. The principal difficulty is encountered in lengthening the spermatic vessels sufficiently to permit the testis to rest easily in the bottom of the scrotum.

It is usually convenient to open the hernial sac in its midportion. Great care must be taken to cut only into a portion of the sac which is not attached to blood vessels or the ductus deferens. Under vision, the hernial sac can be opened distally to its extremity, again with care to avoid injuring any extension of the ductus deferens onto the distal portion of the sac wall. The ductus may resemble a meandering tiny white thread, and must be watched for carefully. The sac is now opened proximally to a point about 1 inch from the internal inguinal ring, and with a sharp-pointed mosquito clamp a plane of dissection is developed between the hernial sac and the other components of the cord, sticking very close to the hernial sac. This is a tedious part of the dissection but should be done with great care, so that structures are not damaged.

It has been suggested that a bleb of saline be injected under the layer of the hernial sac to lift it from the other structures of the cord. This merely distorts the tissues and prolongs the procedure, in my opinion. Still another recommended method is to take a No. 15 (smallest) scalpel blade and cut directly across the sac at a very superficial level, and then dissect the sac away from the vessels by blunt and sharp dissection. This method has the danger that blood vessels may be cut during the dissection.

Once the hernial sac has been separated from the remainder of the cord, the sac can be cut across at a point approximately 1 inch distal to the internal inguinal ring, and the blood vessels and ductus deferens teased away from the lateral side of the upper part of the sac. This must be done very carefully, lest the sac be torn. If the sac begins to tear at this point, it is difficult to retrieve the damage in tiny children, in whom the peritoneal layer is diaphanous. The hernial sac must be completely separated from the ductus deferens and the blood vessels of the cord, and the dissection of the ductus deferens carried far down behind the peritoneum, at least halfway to the seminal vesicle.

Attention is then turned to the spermatic vessels, which are dissected by blunt and sharp dissection, away from the peritoneum and upward into the retroperitoneal space to a distance of about 4 inches. Care must be taken not to cut into the peritoneum at the superior portion of the incision, where the peritoneum runs laterally and above the cord and can very easily be accidentally cut during efforts to free the cord superiorly. It will be obvious, at this point, that there is a band of unnecessary tissue between the blood vessels of the cord and the ductus deferens. This strand of connective tissue may be cut with impunity. The dissection is now carried down along the ductus deferens until it is free and has been liberated from the tightly adherent bands and tiny blood vessels which often accompany it. Rarely, a short ductus deferens limits the distance the testis can be brought down.

The vessels of the spermatic cord can now be separated by blunt and sharp

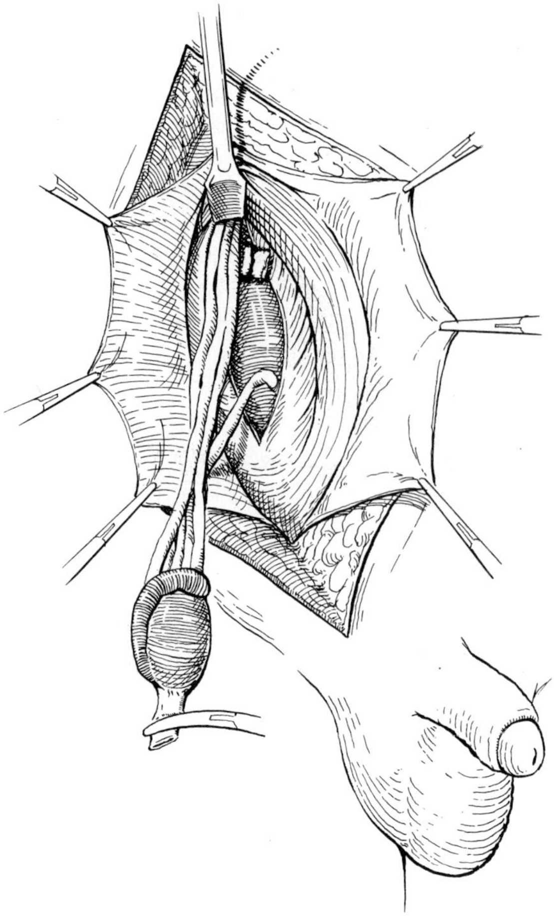

FIGURE 1. The spermatic cord has been dissected out well up beyond its trifurcation into hernial sac, spermatic vessels, and ductus deferens. The hernial sac is closed.

dissection from their attachments to the peritoneum and the lateral body wall, to whatever height is necessary to give the length required for the testis to reach into the scrotum. Prentiss has pointed out that the vessels are held in a slightly lateral position by a leaf of fascia. If this fascia is divided, the vessels can drop medially and come anteriorly with slightly more freedom. This change in position adds to their length. Tight bands within the leash of spermatic blood vessels can be detected by stretching the vessels slightly over the finger tip and feeling for the tautest areas. These can be divided individually. Sometimes another half inch is thereby added to the length of the cord. If measurements of the cord down toward the scrotum still show insufficient length, the floor of the inguinal canal may be dissected with impunity, including the division and ligation of the inferior epigastric artery and vein. The best effect of incising the floor of the inguinal canal is that it permits the hand of the operator to be passed further upward and cephalad behind the peritoneum and lateral to it, in order to dissect out the blood vessels to their origins on the great vessels, at the level of the kidney pedicles. This maneuver is not necessary in most cases, but if it is done, the margins of the transversalis fascia which form the floor of the inguinal canal should be tagged with black silk sutures to facilitate finding the proper layer when closure is begun.

Transfer of the Testis to the Scrotum

It is our practice to leave the redundant opened distal hernial sac adherent to the cord in order to provide more bulk in the scrotum and thus add more weight during the healing period. When the cord has been dissected to a sufficient length for the testis to reach into the bottom of the scrotum, the hernial sac is closed with a running suture of 00 chromic atraumatic catgut (Fig. 1). The finger then burrows downward into the scrotum to its most dependent point (Fig. 2). This does not mean a point far back toward the anus, nor a point far toward the penis, but, instead, a point exactly in between, where traction on the bottom of the scrotum

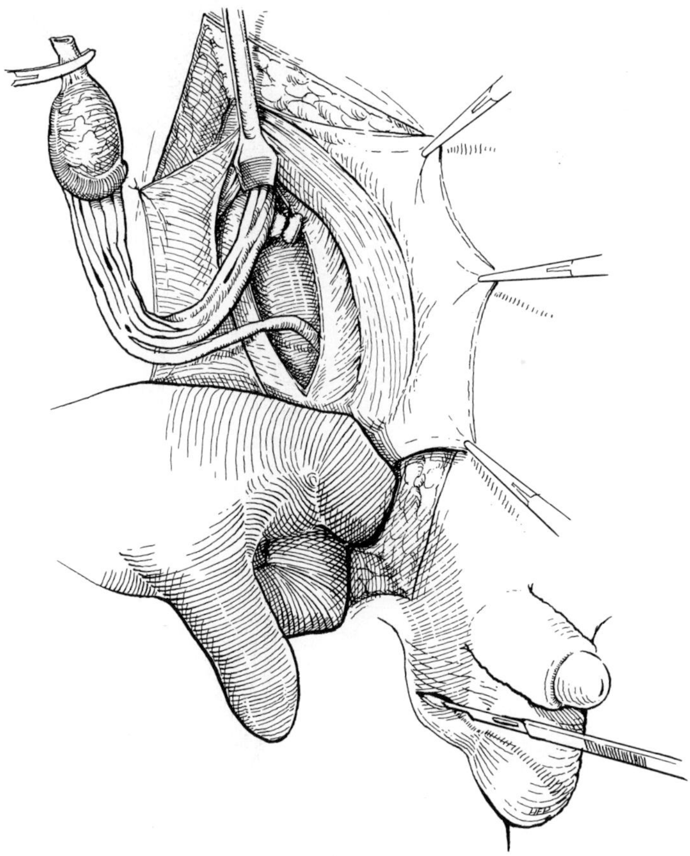

FIGURE 2. A scrotal pouch is formed by passing the finger downward into the scrotum. The bottommost portion of the scrotum is grasped with an Allis clamp, at the midline. The dissecting finger enlarges a pocket in this area, in the bottom of the scrotum, and with the scalpel a 2 cm. incision is made in the side of the scrotum approximately 1 cm. above the lowest portion.

with an Allis clamp produces the greatest downward stretch. A new, 2 cm. transverse incision is made approximately 1 cm. above the lowest point of the scrotum. Through a superficial skin incision a sharp-pointed mosquito clamp is used to dissect through the underlying layers of dartos fascia and cremaster muscle. This cavity is expanded by the use of a large Kelly clamp which is passed through these layers and spread apart vigorously. This dissection must be carried in all directions, downward, laterally, upward, and medially, and all septa and partitions broken down, to provide room for the testis and its tunics (Fig. 3). I wish to emphasize that a *large* subcutaneous pocket must be made.

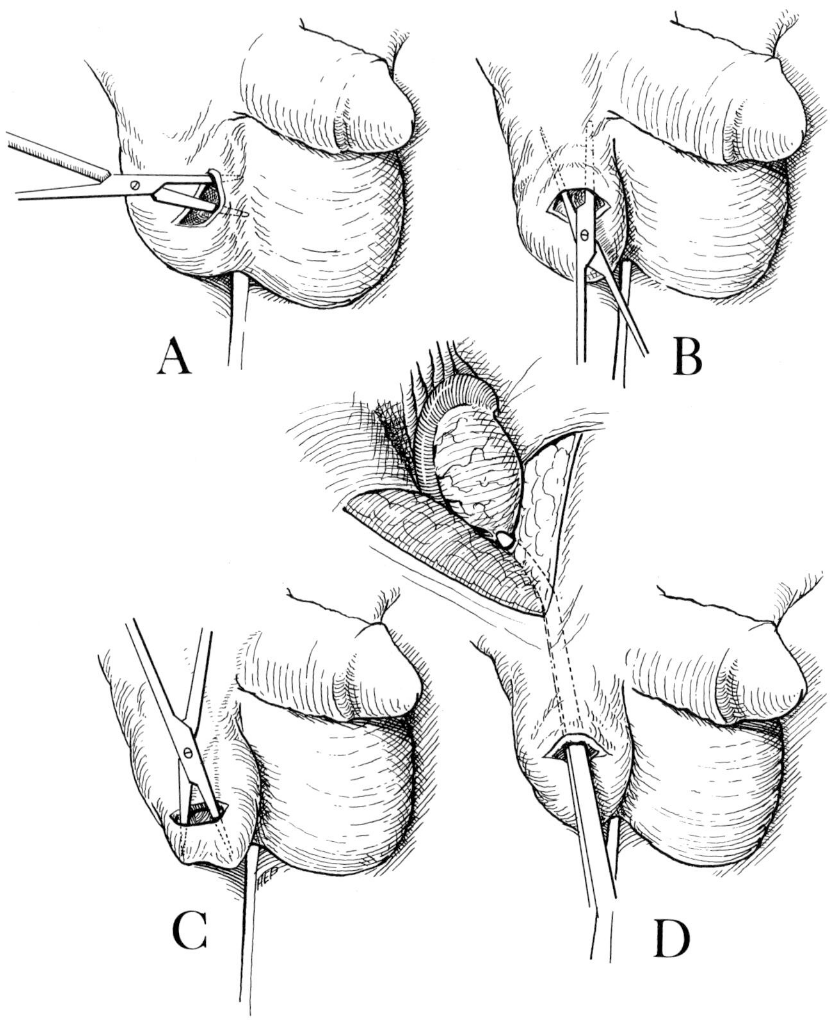

FIGURE 3. Through the small incision in the scrotum, the subcutaneous pocket is enlarged in all directions as in *A*, *B*, and *C*. The testis is drawn down into this pocket by a clamp passed upward into the wound (*D*).

A clamp is passed upward into the wound, and the testis is brought down through the upper portion of the scrotum and out through the incision in the side wall of the scrotum, care being taken to avoid twisting the vessels. A 3–0 black silk suture on a round intestinal needle is passed through the junction of the epididymis and the testis, catching a small amount of tunica albuginea (Fig. 4). Next, straight needles are placed on both ends of the suture, which has not been tied to the testis, and are passed downward and out through the bottommost point of the scrotum. The traction suture is never brought out through the lateral scrotal incision, lest it pull the entire testis out through the incision during the ensuing days of traction. The traction suture is tied to a small rubber band, which is fixed to a safety pin implanted in adhesive tape near or just above the opposite knee (Fig. 5). A point is selected which will afford a fairly direct pull in the axis of the newly located spermatic cord. The traction is not tight. It is only snug, and can be loosened if the patient moves his leg slightly. Nevertheless, during the day, several sharp tugs on the testis will be experienced, in the normal course of activities. If the tension is too severe, atrophy of the testis, preceded by edema, will follow.

The incision in the scrotum is closed with interrupted sutures of 5–0 chromic

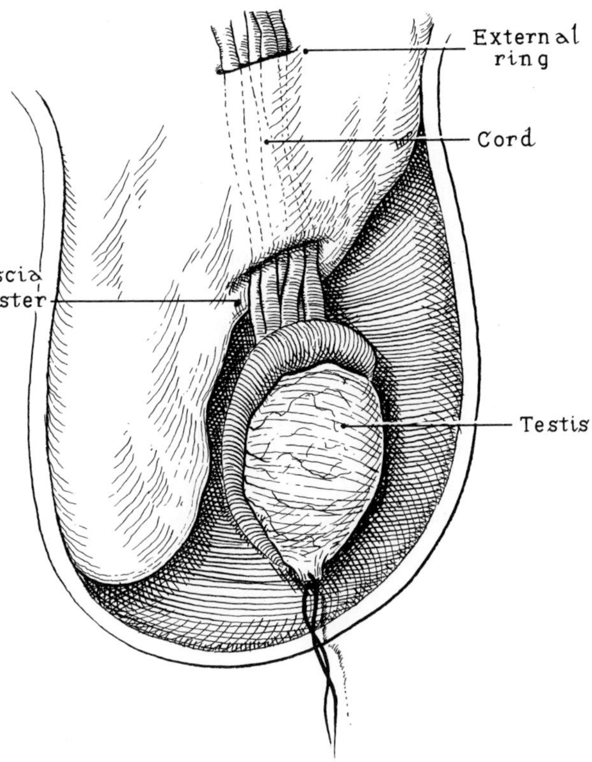

FIGURE 4. A 3–0 black silk suture with a needle on each end is passed through the tunica albuginea and both ends are brought out through the very bottom of the scrotal skin, leaving the testis within the subcutaneous pocket.

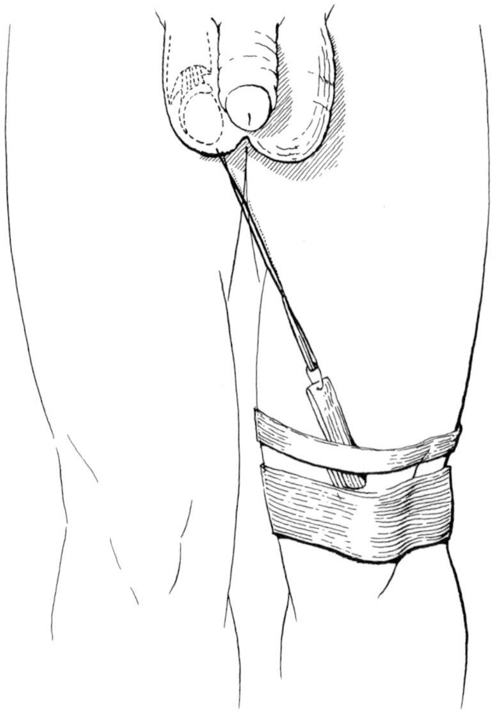

FIGURE 5. A small brand-new rubber band is tied to the black silk suture within 1 inch of the scrotum, and stretched downward to reach a safety pin which is fastened to tape at or near the opposite knee.

atraumatic catgut, and the layers of the abdominal wound approximated carefully over the cord, which exits from a site beneath the conjoined tendon, down through the inguinal canal for about an inch, and then down into the scrotum.

We leave the rubber band traction suture on the testis for 10 days postoperatively, and do not allow the patient to get out of bed for this time. With this routine, the amount of traction can be more carefully controlled and the suture will not tear out. The patients do not mind being kept in bed. It is our present practice to give 500 units of gonadotropic hormone each day during the 10 days the patient is in the hospital with traction on the testis. This has added length to the spermatic cord in several cases. The patient is instructed to pull on the testis ten times, morning and night, for six months after the operation. Use of the scrotal pouch appears to lessen the likelihood of spontaneous retraction of the testis.

Reference

LATTIMER, J. K. Scrotal pouch technique for orchidopexy. *J. Urol.* 78:628, November 1957.

124. Hydrocelectomy

JOHN K. LATTIMER

FOR HYDROCELE OPERATIONS, either a vertical or a transverse incision is appropriate. A vertical incision, however, allows extension in case a communicating channel is discovered going upward along the cord. The principal point of technique to be observed in operating upon hydroceles is to divide all the outer layers of the hydrocele sac until only the very thin layer remains, containing the fluid (Fig. 1A, B). It is surprising how many layers can be divided and stripped

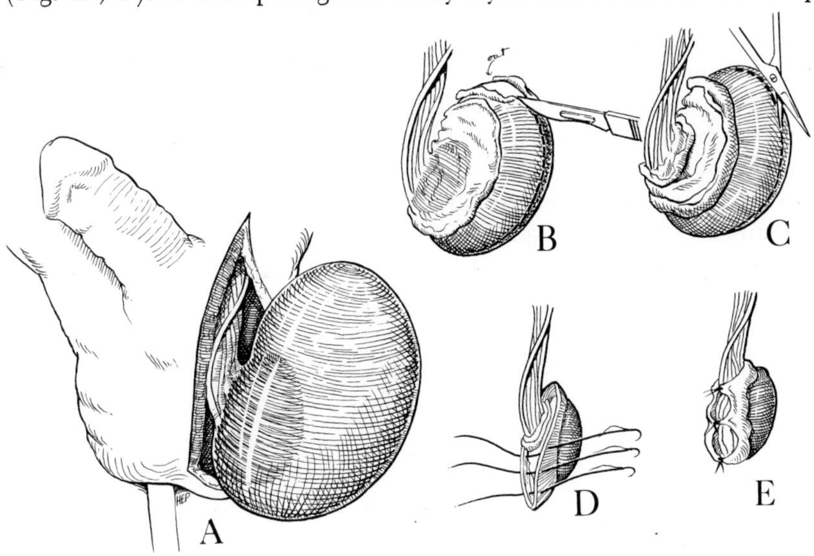

FIGURE 1. Hydrocele eversion. (A) The hydrocele is freed from the scrotum completely, and the tissues wiped away from the blood vessels where they enter the mass. (*B*) The layers of the hydrocele are divided by sharp dissection, one by one, and peeled back. (*C*) The final layer is a thin blue membrane which is punctured so that the fluid can be aspirated. It is then opened completely, from end to end, with scissors. (*D and E*) The excess part of the sac is trimmed away and the margins sutured back to back around the epididymis, very loosely. It is not necessary to remove all of the redundant sac, nor is it recommended, in view of the bleeding that will occur from the many tiny vessels which are transected. The sutures must be very loose, and the edges of the sac do not have to be approximated.

back before the innermost layer is reached and perforated (Fig. 1C). The thinner the last layer, the easier it is to fold back the sac. In the great majority of hydroceles the sac can be reduced to a very thin layer which is then divided upward and downward to the limits of the hydrocele, care being taken in the lower portion not to divide the ductus deferens if it comes around onto the sac wall.

Meticulous hemostasis must be obtained with fine catgut ligatures (usually 4–0 plain catgut is sufficient). Then the two edges of the enlarged tunica vaginalis are turned backward around the epididymis and the lower portion of the spermatic cord, and sutured loosely together with two or three sutures of plain 00 catgut (Fig. 1D, E). These sutures should not be drawn so tightly that they constrict the cord at any point. The sac is usually redundant, but if it should not reach easily around the epididymis, a gap may be left between the two edges of the sac, and be bridged by the plain catgut suture, which is under no tension. There is then no chance that the circulation of the testis or epididymis will be impaired by any pressure of a tight ligature across it.

In chronically inflamed hydroceles or those which have been tapped many times, the wall may, on rare occasions, be so thick that it must be excised because it will not fold back easily around the testis. Whenever the sac is cut away, large numbers of tiny vessels are transected and an infinite amount of tying of these bleeding points is required. This must be done or a very large scrotal hematoma could result. It is certainly preferable to avoid excising the hydrocele sac. As long as the secreting surfaces of the tunica vaginalis are turned outward so that no fluid can be trapped, even when secreted, the hydrocele will be cured.

It is our practice to place a small soft rubber tube into the scrotal wound after hydrocelectomy, as a drain. This is left in for two or three days, until copious drainage ceases, and is then withdrawn. We suture the scrotum in two layers of interrupted sutures of 00 plain catgut, which do not have to be removed from the tender scrotal tissues. A single layer is not enough to withstand the edema of the scrotal tissues which sometimes occurs after hydrocelectomy.

XXIII. PEDIATRIC SURGERY

125. *Tracheoesophageal Fistula and Esophageal Atresia*

JERROLD M. BECKER AND
KEITH M. SCHNEIDER

H-Type Tracheoesophageal Fistula

Three per cent of congenital esophageal anomalies are tracheoesophageal fistula without atresia (H-type tracheoesophageal fistula; isolated tracheoesophageal fistula). This fistula runs from the esophagus to the trachea in an anterior and cephalad direction. It may exist at any level between the pharynx and the carina, and thus the surgical approach may be cervical or thoracic.

Esophagrams performed with the infant in the prone position are more likely to visualize the fistula than studies of the infant in the usual supine position. It is important to take oblique films in addition to routine anteroposterior and lateral views. If the fistula is not demonstrated, cinefluororadiography of the swallowing process is performed. This is a definitive method of making or excluding the diagnosis.

We do not recommend the use of endoscopic diagnostic techniques. The laryngeal and pharyngeal structures in infants are small and there is a risk of respiratory obstruction following these procedures. Moreover, the fistula is usually only a few millimeters in diameter and is rarely visualized by esophagoscopy or bronchoscopy.

In 1938 Imperatori performed the first successful repair of an isolated tracheoesophageal fistula, utilizing a transtracheal approach. Haight in 1946 reported the second successful closure, using a thoracic approach. From 1946 to 1958 all reported cases were repaired through the chest. Miller in 1958 reported the first transcervical approach.

A review of the literature reveals that of the 39 reported cases in which surgery was performed, 29 were explored through the thorax and 10 through the neck. Thoracotomy has been associated with a high mortality and morbidity. When surgery has been performed through the chest, fistulas lying within the neck have been missed and recurrences have been more frequent than with the transcervical approach.

Over 60 per cent of the fistulas have been located at the level of the second thoracic vertebra or higher. We feel that fistulas occurring in these locations are more easily and safely repaired transcervically than by other approaches.

In the four infants reported with double fistulas, only a cervical approach would have visualized the upper communication. All these patients died because the upper fistula was missed.

Since hypothermia can lead to respiratory arrest in infants, it is important to maintain body temperature during the operative procedure. This can most easily be accomplished by the use of the water blanket. However, wrapping the extremities and placing warm water bags under the patient will also conserve body heat. A recording thermometer is inserted into the rectum and the temperature is monitored.

We have routinely performed repair of the H-type tracheoesophageal fistula under general endotracheal anesthesia, leaving the choice of agent to the anesthetist.

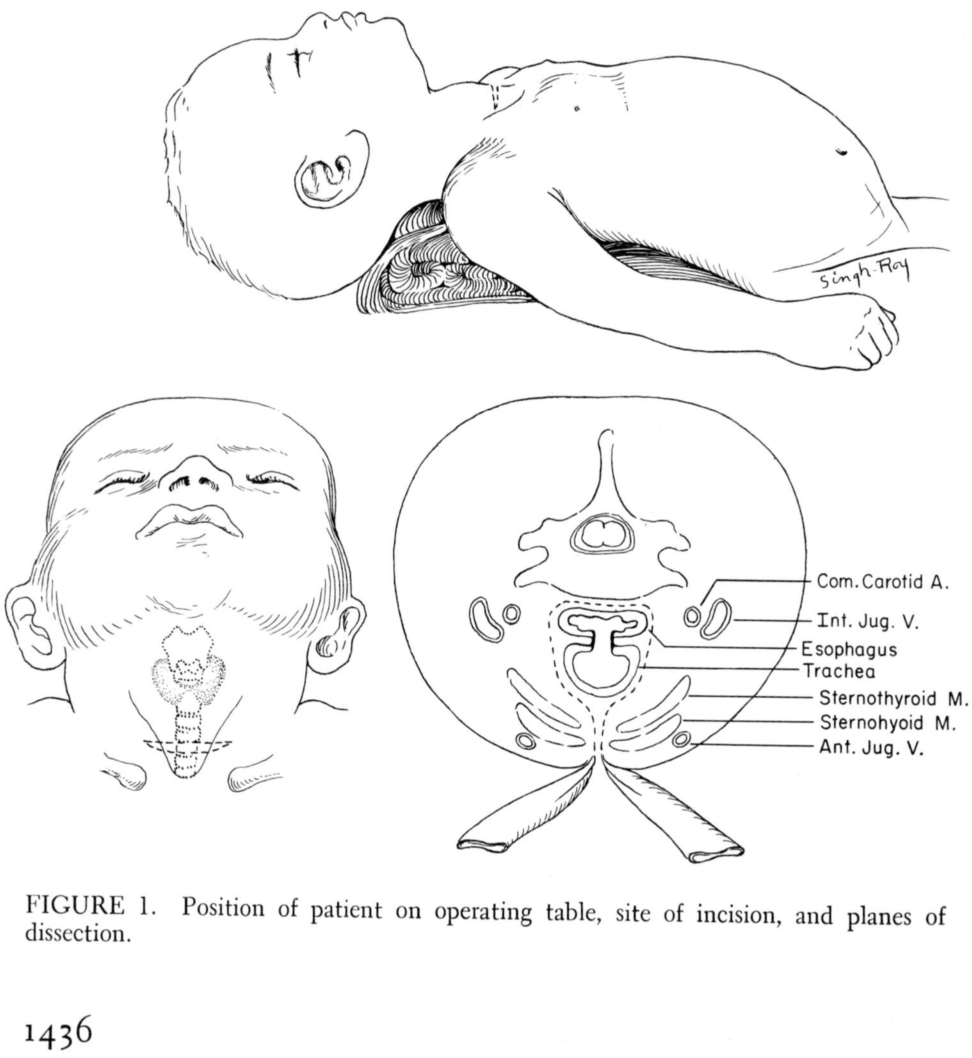

FIGURE 1. Position of patient on operating table, site of incision, and planes of dissection.

Technique

TRANSCERVICAL APPROACH. In the transcervical approach the infant is placed in the supine position with the neck markedly extended (Fig. 1). A transverse skin-crease incision is made about one fingerbreadth above the sternal notch. The incision is carried down to the deep cervical fascia, and flaps are mobilized by sharp and blunt dissection, as in thyroid surgery. The strap muscles are separated in the midline and retracted laterally, exposing the trachea below the thyroid isthmus. The trachea in infants is soft and may buckle if handled roughly.

Both recurrent laryngeal nerves are then identified, lying in the tracheoesophageal groove. The carotid artery and jugular vein are retracted laterally, and the esophagus is freed from the prevertebral fascia by blunt dissection ("peanut" gauze dissector) until a tape can be passed around the trachea and esophagus.

The groove between the esophagus and trachea is then developed by spreading the points of a dull hemostat until a passage is created. A one-quarter inch

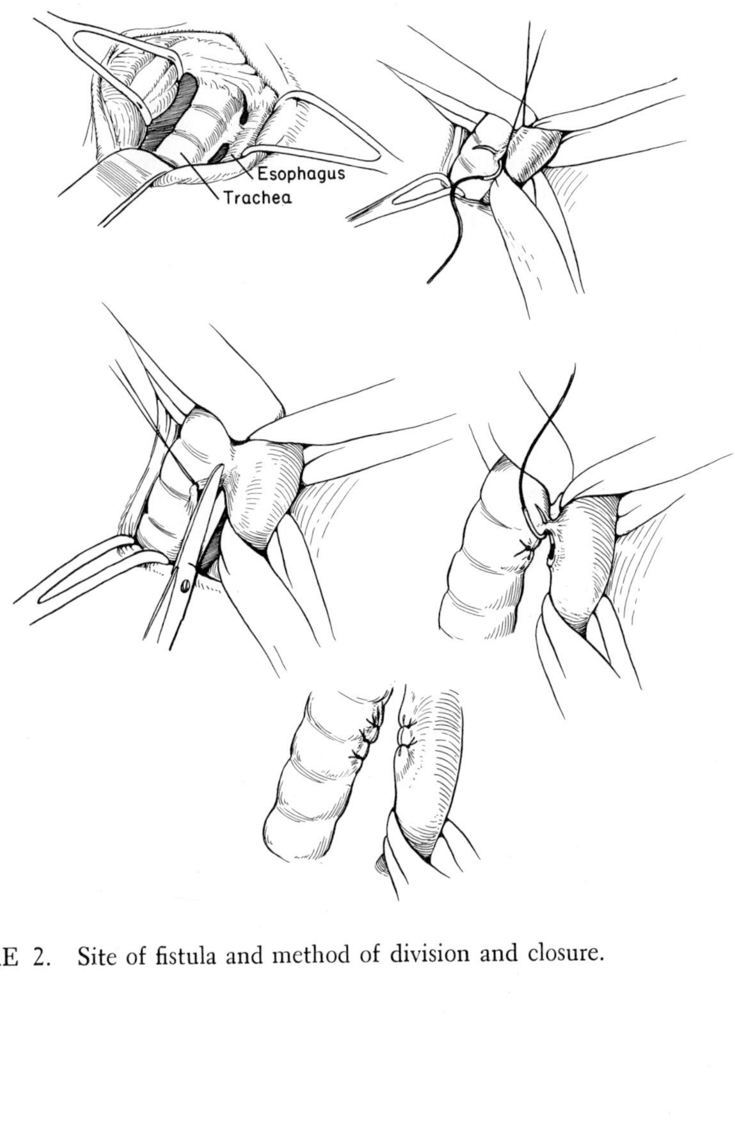

FIGURE 2. Site of fistula and method of division and closure.

Penrose drain is passed around the trachea, and another around the esophagus. The separation of the trachea and esophagus is continued, using small Metzenbaum or blunt iris scissors in a superior and inferior direction, until the fistula is encountered (Fig. 2). Since the posterior aspect of the trachea is noncartilaginous, careful dissection is necessary to avoid perforation.

The fistula is usually 2 to 3 mm. in diameter; however, its muscular coat gives it a broader appearance. After the fistula has been identified, a 0 heavy silk ligature is passed around it. This aids in the complete mobilization of the fistula.

Division of the fistula and closure of the tracheal end are performed as in dealing with a bronchial stump. Sutures of 5–0 arterial silk are alternately placed, the fistula is partially divided, and the sutures are tied. One layer of interrupted silk is sufficient for closure of the trachea.

The esophageal fistula is closed in two layers with 5–0 arterial silk. The first layer consists of interrupted sutures through the full thickness of the esophageal wall; and the second, imbricating sutures, catching just muscularis.

Following complete division of the fistula, the tracheal suture line is cephalad to the esophageal closure. Therefore, we do not interpose any tissue between the esophagus and the trachea.

Closure of the wound is performed without drainage. Chromic catgut 4–0 is used to reapproximate the strap muscles in the midline, and 5–0 plain catgut for platysma and subcutaneous tissue. The skin is closed with interrupted 5–0 silk.

TRANSTHORACIC APPROACH. In repairing fistulas below the second thoracic vertebra, we have utilized a standard right lateral thoracotomy incision through the fourth intercostal space.

The azygos vein is identified, ligated, and divided. The esophagus is located medial to the divided vein. Care in mobilization of the esophagus is necessary to prevent breaking into the contralateral pleural space. A one-quarter inch Penrose drain is then passed around the esophagus. With traction on the drain, the exploration of the tracheoesophageal groove is begun. When the fistula is encountered, usually near the apex of the chest, it is encircled with a heavy 0 silk ligature for traction, and then treated as in the transcervical approach. Closure of the chest is performed in standard fashion. An intercostal tube attached to underwater drainage is left in situ for 24 hours and then removed.

Esophageal Atresia and Tracheoesophageal Fistula

Primary repair of esophageal atresia and tracheoesophageal fistula can be performed using a transpleural or retropleural approach.

The retropleural operation has been performed in two ways. Small posterior segments of the third, fourth, and fifth rib have been resected to gain access to the retropleural region. This technique has been criticized because of increased operating time, increased operative trauma and blood loss, and diminished exposure.

For the past three years we have utilized a retropleural approach in which access to the mediastinum is gained through a subperiosteal resection of the entire fourth right rib. There are important advantages to this approach:

1. The exposure is equal to that achieved transpleurally.
2. The disadvantages of multiple rib resection are avoided.
3. If an anastomotic leak occurs, it will not cause an empyema. If a leak occurs following a retropleural anastomosis, an esophagocutaneous fistula develops which slowly seals itself.

Technique

The patient is anesthetized, positioned, and draped as for the transpleural approach. The same transverse skin incision is used. The incision is carried down through the muscles of the chest wall to expose the fourth rib (Fig. 3A). An incision is made through the periosteum from the costal cartilage anteriorly to a point beyond the paravertebral muscles posteriorly. The periosteum is gently dissected off the rib, using a dental periosteal elevator. The rib is transected anteriorly

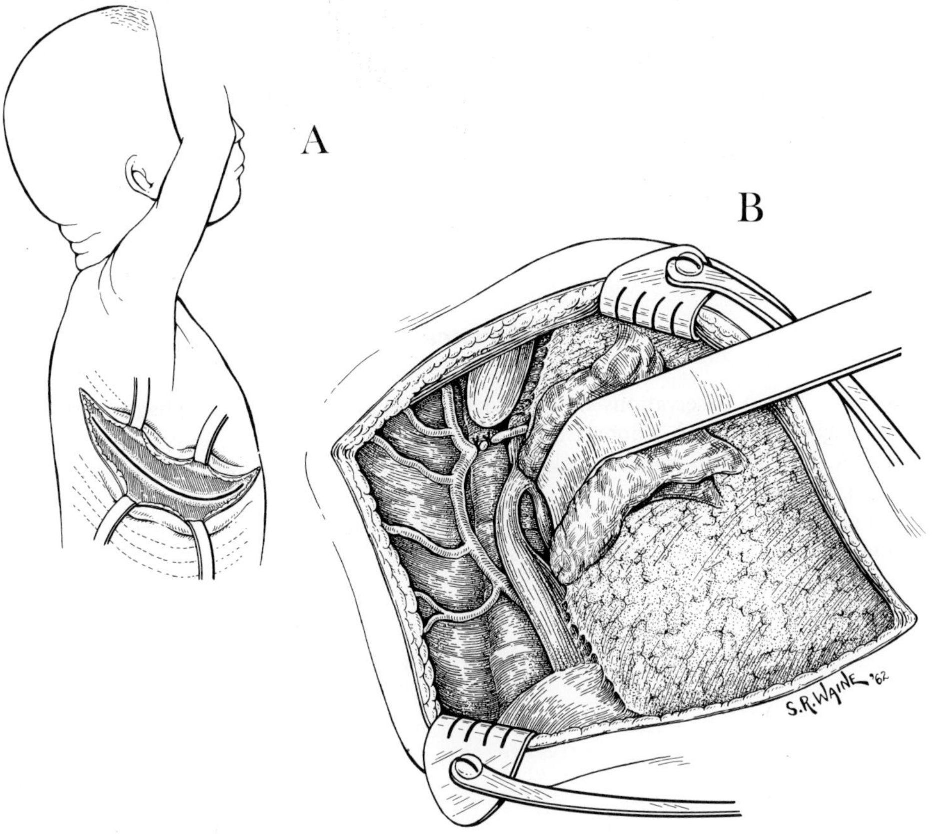

FIGURE 3. (A) Position of patient and site of rib excision. (B) The ample exposure obtained by a retropleural approach through the bed of the fourth rib. Note the ties placed on the azygos vein prior to division.

at the costochondral junction. The entire rib is then removed, separating it from its transverse process and vertebral articulations.

Blunt finger dissection and dissection with a moist "peanut" gauze dissector are used to reflect the pleura from the chest wall and mediastinum for a distance of two or three interspaces superiorly and inferiorly. The ribs are then spread with a "baby" Finochietto rib spreader. The posterior dissection is continued until the azygos vein is cleared. During this dissection the pleura and lung are compressed with a moist sponge and malleable retractors (Fig. 3B). The azygos vein is then divided between ligatures placed as far posterior as possible to preserve length, to interpose it between the tracheal closure and the esophageal anastomosis.

The surgical repair of the tracheoesophageal fistula and esophagoesophagostomy then proceeds in the usual manner. The stump of the azygos vein is interposed between the tracheal and esophageal suture lines, and is sutured to the posterior chest wall.

During the operation the anesthetist inflates the right lung at 20-minute intervals.

A stab wound is made at the level of the fifth interspace in the midaxillary line and a No. 12 French catheter is brought into the retropleural spaces and held with its distal opening 2 cm. from the esophageal anastomosis by means of a suture of 4–0 chromic catgut. The catheter is attached to an underwater drainage bottle.

The chest wall is closed. Three pericostal sutures of 00 chromic approximate the third and fifth ribs. The muscles are approximated with continuous 3–0 chromic atraumatic catgut, and skin edges are approximated with interrupted 4–0 silk.

References

HAIGHT, C. Some observations on esophageal atresias and tracheoesophageal fistulas of congenital origin. *J. Thoracic Surg.* 17:600, October 1948.

MILLER, A. H. H-type tracheoesophageal fistula. *Ann. Otol., Rhin. and Laryng.* 67:1078, December 1958.

SCHNEIDER, K. M., and BECKER, J. M. The H-type tracheoesophageal fistula in infants and children. *Surgery* 51:677, May 1962.

126. *Esophageal Atresia*

WILLIAM B. KIESEWETTER

ESOPHAGEAL ATRESIA is a general term used to designate a developmental condition in which the esophagus ends blindly. It includes a number of anatomical variants. The surgeon usually has to deal with an associated tracheoesophageal fistula, though not always. There is usually enough length of esophageal segments for a primary end-to-end anastomosis, but there may not be. Finally, a normal trachea and esophagus may exist, with only the tracheoesophageal fistula present. All these types of defect are generally included in the terms "esophageal atresia" or "TEF" (tracheoesophageal fistula).

We shall deal with these surgical problems under three headings: (1) Primary Anastomosis; (2) Substitute Esophagus; and (3) H-Type Fistula Repair. Finally, a gastrostomy will be described which may be used in conjunction with all three procedures.

Primary Anastomosis

Though a few surgeons still prefer the retropleural approach to the esophagus in attempting a primary anastomosis, we shall confine ourselves to the points of technique involved in the transpleural approach, which is used by the majority of surgeons today.

The patient is placed in the lateral decubitus position and the fourth intercostal space is opened. The first significant step in the procedure is the development of a pleural flap lateral to the esophagus (Fig. 1). This must be raised in order to preserve it for future sewing over the tracheal end of the tracheoesophageal fistula to lessen the chance of leak or recurrence of the fistula. After the flap has been raised, the upper esophagus is readily identified by having the anesthetist pass a No. 8 or No. 10 French catheter through the nose and into the blind pouch. High dissection is carried out on this tough, hypertrophied muscular segment. A Mixter clamp is helpful in separating the trachea and esophagus down to the tip of the blind pouch, which is almost always intimately adherent to the trachea and must be sharply divided without entering either structure.

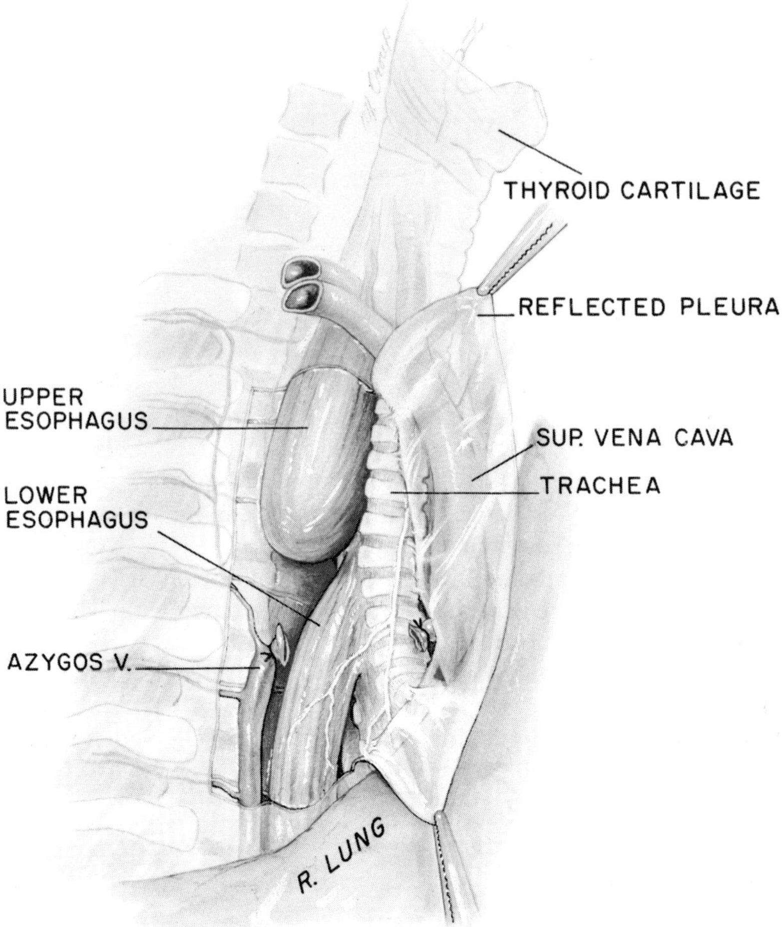

FIGURE 1. The dissected parietal pleura is reflected in such a way as to expose the atresia and tracheoesophageal fistula.

By contrast, the lower esophageal segment is best dissected only as much as is necessary to mobilize it with enough length for anastomosis. We have found that a piece of one-quarter inch Penrose drain is useful to put around the tracheoesophageal fistula for traction. It does not damage tissue that may be needed for the anastomosis. With the fistula clearly delineated, a continuous 5–0 Deknatel vascular suture is used to close the tracheal side. To avoid air leak due to cutting the fistula completely across at once, and to aid visualization of the two edges to be sewn, the fistula is divided serially. A section is divided and closed, then another portion, successively until the esophagus is completely free. A return continuous silk suture reinforces the tracheal closure. The closure is checked for air leak by putting water in the chest and having the anesthetist blow a bit forcefully through the endotracheal tube.

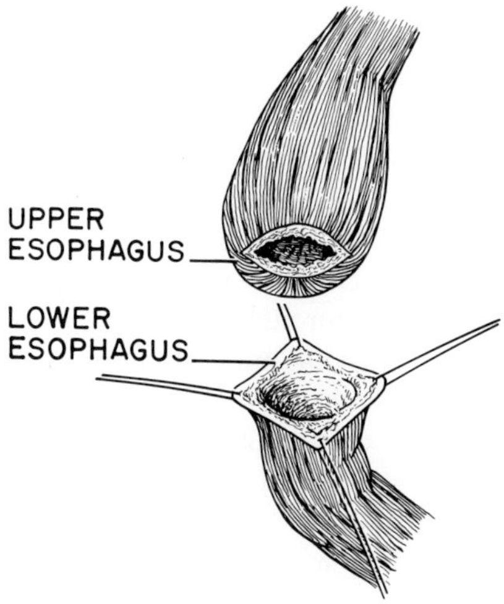

FIGURE 2. The lower esophagus has quadrant stitches placed in it to include the mucosa. The upper pouch has an elliptical segment cut out of it preparatory to anastomosis.

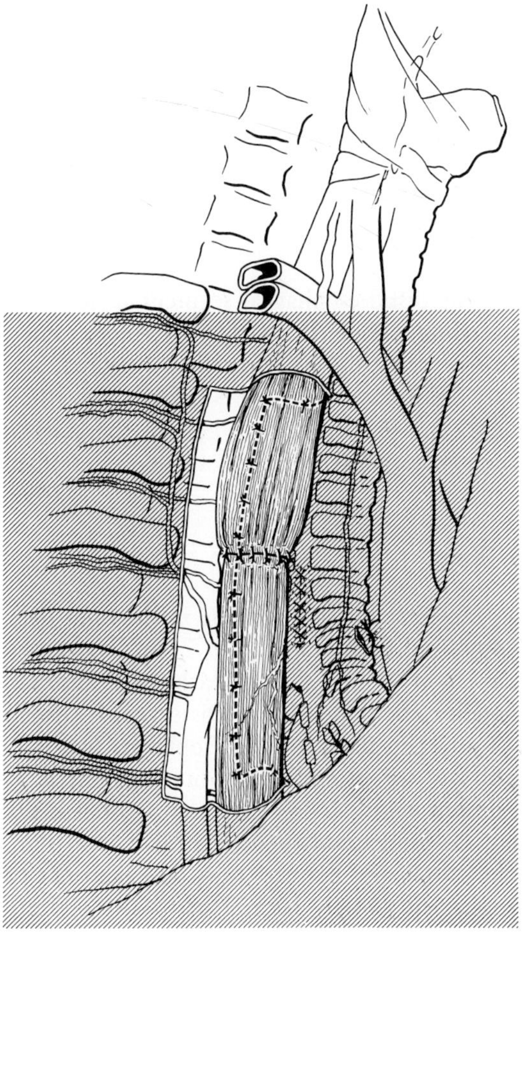

FIGURE 3. The parietal pleural flap is interposed between the tracheal fistula closure and the esophageal anastomosis.

The lower esophagus is trimmed to a point of larger diameter and firmer musculature, but is not shortened so much that the anastomosis will be under tension. This is a matter of balancing the desired length against the caliber and type of tissue. Stitches of 5–0 vascular silk are then placed at the four quadrants; they are one-layer, through-and-through sutures in which the mucosa is clearly included in each bite. A segment that includes all layers is cut out of the esophageal pouch at its most dependent portion (Fig. 2). This is done to prevent the stenosis that often results after merely slitting the pouch. The posterior row of sutures is placed for 180 degrees. These are through-and-through, interrupted silk sutures. Usually five stitches will suffice, and none are tied until all have been placed. After the knots have been tied on the outside of the esophagus, a No. 8 or No. 10 French catheter is threaded through the partial anastomosis from the nose, and the remaining sutures are placed anteriorly. The catheter prevents unintended narrowing or accidental grasping of the posterior mucosa.

Finally, the pleural flap is interposed over the tracheal fistula, and between the esophagus and trachea, as shown in Figure 3.

Substitute Esophagus

A procedure that requires an intestinal segment as a substitute esophagus is necessary if the distance between the upper and lower segments is too great for primary anastomosis.

Primary Stage If Fistula Present by X-ray

When a transthoracic approach is used, the distal esophageal segment is detached from the trachea as described in the preceding section. It is either inverted within a purse-string suture or doubly tied with 4–0 black silk ligatures. The proximal segment is dissected as freely as for primary anastomosis. A long 4–0 black silk stitch is placed through the tip of the segment, and it is tucked up behind the clavicle and sternum to facilitate locating it when the cervical incision is made as described in the following section.

Primary Stage If No Fistula Present by X-ray

No intrathoracic work is done. A 2 cm. transverse incision is made in the right neck at the medial edge of the sternocleidomastoid muscle and 1 to 2 cm. above the sternoclavicular junction (Fig. 4). A No. 8 or No. 10 French catheter is inserted through the nose and into the upper pouch to help identify it. Dissection is carried out bluntly between the carotid sheath and the trachea. The esophagus has traction placed upon it by a figure-of-eight guy stitch, and the entire segment is as freely dissected as possible to gain maximum length. Three layers of 5–0 black silk sutures are utilized to sew the esophagus to muscle, subcutaneous tissue, and skin. This is done to prevent retraction of the esophagus, but care must be taken not to tent the trachea up or distort it by esophageal tension, because serious respiratory

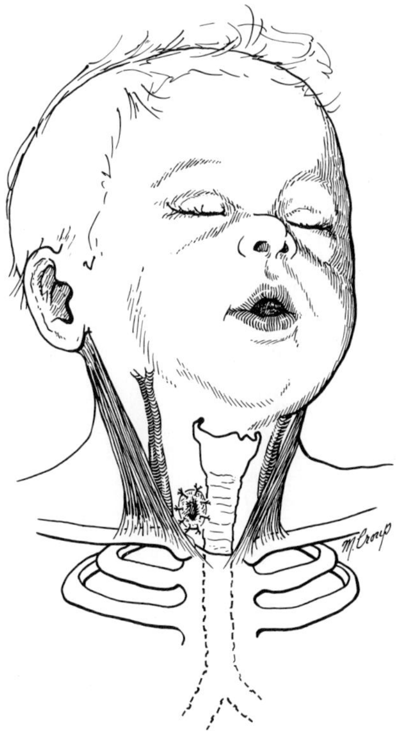

FIGURE 4. The cervical esophagostomy is constructed at the edge of the right sternocleidomastoid muscle and between the carotid sheath and the trachea.

troubles will ensue. The tip of the cervical esophagostomy is opened to allow egress of mucus and permit suturing to the skin.

Secondary Stage

The distal 3 cm. of the ileum, the ascending colon, and the right half of the transverse colon have been found to offer the best interpositional segment for a substitute, isoperistaltic esophagus. The blood supply must be obtained from the middle colic artery, and the marginal arcades must be carefully preserved. The two-layer, catgut and silk, ileocolostomy for intestinal continuity should be completed immediately. Then if the child does not tolerate the procedure at some point, it can be discontinued without ill effects and completed later.

The transverse colon end of the segment should be attached by a two-layer, catgut and silk, anastomosis along the midportion of the greater curvature of the stomach (Fig. 5). A filling stomach tends to block off the segment and prevent reflux.

A fresh incision at the suprasternal notch, with rongeuring of 1 to 2 cm. of the sternum, prepares the way for the development of a substernal tunnel (Fig. 5). This can most easily be done by using the index fingers to sweep away the light mediastinal attachments from the xyphoid and manubrial ends. The cecal end of the "new esophagus" is covered with a rubber glove tied on by umbilical tape. This attempt to prevent bacterial soilage of the mediastinum is abetted by apply-

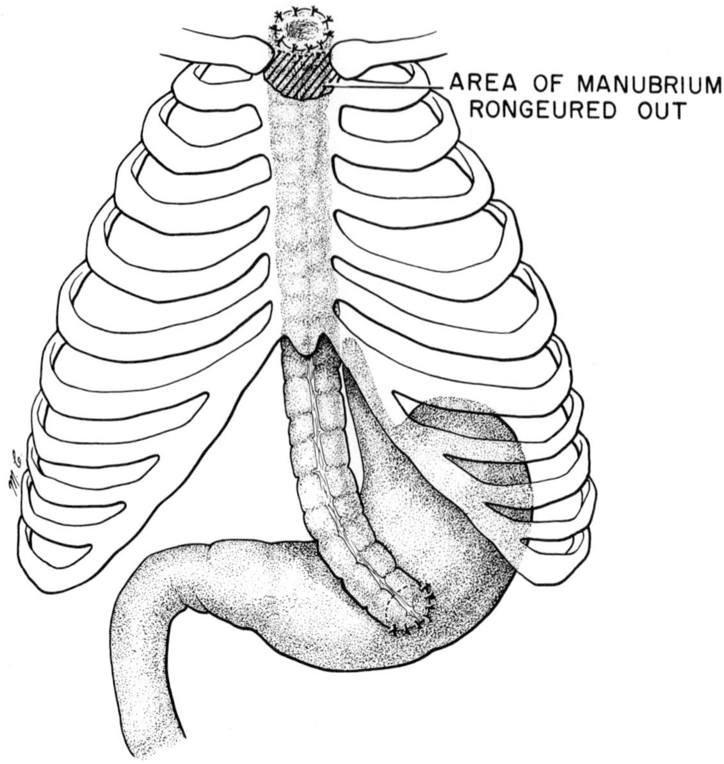

FIGURE 5. The colon as a substitute esophagus is shown attached to the greater curvature of the stomach to prevent reflux. It is brought out at the suprasternal notch, which has been enlarged by rongeuring the manubrium away.

ing lubricating jelly to the segment to facilitate pulling it through the tunnel. A tube is placed in the pulled-through segment from the neck end to prevent distention and consequent necrosis. The rongeuring of the sternum produces a thoracic inlet of sufficient size to prevent pressure necrosis, which we saw in a few of our early cases.

We prefer to wait four to six weeks before attaching the cervical esophagus to the colon, because the disparity in size is not nearly so great when the colon segment has shrunk. If the length of cervical esophagus permits, we do the anastomosis in the cupola of the thorax to avoid the angulation and consequent dysphagia that may occur if the union is made in the neck. Most anastomoses have been done in the neck and have functioned satisfactorily.

H-Type Fistula Repair

In this rather rare type of esophageal anomaly, the rectangular pleural flap described under Primary Anastomosis is developed for the purpose of covering and

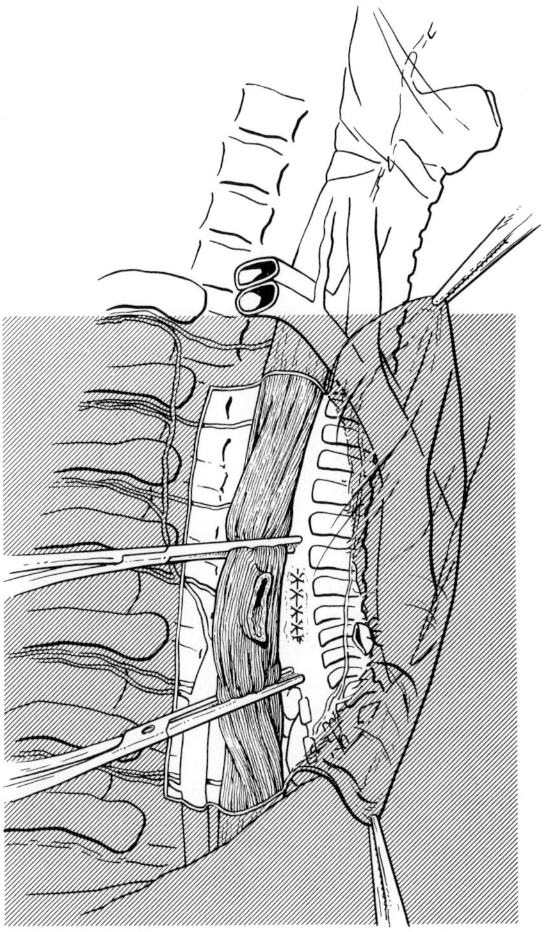

FIGURE 6. Potts clamps have been applied above and below the fistulous opening and rotated to provide better exposure.

separating the divided fistula ends. Careful and adequate mobilization above and below the fistula will allow pieces of Penrose drain to be inserted for traction. With the view thus provided, a continuous 5–0 vascular silk suture is used on the tracheal side and water-tested for leakage. Two Potts patent ductus clamps are then applied to the esophagus above and below the fistula in a manner that allows the opening to be rotated (Fig. 6) 90 degrees for a clearer view of the esophageal side of the fistula. An interrupted, 5–0 silk closure is accomplished as one layer of seromuscular stitches on the esophageal side.

Gastrostomy

A transverse incision centered on the left rectus muscle, with partial division of the central portion of muscle, gives good exposure and size for a No. 14 or No. 16 French Pezzer catheter to be brought out (Fig. 7). With the stomach exposed,

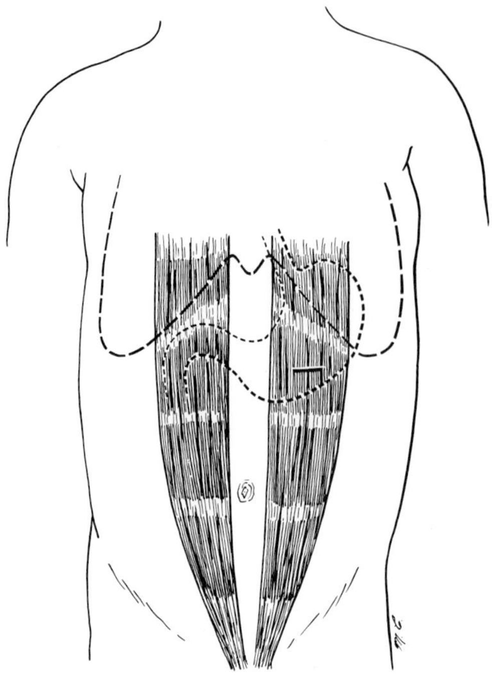

FIGURE 7. The incision is shown for a good gastrostomy position below the middle left rectus muscle.

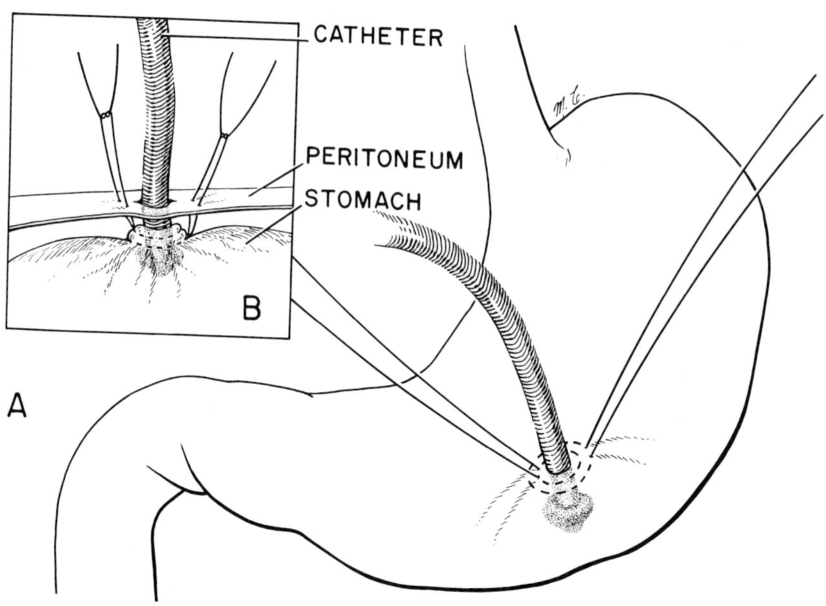

FIGURE 8. (*A*) A Pezzer catheter has been inserted within two purse-string sutures started 180 degrees apart. (*B*) The sutures are being tied down after insertion through the peritoneum in order to bring the stomach up against the abdominal wall.

two purse-string sutures are started 180 degrees apart (Fig. 8A) with 4–0 silk. The anticipated opening should be well up along the greater curvature to prevent any possible initiation of pylorospasm or frank mechanical obstruction by the tube itself. It is perhaps equally important to leave enough space distal to the gastrostomy for a colon interposition anastomosis if a substitute esophagus is needed.

An easy way to open the stomach within the purse-string sutures is to grasp it with a curved hemostat and actually slit it against the countertraction of the clamp. With the tube in place, the sutures are tied and then fastened to the peritoneum (Fig. 8B) in order to bring the stomach up against the peritoneum. This prevents leakage. If the gastrostomy tube should come out within three weeks, a Foley tube should replace it. This will reduce the risk that the stomach will be pushed off the abdominal wall before it has healed solidly. A small amount of Dionosil introduced into the stomach permits confirmation by x-ray that reinstitution of feedings will be safe.

References

Benson, C. D., Mustard, W. T., Ravitch, M. M., Snyder, W. H., Jr., and Welch, K. J. *Pediatric Surgery*. Chicago: Year Book Publishers, 1962. P. 266.

Haight, C. Congenital atresia of the esophagus. *J. Thoracic Surg.* 34:141, August 1957.

Hays, D. M. An analysis of the mortality in esophageal atresia. *Am. J. Dis. Child.* 103:765, June 1962.

Koop, C. E., Kiesewetter, W. B., and Johnson, J. Treatment of atresia of the esophagus by the transpleural approach. *Surg., Gynec. and Obst.* 98:687, June 1954.

Koop, C. E., and Verhagen, A. D. Early management of atresia of the esophagus. *Internat. Abstr. Surg.* 113:103, July 1961.

127. *Pyloromyotomy for Pyloric Stenosis*

C. EVERETT KOOP

THE PROCEDURE here described for pyloromyotomy for congenital hypertrophic pyloric stenosis in infants has been developed (1) to obviate some of the difficulties encountered by general surgeons in exposing the pylorus and performing the pyloromyotomy itself; and (2) to reduce the operating time and the wound complications, both immediate and long-term. Longitudinal incisions extensive enough to permit the surgeon to insert his fingers to extract the pylorus entail long operations, the division of nerves and blood vessels supplying the anterior abdominal wall, and wounds which are neither muscularly strong nor cosmetically acceptable and are prone to infection and disruption because of tissue destruction. The fact that otherwise competent surgeons are frightened (unnecessarily) about the actual pyloromyotomy itself indicates that something must be wrong with our general approach to the division of these few muscle fibers. The procedure to be described avoids these various pitfalls and makes the operation short, easy on the baby, and comfortable for the surgeon.

There is probably no simple operative procedure in which adequate preoperative preparation of the patient pays bigger postoperative dividends. Obviously any baby who has been vomiting, and therefore subject to electrolyte and fluid imbalance, must be brought to surgery only after adequate hydration and correction of his chemical deficit.

General anesthesia is far superior to local for abdominal surgery on infants and should be used for the operative technique to be described.

Technique

The Incision

The incision for a pyloromyotomy need be no longer than is necessary to accommodate the pyloric tumor as it is delivered from the peritoneal cavity. When a small incision such as this is used, the anesthesia must be deeper than that necessary for large incisions. If it is not, respiratory effort alone tends to extrude abdominal viscera through the small opening. The anesthesia need be deep only for those few moments between the opening of the peritoneum and the return of the pylorus to the peritoneal cavity. A transverse incision divides fewer nerves and blood vessels than a longitudinal incision and cosmetically is far superior to any longitudinal or diagonal incision. Being placed in the direction of the lines of skin tension, the transverse incision may grow during childhood to an eventual length one and one-half times that of the original, whereas the longitudinal incision, by adolescence, may extend from over the costal margin to below the umbilicus.

In the anesthetized baby, a careful examination is made to determine the position of the edge of the liver. The skin incision is placed transversely over the rectus muscle 1 cm. cephalad to the palpable liver edge. The incision starts at the midline and moves laterally 3 to 3.5 cm. The entire length of the incision will eventually be used, and it is suggested that once the line of intended incision is drawn, the cut be made from each end toward the middle, with the skin outstretched in a V made by the widely separated index and middle fingers of the surgeon's left hand (Fig. 1). These babies have little subcutaneous fat, and usually bleeding vessels need not be ligated.

A delicate incision is then made transversely across the anterior rectus sheath, which is a tough structure but exceedingly thin. The incision should expose but not traumatize the underlying longitudinal muscle fibers. No retraction will be necessary, thus far in the procedure, if the spread fingers of the surgeon's left hand do their job adequately. Two small right-angle retractors with the retracting blade no deeper than 1.5 cm. are now placed at the upper and lower edges of the wound, and dissecting scissors are inserted into the rectus muscle (Fig. 2) in its midline. The longitudinal muscle fibers are spread medially and laterally by opening the blades of the scissors to expose the peritoneum. While the scissors remains open and the peritoneum is exposed, the retractors are taken from their initial position and placed between the separated rectus muscle fibers. Firm traction is applied both laterally and medially.

The peritoneum is now grasped with two mosquito hemostats, and an incision is made just above the edge of the liver. The peritoneum is incised laterally and medially the length of the skin incision, after which all layers of the wound are retracted superiorly and inferiorly by the insertion of the narrow end of two Parker band retractors.

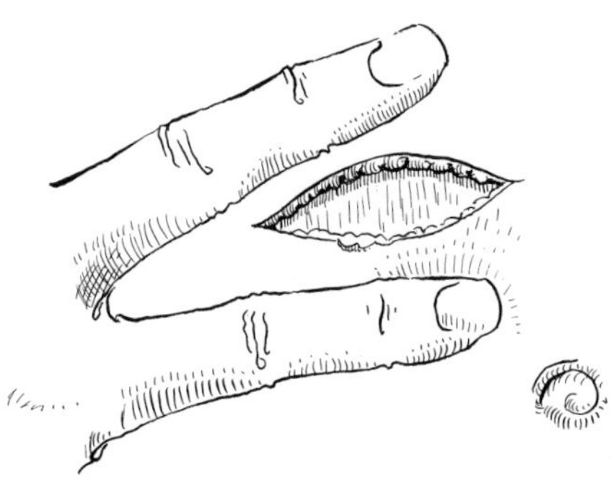

FIGURE 1. The skin of the anterior abdominal wall is stretched superiorly and inferiorly between the surgeon's spread fingers to facilitate the making of a small incision.

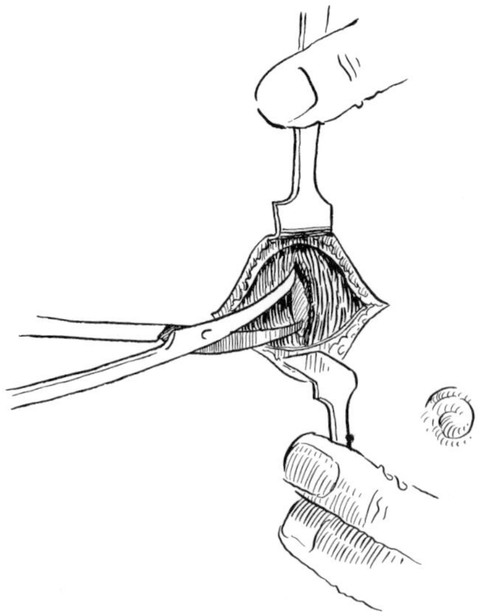

FIGURE 2. The anterior rectus sheath has been divided transversely, and scissors are now inserted between bundles of longitudinal rectus muscle fibers to expose the peritoneum.

If the incision has been properly placed and the wound edges properly retracted, nothing should appear beneath the peritoneum but the anterior surface of the liver (Fig. 3). In this position the liver effectively blocks the extrusion of abdominal viscera through the wound, an advantage which will be more apparent when the peritoneum is being closed after pyloromyotomy. The handle of a tissue forceps is inserted between the liver edge and the lower border of the wound, and by a rotary action of the left wrist the liver edge is elevated to expose the abdominal viscera. It is difficult to find the pylorus or even the stomach, and attempts made blindly with grasping forceps can be hazardous, since a tight clamp will cut through the muscle fibers of the edematous stomach so frequently found in babies with pyloric stenosis. If advantage is taken of anatomical attachments of the viscera and the propensity of the infant's omentum to stick to a sponge, the pylorus can be extracted from the abdomen without insertion of even a finger into the peri-

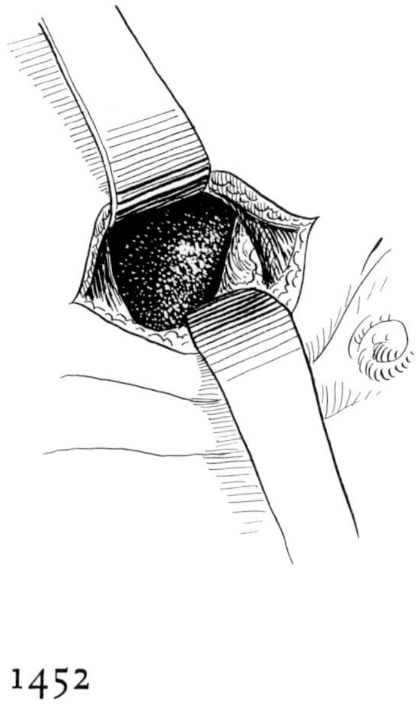

FIGURE 3. The peritoneum is opened and retracted superiorly and inferiorly to expose the liver.

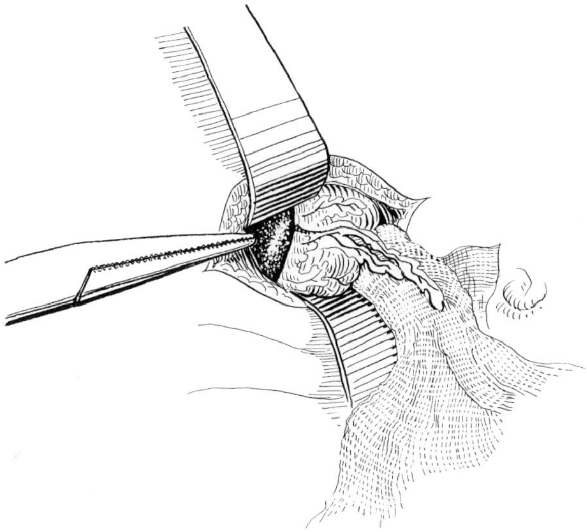

FIGURE 4. Dry gauze inserted into the peritoneal cavity in the direction of the pylorus has been extracted, pulling with it a piece of omentum.

toneal cavity. With the liver edge still slightly elevated by the forceps held in the left hand, a dry, fine gauze sponge held between the prongs of tissue forceps is inserted through the incision in the direction of the pylorus. Both forceps may now be abandoned, and the surgeon can gently pull the gauze sponge out of the abdomen. Almost invariably the youngster's delicate omentum leaves the wound with the sponge (Fig. 4). Gentle traction on the omentum will bring into vision the transverse colon, which can be grasped between thumb and forefinger, and gentle traction on this portion of the colon will bring the greater curvature of the stomach into view. If the colonic traction is applied with the thumb and forefinger of the left hand, the surgeon can grasp the anterior wall of the stomach with Babcock forceps held in the right hand (Fig. 5). The Babcock clamp is closed to the first notch only and is then gently depressed into the peritoneal cavity so that the stomach goes back to its normal position. With the Babcock clamp still attached to the stomach, tissue forceps are used to replace gently the transverse colon and the omentum. The Babcock clamp is then brought through the wound until a portion of the anterior wall of the stomach or its greater curvature bulges slightly through the wound. This traction is done with the Babcock forceps held in the surgeon's right hand, and as soon as there is an ample bulge of stomach the surgeon grasps the stomach wall between the gauze-covered thumb and forefinger of his left hand. Gentle traction with these two fingers on the stomach will bring enough stomach wall into the wound for the surgeon to grasp with his right thumb and index finger a larger segment of that viscus so that it will not slip from his grasp as he extracts the pylorus.

Delivery of the Pylorus onto the Abdominal Wall

The pylorus is delivered through the abdominal incision not by traction toward the ceiling, but by a rotary motion of the surgeon's wrist as its volar surface rests

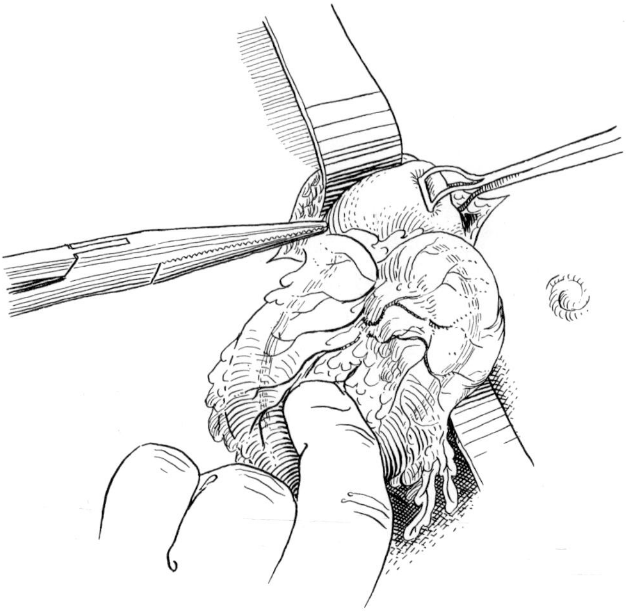

FIGURE 5. Gentle traction on the transverse colon, which has been brought into the wound by traction on the omentum, reveals the anterior surface of the stomach so that a Babcock clamp can be applied.

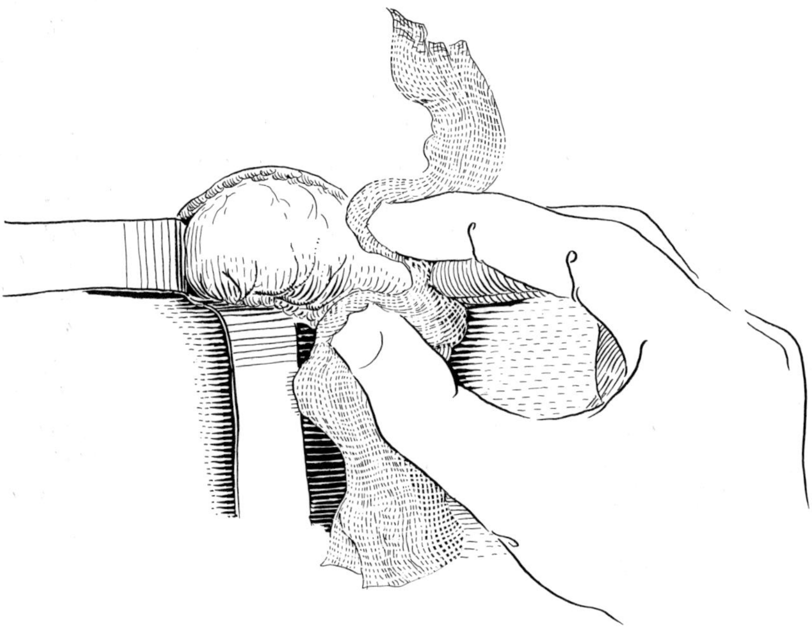

FIGURE 6. The pylorus is delivered after rotary motion of the surgeon's right hand has extracted it through the abdominal wound.

gently on the child's abdomen in the midline, fingers pointed cephalad (Fig. 6). A gentle clockwise rotation will bring the proximal edge of the pylorus to the wound. It may be necessary, however, to shift the position of thumb and forefinger on the stomach once or twice in order to have an adequate purchase for the extraction of the pylorus. If the incision is large enough, further clockwise rotation of the surgeon's hand will roll the pylorus out of the wound. If it is a tight fit, the index finger of the surgeon's hand can push from the area just lateral to the lateral edge of the wound to deliver the pylorus onto the abdominal wall.

The Pylorotomy

The abdominal incision is small enough to keep the pylorus from dropping back into the peritoneal cavity, and traction need not be retained on the stomach. However, it is helpful if the assistant across the table grasps the exteriorized portion of the stomach and holds it out of the surgeon's way, depressing it gently against the infant's abdominal wall. The incision which is to be made in the pylorus for the spreading of the circular muscle fibers is not difficult, but because of the frequency with which the duodenum has been perforated, it is a maneuver that many operators perform with unnecessary emotional tension. Surgeons who work comfortably and safely in far more hazardous areas commonly use for division of the pylorus awkward and inefficient procedures which are little more than fetishes.

The pylorus is rotated so that a relatively avascular portion is pointing toward the ceiling. For the occasional operator it is best to have an assistant hold the anterior stomach wall between two fingers and retract it to the left side. The surgeon can then steady the pylorus with one finger of his left hand by placing the finger tip against the distal edge of the pyloric ring with the anterior duodenal wall interposed.

An incision is made from a point just below the pyloric ring to a point just above it, and deep enough so that the serosa is adequately divided to expose the hypertrophied muscle bundles. A mosquito hemostat is then placed into the groove between two prominent muscle bundles and is gently opened to apply pressure against the edematous muscle fibers (Fig. 7). This hemostat should be held by the surgeon in any position in which it is comfortable. Effort to prevent the point of the hemostat from ever coming into apposition with the pyloric mucosa makes spreading of the fibers difficult and the action of the hemostat inefficient. Three to four gentle excursions of the jaws of the mosquito hemostat may be necessary to establish the line of cleavage from one end of the pylorus to the other. After this has been done, a larger hemostat with a relatively blunt tip is used to complete the spreading until the mucosa is definitely visible in the depths of the spread muscle fibers and actually bulges into the declivity that has been made. The advantage of having the tip of a finger of the left hand against the lower end of the pyloric ring is that it tells the surgeon where the pylorus actually ends, and under direct vision he may look for the change in the appearance of the mucosa where the pylorus joins the duodenum.

If the muscle fibers are gently spread under direct vision, there is no reason

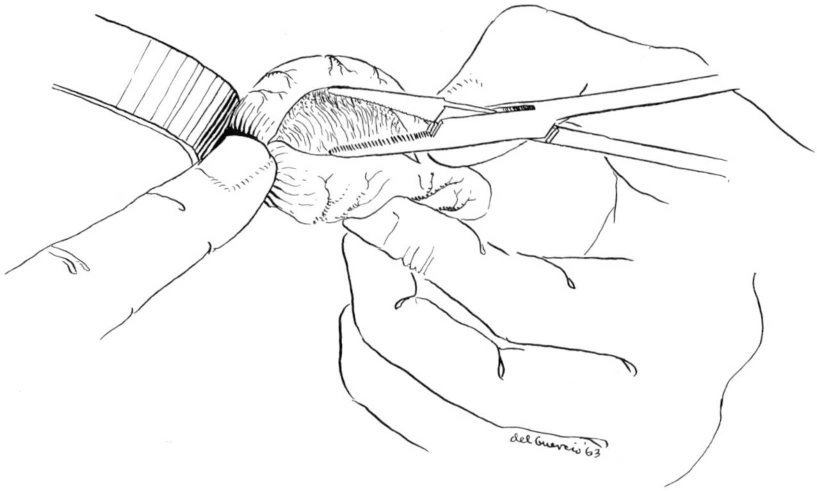

FIGURE 7. Hemostat spreading circular muscle fibers of the pylorus after incision of the serosa.

why the mucosa of the duodenum should be entered. If, however, the mucosa, either of the pylorus itself or of the adjacent duodenum, should be perforated, no effort should be made to close the defect per se with a purse-string suture. Instead, the entire muscular incision should be closed with seromuscular interrupted sutures of fine silk, the entire pylorus rotated 90 degrees, and a new incision made in the serosa and the pyloromyotomy carried out anew.

Attention is turned so frequently to the lower end of the pylorus that the upper end may be inadequately divided. If the serosal incision is carried onto the normal stomach wall, and the pyloric fibers are spread to the point where the junction of the pylorus and stomach can be seen, the division is adequate. Except in the most unusual circumstances, no effort need be made to secure hemostasis. Because of the tightness of the incision, there is some venous congestion of the pylorus at this stage of the procedure; hence, some of the bleeding seen during pyloromyotomy will subside immediately after the pylorus has been replaced into the peritoneal cavity. The pylorus and stomach are replaced in the opposite order to that of their withdrawal.

Closure

If the retractors are then relaxed, the incision should close in such a way that the liver once again lies directly beneath the peritoneal incision and acts like a cork in a bottle to prevent the extrusion of abdominal viscera during closure. The two peritoneal grasping hemostats which were used for opening the peritoneum are still in situ; these are elevated through the wound and additional mosquito hemostats are placed on the lateral and medial edges of the peritoneal incision. The peritoneum is closed with a running 3–0 chromic catgut suture with atraumatic needle, after which it will be seen that the longitudinal division of the rectus muscle still gapes to some extent. A single suture of this same material is used to approximate several muscle fibers lying close to the medial and lateral edges of this gap. The suture is tied in such a way that the gap is closed but any tension on the muscle fiber that might shut off the intrinsic blood supply is avoided.

Four or five interrupted sutures approximate the anterior rectus sheath. These may be of the same 3–0 chromic catgut, or a nonabsorbable suture such as 4–0 silk may be used. Usually there is not enough subcutaneous tissue to warrant separate closure, but if it is appreciable two or three sutures in this layer are advisable. The skin is then closed with four 5–0 white silk subcuticular sutures placed directly in the corium. After the wound edges have been held in apposition between gauze-covered fingers until a fibrinous seal has been achieved, thin collodion is drawn across the wound to keep it waterproof until wound healing has accomplished the same end.

Comments

This operation can be performed comfortably in less than 20 minutes. The child can be started on feedings by mouth three to four hours after reaction from anesthesia, and can be discharged in a few days, depending upon the adequacy of facilities for home care. The wound requires no dressing and no further attention, destruction of any portion of the abdominal musculature is avoided, and the skin incision may not be noticeable after a time.

128. *Duodenal Obstruction in the Newborn*

JERROLD M. BECKER AND

KEITH M. SCHNEIDER

DUODENAL OBSTRUCTION in the newborn can be classified into two forms, intrinsic and extrinsic. Intrinsic duodenal obstruction may be subdivided into complete obstruction (atresia) and incomplete obstruction (stenosis). There are three possible anatomical variations of atresia: (1) an intraluminal membrane causing complete occlusion; (2) a lack of continuity of the duodenum, with no connection between the proximal and distal segments; and (3) a thin fibrous cord connecting the two segments. Duodenal stenosis exists in two forms: (1) a membranous obstruction with a tiny slit-like aperture; and (2) a concentric narrowing of a segment of duodenum.

Extrinsic duodenal obstruction is caused by malrotation of bowel or by annular pancreas. Malrotation is more common. In malrotation, obstruction results from bands which extend from the cecum to the lateral abdominal wall. These bands, called Ladd's bands, course over the anterior aspect of the duodenum and can produce incomplete duodenal obstruction. Of surgical importance is the occasional association of *intrinsic* duodenal obstruction, particularly stenosis, with malrotation.

Annular pancreas, resulting from faulty rotation of the pancreatic anlage, causes partial obstruction by encircling the duodenum with a narrow ring of pancreatic tissue. Intrinsic obstruction may also occur with annular pancreas.

Bile-stained (green) vomitus in the newborn means intestinal obstruction until this condition is ruled out. Infants with duodenal atresia start to vomit during the first day of life. Most obstructions are distal to the ampulla of Vater, and therefore the vomitus is usually green in color. Abdominal distention is frequently not marked, since the proximal duodenum and stomach are decompressed by vomiting.

In duodenal stenosis, malrotation, and annular pancreas, the signs and symptoms are the same as in atresia but their onset may be delayed for days or months, depending on the degree of obstruction.

Maternal polyhydramnios (over 2000 cc. of amniotic fluid) is frequently associated with high intestinal obstruction in the fetus. Infants born of mothers with this condition should have x-rays at 8 to 12 hours of age to rule out obstruction.

Mortality caused by delay in diagnosis is significant. Early diagnosis is important to prevent excessive losses of electrolyte-containing gastroduodenal secretions. Aspiration into the tracheobronchial tree during vomiting is a frequent and serious complication.

Plain films of the abdomen in the supine and erect positions are usually diagnostic of duodenal obstruction. Distention of the stomach and the first and second portions of the duodenum indicates duodenal obstruction. If the obstruction is incomplete, small amounts of gas will be seen in the distal small intestine and colon.

The use of oral radiopaque contrast material in complete high obstruction is unnecessary and time-consuming, and an undue exposure of the infant to x-rays. In incomplete obstruction, oral Hypaque or Gastrografin is used to define the site of obstruction unless this is evident on plain films. Since this contrast material will reach the distal colon in two to three hours, radiopaque enemas are rarely indicated.

Technique

After the diagnosis has been made, a No. 8 French polyethylene nasogastric tube is passed into the stomach and attached to a mild suction. A cutdown is performed in the long saphenous vein at the ankle for administration of intravenous fluids. To conserve body heat, the infant's extremities are wrapped.

The child is placed on the operating table in the supine position with the extremities restrained. All infants under 4 pounds in weight are operated upon using local anesthesia (½ per cent procaine or ¼ per cent Xylocaine) for each layer of the abdominal wall. Five cubic centimeters of anesthetic agent is then introduced into a small opening in the peritoneal cavity through a No. 8 French catheter. Three minutes are allowed to elapse before the peritoneum is widely opened. A quiet operative field can be achieved by this technique.

A transverse incision is made one fingerbreadth above the umbilicus. The incision extends from the midline across the right rectus muscle and out toward the flank (Fig. 1). If necessary, it can be enlarged across the left rectus. On opening the peritoneum, all intestine possible is delivered out of the abdominal cavity.

In duodenal atresia the intestine distal to the atretic area is very narrow. The dilated stomach and first and second portions of the duodenum are identified. The transverse colon is then elevated and the ligament of Treitz located. The proximal jejunum is distended by injecting 20 cc. of saline into its lumen through a No. 24 gauge needle. The saline is then gently milked down through the small and large bowel to rule out the presence of additional sites of obstruction. The hepatic flexure is mobilized medially by cutting its filmy lateral attachments so that an antecolic anastomosis can be made. The colonic mesentery is thin and filmy and must be carefully protected.

A 2 cm. opening is made in the dilated descending duodenum. A similar open-

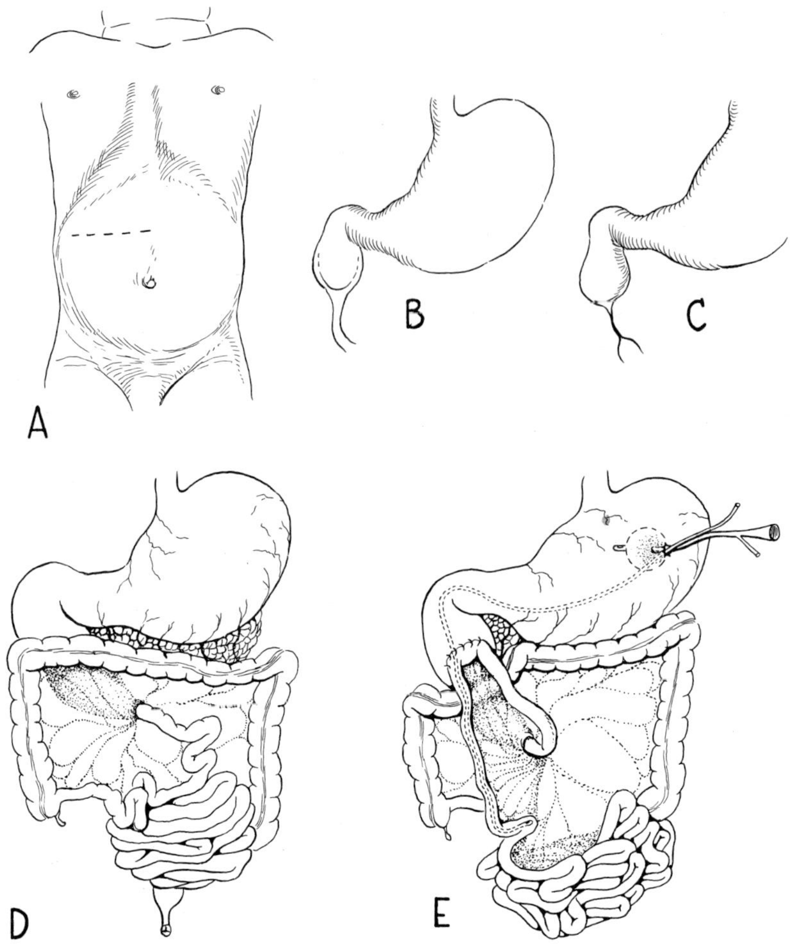

FIGURE 1. Duodenal stenosis and atresia. (A) Site of the incision. (*B, C, and D*) Anatomical findings in atresia and stenosis. (*E*) Antecolic duodenojejunostomy. Note the position of the long polyethylene tube passing through the anastomosis.

ing is made along the antimesenteric border of the jejunum. The use of noncrushing clamps to prevent intestinal secretions from reaching the area of the anastomosis is avoided. These secretions are aspirated as necessary with low pressure suction. The bowel is manipulated with the sutures which are used for the anastomosis rather than with forceps.

A one-layer antecolic duodenojejunostomy is performed, using 5–0 silk sutures. These are passed from mucosa to serosa, serosa to mucosa, starting on the posterior wall of the anastomosis. The knots are tied on the inside. The last two sutures are placed from serosa to mucosa, mucosa to serosa, and tied with the knots on the *outside*. They are then buried with interrupted Lembert sutures.

Prior to the closure of the anterior wall of the anastomosis, the stomach is delivered into the operative field. Two concentric purse-string sutures of 4–0 chromic catgut are placed in its anterior wall. Through a small gastrotomy a No. 5 French (in premature newborns) or No. 8 French (in full-term newborns) polyethylene catheter is threaded through the stomach and past the anastomosis for 6 to 8 inches. The anterior layer of the anastomosis is then completed. A stab wound is then made in the left upper quadrant and a No. 14 French Foley catheter is drawn into the abdominal cavity and inserted into the stomach. The polyethylene tube exits through the same stab wound. The bag of the Foley catheter is inflated with 2 to 3 cc. of saline. The purse-string sutures are then drawn taut and the outer one is sutured to the undersurface of the anterior abdominal wall.

The abdomen is closed with interrupted figure-of-eight No. 32 stainless steel wire, and the skin is approximated with interrupted 5–0 silk sutures. The Foley catheter is then pulled up against the anterior abdominal wall and taped to the polyethylene tube.

The use of gastrostomy and jejunostomy tubes has many advantages. These include (1) avoidance of a nasogastric tube; (2) more effective gastric decompression because of the larger caliber of the gastrostomy tube; (3) a simplification of fluid and electrolyte problems since all drainage from the stomach is instilled into the jejunostomy tube; and (4) alimentation early in the postoperative period. Formula instilled directly into the jejunostomy tube is well tolerated.

The same operation is used for duodenal atresia, duodenal stenosis, and annular pancreas (Fig. 2). The pancreatic ring should not be divided, because of the high incidence of pancreatic fistulas. Dividing the ring, furthermore, will not relieve the obstruction in infants with associated intrinsic stenosis.

In the operative treatment of malrotation, two pathological anatomical features may be present, duodenal obstruction and midgut volvulus (Fig. 3A). In addition to the presence of Ladd's bands, the entire small bowel and right colon are suspended on a narrow mesentery containing the superior mesenteric vessels. There is no fusion of this mesentery to the posterior abdominal wall. Consequently, volvulus of the entire midgut is an important complication of this anomaly.

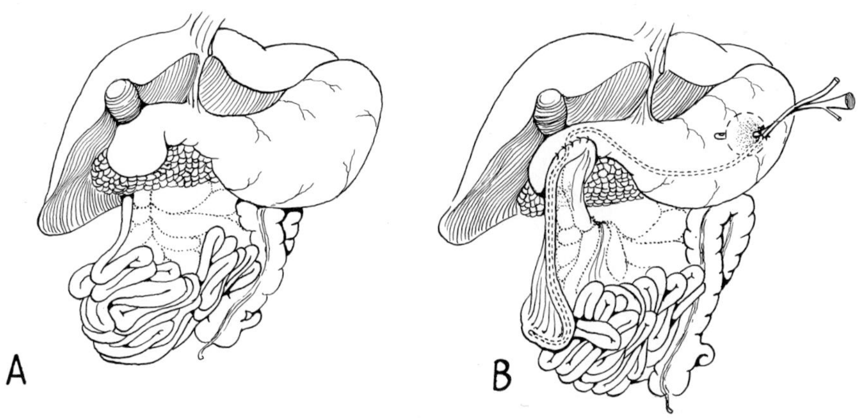

FIGURE 2. Annular pancreas. (A *and* B) Pathological findings and technique of correction. Note the position of the polyethylene tube.

The incision is the same as for other lesions of the duodenum. The entire midgut is delivered from the abdominal cavity. Volvulus is suspected if the entire small intestine is discolored or if one cannot visualize the right half of the colon. The rotation may be one or more full turns and is almost always in a clockwise

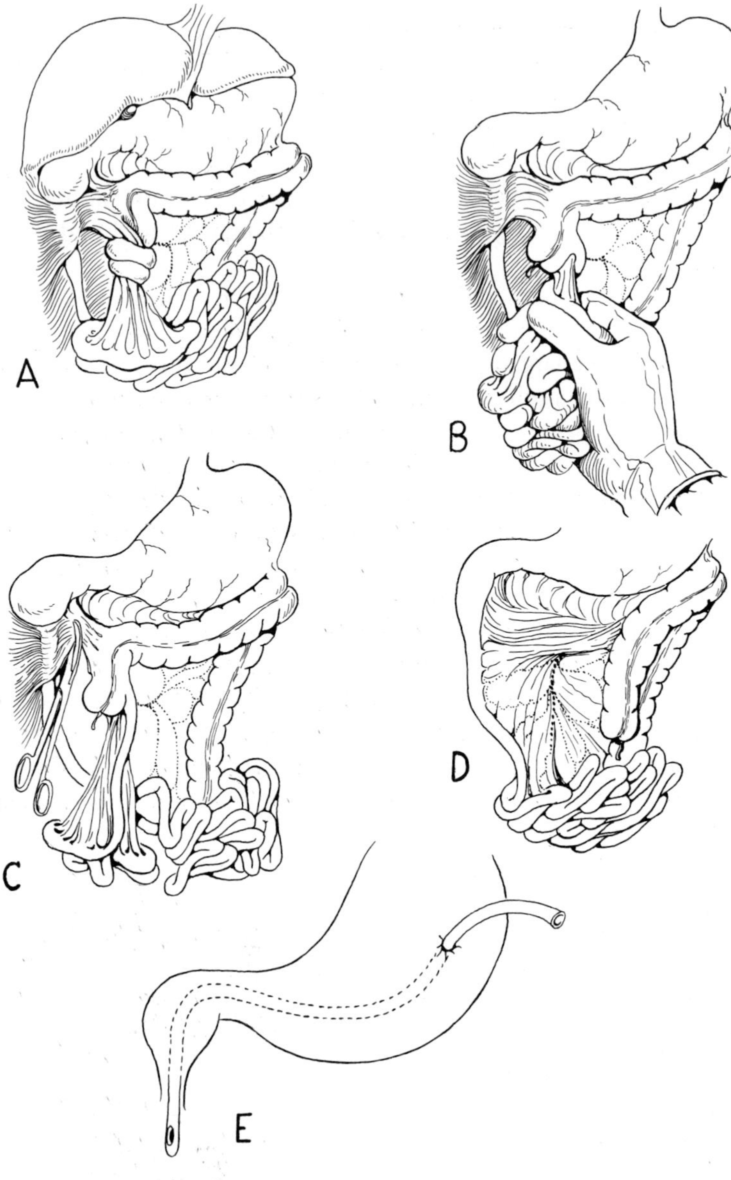

FIGURE 3. Malrotation. (*A*) Malrotation with midgut volvulus. (*B*) Technique of reduction of the volvulus. (*C*) Division of Ladd's bands. (*D*) Appearance of the duodenum and jejunum at the conclusion of the procedure. Note the straight course of the superior mesenteric vessels. (*E*) A No. 22 French catheter is inserted to rule out intrinsic obstruction.

direction. The entire intestinal mass is grasped with both hands and rotated counterclockwise until the volvulus is reduced. The bands between the cecum and lateral abdominal wall are then divided so that the cecum can be placed in the left side of the abdomen. Additional bands are occasionally found distally between loops of small bowel. These can be visualized and divided if the superior mesenteric artery is followed for its entire length. At the completion of the operation, the duodenum runs an unobstructed course straight down the right side of the abdomen to join the jejunum.

Through a gastrostomy incision a No. 20 or No. 22 French catheter is then passed into the upper jejunum. This is done to rule out the presence of intrinsic duodenal stenosis, which is occasionally associated with malrotation. If an obstruction is met, it must be bypassed by a side-to-side duodenojejunostomy. If no obstruction is met, a No. 5 French polyethylene catheter is inserted into the jejunum as previously described, and brought out through the left upper quadrant with a Foley gastrostomy tube.

In operations performed under local anesthesia, an additional 5 cc. of ¼ per cent Xylocaine is instilled into the peritoneal cavity about five minutes before replacement of the viscera. The added relaxation has been a considerable aid in replacement of bowel. Closure is performed as previously described.

Adequate attention must be paid postoperatively to fluid balance, temperature regulation, and administration of antibiotics.

References

BECKER, J. M., and SCHNEIDER, K. M. Tube jejunostomy in the treatment of upper intestinal obstruction in the neonate. *Surg., Gynec., and Obst.* 116:123, January 1963.

EHRENPREIS, T., and SANDBLOM, P. Duodenal atresia and stenosis: twenty cases of intrinsic obstruction. *Acta pediat.* 38:109, 1949.

GLOVER, D. M., and BARRY, F. M. Intestinal obstruction in the newborn. *Ann. Surg.* 130:480, September 1949.

129. *Intussusception*

ROBERT J. IZANT, JR.

THE PHENOMENON of intussusception, whether in adults or infants, is basically in most instances a strangulating small bowel obstruction. If this basic pathophysiological concept is kept in mind, the treatment may be carried out more successfully.

Though there is a place for barium enema reduction of intussusception in infants and children (under 2 to 3 years of age), it is my opinion that the operative treatment is indicated in the following situations: (1) In children over 3 years of age, because of the increasing incidence, with increasing age, of specific pathological lesions: i.e. polyp, inverted Meckel's diverticulum, tumors (lymphosarcoma for example), and duplications. (2) In any age group when symptoms have persisted for more than 24 hours. (3) If definite signs of peritonitis, peripheral vascular collapse, lethargy, or dehydration are present when the patient is first seen. (4) When there is marked abdominal distention, fever over 38°C. (rectally), or marked leukocytosis. Under these circumstances a careful history and physical examination supplemented by plain abdominal flat and upright roentgenograms will in almost every instance give a positive diagnosis without resorting to a time-consuming diagnostic barium enema. The diagnosis of "acute lower small intestinal obstruction" is justified under emergency circumstances and is clearly sufficient evidence to prepare a patient for operative treatment—no matter what the cause.

Preoperative Treatment

Proper preoperative treatment is the sine qua non of a successful outcome. Nasogastric suction (with extra holes in the tubing if necessary) is required. A route for intravenous infusions is essential. If, upon seeing a patient suspected of having an intussusception, doubt arises about the adequacy and dependability of an intravenous needle, a cutdown must be done (under local anesthesia) immediately.

"Priming the pump" with 10 cc. per kilogram of normal saline and 5 per cent dextrose solution (given in 20 to 30 minutes) is an important aid in restoring circulating blood volume of depleted infants and children. This should be followed by appropriate electrolyte solutions—omitting potassium until sufficient urinary output has been established.

Appropriate hematological and electrolyte studies should of course be obtained. Sufficient accurately typed and cross-matched blood must be immediately available. Administration of antibiotics is indicated in patients with advanced obstruction. We prefer intravenous penicillin 15,000 to 25,000 units per kilogram, intravenous chloramphenicol 25 to 50 mg. per kilogram, and intramuscular streptomycin 15 to 20 mg. per kilogram. These drugs can be discontinued or altered appropriately, depending on the finding at surgical exploration. There is now sufficient evidence that the use of such an antimicrobrial regimen reduces the incidence of progressive ischemic changes or anastomotic leaks in obstructed bowel. Appropriate sedation is helpful.

Extremely helpful in determining the optimal time for operative intervention is the use of a "close chart"—a 15-minute record of pulse and respiration and blood pressure, a 30-minute record of temperature and urinary output. These should be recorded graphically on a temperature chart modified for the purpose. Only when the pulse is stable in the 120 beats per minute range, the temperature is stable at 38.4°C. (rectally), the blood pressure is stable, and urine has been produced is the infant patient ready for operation.

Technique

For many practical and surgically sound reasons, only a right transverse incision is used (Fig. 1). This is made just above or just below the level of the umbilicus, depending on the anatomical peculiarities of the individual abdominal wall. The transverse incision can be extended across the abdomen if necessary for further exploration. It heals without as high an incidence of hernia as accompanies the use of a longitudinal incision. The incision is placed over the area of the cecum and terminal ileum—the region where the serious difficulties with reduction occur. It is important to remember that the incision is never made over the intussuscep-

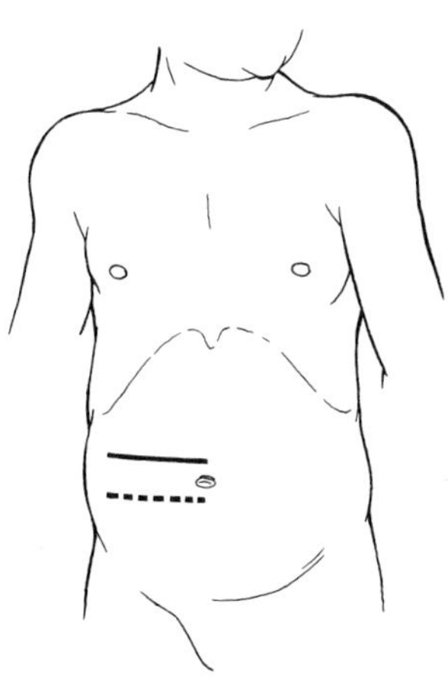

FIGURE 1. The position of the usual transverse incision is shown by the dashed line. The incision also may be made, depending on the abdominal wall proportions, just above the umbilicus.

tion mass—unless it is in the right lower quadrant, where some ileoileal intussusception may present.

If a resection is necessary in a desperately ill infant or small child, a Mikulicz ileostomy or ileocolostomy is the procedure of choice, in our opinion. The Mikulicz loops can be brought out through the lateral edge of the incision close to the lateral abdominal wall, thus largely obviating the chance of internal hernia formation around a more medially placed column of bowel. A long (6 cm.) internal extension of the double barrel is important. Also a deep lip (2 cm.) should be left on the outside because of the chance of retraction. To prevent evisceration, the peritoneum, fascia, and skin must be sewed carefully with 5–0 arterial silk sutures to the loop (Fig. 2A, B, C).

Extraperitoneal closure (Fig. 3) is done 7 to 10 days later after a crushing clamp* (Fig. 2) has been applied to the spur. Occasionally there may be such minimal drainage after the spur has been crushed that the secondary closure can be deferred until weight gain and positive nitrogen balance have occurred. However, in most instances the Mikulicz ileostomy or ileocolostomy drains profusely and produces a severe fluid and electrolyte problem for the first seven days at least.

Extraperitoneal closure of the Mikulicz procedure is a major operation, though a simple one (Fig. 4). An intravenous set should be in place. Blood should be available, because blood loss ranges from 50 to 120 cc. The previously placed black silk sutures on the fascia and peritoneum are a great aid in accomplishing dissection

* Various-sized Mikulicz infant clamps can be obtained from Codman & Shurtleff, Boston, Massachusetts.

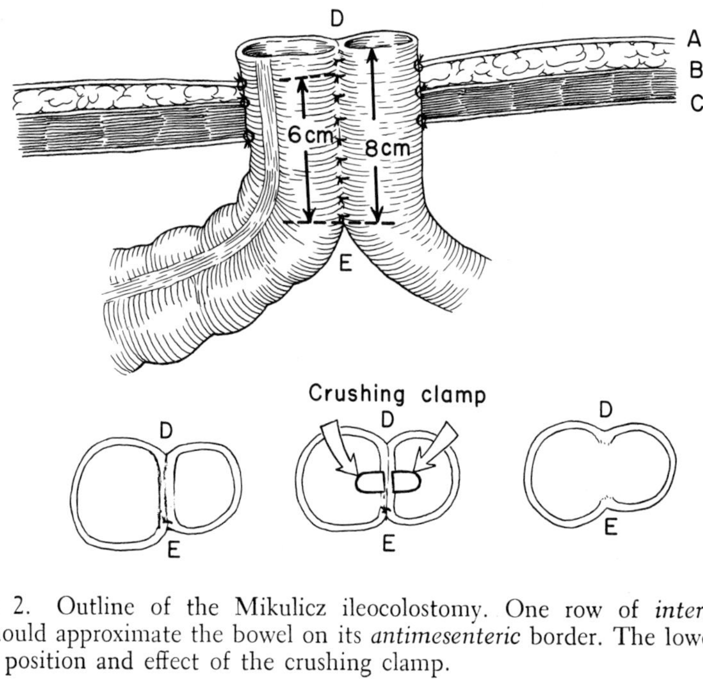

FIGURE 2. Outline of the Mikulicz ileocolostomy. One row of *interrupted* silk sutures should approximate the bowel on its *antimesenteric* border. The lower diagrams show the position and effect of the crushing clamp.

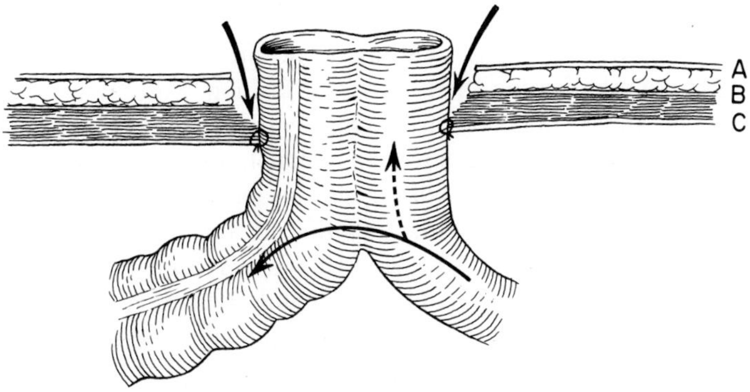

FIGURE 3. Closure of the Mikulicz ileocolostomy. Dissection (heavy arrows) should be carried through the skin (*A*) with the edge near the bowel excised. The fascia previously sutured around the bowel (*B*) is separated. But the peritoneum (*C*) is not opened. The fine (5–0) black silk interrupted sutures that were used in its construction are useful landmarks during the closure of the ileocolostomy. Note that most of the fecal stream (light solid arrow) bypasses the ileostomy.

down to, but not through, the peritoneum (Fig. 3). The edge of the skin and fascia (two layers if possible) should be undermined to reduce tension of the closure and to allow the closed bowel (closed in two layers) to fall loosely to the bottom of the incision. This wound is always drained (subcutaneously) for three days.

Aids to Reduction

Reduction of an intussusception is never done by pulling the intussuscipiens out of the intussusceptum, but rather by pressure from behind or retrograde in the manner of squeezing toothpaste out of a tube (Fig. 5). The operator can facilitate

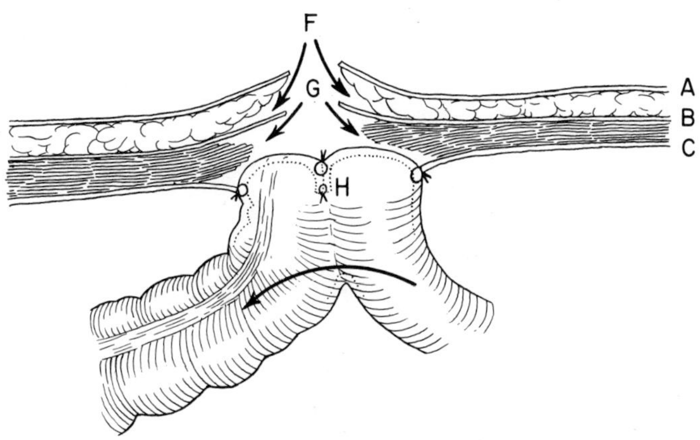

FIGURE 4. Further steps in closure of the Mikulicz ileocolostomy. The skin (*A*) is undermined at *F* to allow for approximation without tension. Even more important is careful dissection of the fascial layers (*B*) at *G* to allow closure (with nonabsorbable suture) at *G*. The bowel is closed in two layers (one may be sufficient) at *H*.

reduction by placing the index and long fingers of one hand across the bowel distal to the intussusception and using them in scissor fashion. Pushing against the intussuscipiens in a proximal direction, as if closing the scissors, helps reduce rectal, rectosigmoid, splenic flexure, and transverse colon lesions.

On rare occasions an intussusception will be lodged below the peritoneal reflection in the rectosigmoid or rectum. A significant aid in reduction of this lesion is the following procedure. (1) After anesthesia has been instituted, the intussuscipiens is reduced as far as possible by digital pressure through the rectum. (2) A large Foley catheter is inserted and the bag inflated. (3) The catheter is connected to a long rubber tube which can be brought out from under the drapes at the foot of the operating table. An enema bag (on an infusion stand) is connected to this catheter. A saline enema (at no more than 30 inches above the operating room table) can then be instituted as a hydrostatic reduction agent when the abdomen is open. By this means the intussuscipiens is brought back to a level at which manual reduction can be easily and safely accomplished.

An aid to reduction of the stubborn intussusception is to straighten the bowel above and below the area of the intussusception. This prevents kinking, which sometimes inhibits reduction. Complete evisceration of the entire area is necessary to accomplish this.

Upon reduction of the usual idiopathic intussusception an edematous lymphoid plaque, which usually is markedly inverted, is apparent as the leading point. The urge to resect or biopsy this plaque, because it "appears to be a tumor," should be resisted. Returning this segment, along with all the remaining eviscerated intestines, to the abdominal cavity and leaving it there for at least 15 minutes (by the clock) is indicated. Upon re-examination, the plaque will be softer and have a less sharp border, and will not have a "tumor-like" appearance. The blood supply and lymphatic drainage are improved by this maneuver enough to change the character of the bowel wall in the region of the lymphoid aggregate.

It is our feeling that a duplication of the terminal ileum or a Meckel's divertic-

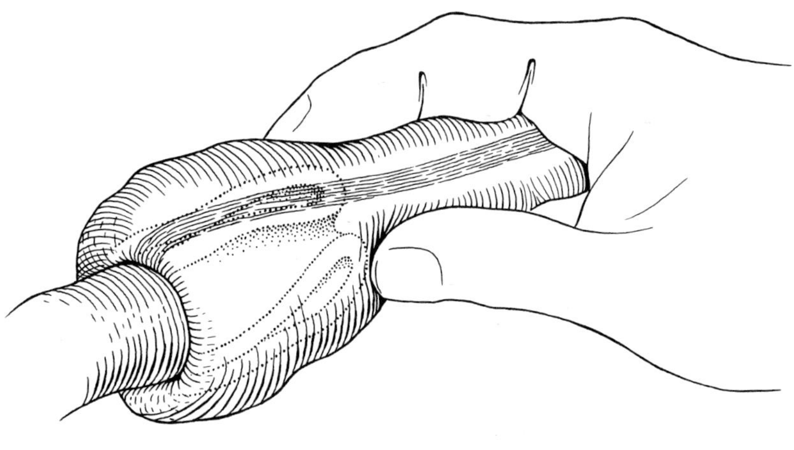

FIGURE 5. The intussuscipiens is milked from the intussusceptum in a retrograde fashion. It is *never* pulled out.

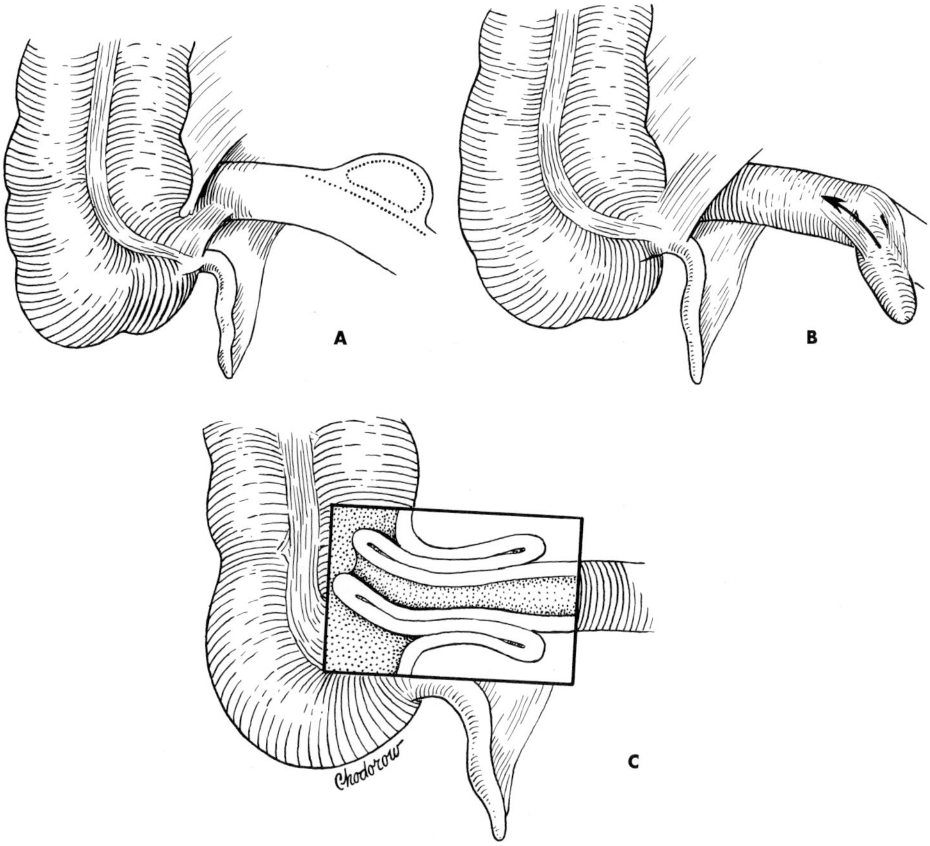

FIGURE 6. A duplication (*A*) and a Meckel's diverticulum (*B*) are the commonest specific causes of an ileoileal or ileocolic intussusception (*C*).

ulum should *not* be resected at the original operation if the bowel is edematous or markedly dilated (Fig. 6). It is better judgment to reoperate within the next 10 to 14 days. The child should not be discharged from the hospital before the second operation can be done. This approach enables a resection of normal bowel which can be prepared, and thus minimizes the chances of poor blood supply, uncertainty as to the extent of a lesion, and disparity at the anastomotic line. Furthermore the patient is under constant observation, an advantage in the rare circumstance of a recurrence in this interim. However, if for any reason the integrity of the duplication or Meckel's diverticulum is in question, it must be resected at the original operation. Intraluminal instillation of 10 to 20 cc. of a 1 per cent neomycin solution in either limb of the anastomosis may be helpful in preparing the bowel locally.

Localized Resection of a Recurrence

One of the most vexing problems of intussusception is the recurrence of idiopathic intussusception. These recurrences are usually of the ileocolic or ileocecal variety.

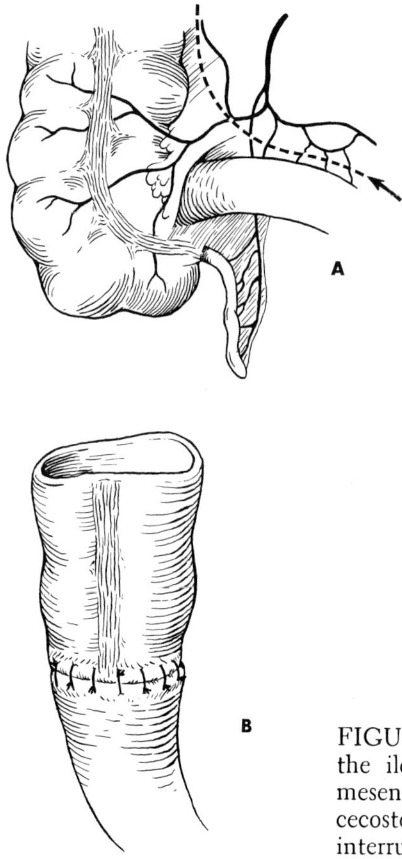

FIGURE 7. (A) Generally accepted blood supply to the ileocecal area (ileocolic artery) and the line of mesenteric resection (dashed line) used for an ileocecostomy. (*B*) End-to-end ileocolostomy. Two-layer interrupted 5–0 or 4–0 silk anastomosis.

One recurrence, accurately documented by either barium enema or a palpable mass with characteristic symptoms, is indication enough for a localized resection of the involved area—nearly always the ileocecal area.

A local resection of the area can be carried out by paying meticulous attention to its blood supply (Fig. 7). With a little care, the resection can be accomplished without an extensive procedure such as a right colectomy. Since there is minimal mesenteric fat in an infant or child, it is not difficult to identify the blood supply to this area, particularly the ileocecal artery. Though variations of the artery are legendary, its origin can be identified rather easily; hence the bowel supplied can be delineated readily once this vessel is temporarily occluded. An end-to-end ileocolostomy is indicated, using a two-layer interrupted 5–0 silk anastomosis.

Fine interrupted silk is used for closing all wounds.

References

GROSS, R. E. *Surgery of Infancy and Childhood*. Philadelphia: W. B. Saunders, 1953.

HIPSLEY, P. L. Treatment of intussusception—by hydrostatic pressure. *M. J. Australia* 2:696, November 24, 1934.

IZANT, R. J., JR., and CLATWORTHY, H. W., JR. Surgical treatment of intussusception. In *Current Surgical Management*. Philadelphia: W. B. Saunders, 1957. P. 357.

RAVITCH, M. M. *Intussusception in Infants and Children*. Springfield (Ill.): Charles C Thomas, 1959.

ZACHARY, R. B. Acute intussusception in childhood. *Arch. Dis. Childhood* 30:32, July 1955.

Index

Index